Introduction to
Public Health

FOURTH EDITION

Mary-Jane Schneider, PhD
Clinical Associate Professor
Department of Health Policy, Management, and Behavior
School of Public Health
University at Albany, State University of New York
Rensselaer, New York

Drawings by Henry Schneider

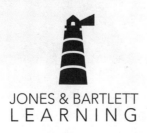

JONES & BARTLETT
LEARNING

World Headquarters
Jones & Bartlett Learning
5 Wall Street
Burlington, MA 01803
978-443-5000
info@jblearning.com
www.jblearning.com

Jones & Bartlett Learning books and products are available through most bookstores and online booksellers. To contact Jones & Bartlett Learning directly, call 800-832-0034, fax 978-443-8000, or visit our website, www.jblearning.com.

Substantial discounts on bulk quantities of Jones & Bartlett Learning publications are available to corporations, professional associations, and other qualified organizations. For details and specific discount information, contact the special sales department at Jones & Bartlett Learning via the above contact information or send an email to specialsales@jblearning.com.

Production Credits
Publisher: Michael Brown
Managing Editor: Maro Gartside
Editorial Assistant: Chloe Falivene
Production Assistant: Alyssa Lawrence
Senior Marketing Manager: Sophie Fleck Teague
Rights & Photo Research Assistant: Amy Rathburn
Manufacturing and Inventory Control Supervisor: Amy Bacus
Composition: diacriTech
Cover Design: Kristin E. Parker
Cover Image: © Bulls Eye/age fotostock
Printing and Binding: Edwards Brothers Malloy
Cover Printing: Edwards Brothers Malloy

To order this product, use ISBN 978-1-4496-9736-5

Library of Congress Cataloging-in-Publication Data
Schneider, Mary-Jane, 1939-
Introduction to public health / Mary-Jane Schneider.—4th ed.
  p. ; cm.
Includes bibliographical references and index.
ISBN 978-1-4496-8887-5 (pbk.)
ISBN 1-4496-8887-X (pbk.)
I. Title.
[DNLM: 1. Public Health. 2. Public Health Practice. WA 100]
362.1—dc23
                                                                2012044440

6048

Printed in the United States of America
17 16 15 14 13   10 9 8 7 6 5 4 3

Contents

Chapter 28

Chapter 29

Chapter 30

Preface

In the Preface to the *First Edition*, I wrote about the public's general ignorance of the field of public health and my own uncertainty about what public health was when, in 1986, I first went to work for the newly established School of Public Health, a collaboration between the University at Albany and the New York State Department of Health. After working with public health professionals from the Department of Health to design curricula for the programs at the school, and after teaching an introductory course in public health for more than 10 years in collaboration with many of the same health department faculty, I feel much more confident about what the term means. After the bioterrorism scare of 2001 and the public health disasters of Hurricanes Katrina and Rita in 2005, I believe that the public has a better sense of the field as well.

This book was written as a text for an introductory course that could be included in the general education curriculum for college undergraduates. As I wrote in the Preface to the *First Edition*, I believe that every citizen of the United States should know something about public health, just as they should know something about democracy, law, and other functions of government. Public health issues are inherently interesting and important to almost everyone. They are featured almost every day on the front pages of newspapers and in the headlines of television news programs, although often they are not labeled as public health issues. One of my goals is to help people put these news stories into context when they occur.

The *Fourth Edition* of this textbook follows the plan of the first three editions, bringing it up to date and including new developments in infectious diseases, injury control, environmental health controversies, the 2010 Census, the reform of the American healthcare system, and many other issues. I have illustrated public health principles by presenting stories that have been in the news; some of these stories have been ongoing sagas that have been supplemented with each edition. Issues that arose since the publication of the *Third Edition* include the fact that poisoning has become the leading cause of injury death, replacing motor vehicle injuries; the controversy over publication of a scientific paper describing how to synthesize the bird flu virus, raising concern that terrorists could use the information to cause a deadly epidemic; the discussion of domestic violence as a cause of injury; and the use of smart phones to help people receive health tips, monitor their health-related behaviors, and be informed about emergency alerts. The *Second* and *Third Editions* focused on political interference with science, but as discussed in this *Fourth Edition*, the Obama administration has vowed to restore honest science as a basis of policy decisions. Other changes in the *Fourth Edition* include a new chapter on mental health and a section describing President Obama's medical care reform plan, the Patient Protection and Affordable Care Act.

I have tried to make this book easily comprehensible to the general reader. One of the things that makes public health fascinating to me is the fact that it is often controversial, depending on political decisions as well as scientific evidence. The politics are frustrating to many practitioners, but it is often the politics that put public health in the headlines. I hope that by describing both the science and the politics, I will contribute to making public health as fascinating to the readers as it is to me.

Prologue: Public Health in the News

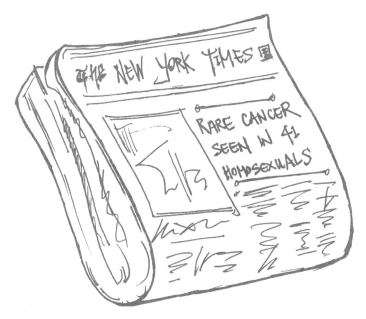

What is public health? It is an abstract concept, hard to pin down. Reports about public health appear in the news every day, but they are not labeled as public health stories, and most people do not recognize them as such. Here in the Prologue are four major public health stories of the modern era that bring the abstraction to life. The ongoing AIDS epidemic, arguably the greatest challenge that the public health community has faced in the past 50 years, illustrates the multidisciplinary nature of the field and the complex ethical and political issues that are often an inherent component of public health. The outbreak of waterborne disease that sickened more than 400,000 people in Milwaukee, Wisconsin in 1993 was the consequence of a breakdown in a routine public health measure that has protected the populations of developed countries for most of the past century. Lest Americans forget that maintaining the health of the population requires constant vigilance, the dramatic decline in all measures of health in Russia presents a cautionary lesson of what can happen to a society that is unable to protect its people in one regard or another. Finally, the terrorist attacks in the Fall of 2001 made it clear that the national security of the United States depends not only on the Defense Department, but also on the American public health system.

AIDS Epidemic

On July 3, 1981, *The New York Times* ran a story with the headline: "Rare Cancer Seen in 41 Homosexuals."[1] The cancer was Kaposi's sarcoma, a form of skin cancer, rare in the United States but more common in equatorial Africa. The victims were young gay men living in New York City or San Francisco, and 8 of the 41 had died within 24 months of being diagnosed. The report noted that several of the victims had been found to have severe defects in their immune systems, but it was not known whether the immune defects were the underlying problem or had developed later. Most of the victims had had multiple and frequent sexual encounters with different partners, the article said, but there was no evidence that the disease was contagious, since none of the patients knew each other.

On August 29, there was another story: "2 Fatal Diseases Focus of Inquiry."[2] A rare kind of pneumonia called pneumocystis had been striking gay men with a 60 percent fatality rate. According to *The New York Times*, 53 cases of pneumocystis had been diagnosed. Also, the number of cases of Kaposi's sarcoma had grown to 47, and 7 patients had both diseases. No one knew why gay men were affected, but there was speculation that there might be a link to their sexual lifestyle, drug use, or some other environmental cause. The article noted without comment that one woman had also been reported to have pneumocystis pneumonia. A scientific task force had been formed at the Centers for Disease Control and Prevention (CDC) to investigate what was going on. There was no further news in *The New York Times* about what would become known as AIDS until May 1982.[3] In that article, the underlying commonality of the immune defect was recognized, and the condition was called gay-related immune deficiency syndrome (GRID). While immune deficiencies had been known and studied previously, most were genetic conditions that afflicted children from birth or were caused by immunosuppressive drugs used to prevent rejection of transplanted organs. The total suppression of the immune system by whatever means leads to many infections, one of which eventually kills the victim. Speculation as to the cause of GRID generally focused on a sexually transmitted infectious agent, although there was a suspicion that multiple factors might be involved, perhaps including drugs or an immune response to the introduction of sperm into the blood through sexual contact.

As the number of reported cases grew, CDC scientists interviewed people with GRID, questioning them about their sexual behavior and partners. The sexual activities of gay men became the focus of scientists and the news media alike—reports of promiscuous and anonymous sex in public baths and use of drugs to enhance sexual pleasure emerged—which tended to worsen many people's already negative view of gay men. Linkages were found that began to confirm that a sexually transmitted infectious agent was responsible. But the investigations were hampered by lack of funding. President Ronald Reagan had been inaugurated in January 1981 on a conservative platform. His administration was not interested in a disease that affected people who behaved in ways so unappealing to the general population. Nor was there much concern on the part of the general public. Most people felt no threat to themselves, although people who lived in New York, San Francisco, Los Angeles, and Miami, where most of the cases had been reported, might have felt more cause for concern.

Since early in the epidemic, however, there had been occasional reports of the immune deficiency in women and heterosexual men, many of them intravenous drug users. By the summer of 1982, cases of the syndrome had also been reported in people with hemophilia who were exposed to blood products used to make a clotting factor and in patients who had received blood transfusions. A study of female sexual partners of men with the syndrome suggested that the disease may also be transmitted by heterosexual relations. A number of babies turned up with a syndrome that resembled GRID, possibly transmitted from their mothers before or at birth. It was clear that the condition was not limited to gay men, and its name was changed to Acquired Immune Deficiency Syndrome (AIDS). The public began to take notice.

By mid-1983, the public began to panic. A report by a pediatrician in New Jersey suggested that AIDS had spread within a family by routine household contact. That scared a lot of people: AIDS was a fatal disease, and people did not want to take any chances of catching it. Inmates in a New York State prison refused to eat meals in a mess hall used by a fellow inmate who had died of AIDS. A New York City sanitation worker with no known risk factors contracted AIDS, perhaps from a syringe protruding from a trash bag. In San Francisco, with its large gay population, the police officers demanded special masks and gloves for handling people suspected of being infected with AIDS. Blood banks reported that blood supplies were critically low because people wrongly feared that they could contract AIDS through donating blood. In New York City, tenants of a cooperative apartment building tried to evict a doctor known for treating people with AIDS. In a few well-publicized incidents, schools refused to allow children with AIDS—usually hemophiliacs—into the classroom. A special telephone information number on AIDS, set up by the federal government, was swamped with 8,000 to 10,000 calls per day. Fundamentalist preachers and conservative legislators fulminated that AIDS was God's punishment for abominable behavior and that people with AIDS deserved their fate. Meanwhile, although controversy still restricted federal funding for AIDS research, biomedical scientists were competing to identify the infectious agent, which most scientists believed would turn out to be a virus. Despite the ill repute of many AIDS patients, the disease was of great scientific interest, and the growing public concern promised to reward with acclaim and financial benefits the scientist who isolated the virus. On April 23, 1984, the Secretary of Health and Human Services convened a press conference to announce that Dr. Robert Gallo of the National Cancer Institute had discovered the virus—now known as the Human Immunodeficiency Virus (HIV)—and that a vaccine would be available within 5 years.[4] While both of those statements proved to be less than accurate—Gallo's priority was disputed and eventually disproved, and after almost 30 years an effective vaccine has still not been developed—the discovery did promise to allow testing of blood for exposure to the virus. Just a year later, blood banks in the United States began screening donated blood, greatly reducing the risk to transfusion recipients and people with hemophilia.

Now, more than 3 decades after the first reports on AIDS were publicized, most of the hysteria has faded, while many of the direst predictions have been realized. By the end of 2008, more than 1 million people in the United States had been diagnosed with AIDS, and 617,000 had died.[5] An estimated 1.1 million Americans are living with HIV. The proportion of women diagnosed with AIDS increased steadily over the first 2 decades and then stabilized at about 25 percent. A great deal more is known about the disease. New drugs have "miraculously" restored health to some dying patients and offer hope that HIV is becoming a chronic, manageable condition rather than a progressively fatal disease. However, there is still no cure, and long-term prospects for HIV-infected individuals are uncertain at best. The only prevention is the avoidance of risky behaviors. The question of how the government should respond to the AIDS epidemic raised some of the most difficult ethical and political issues imaginable in public health. Every new scientific discovery stimulated new dilemmas. Most of the controversies pitted two opposing principles against each other: the protection of the privacy and freedom of the individual suspected of being ill, and the protection of the health of potential victims at risk of being exposed. This conflict is common to many public health problems. Historically, the protection of the public has taken precedence over the rights of the individual. Thus, the principle of quarantining patients with dangerous infectious diseases such as plague, smallpox, or tuberculosis has been generally accepted and upheld by the courts. However, in the case of AIDS, the issues were more complicated.

Because people with AIDS belonged to stigmatized groups who may have been exposed to the virus because of illegal behavior (intravenous drug use or homosexual acts that were still illegal in many states), they bitterly opposed being publicly identified. Gay men, who had only recently achieved a degree of liberation from public oppression, were very well organized politically; they effectively opposed some measures that would have normally been considered standard public health practice, such as reporting the names of diagnosed patients to the health department. They had well-founded fears of being discriminated against for jobs, housing, access to health insurance, and so on. Major political battles erupted over issues such as whether gay bathhouses should be closed and whether AIDS should be declared a communicable disease, which would legally require names of patients to be reported to the local health department. As HIV infection has become more controllable, much of the controversy has subsided.

AIDS is particularly difficult for government to deal with because the only effective way to prevent its spread is to change people's behavior. There are precedents for governmental efforts at promoting behavior change—campaigns to promote smoking cessation, use of bicycle helmets, and healthy diet and exercise—but their success has been modest. Generally, the weight of a law adds significantly to the government's success in promoting healthy behavior, as in the case of seat-belt laws and laws against drunk driving. However, behavior that spreads HIV is very difficult to control by law; intravenous drug use is already illegal everywhere in the United States, and homosexual acts were also illegal in many states until the U.S. Supreme Court declared these laws unconstitutional in 2003. From the beginning, public health officials recognized that AIDS could be prevented only by persuading people to reduce their risk by limiting their exposure, which requires convincing them to control powerful biological and social urges.

Beginning with the earliest attempts at AIDS education, conflict arose between the attempt to communicate effectively with people most likely to be at risk and the likelihood of offending the general public by seeming to condone obscene or illegal acts. Conservatives argued—and still argue—that the only appropriate AIDS education message is abstinence from sex and drugs. C. Everett Koop, President Reagan's Surgeon General, was originally known for his right-to-life views. Later he became an unexpected hero to public health advocates by taking a strong stand in favor of frank AIDS education. While stressing the importance of mutually faithful monogamous sexual relationships and avoiding injected drugs, he nevertheless advocated education about the advantages of condoms and clean needles, and he urged schools to teach children about safe sex. In response, Senator Jesse Helms, a powerful conservative from North Carolina, denounced safe sex materials aimed at gay men as "promotion of sodomy" by the government and sponsored an amendment banning the use of federal funds "to provide AIDS education, information, or prevention materials and activities that promote or encourage, directly or indirectly, homosexual activities."[6(p.218)] Today, television advertising of condoms, the most effective barrier to HIV transmission, while not as restricted as it was 2 decades ago, is still controversial.[7] Despite the abundance of sexually explicit programming and widespread advertising of Viagra and similar drugs, stations still fear the ire of political conservatives and moralists.

Drug regimens introduced in the mid-1990s that are capable of controlling the damage the virus wreaks on the immune system stimulated new medical, ethical, and economic challenges. The drugs have side effects that may prove fatal for some patients and have long-term adverse effects in others. Complicated regimens for taking many pills per day have been simplified, but new problems of viral strains resistant to the drugs have arisen. These strains may be transmitted to others. Moreover, the drugs are expensive, costing an average of $15,475 for a year's supply,[8] well beyond the budget of most patients, although government programs pay for the treatment of many patients. The federal government spent $14.1 billion on HIV-related medical care in the United States in 2011.[9]

The history of the AIDS epidemic vividly illustrates that public health involves both science and politics. It took the science of epidemiology, the study of disease in human populations, to determine the basic nature of the disease and how it is transmitted. The biomedical sciences, especially virology and immunology, were crucial in identifying the infectious agent, determining how it causes its dire effects on the human organism, developing methods to identify virus-infected blood, and devising drugs that can hold the virus at bay. Biostatisticians help to design the trials that test the effectiveness of new drugs and, eventually it is hoped, vaccines—believed to be the greatest hope for controlling the virus. In the meantime, behavioral scientists must find ways to convince people to avoid actions that spread the virus.

The politics of the AIDS epidemic shows the tension between individual freedom and the health of the community. There is a strong tradition of the use of police powers to protect the health of the public in all civilized societies. In the United States, there is also a strong tradition of individual liberty and civil rights. Politics determines the path the government will take in balancing these traditions. Public health is not based on scientific facts alone. It depends on politics to choose the values and ethics that determine how science will be applied to preserve people's health while protecting their fundamental rights.

Cryptosporidium in Milwaukee Water

In early April 1993, an outbreak of "intestinal flu" struck Milwaukee, causing widespread absenteeism among hospital employees, students, and schoolteachers. The symptoms included watery diarrhea that lasted for several days. The Milwaukee Department of Health, concerned, contacted the Wisconsin State Health Department and an investigation began.[10]

Stool samples from the most severely ill patients had been sent to clinical laboratories for testing, and these tests yielded the first clues to the cause of the illness. Two laboratories reported to the city health department that they had identified *Cryptosporidium* in samples from seven adults. This organism was not one that most laboratories routinely tested for, but starting April 7, all 14 clinical laboratories began looking for it in all stool samples submitted to them— and they began finding it. Ultimately, 739 stool samples tested between March 1 and May 30 were found positive for *Cryptosporidium*.

Cryptosporidium is an intestinal parasite that is most commonly spread through contaminated water. In people who are basically healthy, the severe symptoms last a week or so. In addition to the watery diarrhea, the symptoms include varying degrees of cramps, nausea, vomiting, and fever. The infection can be fatal in people with a compromised immune system, such as AIDS patients or people taking immunosuppressive drugs for organ transplants or cancer treatment.

In Milwaukee, public health officials immediately suspected the municipal water supply, which comes from Lake Michigan. They inspected records from the two water treatment plants that supplied the city, and suspicion immediately fell on the southern plant. The inspectors noted that the water's turbidity, or cloudiness, which was monitored once every 8 hours, had increased enormously beginning on March 21, an ominous sign. On April 7, city officials issued a warning, advising customers of the Milwaukee Water Works to boil their water before drinking it. On April 9, they temporarily closed the plant. Looking for evidence that the water was indeed contaminated with *Cryptosporidium*, they discovered that a southern Milwaukee company had produced and stored blocks of ice on March 25 and April 9. Testing confirmed that the organism was present in the ice.

Meanwhile, public health investigators were trying to determine how many people had been made sick by the contaminated water. Reasoning that only the most severely affected patients would go to a doctor and have their stools tested, they began a telephone survey of Milwaukee residents. On April 9, 10, and 12, they called randomly selected phone numbers and asked the first adult who answered whether anyone in the household had been sick since March 1. Of 482 respondents, 42 percent reported having had watery diarrhea, which was considered to be the defining symptom of the illness. In a more extensive telephone survey conducted on 1,663 people in the greater Milwaukee area between April 28 and May 2, 30 percent of the respondents reported having had diarrhea. Half of the respondents whose water came from the southern plant reported the symptoms, while only 15 percent of those whose homes did not get water from the Milwaukee Water Works had been ill. These individuals had probably been exposed at work or from visiting the affected region.[10]

The investigators, who reported the results of their study in the *New England Journal of Medicine*, estimated that at least 403,000 people were made ill by the *Cryptosporidium* contamination of the Milwaukee water supply.[10] The number of deaths has been estimated to be 54; 85 percent of them were AIDS patients, whose compromised immune systems made them especially vulnerable.[11] In discussing how the contamination had occurred, the investigators speculated that unusually large amounts of the organism may have come from cattle farms, slaughterhouses, or human sewage swept into Lake Michigan by heavy spring rains and snow runoff. Flaws in the water treatment process of the southern plant led to inadequate removal of the parasites. After the problem was diagnosed, the southern water treatment plant was thoroughly cleaned, and a continuous turbidity monitor was installed that automatically sounds an alarm and shuts down the system if the turbidity rises above a certain level.

Cryptosporidium contamination is probably much more common than is recognized. It is difficult to control because the organisms are widespread in the environment and they are resistant to chlorination and other commonly used water disinfection methods. *Cryptosporidium* was first recognized as a waterborne pathogen during an outbreak in Texas in 1984 that sickened more than 2,000 people.[12] There may be many other pathogens that could surprise us with waterborne outbreaks; according to a report by the Institute of Medicine, only 1 percent of the organisms associated with disease that might be found in water have been identified.[13]

The United States has one of the safest public water supplies in the world. Nonetheless, according to the CDC, an estimated 4 million to 33 million cases of gastrointestinal illness associated with public drinking water systems occur annually.[14] Many communities are still using water treatment technology dating to World War I, while population growth, modern agricultural technology, toxic industrial wastes, and shifts in weather patterns due to climate change are challenging the aging infrastructure. Updating the infrastructure is expensive; but waterborne disease outbreaks are also expensive. An analysis of the cost of the Milwaukee outbreak in medical and productivity costs, done by scientists from the CDC, the City of Milwaukee Department of Health, the Wisconsin State Division of Public Health, and Emory University yielded an estimate of $96.2 million.[15] These authors estimated that, based on the approximately 7.7 million cases of waterborne disease annually, waterborne disease outbreaks cost $21.9 billion each year in the United States. They recommended that the cost of the outbreaks should be considered when costs of maintaining safe water supplies are calculated. Safe drinking water, one of the most fundamental public health measures, is by no means assured in the United States.

Worst Case Scenario: Public Health in Russia

The Soviet Union set a high priority on public health soon after the Russian Revolution, when the population was suffering from the effects of war, including famine, plague, and a general lack of sanitation. The communist government ran educational campaigns to teach people to practice basic hygiene and prevent disease. It promised free medical care to all; it trained physicians and built hospitals and tuberculosis sanitariums. The incidence of typhus, typhoid fever, and dysentery were dramatically cut. By the 1930s, Western visitors were impressed with the nation's progress in raising the health of the population to near European levels. However, the promise was soon eroded by the abuses of the Soviet system. Progress was choked off by Stalin's suppression of science, the policy of secrecy that concealed bad news, and the Soviet industrial planning process that pushed for continuously increased production at all costs.[16]

The extent of the public health disaster was not known until the late 1980s when Gorbachev began the policy of glasnost, or openness. Westerners—and Russians themselves—learned that infant mortality rates had been rising since the 1970s but were not published because they were embarrassing to the government. The extent of environmental degradation throughout the former Soviet Union, together with increasing rates of cancer, respiratory disease, and birth defects, had become obvious. The corruption and incompetence in the Soviet medical system were also clear: shortages of vaccines, drugs, and medical supplies; unhygienic practices including the reuse of needles for injections and immunizations; poor training of physicians; and shortages of nurses. Alcoholism was rampant.[16]

After the Soviet Union disintegrated in 1991, public health in Russia and other former Soviet states grew dramatically worse. In Russia, death rates increased and birth rates declined so that by the mid-1990s, deaths were almost twice as common as births. While economic and social conditions have improved somewhat since then, the public health has improved only marginally. In 2012, the ratio of deaths to births was approximately 1.5.[17] Life expectancy at birth for Russian men, which was 65.4 years in 1962–1963, fell to 57.3 in 1994 and has recovered only to 60.1 in 2012.[17] Life expectancy for women is longer, at 73.2 years, but women tend to suffer from worse health than men, especially at older ages.[17,18] (In 2012, the life expectancy for American men was 76.0 and 81.0 for American women.[17])

The infant mortality rate fell during the 1990s and 2000s, but still it was 9.9 per 1,000 live births in 2012, compared to 6.0 in the United States.[17] Abortions, the most common method of birth control, were twice as common as childbirth in the early 1990s; recent government efforts to restrict abortions, together with the increased availability of birth control, reduced their number; still, the abortion rate in Russia is among the highest in the world.[19] These factors have led to a decline in the size of the Russian population, which has fallen by 6 million people since 1992 to about 143 million in 2008 and is expected to continue its decline; it is projected to reach below 100 million in 2050.[18] This has negative implications for Russia's future economics, security, and public health.[20] Although many factors contribute to these alarming statistics, much of the blame appears to fall on the economic stress and social breakdown that accompanied the breakup of the former Soviet Union. Middle-aged men have been the group most severely impacted by the changes in the system. They are dying in large numbers from motor vehicle accidents, suicide, homicide, drowning, alcohol poisoning, and cardiovascular disease. Alcohol contributes to many of these deaths; although the official per capita consumption is only marginally higher than in the United States and Western Europe, 75 percent of the alcohol consumed in Russia is in the form of spirits, while Americans and Europeans are more likely to drink beer and wine. There is also a problem in Russia with drinking of alcoholic substances not intended for consumption, such as perfumes and medicines. One-quarter to one-third of all adult male deaths have been directly attributed to alcohol abuse. Among men, deaths from alcohol poisoning, accidents, violence, and cardiovascular disease occur disproportionately on Saturdays, Sundays, and Mondays after binge drinking on weekends.[21]

Although the effects of alcohol are said to outstrip all other health risks, other unhealthy behaviors contribute to the high death rates among adults, especially men. Some 61 percent of Russian men smoke. The rate is much lower—15 percent—for women, but it is increasing. The Russian diet, high in cholesterol-rich animal fats and eggs and low in fruit and vegetables, contributes to abnormally high rates of cardiovascular disease and some cancers. Russians tend to have a sedentary lifestyle and although obesity is less prevalent among Russian men than American men, it is more common in Russian women than Americans.[21]

Infectious diseases, which had been well controlled during the Soviet era, have reappeared, and the CDC warns travelers about hepatitis A, tickborne encephalitis, measles, and rabies, especially in rural areas.[22] Tuberculosis has been a major problem, fed by poverty and social dislocation in the 1990s and overcrowded conditions in prisons, which spreads the disease to communities when prisoners are released. Improper use of antibiotics has led to drug resistance in many of these cases.[23] Infection with HIV, the virus that causes AIDS, has been spreading out of control, contributing to the prevalence of tuberculosis. The United Nations estimates that about 1 million Russians carry the HIV virus, almost as many as in the United States, which has more than double the population.[24] Intravenous drug use is responsible for the majority of infections, although they are expanding in heterosexual populations and are also being seen more in men who have sex with men.

The Russian medical system is vastly underfunded. Doctors and nurses are poorly paid and many hospitals are poorly equipped, especially in rural areas. Although health care is free in principle, many patients must pay under the table for services.[25] According to World Health Organization figures, the Russian government spends $1,038 per person annually on health, which is more than double what it spent in 2000; but this still compares poorly with annual expenditures of $2,784 in the United Kingdom. The United States spends $7,410 per person annually, which is generally regarded as excessive.[26] A 2008 World Bank report on recommendations for healthcare reform in Russia starts with public health strategies that are already widespread in the United States, strategies that will be discussed later in this book. These are the World Bank's recommendations:

1. Control excessive alcohol consumption by targeting supply (e.g., regulation of production, distribution, prices, access, and advertising) and demand (e.g., information, education, and communication campaigns).
2. Control tobacco consumption (e.g., development of policies for smoke-free worksites and public places; taxation; legislation for banning tobacco advertising and promotion, as well as sale to minors).

3. Promote changes in diet and physical activity (e.g., public health policy incentives to promote dietary guidelines for healthier eating; school programs on the importance of health, nutrition, and physical activity).
4. Improve road safety by promoting the use of seat belts and helmets, enforcing laws to prevent accidents due to drunk driving, and retrofitting current road infrastructure with low-cost safety design features (e.g., medians, separation for pedestrians and cyclists) and systematic maintenance to remediate road hazards.[18]

The report then goes on to discuss methods for improving the medical care system.

In addition to all of these issues, environmental pollution contributes to the public health crisis. The Soviet emphasis on industrialization and competitiveness in waging the cold war led to a neglect of environmental protection and civilian public works. A 2007 report, *The World's Worst Polluted Places* by the Blacksmith Institute, an international nonprofit organization, focused on the health effects of industrial pollution in the developing world, found that 10 of the 30 worst places, the "Dirty Thirty," were in the former Soviet Union. At the top of the list was Dzherzhinsk, a city of 300,000 that is still a center of Russian chemical manufacturing and is listed in the *Guinness Book of World Records* as the most chemically polluted city in the world.[27] In cities across the nation, Soviet factories of 1930s vintage still spew black smoke and toxic chemicals into the air, causing asthma, chronic bronchitis, cardiovascular disease, and lung cancer. An analysis by the Environmental Defense Fund, published in 2008, concluded that 10 percent of all deaths in Russian cities could be attributed to air pollution. In the remainder of Russia the data are not as reliable, but the authors estimated that, overall, air pollution caused about the same number of deaths as suicide and homicide combined and double the number from transportation accidents.[28]

Raw sewage and industrial wastes pour into rivers used for drinking water and almost three-quarters of the nation's surface water is polluted. Less than half of Russia's population has access to safe drinking water.[29] Rivers used for irrigation have run dry, leaving contaminated dust to blow in the wind. Soil and water are heavily contaminated by the excessive use of pesticides, many of them banned in the United States because of their toxicity. The accident at the Chernobyl nuclear power station in 1986 poured quantities of radioactive material into the atmosphere that contaminated water and soil over 50,000 square miles of the Ukraine, Belarus, and western Russia. Other less publicized nuclear accidents, as well as atomic tests and deliberate dumping of nuclear materials, have exposed thousands of citizens to dangerous levels of radiation. Genetic damage, caused by exposure to radiation and toxic chemicals, is one hypothesis put forward to explain the dramatic increases in birth defects and other health problems that are taking their toll on the Russian people.[16,27]

There does not seem to be much hope for improvement in the environment in the foreseeable future. The Russian government tends to focus its efforts more on economic development than environmental concerns. Even when local authorities wish to take measures to protect the health of their communities, they tend to be overridden by federal bureaucracies driven by economic concerns.[30] The public health disaster in Russia serves to remind Americans how lucky they are and how wise they have been to—through local, state, and federal governments—take measures to protect the environment and their health. Americans take most public health protections for granted—safe water, clean air, freedom from exposure to dangerous radiation, sterile medical instruments, the availability of effective antibiotics to treat infections, and access to immunizations against formerly common diseases. Most Americans expect to live a long and healthy life. However, the benefits of effective public health measures require continued vigilance. The Russian experience illustrates what can happen if these protections are not maintained. In fact, one expert on Russian public health warns that the United States may be in danger of a similar fate. In Russia, he writes, there was a "massive transfer of resources from its social sector to the military–industrial complex." In the long term, the façade of economic and military success fell away. "Could this be a lesson for the current leaders of the world's remaining superpower, a country that can project its military power globally but still fails to provide health care for all its people?"[31]

Public Health and Terrorism

On September 11, 2001, the United States was struck by foreign terrorists, and Americans entered a new phase of civic life. Four passenger airliners were simultaneously hijacked; three were crashed into buildings filled with people going about their work, and one crashed in an empty field in Pennsylvania, apparently headed for another target but was retaken by passengers.

The immediate public reaction to these disasters was the activation of emergency response plans in the regions where the crashes occurred. Police, firefighters, and ambulances rushed to the scenes; hospital emergency rooms were alerted; extra doctors and nurses were called in. In the New York City area, healthcare facilities in the whole region readied themselves to receive the expected large numbers of people wounded at the World Trade Center. Unfortunately, much of this preparation was not utilized because there were so few injured people who survived.

Although the disaster of September 11 was unprecedented in its magnitude, it was similar in kind to other emergencies and disasters for which communities plan: plane and train crashes, factory explosions, earthquakes, hurricanes, and so on. In New York, public health agencies were concerned not only with coordinating emergency medical care, but also with ensuring the safety of cleanup workers and area residents. Problems with polluted water, contaminated air, spoiled food, infestation of vermin, and so on, had to be dealt with in lower Manhattan just as they must be dealt with after any natural disaster. The longer-term response to September 11 has focused on law enforcement and national defense, with the goal of preventing future hostile acts by terrorists. The federal government has tightened security at airports and borders; it has attacked or warned foreign countries thought to harbor terrorists; and national intelligence agencies have increased their surveillance of persons and groups suspected of being a threat to the United States, to the extent that there are concerns that civil liberties are being eroded. In contrast to the dramatic events of September 11, the second terrorist attack occurring in Autumn 2001 became apparent only gradually. On October 2, Robert Stevens, an editor for a supermarket tabloid, was admitted to a Florida hospital emergency room suffering from a high fever and disorientation. An infectious disease specialist made a diagnosis of anthrax, in part because of heightened suspicions of bioterrorism provoked by the September 11 attacks. The doctor notified the county health department, which notified the state and the CDC. After further tests, the health agencies announced on October 4 that a case of inhalational anthrax had been confirmed. An intensive investigation into the source of exposure began at once. Mr. Stevens died on October 5.[32,33]

On that same day, another case was diagnosed in a worker at the same tabloid office as Robert Stevens. Tests done throughout the building detected a few anthrax spores on Mr. Stevens' computer keyboard and more in the mailroom. The building was closed, and all employees were offered antibiotics to protect them against the development of disease.

On October 9, the New York City Department of Health announced that a newsroom worker at NBC in New York City had developed cutaneous anthrax. She had handled a suspicious letter containing a powder, later identified as anthrax spores. Shortly after, a 7-month-old infant, who had visited his mother's workplace at ABC-TV 2 weeks earlier, was diagnosed with cutaneous anthrax. The child had developed a severe, intractable skin lesion that progressed to severe anemia and kidney failure, but anthrax had not been suspected as a cause of these symptoms.[34] By this time, it was clear that the outbreak was intentionally caused and that a bioterror attack was under way.

On October 15, a staff member working in Senator Tom Daschle's office in Washington, DC opened a letter and noticed a small burst of powder from it. Alert to the threat of anthrax, the aide notified the police and the FBI, and the area was vacated. The letter tested positive for anthrax. Staff and visitors who were potentially exposed were offered antibiotics, as were workers in the Capitol's mail rooms.[35]

The bad news continued. At about the same time that workers in the media and in Congress were being exposed, the disease was breaking out in postal workers in New Jersey, Maryland, and Virginia, although it took days or weeks to recognize what was happening. While it was known by mid-October that anthrax spores were being sent through the mail, they were not believed to escape from sealed envelopes. As it turned out, postal workers were among the most affected by the outbreak. The Brentwood Mail Processing and Distribution Center in the District of Columbia was closed on October 21 after four postal workers were hospitalized with inhalational anthrax; two of these workers died.[36]

All told, a total of 22 cases of anthrax were diagnosed over a 2-month period, of which 11 were the inhalational form. Five of the latter group died, one of whom was a 94-year-old woman in Connecticut whose source of exposure was never verified. It was surmised that a piece of mail received at her home had been cross-contaminated by another piece of mail at a postal facility.[37] The CDC estimated that 32,000 potentially exposed people received prophylactic antibiotic therapy, which may have prevented many more cases.[38] Contaminated buildings, including five U.S. Postal Service facilities, had to be closed and laboriously decontaminated; some of these building could not be reopened for more than a year.[39,40]

Investigation of postal service records determined that letters to the media were mailed in Trenton, New Jersey in mid-September. The letter to Senator Daschle and one to Senator Patrick Lahey, which was not opened until it was irradiated to kill the bacteria, were mailed in Trenton on October 9. A number of hoax letters, similar to the anthrax letters, some containing innocuous white powder, were also mailed to media and government offices from St. Petersburg, Florida. Since they were sent before the news broke about the anthrax letters, they were presumably sent by the same person. The perpetrator of the anthrax mailings was finally identified in 2008 as a scientist working on drugs and vaccines against anthrax at the U.S. Army Medical Research Institute of Infectious Diseases. As the FBI began to close in on him as a suspect, Bruce Ivins committed suicide. Many of his colleagues doubt that he was responsible, and the case will never be proven in court. The Department of Justice released its evidence against him and requested the National Academy of Sciences to conduct a review of the evidence.[41] The Academy's report concluded that the evidence was consistent with Dr. Ivins's lab being the source of the anthrax spores but did not prove it.[42] That is likely to be the last word on the subject.

The anthrax attacks terrorized the population far beyond the actual damage done. They also disrupted the public health and emergency response systems out of proportion to the actual threat. Any encounter with white powder evoked panic, causing people to send samples to public health laboratories for testing. At New York State's Wadsworth Center in Albany, scientists worked around the clock throughout the fall, testing more than 900 samples. Some of the unlikely specimens sent for testing were a pair of jeans, a box of grape tomatoes, a box of Tic Tac® breath freshener, and several packets of cash from automatic teller machines. The largest amount of cash submitted at one time was $8,000, carefully guarded and picked up by police immediately after the anthrax tests proved to be negative (L. Sturman, personal communication).

The events that occurred in the Autumn of 2001 disturbed Americans' sense of security within their borders. The terrorists' hijacking of four airplanes prompted major efforts to strengthen homeland security through more rigorous screening of airline passengers and of international travelers at the borders, precautions that are now routine and are expected to be maintained. The anthrax attacks called attention to the fact that the public health system is America's best protection from bioterrorism. Increased funding for disease surveillance, public health laboratories, and emergency response systems has strengthened the ability of the public health system to respond to bioterrorist attacks as well as to natural disasters and epidemics. These precautions are just as important as other homeland security measures for Americans to be safe in their homeland.

References

1. L. Altman. "Rare Cancer Seen in 41 Homosexuals," *The New York Times*, July 3, 1981.
2. Associated Press. "2 Fatal Diseases Focus of Inquiry," *The New York Times*, August 29, 1981.
3. L. Altman. "New Homosexual Disorder Worries Health Officials," *The New York Times*, May 11, 1982.
4. L. Garrett. *The Coming Plague: Newly Emerging Diseases in a World Out of Balance* (New York: Farrar, Straus, and Giroux, 1994).
5. U.S. Centers for Disease Control and Prevention. "HIV/AIDS: Basic Statistics." http://www.cdc.gov/hiv/topics/surveillance/basic.htm, accessed April 25, 2012.
6. R. Bayer. *Private Acts, Social Consequences: AIDS and the Politics of Public Health* (New York: Free Press, 1989), p. 218.
7. A. A. Newman. "With Condoms in Particular, Local Stations Can Say No," *The New York Times*, July 16, 2007.
8. J. L. Juusola et al. "Cost-Effectiveness of Symptom-Based Testing and Routine Screening for Acute HIV Infection in Men Who Have Sex with Men in the USA," *AIDS* 25 (2011): 1779–1787.
9. Kaiser Family Foundation. "HIV/AIDS Policy Fact Sheet: U.S. Federal Funding for HIV/AIDS: The President's FY 2012 Budget Request," October 2011. http://www.kff.org/hivaids/upload/7029-07.pdf, accessed March 10, 2012.
10. W. R. MacKenzie et al. "A Massive Outbreak in Milwaukee of Cryptosporidium Infection Transmitted Through the Public Water Supply," *New England Journal of Medicine* 331 (1994): 161–167.
11. N. J. Hoxie et al. "Cryptosporidiosis-Associated Mortality Following a Massive Waterborne Outbreak in Milwaukee, Wisconsin," *American Journal of Public Health* 87 (1997): 2032–2035.

12. U.S. Environmental Protection Agency. "Cryptosporidium: Drinking Water Health Advisory," *EPA-822-R-01-009*, March 2001. http://water.epa.gov/action/advisories/drinking/upload/2009_02_03_criteria_humanhealth_microbial_cryptoha.pdf, accessed March 31, 2012.

13. L. Reiter et al., eds. *From Source Water to Drinking Water: Workshop Summary* (Washington, DC: National Academies Press, 2004).

14. U.S. Centers for Disease Control and Prevention. "Notice to Readers: National Drinking Water Week—May 4–10, 2008," *Morbidity and Mortality Weekly Report* 57 (2008): 465–466.

15. P. S. Corso et al. "Cost of Illness in the 1993 Waterborne Cryptosporidium Outbreak, Milwaukee, Wisconsin," *Emerging Infectious Diseases* 9 (2003): 426–431.

16. M. Feshbach and A. Friendly, Jr. *Ecocide in the USSR: Health and Nature Under Siege* (New York: Basic Books, 1992).

17. U.S. Central Intelligence Agency. "The World Factbook." https://www.cia.gov/library/publications/the-world-factbook/index.html, updated weekly, accessed March 23, 2012.

18. World Bank. "Better Outcomes Through Health Reforms in the Russian Federation: The Challenge in 2008 and Beyond," 2008. http://siteresources.worldbank.org/INTRUSSIANFEDERATION/Resources/Outcomes_Health_Reforms_En.pdf, accessed March 23, 2012.

19. United Nations Statistics Division. "Abortion Rates." http://data.un.org/Data.aspx?d=GenderStat&f=inID%3A12, accessed March 23, 2012.

20. P. Marquez et al. "Adult Health in the Russian Federation: More Than Just a Health Problem," *Health Affairs* 26 (2007): 1040–1051.

21. World Bank. "Dying Too Young: Addressing Premature Mortality and Ill Health Due to Non-Communicable Diseases and Injuries in the Russian Federation," 2005. http://siteresources.worldbank.org/INTECA/Resources/DTY-Final.pdf, accessed March 23, 2012.

22. U.S. Centers for Disease Control and Prevention. "Health Information for Travelers to Russia." http://wwwnc.cdc.gov/travel/destinations/russia.htm, accessed March 22, 2012.

23. U.S. Institute of Medicine and Russian Academy of Medical Sciences. "The New Profile of Drug-Resistant Tuberculosis in Russia: A Global and Local Perspective: Summary of a Joint Workshop," 2011. http://books.nap.edu/openbook.php?record_id=13033, accessed March 23, 2012.

24. UNAIDS. *Country Fact Sheet: Russian Federation.* http://www.unaids.org/en/dataanalysis/tools/aidsinfo/countryfactsheets/2010, accessed March 23, 2012.

25. S. Shishkin and V. Vlassov. "Russia's Long Struggle to Come in from the Cold," *BMJ* 339 (2009): 141–143.

26. World Health Organization. "Countries." http://www.who.int/countries/en, accessed March 23, 2012.

27. Blacksmith Institute. "The World's Worst Polluted Places: The Top Ten of the Dirty Thirty." http://www.worstpolluted.org, accessed March 30, 2012.

28. A. Golub and E. Strukova. "Evaluation and Identification of Priority Air Pollutants for Environmental Management on the Basis of Risk Analysis in Russia," *Journal of Toxicology and Environmental Health* Part A, 71 (2008): 86–91.

29. U.S. National Intelligence Council. "The Environmental Outlook in Russia," January 1999. http://www.fas.org/irp/nic/environmental_outlook_russia.html, accessed March 31, 2012.

30. U.S. National Intelligence Council. "Russia: The Impact of Climate Change to 2030: Geopolitical Implications," September 2009. http://www.dni.gov/files/documents/2009%20 Conference%20Report_Russia_The%20Impact%20of%20Climate%20Change%20to%20 2030.pdf, accessed March 31, 2012.

31. M. McKee. "Commentary: The Health Crisis in the USSR: Looking Behind the Façade," *International Journal of Epidemiology* 35 (2006): 1398–1399.

32. U.S. Centers for Disease Control and Prevention. "Update: Investigation of Anthrax Associated with Intentional Exposure and Interim Public Health Guidelines, October 2001," *Morbidity and Mortality Weekly Report* 50 (2001): 889–891.

33. S. G. Stolberg. "Anthrax Threat Points to Limits in Health System," *The New York Times,* October 14, 2001.

34. D. Grady. "Report Notes Swift Course of Inhalational Anthrax," *The New York Times,* February 20, 2002.

35. U.S. Centers for Disease Control and Prevention. "Update: Investigation of Bioterrorism-Related Anthrax and Interim Guidelines for Exposure Management and Antimicrobial Therapy, October 2001," *Morbidity and Mortality Weekly Report* 50 (2001): 909–919.

36. U.S. Centers for Disease Control and Prevention. "Evaluation of *Bacillus anthracis* Contamination Inside the Brentwood Mail Processing and Distribution Center—District of Columbia, October 2001," *Morbidity and Mortality Weekly Report* 50 (2001): 1129–1133.

37. U.S. Centers for Disease Control and Prevention. "Update: Investigation of Bioterrorism-Related Anthrax—Connecticut, 2001," *Morbidity and Mortality Weekly Report* 50 (2001): 1077–1079.

38. U.S. Centers for Disease Control and Prevention. "Update: Investigation of Bioterrorism-Related Anthrax and Adverse Events from Antimicrobial Prophylaxis, 2001," *Morbidity and Mortality Weekly Report* 50 (2001): 973–976.

39. U.S. Centers for Disease Control and Prevention. "Follow-Up of Deaths Among U.S. Postal Service Workers Potentially Exposed *to Bacillus anthracis*—District of Columbia, 2001–2002," *Morbidity and Mortality Weekly Report* 52 (2003): 937–938.

40. I. Peterson. "Postal Center Hit by Anthrax Is Now Clean, Officials Say," *The New York Times,* February 10, 2004.

41. S. Shane. "Portrait Emerges of Anthrax Suspect's Troubled Life," *The New York Times,* January 3, 2009.

42. National Academy of Sciences. "Review of the Scientific Approach Used During the FBI's Investigation of the 2001 Anthrax Letters." http://www.nap.edu/opebook.php?record_id=13098&pages=R1, accessed March 31, 2012.

What Is Public Health?

Public Health: Science, Politics, and Prevention

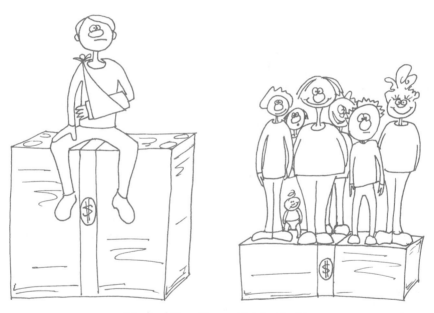

Medical Care Versus Public Health

One expectation about living in a civilized society is that the living conditions will be basically healthy. Unless something unusual happens, like the outbreak of *Cryptosporidium* in the Milwaukee water supply, people assume that they are basically safe: their water is safe to drink; the hamburger they buy at the fast food restaurant is safe to eat; the aspirin they take for a headache is what the label says it is; and they are not likely to be hit by a car—or a bullet—if they use reasonable caution in walking down the street. Even after the attacks in the fall of 2001, which severely disrupted their sense of security, most Americans regained a sense of trust in the safety of their environment.

In historical terms, this expectation is a relatively recent development. In the mid-19th century, when record-keeping began in England and Wales, death rates were very high, especially among children. Of every 10 newborn infants, two or three never reached their first birthday. Five or six died before they were 6 years old, and only about 3 of the 10 lived beyond the age of 25.[1] Tuberculosis was the single largest cause of death in the mid-19th century. Epidemics of cholera, typhoid, and smallpox swept through communities, killing people of all ages and making them afraid to leave their homes. Injuries—often fatal—to workers in mines and factories were common due to unsafe equipment, long working hours, poor lighting and ventilation, and child labor.

There are a number of reasons why people's lives are basically healthier today than they were 150 years ago: cleaner water, air, and food; safe disposal of sewage; better nutrition; more knowledge concerning healthy and unhealthy behaviors; and many others. Most of these factors fall in the domain of public health. In fact, the term "public health" refers to two different but related concepts. We can say that the public health has improved since the 19th century, meaning that the general state of people's health is now much better than it was. But the measures that people take as a society to bring about and maintain that improvement are also known as public health.

Although many sectors of the community may be involved in promoting public health, people most often look to government—at the local, state, or national level—to take the primary responsibility. Governments provide pure water and efficient sewage disposal. Governmental regulations ensure the safety of the food supply. They also ensure the quality of medical services provided through hospitals, nursing homes, and other institutions. Laws regulating people's behavior prevent them from injuring each other. Laws requiring immunization of school-aged children prevent the spread of infectious diseases. Governments also sponsor research and education programs on causes and prevention of disease.

What Is Public Health?

Public health is not easy to define or to comprehend. A telephone survey of registered voters conducted in 1999 by a charitable foundation found that over half of the 1234 respondents misunderstood the term.[2] Leaders in the field have themselves struggled to understand the mission of public health, to explain what it is, why it is important, and what it should do. Charles-Edward A. Winslow, a theoretician and leader of American public health during the first half of the 20th century, defined public health in 1920 this way:

> The science and the art of preventing disease, prolonging life, and promoting physical health and efficiency through organized community efforts for the sanitation of the environment, the control of community infections, the education of the individual in principles

> of personal hygiene, the organization of medical and nursing services for the early diagnosis and preventive treatment of disease, and the development of the social machinery which will ensure to every individual in the community a standard of living adequate for the maintenance of health.[3(p.1)]

Winslow's definition is still considered valid today.

Over the following decades, public health had many successes, carrying out many of the tasks described in Winslow's definition. It was highly effective in reducing the threat of infectious diseases, thereby increasing the average lifespan of Americans by several decades. By the 1980s, public health was taken for granted, and most people were unaware of its activities. But there were signs that the system was not functioning well. Government expenditures on health were alarmingly high, but most of the spending was directed toward medical care. No one was talking about public health. At the same time, new health problems were appearing: the AIDS epidemic broke out, concern about environmental pollution was growing, the aging population was demanding increased health services, and social problems such as teenage pregnancy, violence, and substance abuse were becoming more common. There was a sense that public health was not prepared to deal with these problems, in part because people were not thinking of them as public health problems.

A study conducted by the Institute of Medicine and published in 1988 called *The Future of Public Health* refocused attention on the importance of public health and did a great deal to revitalize the field. One of the first tasks the study committee set for itself was to re-examine the definition of public health, reasoning that for it to be effective, public health had to be broadly defined.[4] The committee's report gives a four-part definition describing public health's mission, substance, organizational framework, and core functions.

The Future of Public Health defines the mission of public health as "the fulfillment of society's interest in assuring the conditions in which people can be healthy."[4(p.40)] The substance of public health is "organized community efforts aimed at the prevention of disease and the promotion of health."[4(p.41)] The organizational framework of public health encompasses "both activities undertaken within the formal structure of government and the associated efforts of private and voluntary organizations and individuals."[4(p.42)] The three core functions of public health are these:

1. Assessment
2. Policy development
3. Assurance[4(p.43)]

These core functions were later translated by another committee into a more concrete set of activities called *The Ten Essential Public Health Services*, shown in Table 1-1.

Table 1-1   The Ten Essential Public Health Services

Assessment
1. Monitor health status to identify community health problems
2. Diagnose and investigate health problems and health hazards in the community

Policy Development
3. Inform, educate, and empower people about health issues
4. Mobilize community partnerships to identify and solve health problems
5. Develop policies and plans that support individual and community health efforts

Assurance
6. Enforce laws and regulations that protect health and ensure safety
7. Link people to needed personal health services and assure the provision of health care when otherwise unavailable
8. Assure a competent public health and personal healthcare workforce
9. Evaluate effectiveness, accessibility, and quality of personal and population-based health services

Serving All Functions
10. Research for new insights and innovative solutions to health problems

Source: Reproduced from *The Future of the Public's Health in the 21st Century,* (Washington, DC: National Academy Press, 2002): 99. With permission of the National Academy of Sciences, Courtesy of the National Academies Press.

Public Health Versus Medical Care

One way to better understand public health and its functions is to compare and contrast it with medical practice. While medicine is concerned with individual patients, public health regards the community as its patient, trying to improve the health of the population. Medicine focuses on healing patients who are ill. Public health focuses on preventing illness.

In carrying out its core functions, public health—like a doctor with his/her patient—assesses the health of a population, diagnoses its problems, seeks the causes of those problems, and devises strategies to cure them. Assessment constitutes the diagnostic function, in which a public health agency collects, assembles, analyzes, and makes available information on the health of the population. Policy development, like a doctor's development of a treatment plan for a sick patient, involves the use of scientific knowledge to develop a strategic approach to improving the community's health. Assurance is equivalent to the doctor's actual treatment of the patient. Public health has the responsibility of assuring that the services needed for the protection of public health in the community are available and accessible to everyone. These include environmental, educational, and basic medical services. If public health agencies do not provide these services themselves, they must encourage others to do so or require such actions through regulation.

Public health's focus on prevention makes it more abstract than medicine, and its achievements are therefore more difficult to recognize. The doctor who cures a sick person has achieved a real, recognizable benefit, and the patient is grateful. Public health cannot point to the people who have been spared illness by its efforts. As Winslow wrote in 1923, "If we had but the gift of second sight to transmute abstract figures into flesh and blood, so that as we walk along the street we could say 'That man would be dead of typhoid fever,' 'That woman would have succumbed to tuberculosis,' 'That rosy infant would be in its coffin,'—then only should we have a faint conception of the meaning of the silent victories of public health."[3(p.65)]

This "silence" accounts in large part for the relative lack of attention paid to public health by politicians and the general public in comparison with medical care. It is estimated that only about 3 percent of the nation's total health spending is spent on public health.[5] During the healthcare reform debate of 1993 and 1994, and again in 2008 during the presidential campaign, virtually all of the discussion focused on paying for medical care, while very little attention was paid to funding for public health. However, President Obama's health reform law, passed in 2010, did include provisions and funding for prevention, wellness, and public health.[6]

Effective public health programs clearly save money on medical costs in addition to saving lives. Moreover, public health contributes a great deal more to the health of a population than medicine does. According to one analysis, the life expectancy of Americans has increased from 45 to 75 years over the course of the 20th century.[7] Only 5 of those 30 additional years can be attributed to the work of the medical care system. The majority of the gain has come from improvements in public health, broadly defined as including better nutrition, housing, sanitation, and occupational safety. One responsibility of public health, therefore, as noted in the Institute of Medicine report, is to educate the public and politicians about "the crucial role that a strong public health capacity must play in maintaining and improving the health of the public ... By its very nature, public health requires support by members of the public—its beneficiaries."[4(p.32)]

Public health, like medical practice, is based on science. However, even when public health scientists are certain they know all about the causes of a problem and what should be done about it, a political decision is generally necessary before action can be taken to solve it. When a doctor diagnoses a patient's illness and recommends a treatment, it is up to the patient to accept or reject the doctor's recommendation. When the "patient" is a community or a whole country, it is usually a government—federal, state, or local—that must make the decision to accept or reject the recommendations of public health experts. Sometimes the process starts within the community when, like a patient going to a doctor with a complaint, the people recognize a problem and demand that the government take action. This has occurred in many communities when victims of drunk drivers form organizations such as Mothers Against Drunk

Driving (MADD) to lobby for stricter laws, or when neighbors of pollution-generating factories demand that the government force the industry to clean up the environment.

Politics enters the public health process as part of the policy development function and especially as part of the assurance function. Since the community will have to pay for the "treatments," usually through taxes, they must decide how much "health" they are willing to fund. They also must decide whether they are willing to accept the possible limitations on their freedom that may be required in order to improve the community's health. Among the assurance functions of public health is the provision of basic medical services: how this should be done has been a matter of great political controversy. Public health professionals are often impatient with politics, as the Institute of Medicine report notes, seeming to "regard politics as a contaminant of an ideally rational decision-making process rather than as an essential element of democratic governance."[4(p.5)]

The Sciences of Public Health

The scientific knowledge on which public health is based spans a broad range of professional disciplines. The Institute of Medicine report notes that "public health is a coalition of professions united by their shared mission" as well as by "their focus on disease prevention and health promotion; their prospective approach in contrast to the reactive focus of therapeutic medicine, and their common science, epidemiology."[4(p.40)] The disciplines of public health can be divided somewhat arbitrarily into six areas. Epidemiology and statistics are the basis for the assessment functions of public health, including the collection and analysis of information. Both assessment and policy development need an understanding of the causes of health problems in the community, an understanding that depends on biomedical sciences, social and behavioral sciences, and environmental sciences. As part of the assurance function, public health seeks to understand the medical care system in an area of study generally referred to as health policy and management or health administration, which also includes the administration and functioning of the public health system.

Epidemiology has been called the basic science of public health. As its name suggests, epidemiology is the study of epidemics. It focuses on human populations, usually starting with an outbreak of disease in a community. Epidemiologists look for common exposures or other shared characteristics in the people who are sick, seeking the causative factor.

Epidemiology often provides the first indications of the nature of a new disease. When AIDS was first recognized in the early 1980s, the cause was unknown. Doctors reported cases of this unusual disease to the U.S. Centers for Disease Control and Prevention, and epidemiologists began looking for common characteristics of the patients. Epidemiologic research indicated that it was an infectious disease spread through blood and body fluids and suggested a virus as the cause. This prompted the biomedical scientists to step in and look for the virus.

Epidemiology is important not only for deciphering the causes of exotic new diseases, but for preventing the spread of old, well-understood diseases. Epidemiologists are mainstays of local health departments. In what is commonly known as "shoe-leather epidemiology," they track down, for example, the source of a food-poisoning outbreak and force a restaurant to clean up its kitchen. Or they trace everyone who has been in contact with a college student diagnosed with meningitis in order to administer high doses of antibiotic to prevent further spread of that dangerous disease. Epidemiologic studies have also been important in identifying the causes of chronic diseases such as heart disease and cancer.

Because public health deals with the health of populations, it depends very heavily on *statistics*. Governments collect data on births and deaths, causes of death, outbreaks of communicable diseases, cases of cancer, occupational injuries, and many other health-related issues. These numbers are diagnostic tools, informing experts how healthy or sick a society is, and where its weaknesses are. For example, the fact that the United States ranks 27th in infant mortality among the nations of the world, 24th in life expectancy of men and 25th of women is one indication that the public health in this country is not as good as that in many others.[8]

To understand what the numbers mean, it is necessary to understand certain statistical concepts and calculations. The science of statistics is used to calculate risks from exposure to environmental chemicals, for example. Statistical analysis is an integral part of any epidemiologic study seeking the cause of a disease or a clinical study testing the effectiveness of a new drug.

Both public health and medicine depend on the *biomedical sciences*. A major proportion of human disease is caused by microorganisms. Prevention and control of these diseases in a population require an understanding of how these infectious agents are spread and how they affect the human body. Control of infectious diseases was a major focus of public health in the 19th and early 20th centuries. Biomedical research was very successful in gaining an understanding of the major killers of that period, providing the information and techniques from which successful public health measures could bring these diseases under control.

Biomedical research is still important to the understanding and control of new diseases such as AIDS, which has become the major epidemic of the late 20th century worldwide. It has also contributed increasingly to an understanding of noninfectious diseases such as cancer and heart disease, which have become increasingly important as many infectious diseases have been controlled. Recent progress in understanding human genetics is providing new insights into people's inherent susceptibility to various diseases, raising new hopes of cures as well as concerns about discrimination.

Environmental health science, a classic component of public health, is concerned with preventing the spread of disease through water, air, and food. While it is not strictly a separate science, because it shares concerns about the spread of infectious organisms with biomedical sciences and depends on epidemiology to track environmental causes of disease outbreaks, it is usually considered a separate area of public health. Much of the great improvement in public health in the United States during the 20th century was due to improved environmental health, especially the fact that most Americans have safe drinking water. In its concern with safe water and waste disposal, environmental health depends on engineering to design, build, and maintain these systems.

Despite the fact that the importance of safe air, water, and food has been recognized for so many decades, there are many new challenges to environmental health. Not only do old systems fail, as occurred in Milwaukee, but new problems arise, brought about by modern lifestyles. Thousands of new chemicals enter the environment every year, and little is known about their effects on human health. Chemicals known to be toxic have accumulated in the environment, and methods must be devised to dispose of them safely. Other environmental threats to health include ultraviolet rays in sunlight, an increasing problem as the ozone layer of the earth's atmosphere is depleted, and exposure to other kinds of radiation. Recently it has become apparent that human activities are causing changes in the climate of the earth, changes that are permanently altering our environment and are already having important effects on human health.

Increasingly, public health is concerned with *social and behavioral sciences*. As biomedical and environmental sciences have conquered many of the diseases that killed people of previous generations, people in modern societies are dying of diseases caused by their behavior and the social environment. Heart disease is related to nutrition and to exercise patterns; many forms of cancer are caused by smoking; abuse of drugs and alcohol is a notorious killer. Violence is a significant cause of death in our society and attracts ongoing concern.

Some subgroups of the population have poorer health overall than others, for reasons that, while not completely understood, relate to social and behavioral factors. People with low incomes are less healthy than those with a higher socioeconomic status. Black Americans have lower life expectancy overall than white Americans, even when their incomes are similar. Other ethnic minority groups, including Hispanics, Asians, and American Indians are at increased risk for a variety of health problems.

Social and behavioral sciences involve more unanswered questions than biomedical and environmental sciences do. Very little is known about why racial and ethnic groups differ in their health-related behavior, why many people of all races behave in unhealthy ways, and how to prevent self-destructive behaviors. In the social and behavioral sciences, of all areas, research and application of its findings are most likely to make a difference in the future.

Until the beginning of the 20th century, public health and medicine overlapped substantially in their spheres of interest and activity. Both fields were concerned primarily with understanding the causes and prevention of infectious disease because medicine was relatively powerless to cure them. With the discovery of antibiotics, however, medicine gained the power to work miracles of healing, leading to a period of rapidly growing influence. Meanwhile, because of its less glamorous task of preventing disease, public health faded into obscurity.

Over the past few decades, it has become apparent that our society's emphasis on curing disease rather than preventing it has gone out of control. Medical care has become so expensive that an increasing proportion of the population cannot afford it, and spending for medical care has eaten up resources that could more profitably be used for education, housing, and the environment. Concern about runaway costs, lack of access, and questionable quality of care has led to an increasing interest in studying the medical care system, its effectiveness, efficiency, and equity, leading to a science called health services research. Traditional categorization of public health fields puts this study into the area of *health policy and management* or *health administration.*

Prevention and Intervention

Public health's approach to health problems in a community has been described as a five-step process:

1. Define the health problem.
2. Identify the risk factors associated with the problem.
3. Develop and test community-level interventions to control or prevent the cause of the problem.
4. Implement interventions to improve the health of the population.
5. Monitor those interventions to assess their effectiveness.[6]

Thus, a main task of prevention is to develop interventions designed to prevent specific problems that have been identified either through an assessment process initiated by a public health agency or through community concern raised by an unusual course of events. For example, statistical data may show that a community has a high rate of cancer in comparison with other similar communities. Or a series of fatal crashes caused by drunk driving may mobilize a community to demand action to prevent further tragedies.

Public health has developed systematic ways of thinking about such problems that facilitate the process of designing interventions that prevent undesirable health outcomes. One approach is to think of prevention on three levels: primary prevention, secondary prevention, and tertiary prevention. Primary prevention prevents an illness or injury from occurring at all, by preventing exposure to risk factors. Secondary prevention seeks to minimize the severity of the illness or the damage due to an injury-causing event once the event has occurred. Tertiary prevention seeks to minimize disability by providing medical care and rehabilitation services.

Thus interventions for primary prevention of cancer include efforts to discourage teenagers from smoking and efforts to encourage smokers to quit. In secondary prevention, screening programs are established to detect cancer early when it is still treatable. Tertiary prevention involves the medical treatment and rehabilitation of cancer patients.

This way of thinking was very effective in developing traffic safety programs that, over the past 4 decades, have significantly reduced the rates of injury from motor vehicle crashes. Primary prevention focused on preventing crashes from occurring, for example, by building divided highways and installing traffic lights. Secondary prevention included the design of safer automobiles with stronger bumpers, padded dashboards, seat belts, and airbags. It also included laws requiring drivers and passengers to wear the seat belts. And tertiary prevention required the development of emergency medical services including ambulances, 911 calling networks, and trauma centers.

Another approach to designing interventions is to think of an illness or injury as the result of a chain of causation involving an agent, a host, and the environment. This approach is traditional when thinking of infectious diseases: the agent may be a disease-causing bacterium or virus; the host is a susceptible human being; and the environment includes the means of transmission by which the agent reaches the host, which may be contaminated air, water, or food, or it may be another human being who is infected. Prevention is accomplished by interrupting the chain of causation at any step. Rendering a potential host unsusceptible through immunization, for example, can interrupt the chain. Or the bacterium infecting a host can be killed through the use of antibiotics. Or the environment can be sanitized through the purification of water and food.

The chain of causation model can also be used for other kinds of illnesses or injuries. For example, suicide is the fourth leading cause of death in the age group 15 to 24.[8] In applying the model to prevention of youth suicide, the host is the susceptible young person; the agent is most often a gun or an overdose of pills; the environment includes the young person's whole social environment, including family, school, and the media. A public health intervention could focus on how to make young people less susceptible to self-destructive thinking; it could try to change the messages presented by television and schoolmates that may lead a young person to think he or she is unattractive or otherwise inferior. However, the public health perspective tends to be that the most effective target of intervention for youth suicide prevention is the agent, especially guns. Many adolescents are susceptible to depressed moods and think of killing themselves, but the best predictor of whether they will succeed is whether they have access to a gun.

Public Health and Terrorism

The events in the fall of 2001 disturbed the sense of complacency many people felt about the health and safety of their living conditions. Evidence that there were groups or individuals who not only wanted to cause harm to Americans at home but who had the resources and the will to succeed in that goal forced us to think about how to prevent similar events in the future. While prevention of violent acts such as hijacking airplanes is primarily a responsibility of law enforcement, public health has an important role to play in controlling the damage caused by such events. In other words, primary prevention of terrorist acts may be out of the domain of public health, but secondary and tertiary prevention are very much a part of public health's mission. Success at these services depend on having well-designed plans in place before a disaster occurs.

The crashing of two planes into the World Trade Center triggered the activation of emergency response plans developed for New York City and New York State, plans designed as secondary prevention—minimizing the damage—and tertiary prevention—providing medical care to those injured in the disaster. Most critically important for saving lives was the ability for occupants of the buildings to get out as fast as possible. The fact that all but 2092 of the 17,400 people who were in the towers when the planes hit made it out is evidence that some aspects of the plans were effective.[9] However, studies done later found many flaws in the emergency planning. Plans for providing medical care to survivors were not seriously tested, because the capacity—including the arrival of numerous volunteers—exceeded the number of injured survivors. The greatest problem was a lack of coordination.

The public health response to the terrorism of September 11, 2001 was essentially the same as the response needed for other emergencies and disasters: factory explosions, plane and train crashes, earthquakes, hurricanes (such as Katrina in 2005), and so on. Public health was concerned not only with coordinating emergency medical care, but also with ensuring the safety of cleanup workers and area residents. Problems with polluted water, contaminated air, spoiled food, infestation of vermin, and so on, had to be dealt with in downtown Manhattan just as they must be dealt with after a natural disaster.

The importance of public health became even more obvious in the aftermath of the anthrax mailings. These bioterrorism attacks did not announce themselves in the dramatic fashion of the airplane hijackings. The first signs that a terrorist event had occurred were not recognized as such. No alarm bells rang when a few patients showed up in hospital emergency rooms with hard-to-diagnose illnesses. Anthrax announced itself in the same way that AIDS appeared, as an outbreak of something new that was reported to public health authorities, who then investigated.

The damage done by the anthrax mailings was relatively minor. However, the potential disaster that would result if a more infectious microorganism were used in a bioterror attack forced many sectors of society to pay attention to public health. In speculating about what would happen if a terrorist clandestinely released smallpox virus into a crowd, public health authorities realized that only epidemiologic methods for controlling natural epidemics could even begin to deal with the crisis. Suddenly the media and politicians began talking about public health. Ironically, the threat of bioterrorism did more to teach the public about public health than any educational program. As Robert F. Meenan, dean of the Boston University School of Public Health, is quoted as saying, the anthrax attacks provided "a marketing campaign we could never have bought."[10] It is not clear, however, that the lessons learned about public health during those difficult times will stay with us when the public's attention shifts to the more politically demanding concerns about paying for medical care.

Conclusion

This chapter has shown that public health is a broad term that is difficult to define. It includes a goal—maximum health for all—as well as the means of attempting to achieve that goal. Public health is concerned with the prevention of disease and disability. It is aimed at benefiting the entire population in contrast with medicine, which focuses on the individual.

The functions of public health in a community can be compared with the functions of a physician in caring for a patient. Public health diagnoses and treats the community's ills by way of assessment, policy development, and assurance. It relies on the tools of science and politics. The public health sciences of epidemiology and statistics are applied in assessing a population's health. Policy is developed based on biomedical sciences, social and behavioral sciences, environmental health sciences, and the study of the medical care system. Public health depends on politics for decision making. Decisions on public health interventions to be taken by the community, insofar as they require government action, are reached through politics.

Public health focuses on prevention of disease and disability. Preventive measures can be applied at three levels: primary prevention aims to prevent a disease or injury from occurring at all; secondary prevention aims to minimize the damage caused by the illness or injury-causing event when it occurs; and tertiary prevention seeks to minimize any ensuing disability by providing medical care and rehabilitation.

Public health prevention programs function through interventions designed to interrupt the chain of causation that leads to an illness or an injury. Interventions can be directed toward eliminating or suppressing the agent that causes an illness or injury, strengthening the resistance of the host to the agent, or changing the environment in such a way that the host is less likely to encounter the agent.

Public health is an abstract concept that is not well understood and is often neglected. The dramatic events in the fall of 2001 forced the government and the media to pay attention to the importance of public health, both in mitigating the effects of obvious disasters, and in recognizing and controlling the more insidious effects of bioterrorism, although it is not clear whether that understanding will endure.

References

1. T. McKeown, *The Role of Medicine: Dream, Mirage or Nemesis?* (Oxford, England: Basil Blackwell, 1979).
2. U.S. Centers for Disease Control and Prevention, "Public Opinion About Public Health— United States, 1999," *Morbidity and Mortality Weekly Report* 49 (2000): 258–260.
3. C.-E. A. Winslow, *The Evolution and Significance of the Modern Public Health Campaign* (New Haven, CT: Yale University Press, 1923); reprinted by the *Journal of Public Health Policy*, 1 (1984).
4. U.S. Institute of Medicine, Committee for the Study of the Future of Public Health, *The Future of Public Health* (Washington, DC: National Academy Press, 1988).
5. A. L. Sensenig, "Refining Estimates of Public Health Spending as Measured in National Health Expenditures Accounts: The United States Experience," *Journal of Public Health Management and Practice* 13 (2007): 103–114.
6. Kaiser Family Foundation, "Focus on Health Reform: Summary of New Health Reform Law," April 15, 2011. http://www.kff.org/healthreform/upload/8061.pdf, accessed May 8, 2012.
7. U.S. Public Health Service, *For a Healthy Nation: Returns on Investment in Public Health* (Washington, DC: U.S. Government Printing Office, 1994).
8. U.S. National Center for Health Statistics, *Health, United States, 2008* (Hyattsville, MD: Public Health Service, 2009), Tables 24, 25.
9. R. R. M. Gershon, "Factors Associated with High-Rise Evacuation: Qualitative Results from the World Trade Center Evacuation Study," *Prehospital and Disaster Medicine* 22 (2007): 165–173.
10. J. S. Smith, "Personal Predicament of Public Health." *Chronicle of Higher Education,* June 27, 2003.

Why Is Public Health Controversial?

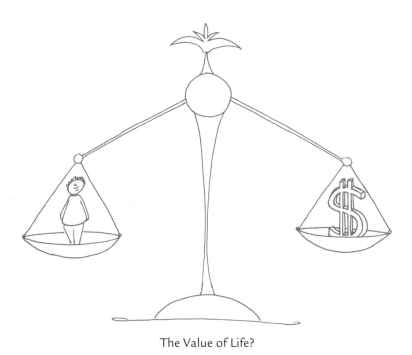

The Value of Life?

The mission of public health as defined by the Institute of Medicine report, *The Future of Public Health*—"fulfilling society's interest in assuring conditions in which people can be healthy"[1(p.40)]—is very broad. The conditions include many factors that might not normally be thought of as relevant to public health. For example, the factor most significant in determining the health of a community is its economic status: people with higher incomes tend to be healthier for a variety of reasons. This expansive view of public health is not new. Winslow's 80-year-old definition specifically includes as part of public health's role, "the development of the social machinery which will ensure to every individual in the community a standard of living adequate for the maintenance of health."[2(p.1)]

Indeed, the early history of U.S. public health was closely tied to social reform movements. In addition to sanitary science and public hygiene, 19th-century reformers campaigned for improved housing, trade unions, the abolition of child labor, maternal and child health, and temperance. Winslow thought of public health as a military-style campaign and wrote of "whole populations mobilized for the great war against preventable disease."[3(p.27)]

Public health can be viewed as a broad social movement. Dan E. Beauchamp, a noted public health philosopher, has written that "public health should be a way of doing justice, a way of asserting the value and priority of all human life."[4(p.8)] In an influential 1974 paper entitled, "Public Health as Social Justice," Beauchamp calls on public health to challenge the ideology that prevails in the United States, an ideology that he calls "market justice." Market justice, he writes, emphasizes individual responsibility, minimal obligation to the common good, and the "fundamental freedom to all individuals to be left alone."[4(p.4)] Under market justice, powerful forces of environment, heredity, and social structure prevent a fair distribution of the burdens and benefits of society. Social justice, on the other hand, suggests that minimal levels of income, basic housing, employment, education, and health care should be seen as fundamental rights. According to Beauchamp, "The historic dream of public health that preventable death and disability ought to be minimized is a dream of social justice."[4(p.6)]

Political conservatives have tended to resist this broad vision of public health. They would prefer to limit public health to a technical enterprise focused on controlling communicable disease or as a safety net that provides medical care to the indigent. This restricted view of public health was encouraged by physicians, concerned about government encroachment on their economic and professional independence; their political power helped to limit federal health funding in the 1930s and 1940s to programs, run by local health departments, which were narrowly focused on providing services for child health, venereal disease control, tuberculosis, and dental health.

Concerns about health threats from environmental pollution that arose in the 1960s were addressed independently of the traditional public health system, and separate agencies were set up to deal with them. Similarly, social problems such as homelessness, drug abuse, and violence were not thought of as public health problems, although they had adverse health consequences. It was this fragmentation of public health that led the Institute of Medicine committee to conclude in 1988 that public health was "in disarray"[1(p.19)] and to affirm the comprehensive view of public health expressed by Winslow and Beauchamp.

The broad view of public health's scope generates considerable controversy in America's individualistic, market-oriented society. The notion that government has an obligation to provide healthy conditions for citizens who are unwilling or unable to provide such conditions for themselves—and indeed to provide medical care for those who need it, as most other industrialized countries do—has often been attacked as socialist. Conservative politicians have won office by campaigning against taxes, starving governments of funds that could provide health services for all. Many Americans reflexively oppose being told what to do and resist the idea of governmental restrictions on their behavior even when the intent is to protect their own health and that of others. Moreover, many health problems have their roots in unhealthy behaviors that are so personal and intimate that moralists oppose even discussing them. Three issues—economic, libertarian, and moral—tend to come up repeatedly in any debate over public health actions or activities.

Economic Impact

Most public health measures have a negative economic impact of some kind on some segment of the population or on some industry. Consequently, any new proposal for a public health regulation is likely to inspire opposition from some quarter, on the grounds that it might cost jobs, add to the price of a product, or require a tax increase. It might also cut into a company's profits. Consequently, industries resist change: milk producers resisted pasteurization, landlords resisted building codes, automobile manufacturers resisted design changes to improve safety. There are several reasons why these conflicts are particularly difficult to resolve.

The difficulty in dealing with the economic impact of public health measures has been illustrated by conflicts with the tobacco industry. Tobacco is clearly harmful to health, causing thousands of deaths and millions of dollars in medical costs annually. Yet, until recently, only mild restrictions and regulations were instituted to discourage use of the product. Tobacco is a major industry in the South, supporting jobs and providing profits for tobacco companies. Cigarette sales also are a significant source of income for many small businesses. Owners of bars and restaurants have fought laws restricting smoking on their premises, fearing that they would lose the patronage of smokers. Politicians are not eager to institute strong public health measures that would have such a major economic impact. Only in the past 2 or 3 decades, with the shift of public opinion against the tobacco industry, together with the industry's need to protect itself against a potentially bankrupting flood of lawsuits by injured smokers, have federal, state, and local governments begun to take serious measures to control smoking.

In many circumstances, controversy arises because those who pay for a public health measure are not the ones who benefit. Environmental regulations such as restrictions on timber harvesting in the Pacific Northwest are regularly under attack because they may cost jobs in the lumber industry, although they may preserve jobs in the fishing and tourist industries as well as contribute in the long term to a more stable climate. Regulations that protect the health and safety of workers may require expensive protective equipment, thus driving up the costs to consumers.

In times of economic difficulty, people are often unwilling to pay short-term costs in order to obtain a benefit in the long term. In both the fishing and lumber industries, stocks have been dangerously depleted, and there is a risk of killing off all the fish and cutting down all the timber, thereby destroying the industries altogether. Yet few workers in the fishing or lumber industries are willing to voluntarily cut back on their own harvests. Companies resist tough pollution control laws even though less polluting technology may lead to a long-term benefit not only for the environment but also for a company's competitiveness in international markets. This short-sightedness became apparent at a time of high gas prices, when U.S. automobile companies suddenly lost market share and profits because they invested so much of their production into formerly profitable gas-guzzling SUVs that Americans can now no longer afford to drive.

The costs of public health measures are usually much easier to calculate than the benefits. For example, experts may know the cost of reducing smog in Los Angeles to a level that reduces deaths from lung disease by 10 percent. But how do they calculate whether this benefit is worth the cost? It is very difficult to put a dollar value on life and health. Furthermore, it is often difficult to quantify what the risk really is and how to balance it against other risks. People are concerned, for example, about farmers' use of pesticides, which may leave toxic residues on fruits and vegetables. Scientists can estimate the health risks the average person faces by consuming that residue. But fruits and vegetables are an important part of a healthy diet. If the use of pesticides were forbidden, the crops might be less abundant, and the price of the produce might rise, perhaps discouraging some people from eating these nutritious foods. Thus, an effort to protect health might have a negative impact on health overall.

Individual Liberty

One of the primary purposes of government is to "promote the general welfare," as called for in the U.S. Constitution. Health and safety, together with economic well-being, are the major factors that contribute to the general welfare. While the government cannot guarantee health and safety for each individual, its role is to provide for maximum health and safety for the community as a whole. One of the central controversies in public health is the extent to which government can and should restrict individual freedom for the purpose of improving the community's health.

There has long been general agreement that it is acceptable to restrict an individual's freedom to behave in such a way as to cause direct harm to others. Laws against assault and murder are found in the Bible and even in the Babylonian Code of Hammurabi, which dates to the 18th century B.C. When the harm is less direct, however, the issues become more controversial. Most controversial are governmental restrictions on people's freedom to harm themselves.

Government restrictions on behavior that causes indirect harm to others is the way to prevent what Garrett Hardin, in 1968, called the "tragedy of the commons."[5] Hardin describes a pasture open to all herdsmen in a community. The land can support a limited number of

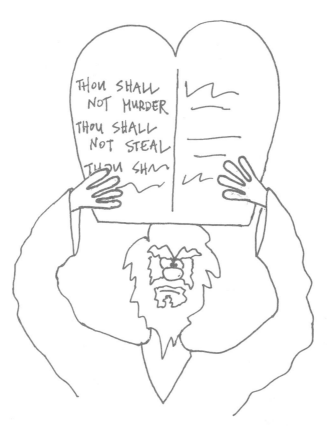

Restricting Individual Freedom

grazing cattle. If each herdsman tries to maximize his gain by keeping as many cattle as possible on the pasture—the commons—the pasture will be overgrazed. The cattle will starve, and the herdsmen will be ruined. The only way for the community to save the pasture is to agree to restrict the freedom of the herdsmen, placing fair and equitable limits on the number of cattle each can keep there.

In the industrialized world of today, the "commons" is the air, water, and other elements of the environment that all people share. Because no individual has the power to control the quality of his or her own personal environment independent of the behavior of his or her neighbors, government action is required to protect these common resources. While the general principle of protecting the "commons" is accepted by most citizens, there is plenty of room for controversy in defining what to include among the protected resources, as well as how extensive the protective measures should be.

The United States has made great progress over the past 40 years in cleaning up air and water through federal legislation. Now questions are being raised as to whether the laws have gone too far in restricting the "freedom" to pollute. Companies have been required to limit emissions from their smokestacks; automobile makers have been required to install emission control devices on every car they manufacture. These regulations may have driven up the costs of automobiles and other products, but they have not limited anybody's freedom. However, California still has a serious air pollution problem. Proposed regulations for the state to meet the federal mandates for clean air have included a ban on gas-driven lawn mowers, elimination of drive-through windows in banks and fast-food restaurants (to cut the pollution that results from idling car engines), and a ban on charcoal lighting fluid. None of these activities on an individual basis—mowing a lawn, sitting in an idling car waiting for a hamburger, or lighting a few chunks of charcoal—contributes in any major way to the pollution of California's air, but when done by thousands of residents each day, they add up to a significant problem. Are Americans willing to accept such significant limitations on their behavior in order to achieve the desirable goal of clean air to breathe?

Most controversial of public health measures are requirements that restrict people's freedom for the purpose of protecting their own health and safety. Examples of such measures include requirements to wear seat belts when traveling in a car and helmets when riding a motorcycle. Such laws inspire allusions to "the tyranny of health"[6] and "the health police," although restrictions on many drugs, such as heroin, cocaine, marijuana, LSD, and—during Prohibition in the early 20th century—alcohol have been generally accepted.

Such restrictions on individual behavior are often criticized as "paternalism." Libertarians, in the words of John Stuart Mill, argue that "the only purpose for which power can be rightfully exercised over any member of a civilized community, against his will, is to prevent harm to others ... In the part [of his conduct] which merely concerns himself, his independence is ... absolute."[7(p.90)] The one form of paternalism that is generally accepted is that children and young people can be restricted in their behavior on the basis that they are not yet mature enough to make considered judgments as to their own best interests. Thus, there are laws that prevent juveniles from buying tobacco and alcohol, that require them to wear bicycle helmets and seat belts (even where adults are not required to wear them), and that require parental permission to obtain birth control information or an abortion, or to go skydiving.

According to the libertarian view, which has a strong tradition in the United States, it is acceptable to outlaw drunk driving but not drunkenness itself. Similarly, smoking in indoor public places can be outlawed because the smoke bothers others (although there is still strong resistance in many places), while smoking itself cannot be regulated in adults.

Restrictions on individual liberty are sometimes justified on the basis that their purpose is really to protect others, even when the argument is a bit strained. For example, unhelmeted motorcyclists could be a threat to others because of the possibility of their losing control if hit by flying debris. Unhelmeted cyclists and unbelted motorists, severely injured in road accidents, drive up insurance rates for others and in extreme cases may become expensive wards of the state. Alcoholics and drug users bring harm to their families and are a nuisance to their neighbors.

Most public health advocates believe that there are more fundamental justifications for restrictions on individual behavior for the sake of the public health. Beauchamp, the philosopher, explores the reasons in his book, *The Health of the Republic*, arguing that such laws are needed most for behaviors that are common and carry small risks. Consistent use of seat belts, for example, prevents thousands of deaths and injuries in the population as a whole, although the risk people face on any one trip, when they must decide whether to buckle up, is quite small. While each individual's choice to take the risk of driving unbuckled may be rational, society's interest in preventing the thousands of deaths and injuries outweighs the minor inconvenience of obeying the seatbelt law.

Beauchamp's argument in favor of limiting individual liberty for the common good is consistent with his view of public health as social justice. Death and disability are collective problems, he says, and collective action is needed to promote the common welfare. The U.S. tradition of supporting private liberty above all is wrong, as noted by that early critic of the American character, Alexis de Tocqueville, in that it "disposes [citizens] not to think of their fellows and turns indifference into a sort of public virtue."[8(p.16)]

Moral and Religious Opposition

Public health often arouses controversy on moral grounds, most often when it confronts sexual and reproductive issues. AIDS, other sexually transmitted diseases, teenage pregnancy, and low birth-weight babies are major public health problems in the United States. The public health approach to these problems includes sex education in schools and the provision of contraceptive services, especially condoms. These measures are often vigorously opposed by members of certain religious groups who believe that they promote immoral behavior. Safe and legal abortion to terminate unwanted pregnancy is even more controversial. While there is no question that the safest and healthiest lifestyle is to abstain from sexual activity before marriage and then to be faithful to one's spouse, experience has long shown that preaching morality has limited efficacy in preventing sexually transmitted diseases and unwanted pregnancy.

AIDS has been an especially divisive issue because so many people with AIDS contracted the disease through behavior that is widely regarded as immoral—homosexual acts and intravenous drug use. Consequently, AIDS-related policy has often been confounded by moral revulsion against the disease and its victims. While not supported by the evidence, it is commonly believed that education on how to protect oneself against contracting the virus that causes AIDS may encourage homosexuality and promiscuous sexual behavior in general. Similarly, moralists frown on the practice of providing clean needles to drug addicts because, while it is effective in reducing the spread of the virus, they believe it condones the use of intravenous drugs.

Moralism also enters into discussions of alcohol and drug policy. Libertarians could argue against regulation of alcohol and bans on addictive drugs on the basis that consumption of drugs is private behavior that does not directly hurt others. In fact, however, most citizens accept the validity of such regulation. The power of government to limit drug and alcohol consumption is well established in the United States and corresponds with the tradition of limiting individual behavior for the common good.

While regulation for the common good is valid, trying to legislate morality has often proven to be ineffective, self-defeating, and a threat to liberty, in part because people differ in what they view as moral. When morality is the justification for banning certain behaviors, rational discussion is often impossible. Free speech is repressed, victims are demonized, practitioners of the behavior are driven underground, and the "epidemic"—whether AIDS, drug abuse, or teenage pregnancy—spreads more easily.[4]

Moral and religious concerns may interfere with scientists' studying how to prevent the spread of the human immunodeficiency virus (HIV) and other diseases and conditions caused by unhealthy behavior. Up to half of the deaths in the United States are preventable, many of them caused by unhealthy behavior. Yet a small fraction of the research funded by the federal government is devoted to understanding why people behave in unhealthy ways and how to encourage them to change these behaviors. Such research tends to be highly controversial and is vulnerable to attacks by conservative groups. For example, in the fall of 2003, a group called the Traditional Values Coalition drew up a list of projects funded by the National Institutes of Health and requested that a congressional committee investigate why taxpayer money was being "wasted" on these studies, which involved HIV transmission and sexual behavior.[9] Although the investigation did not lead to withdrawal of funding from any of these projects, such episodes do have the effect of discouraging scientists and funding agencies from conducting research on many important public health problems.

Political Interference with Science

While there are legitimate differences of opinion on how to weigh the competing interests in making policy that affects public health, these decisions should be informed by science to the extent possible. The George W. Bush administration was notorious for going beyond previous political practices in manipulating and distorting scientific evidence to fit its political agenda. In February 2004 the Union of Concerned Scientists (UCS), a nonprofit advocacy group, released a report called "Scientific Integrity in Policymaking," which was signed by more than 60 leading scientists, including 20 Nobel-Prize winners.[10] The report documented many instances of the administration's misrepresentation or suppression of scientific information and stacking of scientific advisory committees to obscure the fact that policy decisions were based on its political agenda, which usually favored right-wing constituencies and large corporations.

One example cited by the UCS report was pressure on the Centers for Disease Control and Prevention (CDC) to promote abstinence-only programs for preventing teen pregnancy. The CDC was required to remove from its Web site information on "Programs that Work," five sex education programs for teenagers that had been found effective in scientific studies. Similarly, the CDC replaced information on the effectiveness of condoms in preventing the spread of HIV/AIDS with a document that emphasizes condom failure rates and the effectiveness of abstinence. While there is no dispute that abstinence is the most effective way to prevent pregnancy and HIV transmission, scientific studies have found abstinence-only programs to be ineffective. In 2003, *The New York Times* reported that the National Cancer Institute's Web site contained information suggesting that having an abortion increased a woman's risk of breast cancer. This issue had long been discredited by a number of epidemiologic studies, and the publicity forced the Institute to remove the inaccurate information.[11]

Since the publication of the UCS report, the organization has maintained an ongoing "Integrity in Science Watch," documenting instances of political interference with government scientists as well as conflicts of interest by scientists and organizations with ties to industry.

Global warming was an issue on which the Bush administration especially sought to suppress information and to discredit scientific evidence. According to the UCS, the political environment over this issue was so hostile that the Environmental Protection Agency decided to omit an entire climate change section from a major report on the environment rather than compromise its credibility by misrepresenting the scientific consensus. A scientist from the National Oceanic and Atmospheric Administration reported that, when he organized a conference on carbon dioxide, he was told that the words "climate change" could not be used in the title of any presentation.

Another way the administration sought to distort scientific information, according to the UCS report, was by packing scientific advisory committees with ideologues and industry representatives. For example, the President's Council on Bioethics was created to consider research on embryonic stem cells, which offers the hope of curing many degenerative diseases, but has been strongly opposed by abortion opponents. In early 2004, President Bush dismissed two of the members, scientists who were supporters of such research. "It seems like an act of desperation to keep the bioethics commission from coming up with advice [the president] doesn't want to hear," said a Nobel-prize winning geneticist.[12] An advisory committee on childhood lead poisoning prevention was about to recommend that the CDC issue a stricter federal standard for exposure to lead, which damages children's brains and nervous systems, when the Secretary of Health and Human Services replaced highly qualified scientists on the committee with members who had financial ties to the industry. "The Bush administration has the right to implement the policies it chooses," said one of the signers of the UCS statement. "We object to the administration pretending the science supports these policies, when in fact it doesn't."[12]

President Barack Obama has promised to restore scientific integrity to federal policy making. His science advisor, physicist John Holdren, was one of the original signers of the UCS's report.[13] President Obama issued a scientific integrity directive in 2010, which was praised by the UCS, but the organization continues to monitor federal policymaking, tracking the Obama administration's progress—and missteps—toward restoring scientific integrity.[14] Although the Obama administration appears to be more inclined to make policy decisions based on honest science, it is still susceptible to pressure from Congress and business interests to eliminate "unnecessary regulation" and weaken safety protections for economic reasons.[15]

Conclusion

Public health is controversial because, depending upon how it is defined, it may challenge people's values and demand sacrifices. The battle between an expansive and a restrictive view of public health is ongoing. The expansive view asks people to give up a degree of personal liberty for the common good.

At its most idealistic, public health is a broad social movement, a campaign to maximize health for everyone in the population through distributing benefits and responsibilities in an equitable way. Health is therefore "a political endeavor as much as, or at times even more than, a medical one."[16(p.15)]

Public health measures are often controversial because they have an economic impact. The people or industries that must pay the price may not be the ones that will benefit from the new protections. Costs are usually more concrete than benefits. Moreover, the price may need to be paid sooner while the benefit may not be achieved until later.

Public health may be affected by personal and intimate behaviors, which are often embarrassing and even offensive to discuss. Thus some public health measures are controversial because they arouse moral or religious objections.

Although there are legitimate differences of opinion on how to weigh competing interests in making public health policy, concerns were raised that the Bush II administration misused and distorted scientific evidence to pretend that its policies were based on science when they really were not.

References

1. U.S. Institute of Medicine, Committee for the Study of the Future of Public Health, *The Future of Public Health* (Washington, DC: National Academy Press, 1988).

2. C.-E. A. Winslow, *The Evolution and Significance of the Modern Public Health Campaign* (New Haven, CT: Yale University Press, 1923); reprint, *Journal of Public Health Policy*, (1984): 1.

3. C.-E. A. Winslow, "The Contribution of Hermann Biggs to Public Health: The 1928 Biggs Memorial Lecture," *The American Review of Tuberculosis* 20 (1929): 1–28.

4. D. E. Beauchamp, "Public Health as Social Justice," *Inquiry* 13 (1976): 1–14.

5. G. Hardin, "The Tragedy of the Commons," *Science* 162 (1968): 1243–1248.

6. F. T. Fitzgerald, "The Tyranny of Health," *New England Journal of Medicine* 331 (1994): 196–198.

7. J. S. Mill, "On Liberty," quoted in D. E. Beauchamp, *The Health of the Republic: Epidemics, Medicine, and Moralism as Challenges to Democracy* (Philadelphia: Temple University Press, 1988), 90.

8. A. de Toqueville, *Democracy in America*, quoted in Beauchamp, *The Health of the Republic* 16.

9. J. Kaiser, "NIH Roiled by Inquiries Over Grants Hit List," *Science* 302 (2003): 758.

10. Union of Concerned Scientists, "Scientific Integrity in Policy Making," March 2004. http://www.ucsusa.org/scientific_integrity/interference/reports-scientific-integrity-in-policy-making.html, accessed September 21, 2012.

11. Union of Concerned Scientists, "Scientific Knowledge on Breast Cancer Distorted," http://www.ucsusa.org/scientific_integrity/abuses_of_science/breast-cancer.html, accessed April 25, 2012.

12. American Public Health Association, "Politics Outweighing Science in Policy Decisions, Report Says," *Nation's Health* (April 2004): 1.

13. Union of Concerned Scientists, Press Release, "John Holdren Could Strengthen Federal Science," December 19, 2008. http://www.ucsusa.org/news/press_release/john-holdren-could-strengthen-0180.html, accessed September 21, 2012.

14. Union of Concerned Scientists, "The White House's Scientific Integrity Directive," December 22, 2010. http://www.ucsusa.org/scientific_integrity/solutions/big_picture_solutions/SI-directive.html, accessed April 25, 2012.

15. Union of Concerned Scientists, "New Executive Order Could Limit Ability of U.S. Science Agencies to Protect the Public," May 2, 2012. http://blog.ucsusa.org/new-executie-order-could-limit-ability-of-u-s-science-agencies-to-protect-the-public, accessed May 10, 2012.

16. L. Wallack et al., *Media Advocacy and Public Health: Power for Prevention* (Newbury Park, CA: Sage Publications, 1993), 15.

Powers and Responsibilities of Government

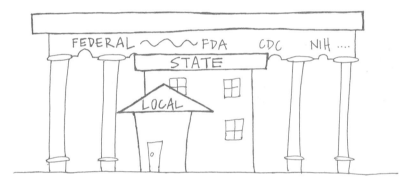

Federal, State, Local . . .

Governments ultimately have the responsibility of making the organized community efforts necessary to protect the health of the population, although many other organizations and community groups are also important participants. Government's role is determined by law; that is, government's public health activities must be authorized by legislation at the federal, state, or local levels. The public health law is further defined by decisions of the courts at the various levels of government. The broad decisions of the legislative and judicial branches of government are worked out in detail by the executive branch, usually the agencies which issue regulations and carry out public health programs. The ultimate authority that allows the laws to be written is the constitution or charter, whether federal, state, or local. Thus the body of public health law is massive, consisting of all the written statements relating to health by any of the three branches of government at the federal, state, and local levels.

Many nongovernmental organizations play an important role in public health, especially through educational programs and lobbying. In recent years, stimulated in part by the Institute of Medicine's *The Future of Public Health*,[1] there has been increasing emphasis on community involvement in public health planning and in generating support for and participation in public health activities. This process expands the concept of the public health system to include, for example, hospitals, businesses, and charitable and religious organizations.

Federal Versus State Authority

The U.S. Constitution does not mention health. Because the Tenth Amendment states that "the powers not delegated to the United States by the Constitution . . . are reserved to the States respectively," public health has been a responsibility primarily of the states. Most state constitutions provide for the protection of public health, and the original states already had laws concerning health before the Constitution took effect.[2]

All states have laws such as mandates to collect data about the population, to immunize children before they enter school, to regulate the environment for purposes of sanitation, and to regulate safety. To a varying extent, responsibility for some public health activities may be delegated by the state to local governments. Figure 3-1, an organization chart of a small state health department, shows public health activities typically provided for in state law.

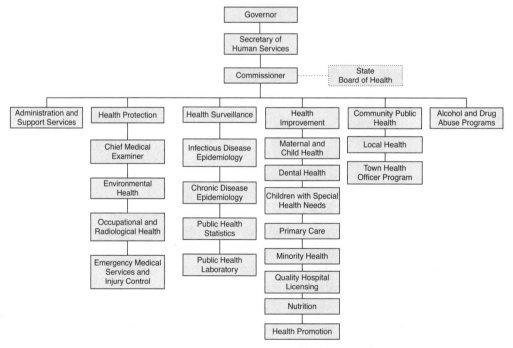

FIGURE 3-1   Organization Chart of a State Health Department. *Source:* Anonymous.

The Constitution, in the Preamble, includes among the fundamental purposes of government, "to promote the general welfare." It gives the federal government authority to regulate interstate commerce and to "collect taxes . . . to pay the debts and provide for the common defense and the general welfare." These powers are the basis for the federal role in public health.

The interstate commerce provision, for example, justifies the activities of the Food and Drug Administration (FDA), which oversees extensive federal regulation of foods, drugs, medical devices, and cosmetics, most of which are distributed across state lines. It is obviously more efficient and economical for the industries that produce these products to be bound by uniform national rules rather than having to comply with 50 different sets of state regulations.

The power to tax and spend is a way for the federal government to achieve goals that it may lack the authority to achieve directly. It can provide funds to the states subject to certain requirements. For example, in 1967 the federal government mandated that, as a precondition for receiving highway construction funds, states must pass laws requiring motorcyclists to wear helmets. The effectiveness of the mandate was demonstrated by the fact that, by 1975, 47 states had passed such laws, with the result that motorcyclist deaths declined by 30 percent in these states.[3] Another example of federal influence over state health programs is the Medicaid program of providing health care for the poor. The federal government provides 50 to 80 percent of the funding for Medicaid. States and counties administer the Medicaid program, providing the remaining funds, and must follow the guidelines established by Congress.[2]

Since World War II, the federal government has used these powers to steadily widen its role in public health, among other matters. That trend began to reverse in the 1980s. In a political climate hostile to government, especially the federal government, there was a strong movement in Congress and the Supreme Court to cut government regulation and return more powers to the states. In an early example of the reversal, in 1976 Congress removed the financial penalty for lack of motorcycle helmet laws. By 1980, 27 states had repealed their helmet laws, and motorcycle deaths rose in those states by 38 percent.[3] The Medicaid program, which has grown enormously expensive since it was established in 1965, has also been a target of Congress, which for some time has threatened, so far without success, to hand it over to the states entirely.

In the 1990s, the U.S. Supreme Court under Chief Justice William Rehnquist, began a trend known as the new federalism, which limited Congress's powers and returned authority to the states. For example, in 1995, the Court struck down a law making gun possession within a school zone a federal offense, rejecting the argument that gun possession was a matter of interstate commerce.[4] In 2001, it decided that the Americans with Disabilities Act could not be enforced against a state, ruling that a woman who was fired from her state job because she had breast cancer could not sue the state of Alabama.[5] However, the new federalism lost much of its momentum after 9/11 when, as *New York Times* reporter Linda Greenhouse noted, "suddenly the federal government looked useful, even necessary." In 2003, Rehnquist "gave up and moved on," writing the majority ruling that state governments could be sued for failing to give their employees the benefits required by the Family and Medical Leave Act.[6] In 2005, the Supreme Court affirmed the priority of federal law over state law in a controversial decision ruling that patients in California could be criminally prosecuted by federal authorities for using marijuana prescribed by a physician according to California's medical marijuana law.[7]

How the Law Works

Governments have broad power to act in ways that curtail the rights of individuals. These police powers of governments are basic to public health, and are the reason why public health must ultimately be government's responsibility.[8] Police powers are invoked for three reasons: to prevent a person from harming others; to defend the interests of incompetent persons such as children or the mentally retarded; and, in some cases, to protect a person from harming himself or herself.[9]

Laws have been used to enforce compliance in health matters for over a century. In 1905, a precedent was set for the state's police power in the area of health when the Massachusetts legislature passed a law that required all adults to be vaccinated against smallpox. A man named Jacobson refused to comply and went to court, arguing that the law infringed on his personal liberty. The trial court found that the state was within its power to enforce the law. Jacobson appealed his case all the way to the U.S. Supreme Court. He lost: the Supreme Court upheld the right of the state to restrict an individual's freedom "for the common good."[4]

The public health law has become more complex over the years, but it follows the same pattern. At any level of government, a legislature, perceiving a need, passes a statute. The statute may be challenged in court and the decision of the court may be appealed to higher courts. Generally, on issues of constitutionality, a state court may overturn a local law or court decision, and a federal court may overturn a state law or court decision.

Since public health increasingly involves complex technical issues, legislatures at the several levels of government generally set up administrative agencies to perform public health functions. The legislature, recognizing that it lacks the necessary expertise, authorizes these agencies to set rules that define in detail how to accomplish the purpose of the legislation. The courts may then be called on to interpret the authority of the agencies under the laws and to determine whether certain rules or decisions of an agency are within its legal authority.

As an example of the interplay of legislation, agency rule making, and the role of the courts, consider the Occupational Safety and Health Act, passed by Congress in 1970. The legislation stated that "personal injuries and illnesses arising out of work situations impose a substantial burden upon . . . interstate commerce," and thus used the federal government's authority over interstate commerce to pass a public health statute.[10(p.180)] The law established the Occupational Safety and Health Administration (OSHA) within the Department of Labor. OSHA was authorized, among other things, to set standards regulating employees' exposure to hazardous substances. Representatives of industry challenged the constitutional authority of Congress to pass the law but were unsuccessful.

Industries that feel economically harmed by OSHA's standard setting have used other routes to weaken the agency's power. One of the substances that OSHA decided to regulate was benzene, which caused a variety of toxic effects among workers in the rubber and petrochemical industries. In 1971, OSHA set a standard limiting benzene exposure to 10 parts per million (ppm) in air, averaged over an 8-hour period. Epidemiologic evidence indicated, however, that exposure to lower concentrations of benzene over time might increase the risk of leukemia, and there was laboratory evidence to support those studies. Therefore, in 1978, OSHA lowered the standard to 1 ppm over an 8-hour period. Representatives of the affected industries appealed the new regulations in court, claiming that evidence that benzene causes leukemia was not sufficiently strong, and that complying with the new standard would be too expensive. The court, in a ruling upheld later by the Supreme Court, agreed that OSHA did not have sufficient evidence to support the need for the new standard and thus had exceeded its authority in issuing the regulation.[10] The standard remained at 10 ppm until 1987, when evidence for the carcinogenicity of benzene was deemed convincing enough to justify the lower value.[11]

The courts did not rule on whether the cost of complying with a standard should be considered in the process of setting it. The act had specified that standards should ensure the health of workers "to the extent feasible."[10(p.180)] Industry argued that OSHA should have done a cost-benefit analysis before issuing the regulation. This issue was decided in another case, in which the courts determined that a formal cost-benefit analysis was not required in the law.[10] Usually, the expected cost of implementing regulations is considered together with the potential benefits when decisions are made. However, there is plenty of room for controversy over the relative magnitudes of the costs and benefits.

Since regulatory activities of federal and state governments are so fundamental to public health, they will often be discussed throughout this text.

How Public Health Is Organized and Paid for in the United States

Local Public Health Agencies

The organization of public health at the local level varies from state to state and even within states. The most common local agency is the county health department. A large city may have its own municipal health department, and rural areas may be served by multicounty health departments. Some local areas have no public health department, leaving their residents to do without some services and to depend on state government for others.

Local health departments have the day-to-day responsibility for public health matters in their jurisdiction. These include collecting health statistics; conducting communicable disease control programs; providing screening and immunizations; providing health education services and chronic disease control programs; conducting sanitation, sanitary engineering, and inspection programs; running school health programs; and delivering maternal and child health services and public health nursing services. Mental health may or may not be the responsibility of a separate agency.

In many states, laws assign local public health agencies the responsibility for providing medical care to the poor. While this task may be considered part of the assurance function defined in *The Future of Public Health*,[1] the Institute of Medicine found that this role tends to consume excessive resources and distract local health departments from performing their assessment and policy development functions. The provision of medical services by public health clinics has often been a source of friction with the medical establishment. Functions of a typical county health department are shown in the organizational chart, Figure 3-2.

The source of funds for local health department activities varies widely among states. Some states provide the bulk of funding for local health departments while others provide very little. The federal government may fund some local health department activities directly, or federal funds may be passed on from the states. A portion of the local health budget usually comes from local property and sales taxes, and from fees that the department charges for some services. The extent to which local health departments are responsive to mandates from the state and federal government is likely to depend on how much of the local agency's budget is provided by these sources. When the bulk of a local health department's budget is determined by a city council or county legislature, the local agency's capacity to perform core functions may depend on its ability to educate the legislative body about public health and its importance.

State Health Departments

The states have the primary constitutional responsibility and authority for the protection of the health, safety, and general welfare of the population, and much of this responsibility falls on state health departments. The scope of this responsibility varies: some states have separate agencies for social services, aging, mental health, the environment, and so on. This may cause problems, for example, when the environmental agency makes decisions that impact the population's health without consulting the health agency, or—in one example described by the Institute of Medicine—when the Indian Health Service, the state health agency, and the state mental health agency argued about which was responsible for adult and aging services.[1] Some state health departments are strongly centralized, while others delegate much of their authority to the local health departments. State health departments depend heavily on federal money for many programs, and their authority is thus limited by the strings attached to the federal funds.

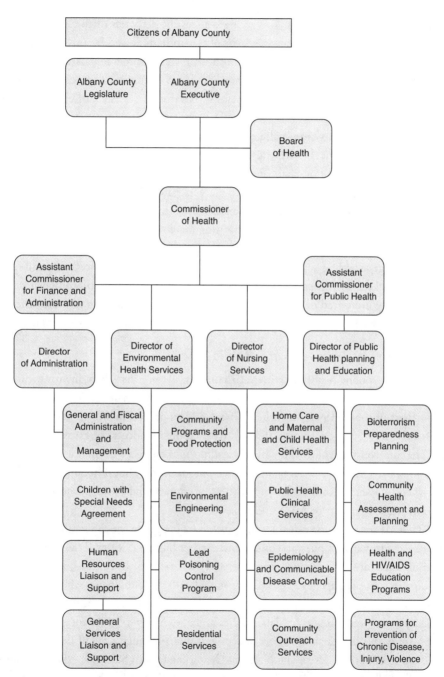

FIGURE 3-2 Organization Chart of a County Health Department. *Source:* Courtesy of the Albany County Department of Health.

State health departments define to varying degrees the activities of the local health departments. The state health department may set policies to be followed by the local agencies, and they generally provide significant funding, both from state sources and as channels for federal funds. The state health department coordinates activities of the local agencies and collects and analyzes the data provided by the local agencies. Laboratory services are often provided by state health departments.

State health departments are usually charged with licensing and certification of medical personnel, facilities, and services, with the purpose of maintaining standards of competence and quality of care. An organization chart of a typical state health department is shown in Figure 3-1.

People who lack private health insurance are generally the concern of state health departments, although many states pass this responsibility on to localities. Some of these people are covered by Medicaid, the joint federal–state program for the poor. States have significant—though not total—flexibility in how to administer the Medicaid program, determining eligibility rules for coverage as well as setting payment amounts for the doctors, hospitals, and other providers of medical care. Most states also provide some kind of funding to hospitals to reimburse them for treating uninsured patients who arrive in the emergency room and must be treated.

Funding for state health department activities comes mostly from state taxes and federal grants.

Federal Agencies Involved with Public Health

Most traditional public health activities at the federal level, other than environmental health, fall under the jurisdiction of the Department of Health and Human Services (HHS). The organization chart of the HHS is shown in Figure 3-3. The predominant agencies are the Centers for Disease Control and Prevention (CDC), the National Institutes of Health (NIH), and the FDA. The Surgeon General is the nation's leading spokesperson on matters of public health. The position does not in itself carry much direct line authority, but it became very visible in the 1980s when C. Everett Koop spoke out with great courage and moral authority on the politically controversial subjects of AIDS and tobacco.

The CDC is the main assessment and epidemiologic agency for the nation. The mission of the CDC is, as its name implies, to control and prevent human diseases. Traditionally, the CDC focused on infectious diseases and was therefore crisis-oriented. In contrast, the NIH holds the longer view of a research agency. The CDC is staffed with epidemiologists who travel throughout the country and the world to detect outbreaks of disease, to track down the causes of epidemics, and to halt their spread. It also has laboratories at its headquarters in Atlanta, where biomedical scientists study the viruses and bacteria linked with the epidemics. One of the 12 centers, institutes, and offices in the CDC is the National Center for Health Statistics, which is the national authority for collecting, analyzing, and disseminating health data for the United States.

The CDC has expanded its mission over recent decades to include chronic diseases, genetics, injury and violence, and environmental health. The CDC's change in focus is justified by

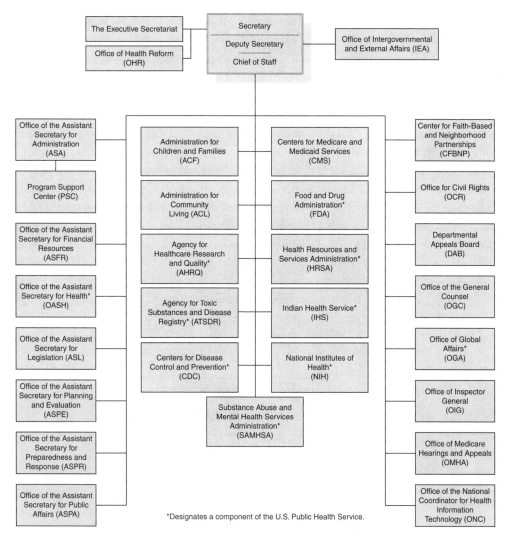

FIGURE 3-3 HHS Organizational Chart. *Source:* Reproduced from U.S. Department of Health and Human Services (2012). HHS Organizational Chart. http://www.hhs.gov/about/orgchart/, accessed October 1, 2012.

the argument that infectious diseases no longer are the leading causes of death and disability in the United States and that these other problems must be addressed in order to make further progress in preventing and controlling disease. However, the CDC's involvement in programs to prevent noninfectious diseases, injury, and violence is more controversial politically, in that it embroils the agency in discussions of health-related behavior, as well as of industries, such as tobacco and firearms, that have supporters in Congress.

Figure 3-4 shows the organization chart of the CDC. The CDC issues a weekly publication called *Morbidity and Mortality Weekly Report (MMWR)*, which is widely distributed in print and electronically via the Internet. *MMWR* reports on timely public health topics that the CDC deals with, such as outbreaks of infectious diseases and new environmental and behavioral health hazards. The first published report that heralded the onset of the AIDS epidemic appeared in *MMWR* on June 4, 1981.[12] The CDC's journal *Emerging Infectious Diseases*, published in print and online, discusses new infectious disease threats that occur naturally as well as potential bioterrorist threats.

The NIH is the greatest biomedical research complex in the world, with its own research laboratories, most of which are located in Bethesda, Maryland, as well as a program that provides grants to biomedical scientists at universities and research centers throughout the United States. The NIH supports research ranging from basic cellular processes to the physiological errors that underlie human diseases. The NIH's Clinical Center in Bethesda is a research hospital where

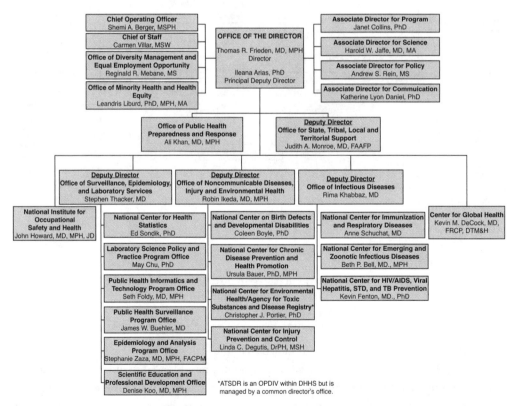

FIGURE 3-4   CDC Organizational Chart. *Source:* Reproduced from the Centers for Disease Control and Prevention (2012). CDC Organizational Chart, updated July 23, 2012. http://www.cdc.gov/maso/pdf/CDC_Chart_wNames.pdf, accessed October 1, 2012.

medical researchers test experimental therapies. The NIH also includes the National Library of Medicine, which serves as a reference library for medical centers around the world. Its computerized bibliographic service can be accessed on the Internet. The organization chart of the NIH is shown in Box 3-1.

Box 3-1

National Institutes of Health; Institutes, Centers, and Offices

- Office of the Director
- National Cancer Institute
- National Eye Institute
- National Heart, Lung, and Blood Institute
- National Human Genome Research Institute
- National Institute on Aging
- National Institute on Alcohol Abuse and Alcoholism
- National Institute of Arthritis and Musculoskeletal and Skin Diseases
- National Institute of Biomedical Imaging and Bioengineering
- Eunice Kennedy Shriver National Institute of Child Health and Human Development
- National Institute on Deafness and Other Communication Disorders
- National Institute of Dental and Craniofacial Research
- National Institute of Diabetes and Digestive and Kidney Diseases
- National Institute on Drug Abuse
- National Institute of Environmental Health Sciences
- National Institute of General Medical Sciences
- National Institute of Mental Health
- National Institute on Minority Health and Health Disparities
- National Institute of Neurological Disorders and Stroke
- National Institute of Nursing Research
- National Library of Medicine
- Center for Information Technology
- Center for Scientific Review
- John E. Fogarty International Center for Advanced Study in the Health Sciences
- National Center for Complementary and Alternative Medicine
- National Center for Advancing Translational Sciences
- NIH Clinical Center

Source: Modified from National Institutes of Health, www.nih.gov/icd, accessed October 1, 2012.

NIH has enjoyed strong Congressional support over the years. Research aimed at curing human diseases is a popular cause and, for the most part, is generally agreed to be a proper activity for the federal government. States and private companies could not afford to do biomedical research, except to a limited extent, and until recently the prospects for corporate profit in this field were not great. Even periodic budgetary constraints have usually spared NIH the worst of the axe.

Regulation of the food and drug industries has been difficult and controversial since Massachusetts passed the first American pure-food law in 1784. As recently as the late 19th century, milk was commonly watered down, then doctored with chalk or plaster of Paris to make it look normal.[13] The Pure Food and Drugs Act of 1906 was opposed by the food-canning industry, drug and patent medicine manufacturers, whiskey interests, and, of course, the meat-packing industry. That law was passed soon after the publication of Upton Sinclair's best selling novel, *The Jungle*, an exposé of brutal and filthy conditions in the Chicago stockyards.

The modern FDA was established in 1931, and the current law provides for the agency, in addition to ensuring that the food supply is safe and nutritious, to evaluate all new drugs, food additives and colorings, and certain medical devices, approving them only if they are proven safe and, in the case of drugs, effective. The agency also regulates vaccines and diagnostic tests, animal drugs, and cosmetics. Because FDA regulations affect major segments of the U.S. economy, it is frequently under attack, either for being too restrictive or, when an approved product is found to cause harm, too lenient.

Other components of the HHS include the Centers for Medicare and Medicaid Services and the Agency for Healthcare Research and Quality, which supports research on healthcare quality and cost. The Indian Health Service operates hospitals and health clinics for Native Americans.

Responsibility for environmental health is scattered throughout the federal government, including the CDC's Center for Environmental Health and the NIH's National Institute of Environmental Health Sciences. The prime agency for the environment is the Environmental Protection Agency (EPA), established in 1970 to carry out programs dealing with water pollution, air pollution, toxic substances control, and other issues of environmental contamination. The EPA is one of the most controversial federal public health agencies. It has often been attacked by Congress and its policies were often watered down by the Bush II White House.

Many other federal agencies have public health responsibilities. For example, although meat safety concerns were a major factor in the establishment of the FDA, standards of meat safety are the province of the Department of Agriculture. The Department of Agriculture also oversees food and nutrition programs, including food stamps and school lunches. The Department of Education supervises health education and school health and safety programs. Among the responsibilities of the Department of Transportation is traffic safety, the purview of the National Highway Traffic Safety Administration, which has had great success in reducing deaths caused by motor vehicles. The Department of Labor has OSHA, which is concerned with occupational health and prevention of occupational injury. The Department of Veterans Affairs administers its own health and medical services. The Department of Defense, which provides medical care for the armed forces, has long had to deal with public health concerns relating to threats from infectious diseases in foreign climates as well as health effects from toxic chemicals and radiation. The Department of Homeland Security was created in 2003 to protect the public from acts of terrorism, natural disasters, and other emergencies.

Nongovernmental Role in Public Health

While government bears the major responsibility for public health, many nongovernmental organizations play important roles, especially in education, lobbying, and research. Organizations that focus on specific diseases, such as the American Heart Association, the American Cancer Society, the Alzheimer's Disease and Related Disorders Association, and the American Diabetes Association, lobby Congress for resources and policies to benefit their causes. They also conduct campaigns to educate the public and may sponsor research concerned with their disease. Professional membership organizations, such as the American Public Health Association, the American Medical Association, and the American Nurses Association also are active in lobbying Congress in support of public health issues such as research related to the health effects of smoking. However, the American Medical Association is also known for its opposition to some public health-related programs such as President Clinton's universal healthcare proposal of 1994 and the possibility of a government-sponsored insurance option in President Obama's 2009 health reform plan (both of which failed). Other organizations that will play an important role in defining the future of public health include the National Association of City and County Health Officers, the Association of State and Territorial Health Officers, and the Association of Schools of Public Health.

Several major philanthropic foundations provide funding to support research or special projects related to public health. For example, the Rockefeller Foundation focuses on world population issues; the Robert Wood Johnson Foundation on providing health care to the poor as well as on AIDS, alcoholism, and drug abuse; the Pew Charitable Trusts on health, AIDS, and drug abuse; the Kaiser Family Foundation on health and public policy; and the Commonwealth Fund also on health and public policy, especially concerning minorities, children, and elderly people. Bill Gates of Microsoft has endowed the Bill and Melinda Gates Foundation, the mission of which is to improve global health.

Consumers groups organized around specific issues have sometimes had a major impact on national or regional policy related to public health. For example, Ralph Nader's traffic safety campaign in the 1960s forced Congress to pass legislation requiring the automobile industry to build safer cars. The Gay Men's Health Crisis played a critical role in the 1980s in starting up community health services for AIDS victims in New York City.

One of the lessons of the Institute of Medicine report was that governments alone cannot achieve the objectives of public health. Organized community efforts to prevent disease and prolong life must involve all sectors of the community, including providers of healthcare services, local business, community organizations, the media, and the general public. In the words of one public health leader, "Public health, unlike virtually all other important social efforts, is dependent on its ability to obtain the participation of other agencies to solve its problems."[14(p.399)] Thus, public health leaders must be adept at negotiation and coalition building.

Some efforts—led by the federal government with the participation of other governmental and nongovernmental organizations—of the past decades are discussed elsewhere to develop a framework for public health planning and action that involves all sectors of the community at the local, state, and national levels.

Conclusion

As an organized community effort, public health is primarily the responsibility of government, although a successful public health enterprise must involve all sectors of the community. Because the U.S. Constitution does not mention health, the states have the primary legal responsibility for public health. In turn, local governments, as the level of government closest to the people, provide the bulk of public health services. Despite the lack of explicit constitutional authority, the federal government has established a significant presence in public health. Federal agencies establish and enforce laws and regulations on issues that need a national scope. Through its authority to tax and spend, the federal government leads and assists state and local governments in providing public health services.

References

1. U.S. Institute of Medicine, Committee for the Study of the Future of Public Health, *The Future of Public Health* (Washington, DC: National Academy Press, 1988).
2. T. Christoffel, *Health and the Law: A Handbook for Health Professionals* (New York: The Free Press, 1982), 51–52.
3. G. S. Watson et al., "The Repeal of Helmet Use Laws and Increased Motorcyclist Mortality in the United States, 1975–1978," *American Journal of Public Health* 70 (1980): 579–585.
4. L. O. Gostin, "Public Health Law in a New Century, Part II: Public Health Powers and Limits," *Journal of the American Medical Association* 283 (2000): 2979–2984.

5. W. E. Parmet, "After September 11: Rethinking Public Health Federalism," *Journal of Law, Medicine & Ethics* 30 (2002): 201–211.
6. L. Greenhouse, "2,691 Decisions," *The New York Times*, July 13, 2008.
7. L. O. Gostin, "Medical Marijuana, American Federalism, and the Supreme Court," *Journal of the American Medical Association* 294 (2005): 842–844.
8. L. O. Gostin, "Public Health Law in a New Century, Part I: Law as a Tool to Advance the Community's Health," *Journal of the American Medical Association* 283 (2000): 2837–2841.
9. L. O. Gostin, "Public Health in a New Century, Part III: Public Health Regulation: A Systematic Evaluation," *Journal of the American Medical Association* 283 (2000): 3118–3122.
10. K. R. Wing, *The Law and the Public's Health* (Ann Arbor, MI: Health Administration Press, 1990), 180.
11. I. L. Feitshans, "Law and Regulation of Benzene," *Environmental Health Perspectives* 82 (1989): 299–307.
12. U.S. Centers for Disease Control and Prevention, "Pneumocystis Pneumonia—Los Angeles," *Morbidity and Mortality Weekly Report* 30 (1981): 1–3.
13. R. M. Deutsch, *The New Nuts Among the Berries: How Nutritional Nonsense Captured America* (Palo Alto, CA: Bull Publishing, 1977).
14. G. Pickett, "Book Review: The Future of Public Health," *Journal of Public Health Policy* (Autumn 1989): 397–401.

Analytical Methods of Public Health

Epidemiology: The Basic Science of Public Health

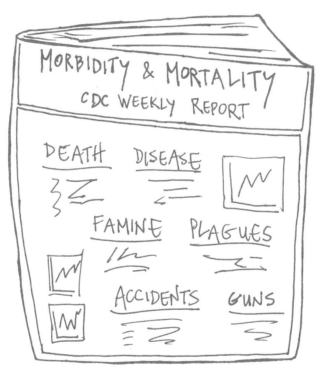

Epidemiological Surveillance

C.-E. A. Winslow, the great public health leader of the early 20th century, called epidemiology "the diagnostic discipline of public health."[1(p.vii)] Epidemiologic methods are used to investigate causes of diseases, to identify trends in disease occurrence that may influence the need for medical and public health services, and to evaluate the effectiveness of medical and public health interventions. Epidemiology is used to perform public health's assessment function called for in the Institute of Medicine's *The Future of Public Health.*[2]

Epidemiology studies the patterns of disease occurrence in human populations and the factors that influence these patterns. The term is obviously related to epidemic (derived from the Greek word meaning "upon the people"). An epidemic is an increase in the frequency of a disease above the usual and expected rate, which is called the endemic rate. Thus, epidemiologists count cases of a disease, and ask who, when, and where questions: Who is getting the disease? Where and when is the disease occurring? From this information, they can often make informed guesses as to why it is occurring. Their ultimate goal is to use this knowledge to control and prevent the spread of disease. The science of epidemiology is examined in more detail elsewhere. This chapter aims to give a more intuitive sense of what epidemiology is and does.

How Epidemiology Works

The first example of the use of epidemiology to study and control a disease occurred in London between 1853 and 1854, and it stands as an illustration of what epidemiology is and how it works. It was conducted by a British physician, John Snow, who is known as the father of modern epidemiology.

Snow was concerned about a cholera epidemic that had struck London in 1848. He noticed that death rates were especially high in parts of the city with water supplied by two private companies, both of which drew water from the Thames River at a point heavily polluted with sewage. Between 1849 and 1854, the Lambeth Company changed its source to an area of the Thames that was free of pollution from London's sewers. Snow noticed that the number of cholera deaths declined in the section of London supplied by the Lambeth Company, while there was no change in the sections supplied by the Southwark and Vauxhall Company. He formulated the hypothesis that cholera was spread by polluted drinking water.[3]

In 1853, there was a severe outbreak of cholera concentrated in the Broad Street area of London, in which some houses were supplied by one water company and some by the other. This provided an opportunity for Snow to test his hypothesis in a kind of "natural experiment," in which "people of both sexes, of every age and occupation, and of every rank and station . . . were divided into two groups without their choice, and, in most cases, without their knowledge . . ."[4(p.6–7)] Snow went to each house in which someone had died of cholera between August 1853 and January 1854 to determine which company supplied the water. When he tabulated the results, he found that in 40,046 houses supplied by the Southwark and Vauxhall Company, there were 1263 deaths from cholera. By comparison, in 26,107 houses supplied by the Lambeth Company, only 98 deaths occurred. The rate of cholera deaths was thus 8.5 times higher in houses supplied by the Southwark and Vauxhall Company than those supplied by the Lambeth Company. This was convincing evidence that deaths from cholera were linked with the source of water (see Table 4-1).

Table 4-1 Deaths from Cholera by Company Supplying Water to the Household

Water Company	Number of Houses	Deaths from Cholera	Deaths per 10,000 Houses
Southwark and Vauxhall Company	40,046	1263	315
Lambeth Company	26,107	98	37
Rest of London	256,423	1422	59

Source: Data from J. Snow, "On the Mode of Communication of Cholera" (London: John Churchill, New Burlington Street, England, 1855).

Snow would not have been able to test his hypothesis without the data on cholera deaths, which had been collected by the British government as part of a system for routine compilation of births and deaths, including cause of death, since 1839. Now, the governments of all developed countries collect data on births, deaths, and other vital statistics. These data are often used for epidemiologic studies.

Because it is preferable to recognize that an epidemic is occurring before many people start dying, governments also use a system called epidemiologic surveillance, requiring that certain "notifiable" diseases be reported as soon as they are diagnosed. These are usually infectious diseases whose spread can be prevented if the appropriate actions are taken. In the United States, approximately 60 diseases have been identified by law as notifiable at the federal level, including, for example, tuberculosis, hepatitis, measles, and syphilis. Some states require reporting of additional infectious diseases. There may also be requirements for reporting birth defects, cancer, and other noninfectious conditions. All physicians, hospitals, and clinical laboratories must report any case of a notifiable disease or condition to their local health department, which in turn reports to the state health department and the Centers for Disease Control and Prevention (CDC). The timely reporting of cases of notifiable diseases allows public health authorities to detect an emerging epidemic at an early stage. Measures can then be taken to control the spread of infectious diseases, as discussed later in this chapter. Reporting of chronic diseases is less widespread, but some public health agencies have urged a system to monitor conditions such as birth defects, Alzheimer's disease, asthma, and a variety of cancers.[5] Such a system would help to identify causes of these diseases, including environmental causes that could be controlled or eliminated, preventing further harmful effects.

While the surveillance system was created to control the spread of known diseases, the established network of reporting can facilitate the recognition that a new disease may be emerging. The first step in recognizing that a community is facing a new problem is usually a report to the local or state health department or the CDC by a perceptive physician who notices something unusual that he or she thinks should be investigated further. This is how AIDS came to be recognized early in the epidemic.

A Typical Epidemiologic Investigation—Outbreak of Hepatitis

Hepatitis A is a notifiable disease in all 50 states. Because it is caused by a virus that contaminates food or water, it is important to identify the source of any outbreak so that wider exposure to the virus can be prevented. Although hepatitis is not usually fatal to basically healthy people, it can make people quite sick for several weeks and can sometimes require hospitalization.

Because hepatitis is a notifiable disease, the local public health department is able to recognize when an outbreak occurs. A county may normally record only a few cases of hepatitis each year. This is the endemic level, the background level in a population. A sudden increase in the number of cases signifies an epidemic and calls for an epidemiologic investigation to determine why it is occurring.

The investigation requires asking the who, where, and when questions. This kind of medical detective work is nicknamed "shoeleather epidemiology." The investigator starts with the reported cases—the who—although other, unreported cases may turn up once the investigator starts asking questions. Each victim must be interviewed and asked the when question: on what date did the first symptoms appear? Knowing that hepatitis has an incubation period of about 30 days, it is possible to work back to an estimated date of exposure. The where question is the hardest: where did the victims obtain their food and water during the period of likely exposure and what sources did they have in common?

It may be that they all had eaten at the same restaurant. The epidemiologist would visit the restaurant and might find that the chef had developed hepatitis about a month earlier and been hospitalized; so the contamination of the food had stopped, and the epidemic would also stop. Alternatively, the chef may have had only a mild, perhaps unrecognized case and continued to work, thereby continuing to spread the infection. The health department might have to close the restaurant down, if necessary, until the chef is declared healthy.

Such investigations are a frequent task of epidemiologists at local health departments. A large number of these investigations deal with food poisoning outbreaks caused by contamination with *Salmonella* or *Shigella*, bacteria that commonly infect carelessly prepared or preserved food, both of which cause notifiable diseases. The Milwaukee cryptosporidiosis outbreak was solved by such an epidemiologic investigation. Although cryptosporidiosis was not a notifiable disease, the epidemic was recognized because it was so severe and widespread. If the disease had been notifiable, it might have been recognized and halted earlier. Cryptosporidiosis was added to the national list of notifiable diseases in 1995. Table 4-2 gives a list of diseases that were reportable at the national level in 2007.

Table 4-2   Infectious Diseases Designated as Notifiable at the National Level and Number of Cases Reported During 2009

Anthrax	1
Arboviral diseases	
California serogroup virus disease	
Neuroinvasive	46
Nonneuroinvasive	9
Eastern equine encephalitis virus disease	
Neuroinvasive	3
Nonneuroinvasive	1
Powassan virus disease, neuroinvasive	6
St. Louis encephalitis virus disease	
Neuroinvasive	11
Nonneuroinvasive	1
West Nile virus disease	
Neuroinvasive	386
Nonneuroinvasive	334
Botulism, total	118
Foodborne	10
Infant	85
Other	25
Brucellosis	115
Chancroid	28
Chlamydia trachomatis, genital inf.	1,244,180
Cholera	10
Coccidioidomycosis	12,926
Cryptosporidiosis, total	7654
Confirmed	7393
Probable	261
Cyclosporiasis	141
Ehrlichiosis/Anaplasmosis	
Ehrlichia chaffeensis	944
Ehrlichia ewingii	7
Anaplasma phagocytophilum	1161
Undetermined	155
Giardiasis	19,399
Gonorrhea	301,174
H. influenzae, invasive disease, all ages, serotypes	3022
Age <5 years	
Serotype b	38
Nonserotype b	245
Unknown serotype	166
Hansen disease (Leprosy)	103
Hantavirus pulmonary syndrome	20
Hemolytic uremic syndrome, postdiarrheal	242

(Continued)

Table 4-2   Infectious Diseases Designated as Notifiable at the National Level and Number of Cases Reported During 2009 (*Continued*)

Hepatitis viral, acute	
A	1987
B	3405
C	782
HIV diagnosis	36,870
Influenza-associated pediatric mortality	358
Legionellosis	3522
Listeriosis	851
Lyme disease, total	38,468
Confirmed	29,959
Probable	8509
Malaria	1451
Measles, total	71
Indigenous	51
Imported	20
Meningococcal disease, all serogroups	980
Mumps	1991
Pertussis	16,858
Plague	8
Poliomyelitis, paralytic	1
Psittacosis	9
Q fever	113
Acute	93
Chornic	93
Rabies, animal	5343
Human	4
Rocky Mountain spotted fever, total	1815
Confirmed	151
Probable	1662
Rubella	3
Rubella, congenital syndrome	2
Salmonellosis	49,192
Shiga toxin-producing E. coli (STEC)	4643
Shigellosis	15,931
Streptococcal disease, invasive, group A	5279
Streptococcal toxic-shock syndrome	161
Streptococcus pneumoniae, invasive disease	
Drug resistant	
All ages	3370
Age <5 years	583
Nondrug-resistant, age <5 years	1988
Syphilis, total, all stages	44,828
Congenital (age <1 year)	427
Primary and secondary	13,997

Tetanus	18
Toxic-shock syndrome	74
Trichinellosis	13
Tuberculosis	11,545
Tularemia	93
Typhoid fever	397
Vancomycin-intermediate *Staphylococcus aureus* (VISA)	78
Vancomycin-resistant *Staphylococcus aureus* (VRSA)	1
Varicella (chicken pox)	
Morbidity	20,489
Mortality	2
Vibriosis	789

No cases of diphtheria; poliovirus infection, nonparalytic; Powassan virus disease, nonneuroinvasive; severe acute respiratory syndrome-associated coronavirus disease (SARS-CoV); smallpox; western equine encephalitis virus disease; and yellow fever were reported in 2009.

Source: Reproduced from the Centers for Disease Control and Prevention, *Morbidity and Mortality Weekly Report* 58, (2011): 30–31. http://www.cdc.gov/mmwr/PDF/wk/mm5853.pdf, accessed October 1, 2012.

With some diseases, even a single case amounts to an epidemic. Measles, which is highly contagious, is preventable by vaccination. Although measles immunization for children was required by all states beginning in the 1970s, a number of measles epidemics occurred between 1989 and 1991 on college campuses. A reported case triggered a need for mass immunizations on campus. When epidemiologists found that many of the affected students had been immunized as infants, they concluded that a second vaccination was necessary for teenagers. The new policy put a halt to measles epidemics on campuses.

Since the bioterror attacks in the fall of 2001, the CDC has added to the list of notifiable diseases several infectious diseases caused by potential agents of bioterrorism. The first sign of a bioterror attack could be the report of a single case identified in a hospital emergency room.

Legionnaires' Disease

In July 1976, the American Legion held a 4-day convention in Philadelphia. Before the event was over, conventioneers began falling ill with symptoms of fever, muscle aches, and pneumonia. By early August, 150 cases of the disease and 20 deaths had been reported to the Pennsylvania Department of Health, and the CDC was called in to help determine what was causing the epidemic. The investigation determined that the site of exposure was most likely the Hotel Bellevue-Stratford, one of four Philadelphia hotels where convention activities were held.[6,7] Delegates who stayed at the Bellevue-Stratford had a higher rate of illness than those who stayed at other hotels, and many of those who fell ill had attended receptions in the hotel's hospitality suites. However, cases also occurred in people who had only been near, not in, the hotel, suggesting that exposure could have occurred on the streets or sidewalks nearby. The evidence suggested that the causative agent was airborne, but it did not appear to spread person-to-person to the patients' families.

While the epidemiologists were conducting their investigation, they enlisted the help of the CDC's biomedical scientists to look for evidence of viruses or bacteria in the body tissues of the victims. They also considered the possibility of a toxic chemical, but no evidence of a cause could be found. It was not until the following January that the biomedical scientists found the bacteria that were responsible for the epidemic, which by then was called Legionnaires' disease. The hotel was searched for the source of the bacteria. It was eventually found in the water of a cooling tower used for air conditioning. *Legionella* bacteria had been pumped into the cooled air and inhaled by the victims.

Once the *Legionella* bacteria were identified, they were found to be responsible for a number of other outbreaks of pneumonia around the country. The bacteria were also identified in preserved blood and tissue samples collected in 1965 from victims of a previously unsolved outbreak of pneumonia which affected some 80 patients at St. Elizabeth's psychiatric hospital in Washington, D.C., killing 14 of them.[7] Thus Legionnaires' disease had probably been around but had gone unrecognized as a specific disease at least since the invention of air conditioning. Federal air-conditioning standards were changed after the Philadelphia epidemic; stringent requirements for cleaning of cooling towers and large-scale air-conditioning systems were introduced. Legionellosis is now a notifiable disease.

Eosinophilia-Myalgia Syndrome

Although infectious agents are usually suspected first in any outbreak of a new disease, epidemiologists must also consider exposure to a toxic substance as an alternative cause. Physicians and epidemiologists found this to be the case in a puzzling outbreak first reported in New Mexico. In October 1989, several Santa Fe doctors were comparing notes on three patients suffering from a novel condition involving fatigue, debilitating muscle pain, rashes, and shortness of breath. Blood tests on all three had revealed very high counts of white blood cells called eosinophils. The doctors knew of no known condition that could explain these findings. However, they were struck by the fact that all three patients, when questioned about drugs or medications they were taking, had mentioned a health food supplement called L-tryptophan. L-tryptophan is a "natural" substance, a component of proteins, that had been publicized as a treatment for insomnia, depression, and premenstrual symptoms. Believing that more than coincidence was involved in these three cases, the doctors reported them to the New Mexico State Health Department.[8]

The Health Department reported the cases to the CDC and began an investigation to determine whether additional cases existed and whether there was a consistent link with L-tryptophan. By searching the records of clinical laboratories in Santa Fe, Albuquerque, and Los Alamos, they discovered 12 additional patients whose blood had exhibited high white-cell counts since May 1. A team of health department investigators interviewed these 12 people and found that they all had used L-tryptophan. They also interviewed 24 people of the same age and sex as the patients who lived in the same neighborhoods—a control group—and found that only two had taken the supplement. This strongly suggested that there was a link between L-tryptophan exposure and the illness. The CDC notified other state health departments, which conducted their own investigations, and by November 16 the CDC received reports from 35 states of 243 possible cases of the new disease, called eosinophilia-myalgia syndrome (EMS). On November 17, the Food and Drug Administration announced a nationwide recall of products containing L-tryptophan. The publicity brought forth a flood of new reports of the syndrome, but then new cases began to drop off. By August 1, 1992, 1511 cases had been reported by all 50 states. Many patients were left with permanent disabilities and 38 people had died, but the epidemic was over.[9]

Why had this natural substance caused such severe consequences? L-tryptophan is an amino acid, present in many foods including meat, fish, poultry, and cheese. It is also added to infant formulas, special dietary foods, and intravenous and oral solutions administered to patients with special medical needs. No cases of EMS had been reported from these products. Tests on the recalled tablets indicated that a toxic contaminant, formed as a result of a recent change in one factory's method of production, may have been responsible for the epidemic of 1989. However, there is evidence that earlier, unrecognized cases had occurred since the product was introduced in 1974.[10] The fact that many people took the supplements with no apparent harm suggests that individual variations in susceptibility may exist.

Serious outbreaks of illness caused by toxic contamination of food, through production errors, or outright fraud, have occurred a number of times over the past few decades. It is usually epidemiologists who identify the source of the problem. To many public health experts, the EMS epidemic of 1989 resembled an illness with similar symptoms that affected some 20,000 people in Spain in 1981, killing more than 300 of them within a few months. An infectious agent had first been suspected, but epidemiologists noted an odd geographical distribution of the outbreak. Patients lived either in a localized area south of Madrid or in a corridor along a road north of the city. The epidemiologists found that the affected households had bought oil for cooking from itinerant salespeople, who were illegally selling oil that had been manufactured for industrial use.[11] Laboratory scientists investigating the nature of the contaminants and how they might have caused the symptoms have not specifically identified a single chemical as being responsible. They now suspect that a range of chemicals, even at very low concentrations, may induce autoimmune responses in susceptible people, causing the body's immune system to attack its own tissues. Such outbreaks caused by toxic contamination of foods and drugs may be much more common than is generally recognized.[12] In the cases of toxic oil syndrome and EMS, government action to remove the contaminated product put an end to the epidemic. However, survivors still suffer from symptoms.

Epidemiologic surveillance is a major line of defense in protecting the public against disease. It is the warning system that alerts the community that something is wrong, that a gap has opened in the protective bulwark against preventable disease or that a new disease has appeared on the horizon. The sooner the surveillance system kicks in, the sooner action can be taken to stop the epidemic. Before the health department is notified, individual doctors are trying to cure individual patients, often unaware that the problem is more widespread. After the epidemic is recognized, all the resources of the community—local, state, or national—can be mobilized to prevent the disease's spread. Whether it uses vaccination campaigns against measles, isolation of hepatitis-infected food workers, new regulations on air conditioning systems, or recall of contaminated food or drugs, the government must act to protect the health of the public. Epidemiologic surveillance has become even more important as concerns about bioterrorism have increased.

Epidemiology and the Causes of Chronic Disease

Epidemiology has had a different role to play in investigating the causes of the diseases common in older age, such as cancer and heart disease, which are quite different from infectious diseases or acute poisoning. Until the mid-20th century, these conditions were thought of as a natural part of aging, and no one thought to look for causes or tried to prevent them.

Cancer, heart disease, and other diseases of aging do not have single causes. They tend to develop over a period of time, are often chronic and disabling rather than rapidly fatal, and cannot be prevented or cured by any vaccine or "magic bullet." The best hope for protecting the public against these diseases is to learn how to prevent them, or at least how to delay their onset. Prevention, however, requires an understanding of the cause or causes of a disease and the factors that influence how it progresses. Epidemiology has made major contributions to the current understanding of the causes of heart disease and some cancers and what can be done to prevent them. Epidemiologic studies will continue to yield information on how people can protect themselves against cancer, Alzheimer's disease, and other afflictions of aging.

Epidemiologic studies of these chronic diseases are much more complicated and difficult than investigations of acute outbreaks of infectious diseases or toxic contamination. Except for the clear link between smoking and lung cancer (discussed later in this chapter), most chronic diseases cannot be attributed to a single cause. There may be many different factors that play a part in causing a disease, factors that epidemiologists call "risk factors." The long period over which these diseases develop also contributes to the difficulty of determining the causative

factors. Epidemiologists must determine which of a person's many experiences over the previous decades are relevant, and what significant exposures might have occurred 10 or 20 years ago
that may have increased the person's risk of developing the disease today.

Epidemiology has developed a number of methods to study chronic diseases and to try to
answer the difficult questions. This chapter describes a few of the best-known studies that have
had major impacts on understanding the causes of heart disease and cancer.

Heart Disease

Since the 1920s, when infectious disease mortality had dropped to approximately its current
low levels, heart disease has been the leading cause of death in the United States for both
men and women. Deaths from heart disease increased dramatically during the first half of the
20th century, as seen in **Figure 4-1**. After World War II, one in every five men was affected
with heart disease before the age of 60, and little was known about why. In 1948, an epidemiologic study was launched in Framingham, Massachusetts, to investigate factors that might
be causing the problem. It was the first major epidemiologic study of a chronic disease. More
than half of the middle-aged population of the town, more than 5000 healthy people, were
examined, and data were recorded on their weight, blood pressure, smoking habits, the results

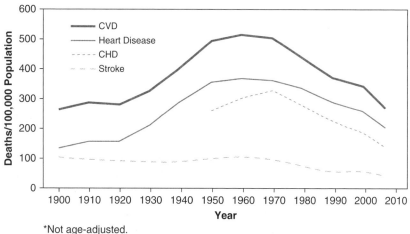

*Not age-adjusted.
Source: Vital statistics of the United States, NCHS.

FIGURE 4-1   Death Rates for Cardiovascular Diseases, U.S., 1900–2008.
Source: Reproduced from National Heart, Lung, and Blood Institute 2011 Fact Book,
p. 37. http://www.nhlbi.nih.gov/about/factbook/FactBook2011.pdf, accessed
October 1, 2012.

of various blood tests, and other characteristics. Two years later, the same people were examined again, and these tests have been and continue to be repeated every 2 years for the rest of their lives.[13]

As early as 10 years later, the Framingham Heart Study had revealed a great deal about how to predict which of their subjects were likely to develop heart disease. The study identified three major risk factors: high blood pressure, high blood cholesterol, and smoking. As a result of the findings, concepts of "normal" blood pressure and cholesterol levels changed significantly. Doctors had previously believed that blood pressure naturally increased as people aged and that the increase was normal and healthy. The Framingham Study found that some people maintained their youthful blood pressure and cholesterol values as they got older and that these people remained healthier. Weight gain and lack of exercise were found to be associated with increased blood pressure and cholesterol values and with an increased risk of heart disease.[14]

Remarkably, the Framingham findings had a major impact on the course of the heart disease epidemic. Publicity on the information gained by the study, confirmed and supported by other studies, persuaded some people to change their behavior and formed the basis of public health programs to encourage others to do the same. By the 1970s, it was clear that death rates from heart disease were falling in the United States. The Framingham Study itself found in 1970 that the death rate over the previous 10 years had declined by 60 percent since 1950.[14] This improvement was associated with a decline in risk factors: in 1970, blood cholesterol levels were lower; blood pressure was lower; and smoking was less common. These beneficial trends have continued. In 2008, the age-adjusted death rate from heart disease in the United States was 72 percent lower than it was in 1950.[15]

Meanwhile, the Framingham Study has continued and expanded, and much more has been learned. For example, a smoker's risk of heart disease rapidly drops back to that of nonsmokers soon after the smoker quits; but low-tar, low-nicotine cigarettes are no better than the old-fashioned kind in their effects on risk of heart disease.[14] Various forms of cholesterol have been identified, including high-density lipoprotein (HDL) cholesterol—the "good" kind that is protective—and low-density lipoprotein (LDL) cholesterol—the "bad" kind. Drinking alcohol in moderation has been found to increase HDL cholesterol and to protect against heart disease. Exercise also raises HDL levels. The scope of the Framingham Study has expanded: in 1978, the subjects began to be given neurological examinations in addition to tests for cardiac risk factors. The investigators are watching for the development of Alzheimer's disease in the aging study population, hoping that they will be able to detect risk factors for this increasingly common and tragic condition.[16]

An offshoot of the original study, the Framingham Offspring Study, was created in 1971; it included about 5000 children of the original participants and their spouses. Investigators use comparisons of risk factors within families and across generations, hoping to sort out the roles of genetics and environment in heart disease and other common disorders. The younger study population is being tested with more advanced medical technologies and more sophisticated blood tests, including genetic tests. In 1994, a more diverse sampling of Framingham residents, called the Omni Cohort, was added. Another expansion to form the Third Generation Study, which enrolled grandchildren of the study's original participants, was added in 2002 and a Second Generation Omni Cohort, as well as a New Offspring Spouse Cohort, in 2003. The diseases now being studied include diabetes, lung disorders, osteoporosis, arthritis, eye diseases and hearing disorders.[13]

Lung Cancer

Epidemiologic studies seeking causes of cancer began soon after the Framingham Study. However, studies of most kinds of cancer had much less success than the studies of heart disease; epidemiologists had few strong clues about possible causes or risk factors.

An exception was the link between smoking and lung cancer. Mortality from lung cancer had been increasing dramatically since the 1930s, as shown in Figure 4-2. Because it was

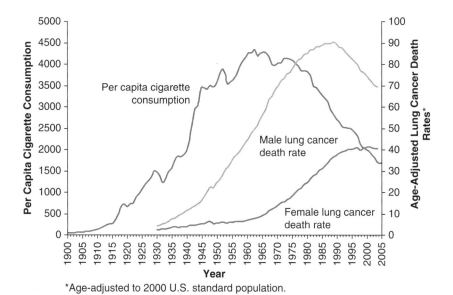

*Age-adjusted to 2000 U.S. standard population.

FIGURE 4-2   Cigarette Consumption and Lung Cancer Deaths in the U.S., 1900–2005. *Source:* Reproduced from Cancer Statistics 2012: A Presentation from the American Cancer Society. Slide 23. Reprinted by the permission of the American Cancer Society, Inc., from www.cancer.org. All rights reserved.

logical to suppose that the cause might be something that was inhaled, the two main hypotheses proposed to explain this increase were tobacco smoking and air pollution, both having increased during the same period that lung cancer was rising. Several early studies conducted in England and the United States beginning in the late 1940s questioned lung cancer patients about their smoking habits. All of these studies found that a high proportion of these patients were heavy smokers.

In late 1950 and early 1952, two major epidemiologic studies were started that convincingly established a link between lung cancer and tobacco smoking. The British epidemiologists Richard Doll and A. Bradford Hill sent out a questionnaire to all physicians in the United Kingdom, asking whether they were smokers, past smokers, or nonsmokers. Smokers and ex-smokers were asked to provide additional information on their age at starting to smoke and the amount of tobacco smoked, and ex-smokers were asked when they had quit smoking. Over 40,000 doctors responded to the survey.[17]

During the following years, Doll and his collaborators, by arrangement with the British Medical Association and the Registrar General of the United Kingdom, gathered information on which doctors had died each year and what was the cause of death. A little over 4 years after the survey began, several important conclusions were apparent: First, the death rate from lung cancer was about 20 times higher among smokers than among nonsmokers, increasing as the amount smoked increased. Second, the death rate among ex-smokers was lower than that of smokers and declined as the length of time increased since the doctor had quit smoking. Third, the contrast in lung cancer mortality between smokers and nonsmokers was the same whether the doctors lived in rural or urban areas. Therefore, the difference could not be attributed to air pollution. Fourth, deaths from heart attacks were also significantly higher among heavy smokers aged 35 to 54 than among nonsmokers.[18]

A similar study on a much larger group of people was conducted in the United States by epidemiologists E. Cuyler Hammond and Daniel Horn. They obtained smoking histories from almost 188,000 men and followed them over a period of 3 years and 8 months. For all the study participants who died, they obtained the cause of death from death certificates. Their findings confirmed and extended the results of the Doll and Hill study of British doctors. First, cigarette smokers were more than 10 times more likely to die of lung cancer than nonsmokers. Second, cigarette smokers were about five times more likely to die of cancer of the lip, tongue, mouth, pharynx, larynx, and esophagus as nonsmokers. Several other types of cancer were also more common among smokers. Third, heavy smokers (two or more packs per day) were 2.4 times more likely to die of heart disease than nonsmokers.[19]

The British study continued until 1971, tracking all the doctors for 20 years, by which time about 33 percent of them had died. The longer period of observation confirmed the results obtained earlier. An interesting finding was that many physicians reacted to the earlier reports by quitting smoking. By 1971, the average number of cigarettes smoked per day by the physicians in the study was less than half what it had been in 1951, and as a result, lung cancer became relatively less common as a cause of death in this group.[18]

The Framingham Study and the two lung cancer studies are examples of prospective cohort studies, following large numbers of people over extended periods of time. These are considered among the most reliable kinds of epidemiologic studies for investigating causes of chronic diseases. Other such studies have been done and continue at present, many of them seeking causes of various kinds of cancer.

Conclusion

Epidemiology is an important component of the assessment function of public health. Epidemiologists investigate epidemics of known and unknown diseases by counting the number of cases and how they are distributed by person, place, and time. Using this information, they can often determine a probable cause of a new disease or a reason for an outbreak of a previously controlled disease. This knowledge allows public health workers to institute measures that prevent and control the spread of the disease.

An early achievement of epidemiology was the recognition in the 19th century that cholera was spread by polluted water. In 1993, similar epidemiologic methods determined that polluted water had caused an outbreak of cryptosporidiosis in Milwaukee. The same approach has been successful in halting outbreaks of illness caused by toxic contaminations. "Shoeleather epidemiology" by local health departments provides the front line of defense against acute diseases. Epidemiologic surveillance, including mandatory reporting of notifiable disease, alerts a local health department that an epidemic is beginning in time for an agency to investigate the reasons and take preventive action.

Epidemiology also provides information on the causes of chronic disease. Formal long-term studies of heart disease and lung cancer provided the earliest information on the risk factors that contributed to these diseases. The Framingham Study, which has tracked citizens of Framingham, MA for over 6 decades, identified high blood pressure, high blood cholesterol, and smoking as risk factors for heart disease. Two epidemiologic studies conducted in the 1950s—one on the smoking habits of British doctors and a similar study on a group of 188,000 American men—indicated a clear link between smoking and lung cancer.

Epidemiology's role in identifying causes of disease leads directly and indirectly to prevention and control. In some cases, regulatory action by a local government is necessary to eliminate the conditions that are causing disease. Sometimes simply publicizing the results of a study allows people to modify their behavior to avoid risk factors for a disease. For example, information released in the 1950s on results from the Framingham Study and the studies regarding smoking and lung cancer contributed to a significant decline in smoking in the United States, accompanied by a drop in mortality from both heart disease and lung cancer since the 1950s. To achieve additional improvements in public health, health agencies build on epidemiologic information to develop policy and plan programs aimed at reducing risk and promoting health in the population.

References

1. C.-E. A. Winslow et al., quoted in R. C. Brownson and D. B. Petitti, eds., *Applied Epidemiology: Theory to Practice* (New York: Oxford University Press, 1998), vii.
2. Institute of Medicine, *The Future of Public Health* (Washington, DC: National Academy Press, 1988).
3. C. J. Hennekens and J. F. Buring, *Epidemiology in Medicine* (Boston: Little, Brown, 1987).
4. J. Snow, "On the Mode of Communication of Cholera" (London: Churchill, 1955). Quoted in Hennekens and Buring, *Epidemiology in Medicine* (Boston: Little, Brown, 1987).
5. P. J. Hilts, "Panel Urges Monitoring of Chronic Diseases," *New York Times* September 12, 2000.
6. D. W. Fraser et al., "Legionnaires' Disease," *New England Journal of Medicine* 297 (1977): 1189–1197.
7. L. Garrett, *The Coming Plague: Newly Emerging Diseases in a World Out of Balance* (New York: Farrar, Straus, and Giroux, 1994).
8. U.S. Centers for Disease Control, "Eosinophilia-Myalgia Syndrome—New Mexico," *Morbidity and Mortality Weekly Report* 38 (1989): 765–767.
9. S. L. Nightingale, "Update on EMS and L-Tryptophan," *Journal of the American Medical Association* 268 (1992): 1828.
10. T. A. Medsger, Jr., "Tryptophan-Induced Eosinophilia-Myalgia Syndrome," *New England Journal of Medicine* 322 (1990): 926–928.
11. E. M. Kilbourne et al., "Clinical Epidemiology of Toxic-Oil Syndrome: Manifestations of New Disease," *New England Journal of Medicine* 309 (1983): 1408–1414.
12. M. Posada de la Paz et al., "Toxic Oil Syndrome: The Perspective After 20 Years," *Epidemiology Reviews* 23 (2001): 231–247.
13. National Heart, Lung, and Blood Institute, "Framingham Heart Study." http://www.framinghamheartstudy.org/, accessed May 11, 2012.
14. W. B. Kannel, "The Framingham Experience," in M. Marmot and P. Elliott, eds., *Coronary Heart Disease Epidemiology: From Aetiology to Public Health* (New York: Oxford University Press, 1992).
15. National Heart, Lung, and Blood Institute, "Morbidity & Mortality: 2012 Chartbook on Cardiovascular, Lung, and Blood Diseases," February 2012 http://www.nhlbi.nih.gov/resouces/docs/2012_Chartbook_pdf, accessed May 11, 2012.
16. D. L. Backman et al., "Incidence of Dementia and Probable Alzheimer's Disease in a General Population: The Framingham Study," *Neurology* 43 (1993): 515–519.

17. R. Doll and A. B. Hill, "Smoking and Carcinoma of the Lung: Preliminary Report," *British Medical Journal* (September 30, 1950): 739–748.

18. R. Doll and R. Peto, "Mortality in Relation to Smoking: 20 Years' Observations on Male British Doctors," *British Medical Journal* 2 (1976): 1525–1536.

19. E. C. Hammond and D. Horn, "Smoking and Death Rates—Report on Forty-Four Months of Follow-up of 187,783 Men," *Journal of the American Medical Association* 166 (1958): 1294–1308.

Epidemiologic Principles and Methods

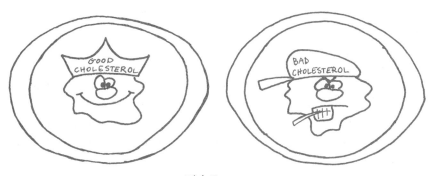

Risk Factors

This chapter examines epidemiology more closely, defining some of its basic terms and describing how epidemiologists use the terms to describe the patterns of disease occurrence. The chapter also explains the different kinds of epidemiologic studies, with examples of the types of information each form of epidemiologic study can provide.

Epidemiology is defined as "the study of the *distribution* and *determinants* of *disease frequency in human populations*," (emphasis added).[1(p.1)] Each of these terms must be clearly understood.

First, the epidemiologist must define the disease in a clear way so that there is no doubt about whether an individual case should or should not be counted. Some diseases are easier to identify than others. In a hepatitis outbreak, the symptoms are fairly nonspecific, and not every patient who comes to an emergency room with vomiting and diarrhea has hepatitis. Therefore, the epidemiologist must include the results of blood tests for liver function in his/her case definition. In a study of deaths from gunshot wounds, on the other hand, the cases are fairly easy to count since virtually 100 percent of deaths are reported, and the cause of death is usually identified easily and listed on the death certificate. With a new disease like eosinophilia-myalgia syndrome, working out the case definition might be the most important part of the investigation.

In defining a disease to be studied, epidemiologists use the term "disease" broadly: "health outcome" is a more accurate but cumbersome description of what is to be studied. For example, epidemiologists might study the frequency and distribution of high blood cholesterol, which is not a disease but is related to the risk of heart attack, or they might study injuries due to traffic accidents, which are not diseases but are certainly significant to health. In both cases, an epidemiologic study may point to ways of preventing the negative health outcome.

In measuring disease *frequency*, it is necessary not only to count the number of cases but to relate that number to the size of the population being studied, yielding a *rate*. Six cases of Legionnaires' disease among 1,000 vacationers on a cruise ship, as happened in June 1994, is of much greater concern than if the same number of cases were diagnosed in the whole country. In calculating a rate, the denominator is generally the *population at risk*. The rate of ovarian cancer in a city of one million, for example, would be calculated by dividing the number of cases by the female population, not the total population of the city.

Two kinds of frequency measures are commonly used in epidemiology: incidence rates and prevalence rates. *Incidence* is the rate of new cases of a disease in a defined population over a defined period of time. For notifiable diseases, it is ascertained by counting cases reported to the local or state health departments and dividing by the population at risk. Incidence measures the probability that a healthy person in that population will develop the disease during that time. Incidence rates are useful in identifying causes of a disease. For example, the incidence of birth defects in Europe rose dramatically in 1960 after the introduction of thalidomide, a drug used in sleeping pills. This sudden increase and its timing aroused suspicions that thalidomide use by pregnant women was the cause of limb deformities in their infants, a suspicion that was soon confirmed by epidemiologic studies.[2]

Prevalence is the total number of cases existing in a defined population at a specific time. It would generally be measured by doing a survey. Incidence and prevalence are related to each other, but the relationship depends on how long people live with the disease. A disease with high incidence could have a low prevalence if people recover from it rapidly, or if they die from it in a short period of time. However, for chronic diseases that are not lethal—arthritis, for example—the prevalence will be much higher than the incidence. For most diseases, prevalence rates change slowly and are less useful for epidemiologic studies. They are most useful in assessing the societal impact of a disease and planning for healthcare services.

Death rates, or mortality rates (the incidence of death), are often used as a measure of frequency for diseases that are usually fatal. Death rates are close to incidence rates for the most lethal diseases, such as pancreatic cancer. For diseases such as breast cancer, which many women survive, the mortality rate will be much smaller than the incidence rate. Death rates are not at all useful as a measure of frequency for diseases that are rarely fatal, such as arthritis.

The *distribution* of disease is comprised of the answers to the *who*, *when*, and *where* questions. The *who* question characterizes the disease victims by such factors as age, sex, race, and economic status. For example, the incidences of cancer and heart disease are greater in older people; measles and chicken pox occur more often in the young. Old women and young men are more likely to suffer broken bones than old men and young women. During the early months of the AIDS epidemic, the answer to the *who* question was gay men and intravenous drug abusers. This information led to some obvious hypotheses as to how the disease was transmitted.

The *when* question looks for trends in disease frequency over time: is the incidence increasing, decreasing, or remaining stable? The incidence of lung cancer in American men, for example, increased steadily from the 1930s to about 1990, when it peaked and began to decrease. Meanwhile, the incidence of stomach cancer has been declining. Posing another kind of when question, epidemiologists look for seasonal variations in incidence. The incidence of respiratory infections is always higher in the winter.

The *when* question is crucial in tracking an outbreak of infectious diseases such as hepatitis and legionellosis. Epidemiologists construct *epidemic curves*, like those shown in Figures 5-1 and 5-2, by plotting the number of cases identified over a period of time. Figure 5-1 shows the epidemic curve for the 1976 outbreak of Legionnaires' disease in Philadelphia. It is clear from the epidemic curve that most of the victims were exposed to the virus at about the same

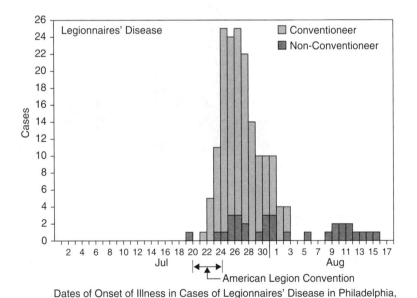

Dates of Onset of Illness in Cases of Legionnaires' Disease in Philadelphia,
July 1–August 18, 1976. (Dates of onset of two cases are unknown.)

FIGURE 5-1   Epidemic Curve for Legionnaires' Disease Outbreak. *Source:* Reproduced from the Centers for Disease Control and Prevention, Steps of an Outbreak Investigation, 2004. http://www.cdc.gov/excite/classroom/outbreak/steps.htm#step5, accessed January 17, 2013.

time, and therefore, probably from the same source. Comparing the dates of onset with the dates of possible exposure, epidemiologists calculated an incubation period of 2 to 10 days. An epidemic curve such as the one shown in Figure 5-2 is typical of a disease that has been passed from one person to another.

The *where* question looks at comparisons of disease frequency in different countries, states, counties, or other geographical divisions. It may also look at comparisons between urban and rural populations. The hypothesis that fluoride protects against tooth decay arose from the observation that dental cavities were less common in children who lived in parts of the country that had high concentrations of fluoride in the water. Statistics on causes of death in different countries can be very suggestive in generating hypotheses about the causes of disease. The wide

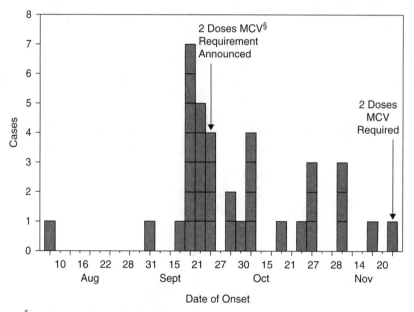

§Measles-containing vaccine.

FIGURE 5-2 Number of Confirmed* Measles Cases, by Date of Rash Onset, by 3-Day Interval—Anchorage, Alaska, August 10–November 23, 1998. *Source:* Reproduced from U.S. Centers for Disease Control and Prevention, *Morbidity and Mortality Weekly Report* 47 (1999): 1110. www.cdc.gov/mmwr/preview/mmwrhtml/00056144.htm, accessed September 22, 2012.

*A confirmed case was laboratory confirmed or met the clinical case definition and wasepidemiologically linked to a confirmed case. A clinical case was defined as an illness characterized by generalized rash lasting ≥ 3 days; temperature ≥ 101°F (≥38.3°C);and either cough, coryza, or conjunctivitis, n = 33.

international variation in death rates from heart disease has been interpreted in a variety of ways, including that diet is a factor and that the pressures of urban life have a negative effect on health.

Thus, information on the *distribution* of disease gives clues about the *determinants* of disease. International comparisons of cancer incidence, such as those shown in Figure 5-3, have led to hypotheses on causes of various kinds of cancer. For example, cancer of the colon and rectum is much more common in industrialized countries than in developing countries, which has led to the hypothesis that the difference is due to differences in diet: Americans eat meals rich in fat, meat, and dairy products, while diets in China are traditionally high in fiber, cereals, and vegetables. Evidence that environmental factors rather than genetics are to blame comes from studies of people who move from a low-rate country to a high-rate country. They tend to develop higher rates of the disease as they acquire the habits of the host country. In Japan, the rates of colorectal cancer more than doubled between the 1950s and the 1990s as Japanese adopted more Western-style diets.[3] International patterns of breast cancer are somewhat similar to those of colorectal cancer, suggesting that similar dietary factors may play a role.[4,5] However, as more is learned about other risk factors for breast cancer, such as hormonal and reproductive history, it has become clear that diet is not the whole story.[5] The incidence of breast cancer in Japan is only about half the rate in the United States. Rates of stomach cancer are much higher in China and Japan than in the United States, evidence that different dietary factors may be involved; diets high in smoked foods, salted meat or fish, and pickled vegetables increase the risk of stomach cancer. However *H. pylori*, the bacteria that cause ulcers, also play an important role in causing stomach cancer.[4]

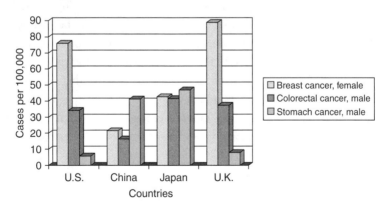

FIGURE 5-3   Cancer Rates in Four Countries, 2008. Age standardized incidence rates, cases per 100,000 population, 2008. *Source:* Data from International Agency for Research on Cancer. http://globocan.iarc.fr/factsheets, accessed October 1, 2012.

The relevance of the *who* and *when* questions is clearly illustrated in the evidence that smoking is a determinant of lung cancer. Men began smoking cigarettes early in the 20th century, and lung cancer rates began rising 20 years later. Women did not begin smoking in large numbers until the 1940s and 1950s. Lung cancer rates for women did not begin to rise sharply until the 1960s.

Why are broken bones in young people more common in males, while among the elderly, they are more common in females? This question leads to an investigation of the determinants of broken bones. It turns out that these injuries in boys and young men are usually the result of accidents stemming from reckless behavior, which males are more likely to engage in than females. In the elderly, however, broken bones are usually the result of osteoporosis, or weakening of the bones, which is more common in females.

Epidemiology studies *human populations*, usually using observational rather than experimental methods. The alternative approach to investigating causes of disease is the biomedical approach, often using animal models of the disease. There are advantages and disadvantages to each approach. Experiments done on animals can yield clear answers as to cause and effect, while for ethical reasons experiments cannot usually be done on humans. However, there are always uncertainties about the relevance of animal studies to humans and whether the findings on "animals can be extrapolated to people."

Kinds of Epidemiologic Studies

Answers to the who, when, and where questions provide clues about the causes of a disease or the source of an outbreak. This type of analysis is called descriptive epidemiology. The hypotheses generated by descriptive epidemiology are tested by formal epidemiologic studies, designed to confirm or disprove the hypothesis. For example, in investigating the eosinophilia-myalgia syndrome (EMS) outbreak in New Mexico, epidemiologists found an apparent link with the use of L-tryptophan. To test the hypothesis, they conducted a study comparing 12 cases of EMS with 24 controls, a case-control study (described later in the chapter) that confirmed the link.[6]

Epidemiologic studies are sometimes referred to as being prospective or retrospective. Prospective studies start in the present and monitor groups of people into the future, or they may start at a point in time in the past and look forward from there. Retrospective studies look into the past for causes of diseases from which people currently suffer. In both cases, investigators are looking for associations between exposure to the suspected causative factor and disease (or other health outcome).

Intervention Studies

Intervention studies are the exception to the rule that epidemiologists do not do experiments. These studies are conducted in very much the same way as those of laboratory experiments on animals. They are usually done to test a new treatment for a disease, such as a chemotherapy drug for cancer, or a preventive measure, such as a vaccine. In a clinical trial, one group is exposed to the intervention, while a *control group* is not exposed. The investigators then watch and wait to see whether the response of the treatment group is different from that of the control group. Of course, only a limited number of interventions lend themselves to being tested in clinical trials for ethical reasons or because a trial is too difficult to conduct. In testing treatments for serious diseases, there must be enough doubt about the effectiveness of the intervention to justify withholding it from people who could be helped and enough evidence that it will not harm the people on whom it is tested.

The control group may be given a *placebo*—an inactive substance similar in appearance to the drug or vaccine being tested. When a treatment for a disease is already known to exist, trials may compare the new treatment with the existing treatment. The purpose of the placebo is to prevent subjects from knowing whether they are receiving the intervention. Many trials over the years have found that up to a third of patients respond to a placebo as if it were the intervention, reporting that they feel better or that they suffered side effects. This is the placebo effect. The drug being tested must show a higher response rate than the placebo if it is to be considered effective.

The most convincing clinical trials are conducted in a *randomized, double-blind* manner. *Randomized* means that each subject is assigned to the treatment group or the control group at random. This helps to equalize the groups with respect to unknown and known factors that might affect the results. *Double-blind* means that both the patient and the doctor are blind as to whether the patient is receiving the drug or a placebo. One reason that the doctor should also be blinded is that studies have shown patients to respond more favorably to a treatment that the doctor believes in. Another reason is to prevent the possibility that doctors might interpret the patient's condition differently if they know how the patient is being treated.

In a therapeutic clinical trial, both the experimental group and the control group are composed of patients who have the disease for which a therapy is being tested. Thousands of therapeutic trials are being conducted each year by pharmaceutical companies testing new drugs. The Food and Drug Administration (FDA) requires that the safety and effectiveness of any new drug must be demonstrated in a properly conducted clinical trial before it can be approved for marketing.

A classic example of a randomized, double-blind clinical trial of a preventive intervention is the field trial of the polio vaccine in 1954. Polio, then a greatly dreaded disease in the United States, killed and paralyzed children and adults. President Franklin Roosevelt, for example, had paralysis of the legs from polio, which he had contracted at the age of 39 when he was already active in politics and public service.[7] In 1952, 21,269 cases of paralytic polio were reported in the United States.[8] The development of a vaccine by Jonas Salk offered great hope for prevention of this scourge. Preliminary tests had shown the vaccine to be safe and to stimulate disease-fighting antibodies in the blood of people who had been vaccinated. Before the vaccine could be approved for widespread use, however, it had to be tested in a clinical trial to determine if it really could protect a large number of people against the disease. In 1954, some 400,000 school children in 11 states were given the Salk vaccine or a "dummy" vaccine (the placebo); they were then tracked through the end of the year to see whether they became ill with polio. The incidence of polio among the children who had received the vaccine turned out to be less than half that of those given the placebo vaccine.[9] This result demonstrated that polio immunization could reduce the incidence of disease; in fact, the use of the vaccine (or an oral vaccine developed by Albert Sabin in the 1960s) has virtually eliminated polio in the United States.

Another randomized controlled trial of a preventive intervention is the Physicians' Health Study, in which 22,000 American physicians participated. Two hypotheses were being tested: whether aspirin reduced mortality from heart disease and whether beta carotene decreased the incidence of cancer. The physicians were randomly divided into four groups: those who took aspirin and beta carotene, those who were given one or the other and a placebo, and those who were given placebos only. The trial began in 1983 and was scheduled to run until 1995. The aspirin part of the trial was halted in 1988, however, because it was clear by that time that the physicians taking aspirin had a much-reduced risk of suffering a heart attack.[10] They were only 56 percent as likely to have a heart attack as the group taking the placebo. The beta carotene part of the trial, which continued until 1995, found no significant difference in the incidence of cancer between the group receiving the beta carotene and the placebo group.[11]

The Kingston–Newburgh study of fluoride for the prevention of tooth decay was another form of intervention study—a community trial. Before the study began, the schoolchildren of these two small cities on the Hudson River in New York State were similar in general health and in the prevalence of tooth decay. For the study, fluoride was added to the water supply of Newburgh, beginning in 1945, while Kingston's water was not fluoridated. Ten years later, dental examinations were conducted on the schoolchildren in both cities. The children of Newburgh were found to have approximately half as many decayed, missing, or filled teeth as the children of Kingston had. No adverse health effects were found in the Newburgh children. This evidence was strongly supportive of the value of fluoridation in preventing tooth decay.[12]

Cohort Studies

Since such experiments are not possible for most hypotheses that epidemiologists want to test, methods have been devised by which investigators can link exposures to results by observation alone, without actively intervening in the lives of the study subjects. Probably the most accurate of these methods is the *cohort study*. In a typical cohort study, large numbers of people—all healthy at the time the study begins—are questioned concerning their exposures. They are then observed over a period of time to see whether those who were exposed are more likely to develop the disease than those who were not. This approach is similar to performing an experiment, except that the people themselves have chosen whether they belong to the "exposed" group or the control group.

The Framingham Heart Study is a cohort study, as were the Doll–Hill and Hammond–Horn studies of smoking and lung cancer. Another well-known cohort study, still under way, is the Nurses' Health Study, which since 1976 has been following some 120,000 married female nurses, looking for factors that may be related to the development of breast cancer and other diseases. The participating nurses have been sent questionnaires every 2 years, asking about their diet, drinking and smoking habits, and use of drugs, including oral contraceptives. The study found that nurses had a 50 percent higher risk of breast cancer while they were taking oral contraceptives, but the risk fell back to normal after they stopped taking them. Another finding was that regular consumption of alcohol increases the risk of breast cancer by 10 to 40 percent.[13,14]

Epidemiologic studies are designed to determine not only the existence of an association between an exposure and a disease, but also the strength of that association. The measure of the strength of association obtained by cohort studies and intervention studies is the *relative risk*, which is the ratio of the incidence rate for persons exposed to the factor to the incidence rate for persons in the unexposed group. A relative risk of 1.0 means that there is no association between the exposure and the disease. A value greater than 1.0 indicates an increased risk from exposure, while a value less than 1.0 indicates a decreased risk.

Doll and Hill, in their study of British physicians, found that the relative risk of lung cancer in heavy smokers compared to nonsmokers was 23.7, a major effect.[15] The calculation that led to this conclusion is shown in Table 5-1. In the Nurses' Health Study, the relative risk of breast cancer for current contraceptive use is 1.5, while that for past use is 1.0. These findings are not very dramatic but they do call for further studies.[14] In the Physicians' Health Study, the relative risk of a heart attack for men taking aspirin was 0.56.[10] The decrease was significant enough to recommend that most older men might benefit from this preventive measure, but the recommendation would carry much less weight than a recommendation to stop smoking.

Table 5-1   Relative Risk for Lung Cancer in Heavy Smokers Compared to Nonsmokers

Exposure Category	Lung Cancer Death Rates per 100,000 Persons
Heavy smokers	166
Nonsmokers	7
Relative risk	166/7 = 23.7

Source: Data from R. Doll and A. B. Hill, "Lung Cancer and Other Causes of Death in Relation to Smoking: A Second Report on the Mortality of British Doctors," *British Medical Journal* 2 (1956): 1071–1081.

Case-Control Studies

In contrast with cohort studies, which start out by measuring exposure and watching for the development of disease, *case-control* studies start with people who are already ill and look back to determine their exposure. Case-control studies are much more efficient than cohort studies in that they focus on a smaller number of people and can be completed relatively quickly. In a case-control study, cases—people who have the disease—are compared with controls, healthy individuals chosen to match the cases as much as possible in age, sex, and other factors that might be relevant to the disease. The investigator asks all participants the same questions concerning the extent of their exposure to factors hypothesized to have caused the disease. Small case-control studies are commonly done to follow up a hypothesis generated by "shoeleather epidemiology," as was done in the investigation of EMS and L-tryptophan described previously in this chapter.

An important case-control study conducted in the mid-1980s sought the cause of Reye's syndrome, a deadly disease of children that occurred a few weeks after a child had recovered from a viral infection such as chicken pox. The study tested the hypothesis that the development of Reye's syndrome was linked to medications the child was given during the viral illness.[16] The cases were children who had been diagnosed with Reye's syndrome and reported a previous respiratory or gastrointestinal illness or chicken pox. Controls were children who did not have Reye's syndrome but who had recently been diagnosed with chicken pox or a respiratory or gastrointestinal illness. Parents of the children in both groups were asked about what medications their children had received during the viral illness. Results of the study are shown in Table 5-2.

Case-control studies estimate the strength of the association between exposure and disease by calculating an odds ratio, which is an estimate of what the relative risk would be if a cohort study had been done. The odds ratio is calculated by dividing the ratio of exposed subjects to nonexposed subjects in the case group by the ratio of exposed subjects to nonexposed subjects in the control group. In the Reye's syndrome study, a link was found with the use of aspirin during the initial viral infection. From Table 5-2, the odds ratio is 26:1 divided by 53:87, or 42.7.

Table 5-2   Use of Salicylates and Reye's Syndrome

	Cases of Reye's Syndrome	Controls
Used salicylates	26	53
Did not use salicylates	1	87
Total	27	140

Odds Ratio: $\dfrac{26/1}{53/87} = \dfrac{26 \times 87}{53 \times 1} = \dfrac{2262}{53} = 42.7$

Sources: Reproduced from D. E. Lilienfeld and P. D. Stolley, *Foundations of Epidemiology*, 3rd ed. (New York: Oxford University Press, 1994). Data from E. S. Hurwitz et al., *Journal of the American Medical Association* 257 (1987): 1905–1911.

The study indicates that children who are given aspirin to treat a viral infection are 42.7 times more likely to develop Reye's syndrome than children who did not take aspirin, a very strong association. As a result of this study, the FDA required drug producers to put warning labels on aspirin containers and told pediatricians to advise parents to give their children acetaminophen (Tylenol) rather than aspirin to treat infections.

A number of case-control studies have been done seeking causes of breast cancer, a particularly intractable problem. The results of a British study exploring a possible link between breast cancer and the use of oral contraceptives are shown in Table 5-3. The cases consisted of 351 female breast cancer patients aged 45 years and younger who were interviewed in eight hospitals between 1980 and 1984. The controls were 351 women of similar age who were hospitalized for other conditions during the same period. All of the women were asked whether they had ever taken oral contraceptives and, if so, for how many years. Odds ratios were calculated for various exposures to oral contraceptives. The results indicate that use of oral contraceptives did increase the risk of developing breast cancer for women aged 45 and under and that the risk increases with longer exposure. Women who took oral contraceptives for more than 4 years had more than double the risk of breast cancer compared to those who had never taken oral contraceptives.[16]

The results of the British breast cancer study are fairly consistent with those of the Nurses' Health Study, indicating that oral contraceptives increase the risk of breast cancer. However, the certainty of this conclusion is much smaller than the certainty that aspirin is a risk for Reye's syndrome. A smaller odds ratio (or relative risk) leads to a much less certain conclusion. In fact, a more recent case-control study that included large numbers of women found no increased risk of breast cancer among women who had used oral contraceptives.[17] The study compared 4575 women with breast cancer with 4682 controls and found that the relative risk of breast cancer among current users of oral contraceptives was 1.0; among former users the relative risk was 0.9.

Table 5-3   Relative Risk of Breast Cancer by Duration of Oral Contraceptive Use

Contraceptive Use	Breast Cancer Cases	Hospital Controls	Odds Ratio (Estimated Relative Risk)
No Use	235	273	1.0
<1 year	27	26	1.2
1–4 years	43	29	1.7
>4 years	46	23	2.3

Sources: Reproduced from D. E. Lilienfeld and P. D. Stolley, *Foundations of Epidemiology*, 3rd ed. (New York: Oxford University Press, 1994). Data from K. McPherson et al., *British Journal of Cancer* 56 (1987): 653–660.

Conclusion

Epidemiologists study the distribution and determinants of frequency of disease in humans. Disease frequency is usually expressed as incidence rate—the number of new cases in a defined population at risk over a defined period of time—or prevalence rate—the number of existing cases in a defined population at a single point in time. Incidence rate is most useful in identifying causes of disease.

Descriptive epidemiology looks at the distribution of disease by characteristics of the person (age, sex, ethnicity, personal habits, etc.), the place (variations by geographical areas), and the time (changes in incidence over the long term, seasonal variations, or time since an epidemic began). This information on the distribution of disease may lead to hypotheses about the determinants, or causes, of disease.

Hypotheses generated through descriptive epidemiology can be tested through systematic epidemiologic studies. There are several types of epidemiologic studies. Intervention studies are true experiments in which subjects are assigned to either a test group (people who receive the intervention) or a control group (people who do not receive the intervention). The most common and rigorous type of intervention study is the randomized, double-blind clinical trial used to test new drug treatments or preventive measures.

For most situations in which epidemiologists wish to investigate whether a certain exposure causes a certain disease, it would be unethical to conduct an intervention study. The next best thing is a cohort study, in which subjects are questioned about their exposures and then tracked over time, comparing the exposed group with the unexposed group to see whether the exposed group is more likely to develop the disease. The third major type of study is the case-control study, which begins with cases of the disease and asks questions about what they had been exposed to, comparing their answers with those of a healthy control group.

Epidemiologists study human populations, which limits the types of studies that can be done. However, epidemiology has provided some of the most useful information about factors that affect human health.

References

1. B. MacMahon and D. Trichopoulos, *Epidemiology: Principles and Methods* (Boston: Little, Brown, 1996).
2. C. G. Hennekens and J. F. Buring, *Epidemiology in Medicine* (Boston: Little, Brown, 1987).
3. R. Doyle, "Colorectal Cancer Mortality Among Men," *Scientific American* (January 1996): 27.
4. American Cancer Society, Global Cancer Facts & Figures, 2nd ed., 2012. http://www.cancer.org/Research/CancerFactsFigures/GlobalCancerFactsFigures/global-facts-figures-2nd-ed, accessed September 22, 2012.

5. P. Porter, "'Westernizing' Women's Risks? Breast Cancer in Lower-Income Countries," *New England Journal of Medicine* 358 (2008): 213–216.

6. U.S. Centers for Disease Control and Prevention, "Eosinophilia-Myalgia Syndrome—New Mexico," *Morbidity and Mortality Weekly Report* 38 (1989): 765–767.

7. J. P. Lash, *Eleanor and Franklin: The Story of Their Relationship* (New York: W. W. Norton, 1971).

8. M. B. Gregg and B. M. Nkowane, "Poliomyelitis," in J. Last, ed., *Maxcy-Rosenau Public Health and Preventive Medicine* (Norwalk, CT: Appleton-Century-Croft, 1986), 173–176.

9. G. D. Friedman, *Primer of Epidemiology* (New York: McGraw-Hill, 1994).

10. Steering Committee of the Physicians' Health Study Research Group, "Final Report on the Aspirin Component of the Ongoing Physicians' Health Study," *New England Journal of Medicine* 321 (1989): 129–135.

11. C. H. Hennekens et al., "Lack of Effect of Long-Term Supplementation with Beta Carotene on the Incidence of Malignant Neoplasms and Cardiovascular Disease," *New England Journal of Medicine* 334 (1996): 1145–1149.

12. E. R. Schlesinger et al., "Newburgh-Kingston Caries-Fluorine Study XIII. Pediatric Findings After Ten Years," *Journal of the American Dental Association* 52 (1956): 296–306.

13. R. J. Lipnick et al., "Oral Contraceptives and Breast Cancer: A Prospective Cohort Study," *Journal of the American Medical Association* 255 (1986): 58–61.

14. M. P. Longnecker, "Alcoholic Beverage Consumption in Relation to Breast Cancer: Meta-Analysis and Review," *Cancer Causes and Control* 5 (1994): 73–82.

15. R. Doll and A. B. Hill, "Lung Cancer and Other Causes of Death in Relation to Smoking: A Second Report on the Mortality of British Doctors," *British Medical Journal* 2 (1956): 1071–1081.

16. D. E. Lilienfeld and P. D. Stolley, *Foundations of Epidemiology* (New York: Oxford University Press, 1994), 227–228.

17. P. A. Marchbanks et al., "Oral Contraceptives and the Risk of Breast Cancer," *New England Journal of Medicine* 346 (2002): 2025–2032.

Problems and Limits of Epidemiology

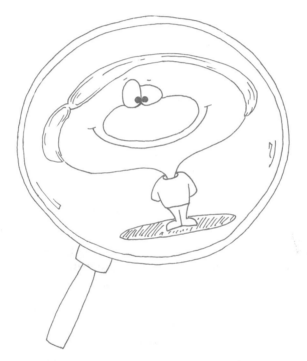

The Study of Humans

The ultimate goal of many epidemiologic studies is to determine the causes of disease. This is generally done first by observing a possible association between an exposure and an illness, second by developing a hypothesis about a cause and effect relationship, and third by testing the hypothesis through a formal epidemiologic study. While the formal study can strongly support the conclusion that a certain exposure causes a certain disease, there are many potential sources of error in drawing such a conclusion. Studies of chronic diseases, which often have multiple determinants and develop over long periods of time, are especially prone to error.

Problems with Studying Humans

All epidemiologic studies have the advantage of studying humans rather than experimental animals; but all are also limited by that fact. Each type of epidemiologic study has its own strengths and weaknesses.

Consider the design of an epidemiologic study to test the hypothesis that a low-fat diet reduces the risk of heart disease. The average American already eats a high-fat diet and has a high risk of heart disease compared with residents of many other countries, so it should be possible ethically to compare the health of people who eat this diet with others who have other dietary patterns.

The randomized controlled trial, the most rigorous form of intervention study, is the most similar in concept to a biomedical scientist's experiment with rats. Suppose researchers choose a group of subjects who have been eating an average American diet and divide them randomly into an experimental group, who will be instructed to eat a strict low-fat diet over the next 5 years, and a control group, who will be told to continue eating normally. Researchers will monitor both groups, watching for signs of heart disease, and they expect that, if their hypothesis is correct, fewer people in the low-fat group will become ill.

In fact, researchers are likely to be disappointed with the results. The problem is that it is impossible to control the behavior of human beings under such circumstances. If the experiment was being conducted using rats, researchers would feed them the assigned diets and could thus be certain of the relative exposures of the two groups. With people, however, even if researchers could find enough of them who would agree to participate in the experiment, it is questionable whether they would remain on the appropriate diet over the necessary length of time. People in the experimental group might succumb to temptation and drop out of the study or lie about what they have eaten. People in the control group might become concerned about their health and voluntarily cut back on the amount of fat they eat. It is unrealistic to expect to succeed at a randomized controlled trial that requires people to alter their behavior over a significant period of time, unless the subjects have a special motivation to participate—if they are suffering from a serious disease, for example—and participation in a trial is their only chance to have access to a new, potentially more effective treatment.

To test the dietary hypothesis, researchers might try, instead of a randomized controlled trial, a cohort study. They would choose a large group of people who are free of heart disease, ask them detailed questions about their diets, and then, over the next 5 years, compare the health of those who already eat a low-fat diet with those who eat an average American diet. This would not require people to change their behavior. The problem with this scenario is that people who have voluntarily chosen to eat a low-fat diet may differ in other respects from the group who eat the average diet. The low-fat group members are likely be more health conscious in general. They may be less likely to smoke and more likely to exercise, for example. These people, therefore, would have a reduced risk of heart disease even if a low-fat diet did not have a protective effect.

The third type of study, the case-control study, has its own difficulties. In this study, researchers would choose a group of people who already have heart disease; perhaps they would go to a hospital and interview patients recovering from a heart attack. A comparable group of people who do not have heart disease would serve as the control group. Researchers would question people in both groups about their diets over the past 5 years and decide whether the diets should be classified as high-fat or low-fat. If the researchers' hypothesis is correct, the patients who have had a heart attack will report a diet higher in fat than the control group. This approach also has obvious problems. People are not likely to remember what they ate in the past, or they might be embarrassed to admit how self-indulgent they have been. The information researchers obtain concerning exposure in the case-control trial may not be reliable.

These difficulties do not mean that no valid conclusion can be drawn from any kind of epidemiologic study. However, they demonstrate the types of errors that different kinds of studies may be prone to and alert researchers about what to watch out for in choosing a study design and in interpreting the results.

Sources of Error

News reports of new health studies can often be confusing. Sometimes there are conflicting reports on the health effects of various substances. Coffee is reported to cause heart disease; then it is reported that there is no such effect. Oat bran is reported to prevent cancer; then it is reported to make no difference. Fish is good for your heart; fish is full of toxic chemicals that may cause harm. All these contradictions tend to make people distrustful of the news and uncertain about how to protect their health. Since most of these news reports are based on epidemiologic studies, it is useful to understand possible sources of error in such studies and how to look for the truth in the reports.

One of the most common reasons for a study to lead to a wrong conclusion is that the reported result is merely a *random variation* and that the association is merely due to chance. As a general rule, epidemiologic studies of chronic diseases require large numbers of subjects to draw valid conclusions. Causes of these diseases are usually complex, and there are usually long periods between exposures to possible causes and the development of illness, making it difficult to draw conclusions about associations between exposure and disease. The cause-and-effect relationship is not obvious—as it is, for example, when a bullet in the heart causes death, or exposure of an unvaccinated child to the measles virus causes the child to develop measles in 10 to 12 days. The weaker the relationship between exposure and disease, the larger the group of people that must be studied for the relationship to be evident. If the group being studied is too small, a cause-and-effect relationship is likely to be missed or a spurious relationship will show up by chance alone. One of the reasons that the Doll–Hill and Hammond–Horn results concerning smoking and lung cancer are so convincing is that they involved such large numbers of subjects.

There are a number of other possible sources of error that well-designed studies may be able to avoid. For example, the cohort study of a low-fat diet proposed previously may be invalidated by the presence of confounding variables, smoking and exercise. *Confounding variables* are factors that are associated with the exposure and that may independently affect the risk of developing the disease. Such an error may have occurred in a 1980s study that suggested coffee drinking could cause pancreatic cancer, a finding that has not been replicated in other studies. Since many heavy coffee drinkers were also smokers, there are suspicions that the cancer was caused by the smoking rather than the coffee.[1] To eliminate the errors caused by smoking as a confounding variable, researchers might conduct the study only on nonsmokers. Alternatively, there are statistical techniques for adjusting the results to compensate for confounding variables as long as the investigator is clever enough to think of possible factors that may affect the result and to take them into consideration when collecting the data and calculating the results. While the investigators in the study of coffee corrected for smoking over the 5-year period before the cancer was diagnosed, the correction may have been inadequate.

An interesting example of confounding occurred in a study, published in 1999 and widely publicized, suggesting that small children were more likely to become myopic—nearsighted—if they slept in a lighted room. In a follow-up study, investigators asked the children's parents about their own vision. It turned out that myopic parents were more likely to leave lights on in their children's rooms than parents with better vision. Their children, therefore, were more likely to be nearsighted because they inherited the condition from their parents, not from the light exposure.[2]

Bias, or systematic error, may be introduced into a study in a number of ways. *Selection bias* is a particular problem in choosing subjects for a case-control study. For example, if the cases of heart disease are chosen from hospitalized patients recovering from heart attacks, and the controls include hospitalized patients being treated for a digestive disorder that causes extreme discomfort from eating fatty foods, the study may suggest an exaggerated effect of dietary fat on heart disease. The results would probably be different if the controls were patients recovering from the effects of motor vehicle crashes, whose diet might be more like the average American's. Selection bias may also occur when there is a systematic difference between people who choose—or are chosen—to participate in a study and those who do not. For example, in a 1988 case-control study that found exposure to high electromagnetic fields (EMF) from power lines increased the risk of childhood cancer, the controls were chosen by a process of telephone random digit dialing until a child was located who matched a case by age and sex. Cases and controls were compared, and cases were found to have had a higher exposure to EMF. However, the cases also were also found to be of lower socioeconomic status; they were more likely to live in areas of high traffic density, and their mothers were more likely to smoke. The random-digit dialing had created a bias: because poor families were less likely to have a telephone, or less likely to have an answering machine and to return calls, the control group was more affluent and consequently was less exposed to confounding poverty-associated factors.[1]

An extreme example of selection bias—one that no well-trained epidemiologist would make—was seen in the report of the author Shere Hite on male and female relationships. Out of 100,000 questionnaires on women's attitudes about men and sex that Hite distributed, only 4500 replies were received. Hite reported that 84 percent of the women in the study were dissatisfied with their intimate relationships, results that were widely publicized. The low response rate suggests that selection bias was operating and that the most dissatisfied women were responding preferentially to the survey.[3]

Cohort studies, which tend to extend over many years, are likely to suffer from a form of bias caused by people dropping out or being untraceable when results are being sought. If people who get sick drop out at a different rate from those who remain healthy, the results will be compromised. Subjects who are lost to follow-up may be more likely than those who are traceable to have entered an institution or to have moved in with family, indicating a serious health problem. A high dropout rate casts doubt on the results of any epidemiologic study.

Reporting bias or recall bias is a common problem in case-control studies. It occurs if the study group and the control group systematically report differently even if the exposure was the same. Subjects' reports of their dietary intake are notoriously unreliable. For example, underweight individuals consistently overreport their fat intake, while obese individuals underreport it.[1] Similarly, studies attempting to relate certain diseases to alcohol consumption may suffer from reporting bias because people who drink heavily tend to underreport their consumption. Case-control studies that attempt to determine causes of birth defects are especially subject to recall bias, since the mother of a child born with a malformation is likely to have thought a great deal about what might have caused the problem, while mothers of healthy children would be less likely to notice an unusual exposure.

Proving Cause and Effect

For the most part, epidemiologic studies, no matter how well designed to avoid error, cannot prove cause and effect. In fact, that is why epidemiologists usually speak of risk factors rather than causes. However, there are several factors that can be combined to make the cause-and-effect relationship almost certain.

First, as discussed previously, a study with a large number of subjects is more likely to yield a valid result than a small study. Second, the stronger the association measured between exposure and disease—the higher the relative risk or odds ratio—the more likely that there is a true cause-and-effect relationship. For example, the Reye's syndrome case-control study found a 42.7 odds ratio from exposure to aspirin during a viral infection. The British case-control study linking birth control pills to breast cancer found only a 2.3 odds ratio, while the Nurses' Health Study—a cohort study—found at most a 1.5 relative risk of breast cancer from oral contraceptives. The much stronger association found in the Reye's syndrome study makes it highly probable that aspirin causes the syndrome in children, while the breast cancer results could possibly be due to some error or alternative explanation. Nevertheless, exposure to hormones is generally accepted as a risk factor for breast cancer, as discussed in the next section.

Third, a dose–response relationship between exposure and risk of disease is evidence supporting exposure as a cause of the disease. Some of the earliest evidence that long-term exposure to low levels of x-rays had adverse health consequences came from a study comparing the mortality rates of physicians exposed to different amounts of radiation. Radiologists had the lowest life expectancy of the three groups of specialists studied. Ophthalmologists and otolaryngologists, who have little exposure to radiation, had the highest life expectancy. Internists, whose exposure was intermediate, had intermediate life expectancy, confirming a dose–response effect—the higher the dose of radiation, the greater the effect on lifespan.[4]

Fourth, epidemiologic evidence is more convincing if there is a known biological explanation for an association between an exposure and a disease. Studies suggesting that EMFs cause leukemia and other forms of cancer have been looked on with skepticism because of the lack of a known mechanism by which such low energy fields could have a biological effect. The question is unresolved. However, a number of other exposures have been identified by epidemiologic studies as causes of disease before a biological explanation was found. For example, strong epidemiologic evidence that cigarette smoking was a major cause of heart disease existed long before there was any biological explanation, and the mechanism is still not well understood.

The most important indication that an epidemiologic result is valid is that it is consistent with other investigations. If several independently designed and conducted studies lead to the same conclusion, it is unlikely that the conclusion resulted from bias or other error. If the reports are conflicting, however, people must be wary of accepting any of the results.

Epidemiologic Studies of Hormone Replacement Therapy—Confusing Results

When women reach menopause at age 50 or so, their natural production of the hormone estrogen drops significantly. Many women at this stage of life begin to have menopausal symptoms that can be troubling: hot flashes that disturb their well-being during the day and their sleep at night and vaginal dryness that causes discomfort and interferes with sexual activity. Prescription of estrogen supplements relieves these symptoms, and this treatment became popular in the 1960s. Estrogen was promoted to help keep women "feminine forever" as promised in a best-selling book of that title by Robert Wilson, published in 1966.[5] Large numbers of postmeno-pausal women took the hormone in the hope that it would keep them looking and feeling younger, improve their memory, and stave off other effects of aging. When evidence appeared in the 1970s that women taking estrogen had an increased risk of uterine cancer, the problem was averted by adding another hormone, progesterone, to the prescription. Progesterone countered the effect of the estrogen on the uterus without appearing to diminish its positive effects on other organs. There was good reason to believe that these female hormones protect women. Rates of cardiovascular disease are well known to be much lower among women than men until middle age, increasing after menopause to match the rates among men. And older women are much more likely to suffer from osteoporosis, thinning of the bones that leads to fractures. It was rea-sonable to think that hormone supplements might also protect women against these problems.

Numerous epidemiologic studies over the years supported the protective role of estrogen for bones and hearts. Most notably, the Nurses' Health Study, the large cohort study, ongoing since 1976, found that women taking hormone therapy had a 61 percent lower risk of heart dis-ease and a 75 percent lower risk of hip fractures.[6] These studies found small increases in breast cancer risk, but the trade-off seemed worthwhile for many women. In 1999, approximately 38 percent of postmenopausal women in the United States were using hormone-replacement therapy (HRT).[7]

Then in July 2002 the news broke that HRT was not as beneficial as it had seemed. The previous positive evidence had all come from observational studies. Meanwhile, a huge clini-cal trial, called the Women's Health Initiative (WHI), had been under way since 1991. The researchers announced in 2002 that the WHI had been stopped early on the basis that the risks had been found to outweigh the benefits.[8] Women randomly assigned to take a combination pill of estrogen plus progesterone were found to have a higher risk of breast cancer than women taking a placebo, which was not surprising. The surprise was that women taking the pill were also found to have a higher risk of heart attack, stroke, and blood clots. The women in the experimental group had fewer hip fractures and fewer cases of colorectal cancer than the control group, but this protective effect was not enough to outweigh the risks.

The news from the WHI study seemed to contradict the overwhelming evidence from cohort studies that HRT protected women against heart disease. However, the WHI was a clinical trial, the gold standard of epidemiologic studies, and thus was much less likely to be subject to bias. Many women stopped taking HRT when the news came out, and the drug's sales fell by 50 percent within 6 months.[9]

Since reports of the study were published, epidemiologists have been struggling to under-stand why the two studies produced such conflicting results. There are still many unanswered questions, but one important factor seems to be selection bias. Women in the observational studies who chose to take hormones were healthier to begin with and had healthier habits than the women who did not take the hormones. Many other factors appear to be involved, including biologic differences between the women in the two types of studies (women in the Nurses' Health Study were younger and thinner than the women in the WHI); there is also a bias stemming from the fact that cohort studies tend to miss adverse events that occur very soon after a therapy is begun, and the cardiovascular risk from HRT is highest during the first year after beginning therapy.[10,11] Evidence supporting some of the WHI conclusions emerged in 2006 when routinely collected cancer data revealed that breast cancer incidence in the United States had dropped significantly in 2003 and 2004, apparently the result of so many women discontinuing use of HRT.[9] Current recommendations call for HRT to be used only short-term for postmenopausal symptoms.

Ethics in Epidemiology

Most epidemiologic studies are observational and have little potential for harm. There are exceptions, however, especially in the conduct of intervention studies. Nowadays, strict ethical limitations apply in any study involving humans. These rules were developed in reaction to abuses such as those by Dr. Joseph Mengele, who conducted medical experiments on concentration camp prisoners during World War II. Ethical abuses have not been limited to Nazi war criminals, however. At one time, medical researchers in the United States were not overly concerned with the rights of the experimental subjects, who were often poor patients or captive populations such as prisoners or inmates of mental institutions. That changed in 1972, when news of the Tuskegee syphilis study shocked the nation.

Syphilis was a dread disease for hundreds of years, inspiring some of the same moral revulsion as AIDS has sometimes done more recently. Spread by sexual contact, syphilis had an unpredictable course that, over a variable number of years, could lead to a range of grim symptoms, including blindness, heart disease, dementia, and paralysis. It was sometimes treated with an arsenic-containing drug called salvarsan, which had been shown to cure syphilis in rabbits but which was not always effective in human patients and sometimes killed them. Some scientists suspected that the disease was not as uniformly dire as its reputation suggested and that the treatment might be worse than the disease. This conclusion was supported by the results of a Norwegian study of untreated syphilis done during the early part of the 20th century, which found that up to 75 percent of the patients were symptom-free after more than 20 years of the disease.[12]

In 1932, the U.S. Public Health Service and scientists from Tuskegee Institute began a similar study of about 400 black men in Macon County, Alabama, where syphilis was rampant: 40 percent of the population suffered from the disease. The purpose was to observe the course of the disease in these men, who were not to receive treatment. In part because it was not common practice at the time, and in part because the subjects were poor, black, and uneducated, the investigators did not try to explain what they intended to do or ask the subjects' permission. The men were told they had "bad blood" and were enticed to participate with free "treatments" and physical examinations, free hot lunches, and free burials. In the 1940s, penicillin was discovered and became standard treatment for syphilis, but the Tuskegee subjects did not receive the antibiotic until after the story broke in 1972.[12]

There is some question about whether the men were physically harmed by the withholding of antibiotic treatment. The course of the disease is complicated, and the surviving subjects were in a late, noninfectious stage by the time penicillin was discovered, perhaps too late to help most of them. However, this study raised a number of ethical issues, the major one being that the men were deceived. They were not told what syphilis was or that they were part of a study, and they were led to believe that they were receiving treatment. Furthermore, one of the tests that was done on the subjects was a spinal tap, a painful procedure that uses a needle to withdraw spinal fluid, which has the potential of causing harmful side effects, including—rarely—paralysis. This treatment would not likely have been tolerated by white, middle-class Americans, and many critics have concluded that the study was racist. In fact, revelations about the study led many African-Americans to distrust medical research. The misconception still lingers that the men were deliberately infected with syphilis.[13]

The outcry that followed the publicity about the Tuskegee study in 1972 led directly to the establishment of rules for the conduct of human experimentation. All institutions that receive federal funds must follow these rules. The rules require that every research subject must be informed of the purpose of a study and its risks and benefits. The subjects must freely consent to participate. In addition, any such study must be approved in advance by an institutional review board, a committee that includes representatives of the community as well as other scientists, who must agree that the study is well designed, that its benefits outweigh its risks, and that the subjects are truly given the opportunity for informed consent. Clinical trials are halted if the treatment group is clearly showing better or worse results than the control group. This was done, for example, in the portion of the Physicians' Health Study that looked at aspirin's effectiveness in preventing heart attacks when it became clear that subjects taking aspirin were suffering fewer heart attacks than those in the placebo group.[14] It was also done in the WHI study of HRT, described earlier in this chapter.

Even with the current strict ethical guidelines, there are a number of controversial issues surrounding clinical trials, including whether such trials should be conducted at all, who should participate, whether informed consent is truly possible, and whether unproven treatments should be available outside of clinical trials.

All of these controversies came to the foreground several years ago in connection with the AIDS epidemic. People with AIDS knew they had a fatal disease that had no known cure, and they were desperate. Many of them were very politically active. People with AIDS argued that they did not have time to wait for clinical trials to test the efficacy of every promising new drug. They wanted immediate access to any new drug that showed promise in the laboratory, because they would prefer to try something—anything that had the slightest chance of working—rather than face certain death. On the other side of the argument is the history of useless therapies that have been employed for years or decades because no one had ever done a scientific test of whether they worked. This is a true ethical dilemma pitting the individual against society. Can we deny today's AIDS patient a treatment that "can't hurt" and might help so that future patients will have access to treatment whose effectiveness is proven? The pressure for untested therapies for AIDS has now been eased somewhat by the development of new drugs that have been found effective in clinical trials.

The use of bleeding by 18th-century physicians as a treatment for almost any illness is well known. The argument for this therapy appears foolish to us today, but the absence of curative power was not obvious to the people of the time. Similarly, tonsillectomies were performed on more than half of all children in the 1930s through the 1950s in the belief that the operation prevented rheumatic fever and other complications of strep throat. In fact, there was no evidence for this benefit. It is now believed that a tonsillectomy may make strep infection more difficult to diagnose and treat.[15] Unfortunately, it is difficult to do a randomized controlled study on a treatment that is already in wide use, because people do not want to risk being randomized to a placebo treatment if they suspect the active therapy is effective.

Such was the case in the 1990s with bone marrow transplant as a treatment for advanced breast cancer. With conventional chemotherapy, a patient had a 40 percent to 45 percent chance of living for 5 more years. A procedure that removed a woman's bone marrow, administered a much higher dose of chemotherapy than usual, and then replaced the bone marrow, in theory gave her a better chance of surviving the cancer. However, the procedure was itself arduous and risky, subjecting the woman to a 5 percent chance of dying of complications of the treatment. It was also expensive, costing up to $200,000. The National Cancer Institute sponsored three large national trials of bone marrow transplants for breast cancer. The trials required women to be randomly assigned to the transplant group or to conventional therapy. Many were reluctant to participate in a trial because they wanted the most aggressive treatment, perceiving that this offered them their last best hope for survival. There were questions whether it was ethical to deny women the chance to choose the procedure, forcing them into a trial. On the other hand, might the practice of offering the transplant outside of a trial be unethical because surgeons and hospitals have a conflict of interest, perhaps influencing patients to choose a treatment from which they—the surgeons and hospitals—stand to profit financially?

Insurance companies were forced through lawsuits and political pressure to pay for these expensive and arduous procedures without evidence that they saved lives.[16]

Fortunately, enough women ultimately enrolled in clinical trials in the United States and in other countries to test the hypothesis. Negative results began to appear in 1999, and an analysis of results from several studies published in 2004 strongly suggested that the intensive procedure did not lead to better survival for women who underwent it and, in fact, led to more treatment-related deaths and adverse side effects than suffered by the controls. As the authors of *False Hope: Bone Marrow Transplant for Breast Cancer*, point out, 23,000 to 40,000 American women with breast cancer had the procedure done outside of clinical trials, while only 1000 were recruited to participate in the clinical trials.[17] "Although there was no deliberate effort to deceive women," they write, "the combined effect of salesmanship by physicians, lawyers, legislators, entrepreneurs, and the press led one of our respondents to say, 'We were all sold a bill of goods.'"[17(p.286)] If the clinical trials had not been completed, bone marrow transplant might have become the standard treatment, although, like bleeding and tonsillectomies, it appears to do more harm than good.

Conflicts of Interest in Drug Trials

Epidemiologic studies are complicated enough, with many opportunities to make honest errors in interpreting them (as described earlier in this chapter), but when millions of dollars are at stake, which is the case with clinical trials of new prescription drugs, it is increasingly obvious that conflicts of interest often affect reported results. Randomized controlled trials are required by the U.S. Food and Drug Administration (FDA) before any new drug can be approved for use in the United States. Pharmaceutical companies conduct these studies to establish the safety and efficacy of a drug and submit the results to the FDA in search of the agency's approval. Often, the results of these studies are also submitted for publication to medical journals; such a publication in a reputable journal adds to the credibility of a drug's effectiveness.

Because randomized controlled trials are considered the best way to test drugs, and because FDA scientists review the results of the companies' studies, FDA approval was generally considered evidence that a drug was indeed safe and effective. However, in the late 1990s and early 2000s a rash of publicity about harm caused by FDA-approved drugs raised questions about the clinical trials that supported their approval. Some of these drugs were removed from the market after news of their harmful side effects came out; others were required to post "black-box warnings" on their packaging, indicating that they should be prescribed with caution. Drugs that were potentially hazardous included the arthritis drugs Vioxx and Bextra and the diabetes drug Avandia, which raised the risk of heart attacks; the cholesterol-lowering drug Baycol, which caused muscle damage; the antibiotic Cipro, which was sometimes associated with the rupture of tendons; the asthma drugs Serevent and Advair, which may lead to severe, sometimes fatal, asthma attacks; and the psychotropic drug Paxil, which increases the risk of suicidal behavior in children and young people.[18]

Harmful side effects may be missed in a clinical trial because they are rare and the number of subjects studied was too small for them to be noted. However, the case of Vioxx demonstrated that a company may purposely suppress negative information about a drug during the approval process. In fact, there is now evidence that companies may purposely bias their studies in ways that make them appear safer and more effective than they are.

Vioxx was the first of a new class of drugs called COX-2 inhibitors to be introduced in the late 1990s. These drugs are a class of nonsteroidal anti-inflammatory drugs (NSAIDs), used for pain relief—especially arthritis pain—and are designed to be less irritating to the digestive system than the established, over-the-counter NSAIDs, such as aspirin, ibuprofen, and naproxen.

Soon after Vioxx was approved by the FDA, the *New England Journal of Medicine* published a report of a clinical trial conducted by drug company scientists that had found a 50 percent reduction of serious gastrointestinal side effects in patients taking Vioxx compared with those taking naproxen.[19] The same article reported that Vioxx caused a five-fold increase in the risk of heart attacks and strokes, but the drug company, Merck, claimed that this was because naproxen protected the heart, as aspirin was known to do. Meanwhile, Pfizer introduced its own COX-2 inhibitors, Celebrex and Bextra. There were high hopes for these drugs, which were also being studied for prevention of colon cancer and Alzheimer's disease. However, the evidence mounted that all the COX-2 inhibitors increased the risk of heart attacks. A later study found that naproxen was not protective of the heart, although it was not harmful either.[20] In 2004, Merck removed Vioxx from the market; Bextra was withdrawn in 2005. Celebrex, and several newer COX-2 inhibitors, are still being sold, although they are required to carry warnings of cardiovascular risk.

These events raised many questions, however, about the way the clinical trials were conducted and reported. The *New England Journal of Medicine* in 2005 published an "Expression of Concern" accusing the Merck authors of providing misleading information in the 1999 article.[21] Information that came out during lawsuits by patients who had been harmed by Vioxx revealed that the scientists knew of three heart attacks and other cardiovascular problems among the subjects taking the drug but had not included them in the data submitted to the journal.

It turns out that there are many tricks used by the pharmaceutical industry to prejudice the conclusions of clinical trials. Marcia Angell, a former editor of the *New England Journal of Medicine* describes them in her 2004 book, *The Truth About the Drug Companies: How They Deceive Us and What to Do About It.*[22] She lists seven strategies the industry uses to bias research. One of the most common is to test a new drug in a clinical trial against a placebo. This seems reasonable, but the results may be misleading if there are older, well-established drugs already in use for the same condition. The new drug will inevitably be more expensive than the older ones—a benefit to the company—but there is no benefit for patients unless the new drug works better, something the trial does not test.

Drug companies use financial influence to ensure that physician-researchers come up with results favorable to the companies. In the extreme case, companies sometimes design clinical trials and seek academic scientists to carry them out, paying the scientists for their work; then the company analyzes and interprets the results and decides what should be published. Even when the scientists conduct their own research, they may be paid as consultants to companies whose products they are studying, or they may become paid members of advisory boards or speakers' bureaus, or they may own stock in the company. These arrangements tend to bias the researchers in favor of the companies' products. One survey found that industry-sponsored research was nearly four times as likely to be favorable to the company's product than NIH-sponsored research.[22(p.106)]

Until recently, when a company sponsored a study, it often had the last word on whether the results could be published at all. This led to strong publication bias: trials with positive results were published, while those with negative results were never revealed. In fact, this tendency was reinforced by the preference of medical journals, which tend not to be interested in publishing articles about treatments that don't work. Beginning in 2005, many reputable journals have adopted a policy of refusing to publish reports of clinical trials unless they had been registered at the beginning in a database of clinical trials, meaning that negative results could not be hidden. The 2007 Food and Drug Administration Revitalization Act now requires registration of all such trials in a public database sponsored by the National Library of Medicine, clinicaltrials.gov.[23]

Conclusion

Epidemiologic studies are susceptible to many sources of error. Confounding factors may influence the results, suggesting an association where none exists. Bias may be introduced in the selection of cases or controls, in the reporting of exposures or outcomes, or in the disproportionate loss to follow-up of exposed and unexposed groups. Nevertheless, epidemiology is the basic science of public health. It is the only science of disease that focuses on human experience.

Epidemiology cannot prove cause and effect. However, certain characteristics of well-designed studies can make them very convincing. Studies with large numbers of subjects are more likely to be valid than smaller studies. A strong measure of association between exposure and disease, in the form of a high relative risk or odds ratio, is likely to indicate a true cause-and-effect relationship. A dose–response relationship that shows increasing risks from higher exposures adds to the validity of a study. A known biological explanation for an association between an exposure and a disease makes epidemiologic evidence more convincing than in situations when there is no known mechanism.

While observational studies have little potential for harming people, many ethical questions have been raised about clinical trials. In response to well-publicized abuses of the past, clinical trials and many other epidemiologic studies are required to be approved by committees, called institutional review boards, which ensure that the subjects' rights are protected. Other ethical concerns have been raised about the availability of treatments that have not been tested in clinical trials. On the other hand, conflicts of interest in the clinical trials for testing safety and efficacy of new drugs, which are required of pharmaceutical companies, have raised questions about the integrity of the research. Drug companies, which have vast amounts of money at stake in the outcomes of these trials, have found ways to manipulate the research to make drugs look better than they are.

Despite its flaws, epidemiology is still of necessity the basic science of public health. Epidemiologic data, when confirmed by repeated, well-designed studies and supported by the results of biomedical experiments in the laboratory, provide the best certainty as to the causes and cures of human disease.

References

1. G. Taubes, "Epidemiology Faces Its Limits," *Science* 269 (1995): 164–169.
2. A. Aschengrau and G. R. Seage III, *Essentials of Epidemiology in Public Health* (Sudbury, MA: Jones and Bartlett, 2003), 286.
3. S. Hite, *Women and Love: A Cultural Revolution in Progress* (New York: Alfred A. Knopf, 1987), described in V. Cohn and L. Cope, *News and Numbers: A Guide to Reporting Statistical Claims and Controversies in Health and Other Fields*, 2nd ed., (Ames, IA: Iowa State University Press, 2001), 154–156.
4. R. Seltser and P. E. Sartwell, "The Influence of Occupational Exposure to Radiation on the Mortality of American Radiologists and Other Medical Specialists," *American Journal of Epidemiology* 81 (1965): 2–22.
5. R. A. Wilson, *Feminine Forever* (New York: M. Evans and Company, 1966).
6. G. Kolata, "Hormone Studies: What Went Wrong?" *The New York Times*, April 22, 2003.
7. J. E. Manson and K. A. Martin, "Postmenopausal Hormone-Replacement Therapy," *New England Journal of Medicine* 345 (2001): 34–40.
8. G. Kolata, "Citing Risks, U.S. Will Halt Study of Drugs for Hormones," *The New York Times*, July 9, 2002.
9. G. Kolata, "Reversing Trend, Big Drop Is Seen in Breast Cancer," *The New York Times*, December 15, 2006.
10. F. Grodstein et al., "Understanding the Divergent Data on Postmenopausal Hormone Therapy," *New England Journal of Medicine* 348 (2003): 645–650.

11. M. Stampfer, "Commentary: Hormones and Heart Disease: Do Trials and Observational Studies Address Different Questions?" *International Journal of Epidemiology* 33 (2004): 454–455.

12. G. E. Pence, *Classic Cases in Medical Ethics: Accounts of the Cases That Shaped and Define Medical Ethics*, 5th ed. (Boston: McGraw-Hill, 2008).

13. S. M. Reverby, "More than Fact and Fiction: Cultural Memory and the Tuskegee Syphilis Study," *Hastings Center Report* (September–October 2001): 22–28.

14. Steering Committee of the Physicians' Health Study Research Group, Final Report on the Aspirin Component of the Ongoing Physicians' Health Study, *New England Journal of Medicine* 321 (1989): 129–135.

15. E. Braunwald et al., eds., *Harrison's Principles of Internal Medicine* (New York: McGraw-Hill, 1987).

16. G. Kolata, "Women Resist Trials to Test Marrow Transplants," *The New York Times*, February 15, 1995.

17. R. Rettig et al., *False Hope: Bone Marrow Transplantation for Breast Cancer* (Oxford, England: Oxford University Press, 2007).

18. U.S. Food and Drug Administration, "Index to Drug-Specific Information." http://www.fda .gov/Drugs/DrugSafety/PostmarketDrugSafetyInformationforPatientsandProviders/ucm111085 .htm, accessed May 17, 2012.

19. C. Bombardier et al., "Comparison of Upper Gastrointestinal Toxicity of Rofecoxib and Naproxen in Patients with Rheumatoid Arthritis," *New England Journal of Medicine* 343 (2000): 1520–1528.

20. D. J. Graham, "COX-2 Inhibitors, Other NSAIDs, and Cardiovascular Risk: The Seduction of Common Sense," *Journal of the American Medical Association* 296 (2006): 1653–1656.

21. G. D. Curfman et al., "Expression of Concern: Bombardier et al., 'Comparison of Gastrointestinal Toxicity of Rofecoxib and Naproxen in Patients with Rheumatoid Arthritis,'" *New England Journal of Medicine* 353 (2005): 1520–1528.

22. M. Angell, *The Truth About the Drug Companies: How They Deceive Us and What to Do About It* (New York: Random House, 2004).

23. J. M. Drazen et al., "Open Clinical Trials," *New England Journal of Medicine* 357 (2007): 1756–1757.

Statistics: Making Sense of Uncertainty

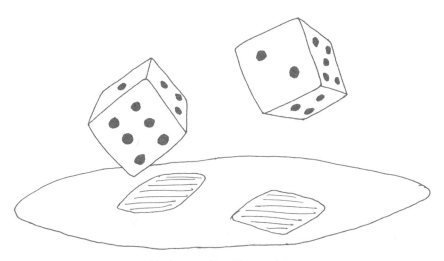

Understanding Uncertainty

The science of epidemiology rests on statistics. In fact, all public health, because it is concerned with populations, relies on statistics to provide and interpret data. The section on the role of data in public health discusses the kinds of data governments collect to assess the need for public health programs and evaluate public health progress. The term statistics refers to both the numbers that describe the health of populations and the science that helps to interpret those numbers.

The science of statistics is a set of concepts and methods used to analyze data in order to extract information. The public health sciences discussed in this book depend on the collection of data and the use of statistics to interpret the data. Statistics makes possible the translation of data into information about causes and effects, health risks, and disease cures.

Because health is determined by many factors—genes, behavior, exposure to infectious organisms or environmental chemicals—that interact in complex ways in each individual, it is often not obvious when or whether specific factors are causing specific health effects. There are ethical and logistical limits to the kinds of studies that can be conducted on human populations and there are limits to the conclusions that can be drawn from biomedical studies on animals. Only by systematically applying statistical concepts and methods can scientists sometimes tease out the one influence among many that may be causing a change in some people's health. Often, however, statistics indicates that an apparent health effect may be simply a random occurrence.

The problems and limits of epidemiology are defined in large part by the uncertainties that are the subject of the science of statistics. This chapter discusses the science of statistics in more detail, describing how it is used to clarify conclusions from a study or a test, to put numbers into perspective so that researchers can make comparisons and discern trends, and to show the limits of human knowledge.

The Uncertainty of Science

People expect science to provide answers to the health questions that concern them. In many cases, science has satisfied these expectations. But the answers are not as definitive as people want them to be. Science has shown that the human immunodeficiency virus (HIV) causes AIDS. But that does not mean that a woman will definitely contract AIDS from having sex with an HIV-positive man. Her chance of becoming infected with the virus from one act of unprotected intercourse is about one in 1000.[1] Similarly, scientific studies show that as a treatment for early breast cancer, a lumpectomy followed by radiation is as effective as a mastectomy. However, a woman who chooses the lumpectomy still has a 10 percent chance of cancer recurrence.[2] Both the woman who had unprotected intercourse and the woman who chose the lumpectomy would dearly like to believe that they will be one of those in the majority of cases who will have a positive outcome, but science cannot promise them that. It can only say, statistically, that if 1000 women like her have unprotected sex with an HIV-positive man, 999 probably will fare well while one will not, and if 100 women with early breast cancer have a lumpectomy with radiation, 90 probably will be cancer-free after 12 years while 10 will have a recurrence.

In many cases, there are not enough data even to give us that degree of certainty, or the data that exist are too ambiguous to allow a valid conclusion. In 1995, the *New England Journal of Medicine* published a report that the Nurses' Health Study (a cohort study), which had monitored 122,000 nurses for 14 years, found a 30 to 70 percent increased risk of breast cancer in women who had taken hormone replacement therapy after menopause.[3] One month later, the *Journal of the American Medical Association* published the results of a case-control study that found no increased risk from the hormones. Some 500 women who had newly diagnosed breast cancer were no more likely to have taken postmenopausal hormones than a control group of 500 healthy women.[4] In *The New York Times* article reporting on the studies, each researcher is quoted suggesting possible flaws in the other study.[5] There was little comfort in these results for women seeking certainty on whether the therapy would improve their health. According to one view, postmenopausal estrogen was clearly worth the possible risk of cancer because it appeared to decrease a woman's risk of heart disease and osteoporosis. In the opposing argument, women could achieve similar benefits without the possible risk through exercise, avoiding smoking, eating a low-fat diet, maintaining a normal weight, and taking aspirin. Now a clinical trial has contradicted some of the findings of each of these studies; hormone replacement therapy has been found to increase cancer risk and not to benefit the heart.

Contradictory results from epidemiologic studies are common. There are many possible sources of error in this kind of research, including bias and confounding, which are factors irrelevant to the hypothesis being tested that may affect a result or conclusion. Later in this chapter, additional factors to be considered in assessing whether to believe a study's conclusions are examined.

People sometimes demand certainty even when science cannot provide it, as occurred in 1997 over the issue of whether women ages 40 through 49 should be screened for breast cancer using mammography. Studies had shown that routinely testing women aged 50 and over with the breast x-rays could reduce breast cancer mortality in the population. However, studies done on younger women had not demonstrated a life-saving benefit overall for this group. Routine screening of these women increases their radiation exposure, perhaps raising their risk of cancer. It also yields many false alarms, leading to unnecessary medical testing, and major expense. The follow-up testing itself may cause complications, and many of the women remain anxious even after cancer is ruled out.[6]

When Dr. Richard Klausner, the director of the National Cancer Institute (NCI), called together a panel of experts in early 1997 to advise him on the issue, the panel concluded that, for younger women, the benefit did not justify the risks and costs, and recommended that each woman make the decision in consultation with her doctor, considering her own particular medical and family history. The public and political response was heated: after a barrage of media publicity, the Senate voted 98 to 0 to endorse a nonbinding resolution that the NCI should recommend mammography for women in their 40s. A letter signed by 39 congresswomen stated that, "without definitive guidelines, the lives of too many women are at risk to permit further delay," assuming that screening could save lives despite the lack of evidence.[7(p.1104)] In the end, director Klausner, with the support of President Clinton and Secretary of Health and Human Services Donna Shalala, recommended that women in their forties should be screened. It seems clear that pressure from politicians eager to get credit for supporting women's health led to a pretense of scientific certainty where none existed.

On this question, further analysis supported the politicians, although the benefit is weaker for the younger age group. While the "melee that followed the meeting will not qualify for a place in the history of public health's most distinguishing scientific or policy moments," in the words of one analyst, there is now a far better understanding of the issue and evidence that screening may be life-saving for some younger women.[8(p.331)] However, because the incidence of breast cancer is lower in women in their 40s, and the effectiveness of mammography is also lower in the denser breasts of the younger women, the benefit of screening is less for them. In a review of the evidence published in 2007, the conclusion seems to echo the NCI's original recommendation that individual women, in consultation with their doctor, should decide whether to be screened. The authors suggest that, "a woman 40 to 49 years old who had a lower-than-average risk for breast cancer and higher-than-average concerns about false-positive results might reasonably delay screening. Measuring risks and benefits accurately enough to identify these women remains a challenge."[9(p.522)]

Remarkably, the whole political uproar was repeated in 2009, when an independent panel of experts, appointed by the Department of Health and Human Services, issued a recommendation that routine breast cancer screening begin at age 50, not 40. Because the recommendation was published in the midst of the public debate over health care reform, conservative politicians cried "rationing." As science reporter Gina Kolata pointed out in a *New York Times* article, the dispute gives many people "a sense of déjà vu."[10] The data hadn't changed much since the earlier debate, except that new evidence was published in 2008 suggesting that some invasive breast cancers may spontaneously regress, supporting the argument that screening may lead to unnecessary treatment.

Many people concerned about how to protect their health find it frustrating when today's news seems to contradict yesterday's. As this example shows, science is a work in progress. In the words of Dr. Arnold Relman, former editor of the *New England Journal of Medicine*, "Most scientific information is of a probable nature, and we are only talking about probabilities, not certainty. What we are concluding is the best opinion at the moment, and things may be updated in the future."[11(p.11)]

Probability

Scientists quantify uncertainty by measuring probabilities. Since all events, including all experimental results, can be influenced by chance, probabilities are used to describe the variety and frequency of past outcomes under similar conditions as a way of predicting what should happen in the future. Aristotle said that, "the probable is what usually happens." Statisticians know that the improbable happens more often than most people think.[11(p.19)]

One concept scientists use to express the degree of probability or improbability of a certain result in an experiment is the *p* value. The *p* value expresses the probability that the observed result could have occurred by chance alone. A *p* value of 0.05 means that if an experiment were repeated 100 times, the same answer would result 95 of those times, while 5 times would yield a different answer. If a person tosses a coin 5 times in a row, it is improbable that it will come up the same—heads or tails—every time. However, if each student in a class of 16 conducts the experiment, it is probable that 1 student will get the identical result in all 5 tosses. The probability of that occurrence is 1 chance in 16, or 0.0625 ($p = 0.0625$). Thus a p value of 0.05 says that the probability that an experimental result occurred by chance alone is less than the probability of tossing 5 heads or 5 tails in a row. A p value of 0.05 or less has been arbitrarily taken as the criterion for a result to be considered statistically significant.

Another way to express the degree of certainty of an experimental result is by calculating a *confidence interval*. This is a range of values within which the true result probably falls. The narrower the confidence interval, the lower the likelihood of random error. Confidence intervals are often expressed as margins of error, as in political polling, when a politician's support might be estimated at 50 percent +/– 3 percent. The confidence interval would be 47 percent to 53 percent.[11]

While p values and confidence intervals are useful concepts in deciding how seriously to take an experimental result, it is wrong to place too much confidence in an experiment just because it yields a low p value or a narrow confidence interval. There may be up to 10,000 clinical trials of cancer treatment under way at any time. If a p value of 0.05 is taken to imply statistical significance, 5 out of every 100 ineffective treatments would appear to be beneficial, errors caused purely by chance.[11] Thus, large numbers of cancer treatments could be in clinical use that are actually not effective. Other reasons that a low-p-value study could lead to an erroneous conclusion could be bias or confounding, which are systematic errors. The results of the study that linked coffee-drinking with pancreatic cancer were statistically significant with a p value of 0.001.[12] The conclusion is thought to be wrong not because of random error but because the cancer was caused by smoking rather than coffee drinking.[13]

The fact that the probable is not always what happens leads to the Law of Small Probabilities.[11] The most improbable things are bound to happen occasionally, like throwing heads 5 times in a row, or even—very rarely—99 times. This means, for example, that a few people with apparently fatal illnesses will inexplicably recover. They may be convinced that their recovery was caused by something they did, giving rise—if their story is publicized—to a new vogue in quack therapies. But because their recovery was merely a random deviation from the probable, other patients will not get the same benefit.

Another consequence of the Law of Small Probabilities is the phenomenon of cancer clusters. Every now and then a community will discover that it is the site of an unusual concentration of some kind of cancer, such as childhood leukemia, and everyone will be highly alarmed. Is there a carcinogen in the air or the drinking water that is causing the problem? Could the cause be electromagnetic fields, which residents blamed for the cluster of six cases of childhood cancer between 1981 and 1988 among the pupils of an elementary school in Montecito, California?[14] Under great political pressure, the local and state government will investigate, but no acceptable explanation will be found. In the case of the electromagnetic fields, it could not be proven that they were *not* responsible for the cluster, but as more studies are done the evidence is still ambiguous. Most such clusters are due to statistical variation, like an unusual run of tails in a coin toss. Such an explanation tends to be unsatisfactory to community residents, who may accuse the government of a cover-up; but after the investigation the number of new cases usually returns to more or less normal levels, and the sense of alarm subsides.

If a cluster is very large, it is likely not to be a random variation—just as in coin tossing, 50 heads in a row is a much less likely outcome than 5 heads unless there is something wrong with the coin. A large number of cases is said to confer *power* on a study. Power is the probability of finding an effect if there is, in fact, an effect. Thus, an epidemiologic study that includes large numbers of subjects is more powerful than a small study, and the results are more likely to be valid, although systematic errors due to bias or confounding can be present in even the largest studies.

In designing studies of any kind, statisticians can calculate the size of the study population necessary to find an effect of a certain size if it exists. Studies with low power are likely to produce *false-negative* results (i.e., to find no effect when there actually is one). *False-positive* results occur when the study finds an effect that is not real (e.g., when a random variation appears to be a true effect). In a study of epidemiologic studies, a statistician examined the power of each of 71 clinical trials that reported no effect. He concluded that 70 percent of the studies did not have enough patients to detect a 25 percent difference in outcome between the experimental group and the control group. Even a 50 percent difference in outcome would have been undetectable in half of the studies.[11] This common weakness in epidemiologic studies is probably one reason for the contradictory results so often reported in the news.

In the review of high dose chemotherapy and bone marrow transplant for advanced breast cancer, the authors addressed the question of whether the studies had enough power to detect a significant improvement in survival for the treated women. They concluded that at least one of the individual studies did have sufficient power, and that the systematic review of all studies combined had the power to detect a 10 percent difference after 5 years.[15] Although some subgroups of women appeared to have benefited slightly from the high dose treatment, further studies would be necessary to demonstrate this, and no such studies are planned. The question remains of how much difference would be clinically relevant. Would it be acceptable for a woman to undergo the arduous treatment if her chance of survival was only 10 percent better? That is a question that cannot be answered by statisticians.

The Statistics of Screening Tests

In public health's mission to prevent disease and disability, secondary prevention—early detection and treatment—plays an important role. When the causes of a disease are not well understood, as in breast cancer, little is known about primary prevention. The best public health measure is to screen the population at risk so as to detect the disease early, when it is most treatable. Screening is also an important component of programs to control HIV/AIDS by identifying HIV-infected individuals so that they can be treated and counseled about how to avoid spreading the virus to others. As discussed later in this volume in the section of genetic diseases, newborn babies are routinely screened for certain congenital diseases that can be treated before permanent damage is done to the infants' developing brains and bodies.

While laboratory tests to be used in screening programs should ideally be highly accurate, most are likely to yield either false positives or false negatives. Tests may be highly *sensitive*, meaning that they yield few false negatives, or they may be highly *specific*, meaning that they yield few false positives. Many highly sensitive tests are not very specific and vice versa. For most public health screening programs, sensitive tests are desirable in order to avoid missing any individual with a serious disease who could be helped by some intervention. However, inexpensive, sensitive tests chosen to encourage testing of as many at-risk individuals as possible are often not very specific. When a positive result is found, more specific tests are then conducted to determine if the first finding was accurate. For example, if a sensitive mammogram finds a suspicious spot in a woman's breast, the test is usually followed up with a biopsy to determine whether the spot is indeed cancerous.

When screening is done for rare conditions, the rate of false positives may be as high as or higher than the number of true positives, leading to a lot of follow-up testing on perfectly normal people. Such a situation occurred in 1987 when the states of Illinois and Louisiana mandated premarital screening for HIV.[16] With the rate of HIV infection in the general, heterosexual population quite low, a great many healthy people were unnecessarily alarmed and subjected to further tests, while very few HIV-positive people were identified. Some couples went to neighboring states to marry to avoid the nuisance. The programs were discontinued within a year. The problem of false positives is also the reason why mammography screening is questionable for women in their 40s, as discussed earlier.

There are other conditions for which screening may not be as beneficial as expected. One of these is prostate cancer, discussed elsewhere in this text. Another is lung cancer screening of smokers. Lung cancer is usually a fatal diagnosis; by the time most patients suffer symptoms, it is too late for medicine or surgery to make a difference. The idea of screening smokers so that cancers can be detected and treated earlier in the course of the disease has been around since the 1970s and 1980s. However, at that time, the only method of screening was to use chest x-rays, and it turned out that cancers detected by x-ray screening were almost always too far advanced to be treatable.

In fall 2006, a paper published in the *New England Journal of Medicine* reported that screening with spiral CT scans (a kind of three-dimensional x-ray) could detect lung cancers early enough that treatment allowed 80 percent of patients to survive for 10 years, compared to a 10 percent survival rate for patients who had been diagnosed the usual way.[17] A few months later, the *Journal of the American Medical Association* published another study, concluding that spiral CT scanning does not save lives and may actually cause more harm than good.[18] An analysis of the findings of the first trial revealed two sources of bias: lead-time bias and overdiagnosis bias.[19] The former may occur in all cancer screening and must be taken into consideration before concluding that screening saves lives. Lead-time bias occurs when increased survival time after diagnosis is counted as an indicator of success. If early detection of a cancer does not lead to a cure, the only result of early diagnosis is that patients will live longer with the knowledge that they are sick before dying at the same time they would have died anyway. This appears to be the case in the *New England Journal of Medicine* study of lung cancer screening. In fact, the effects of the additional diagnostic tests and surgeries that follow the early diagnosis may hasten the patients' death.

Overdiagnosis bias occurs when the tumors that are detected by the screening are not likely to progress to the stage that they cause symptoms and be life-threatening. Such small tumors had also been found in the earlier lung cancer screening trials using x-rays. Overdiagnosis bias is also a problem with prostate cancer screening, and perhaps with breast cancer screening, as discussed earlier in this chapter. The only way to be sure that screening actually saves lives is to conduct randomized controlled trials, comparing mortality among patients who are screened with that of patients who are not screened. Such trials, together with data showing that breast cancer mortality overall has fallen in the United States by 24 percent since 1990, have shown that mammography does save lives.[8,9,20]

Rates and Other Calculated Statistics

Epidemiology makes extensive use of rates in studies of disease distribution and determinants. Rates put the raw numbers into perspective by relating them to the size of the population being considered. Vast quantities of health-related data are collected on the American population, data that are used to assess the people's health and to evaluate the effectiveness of public health programs. For these purposes too, the raw numbers are subjected to statistical adjustments that yield various rates useful in making comparisons and identifying trends.

For example, knowing that a city has 500 deaths per year is not very informative unless the population of the city is known. Death rates are generally expressed as the number of deaths per 1000 people. Thus, 500 deaths per year is a low number for a city of 100,000, while it is high for a city of 50,000. The overall death rate in the United States was 8.0 per 1000 people in 2010.[21] The same data may yield different rates depending on the population referred to. Rates are usually calculated using the population at risk for the denominator. In the case of death rates, the whole population is at risk. Birth rates are an exception; like the death rate, the birth rate is defined as the number of live births per 1000 people. The fertility rate, by contrast, does use the population at risk, giving the number of live births per 1000 women ages 15 to 44. Two communities with the same fertility rate may have quite different birth rates if one contains many young women and the other is older with a higher proportion of men. Both rates

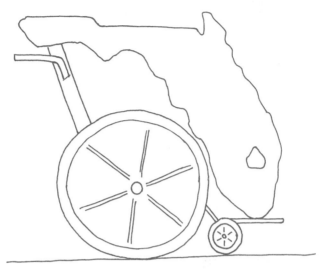

Florida's Population Is Older than Average

start with the same raw number—the number of live births—but use a different population for reference. In 2009, the birth of 4,131,019 babies in the United States led to a birth rate of 13.5 per 1000 people overall. The fertility rate ranged from 58.5 per 1000 non-Hispanic white women to 93.3 per 1000 Hispanic women.[22]

Other rates commonly used as indicators of a community's health are the infant mortality rate and the maternal mortality rate, as discussed later in this text. The infant mortality rate is the number of infants that die before their first birthday in a year, divided by the number of live births in that year. The maternal mortality rate is the number of deaths among women associated with pregnancy and delivery in a year, divided by the number of live births in that year.

For some purposes, the numbers can be made still more useful by converting crude rates into adjusted rates. Death rates are often adjusted for the age of the population. The adjustment uses a statistical calculation to make the populations being examined equivalent to one another. For example, the crude mortality rate in Florida is much higher than the crude mortality rate in Alaska. There is no cause for alarm in Florida, however. Since the average age of the Floridians is significantly higher than the average age of Alaskans—in fact many residents of other states retire to Florida and die there, while people who move to Alaska are likely to be young—it is to be expected that a higher percentage of Floridians die each year. After adjusting the mortality rate to what it would be if the average ages of the two populations were the same, the age-adjusted mortality rate for Alaska is higher than that in Florida, as seen in Table 7-1. Rates may also be adjusted for other factors relevant to health, such as gender, race, ethnicity, and so forth. For example, because males have higher mortality rates at all ages than females, it

Table 7-1   Age-Adjusted Mortality Rates for Florida and Alaska, 2006

	Florida	Alaska
Crude death rate per 100,000	940.1	500.6
Age-adjusted death rate per 100,000	711.3	775.9

Source: Data from "Deaths: Final Data for 2006." *National Vital Statistics Reports* 58, No. 1, National Center for Health Statistics (2009).

may sometimes be useful to calculate a gender-adjusted mortality rate for a population that has a higher proportion than average of one gender.

Rates are also calculated on a group-specific basis. Researchers may calculate rates for males alone or females alone, blacks, whites, Hispanics, members of other racial or ethnic groups, and people in defined age groups. This kind of data informs us, for example, that males have higher mortality rates than females in the same age group, and that blacks have higher mortality rates than whites of the same sex and age. It is common to break down death rates from various causes by age group, revealing that different age groups are more likely to die of different causes. For example, death rates from cancer, stroke, and heart disease increase steadily with age. Death rates from AIDS, however, are highest for the 45 to 54 year age group and fall to almost zero for those older than 75 years.[23(Table 35)] Death rates from firearms injuries and motor vehicle injuries are highest in the 20 to 24 age group, although death rates from motor vehicle injuries are almost as high for people over 75.[23(Tables 37,40)]

Further calculations can be done using age-specific death rates to yield life expectancies, data that is intuitively meaningful in describing the health of a population. Life expectancy is the average number of years of life remaining to people at a particular age, and it reflects the mortality conditions of the period when the calculation is made. Life expectancies may be determined by race, sex, or other characteristics using age-specific death rates for the population with that characteristic. The most common figure used in comparing the health of various populations is the life expectancy at birth. As seen in Table 7-2, life expectancies at birth in the United States have been increasing since 1900. In Russia, however, life expectancies have declined since the fall of the Soviet Union, reflecting many societal ills that have led to poorer health of the population there. Table 7-3 shows the life expectancy at birth for males and females of selected countries.

Another calculated concept that is sometimes used as a measure of premature mortality is years of potential life lost (YPLL). It gives greater weight to deaths of young people, appropriate to the priorities of public health, which has the goal not of eliminating death entirely but of enabling people to live out their natural lifespan with a minimum of illness and disability.

Table 7-2   Life Expectancy at Birth According to Race and Sex in the United States, Selected Years, 1900–2009

Updated data when available, Excel, PDF, and more data years: http://www.cdc.gov/nchs/hus/contents2011.htm#022.

[Data are based on death certificates]

Specified Age and Year	All Races			White			Black or African American[1]		
	Both Sexes	Male	Female	Both Sexes	Male	Female	Both Sexes	Male	Female
At birth				Remaining life expectancy in years					
1900[2,3]	47.3	46.3	48.3	47.6	46.6	48.7	33.0	32.5	33.5
1950[3]	68.2	65.6	71.1	69.1	66.5	72.2	60.8	59.1	62.9
1960[3]	69.7	66.6	73.1	70.6	67.4	74.1	63.6	61.1	66.3
1970	70.8	67.1	74.7	71.7	68.0	75.6	64.1	60.0	68.3
1980	73.7	70.0	77.4	74.4	70.7	78.1	68.1	63.8	72.5
1990	75.4	71.8	78.8	76.1	72.7	79.4	69.1	64.5	73.6
1995	75.8	72.5	78.9	76.5	73.4	79.6	69.6	65.2	73.9
1999	76.7	73.9	79.4	77.3	74.6	79.9	71.4	67.8	74.7
2000	76.8	74.1	79.3	77.3	74.7	79.9	71.8	68.2	75.1
2001	76.9	74.2	79.4	77.4	74.8	79.9	72.0	68.4	75.2
2002	76.9	74.3	79.5	77.4	74.9	79.9	72.1	68.6	75.4
2003	77.1	74.5	79.6	77.6	75.0	80.0	72.3	68.8	75.6
2004	77.5	74.9	79.9	77.9	75.4	80.4	72.8	69.3	76.0
2005	77.4	74.9	79.9	77.9	75.4	80.4	72.8	69.3	76.1
2006	77.7	75.1	80.2	78.2	75.7	80.6	73.2	69.7	76.5
2007	77.9	75.4	80.4	78.4	75.9	80.8	73.6	70.0	76.8
2008	78.1	75.6	80.6	78.5	76.1	80.9	74.0	70.6	77.2
2009	78.5	76.0	80.9	78.8	76.4	81.2	74.5	71.1	77.6

Source: Reproduced from U.S. Centers for Disease Control and Prevention, Health, United States, 2011. Table 22. http://www.cdc.gov/nchs/data/hus/2011/022.pdf, accessed October 1, 2012.

Table 7-3   Life Expectancy at Birth for Males and Females of Selected Countries

Country	Male			Female		
	1980	2009	Rank	1980	2009	Rank
Australia	71.0	79.2	5	78.1	83.9	6
Austria	69.0	77.6	17	76.1	83.2	13
Belgium	70.0	77.3	18	76.8	82.8	15
Canada	71.7	78.0*	14	78.9	82.7*	17
Chile	—	75.6	26	—	80.9	25
Costa Rica	71.9	76.4	23	77.0	80.7	27
Cuba	72.2	75.4	27	—	79.8	31
Czech Republic	66.8	74.2	29	73.9	80.5	28
Denmark	71.2	76.9	19	77.3	81.1	24
Estonia	64.2	69.8	35	74.2	80.1	29
Finland	69.3	76.6	21	78.0	83.5	8
France	70.2	77.7	16	78.4	84.4	5
Germany	69.6	75.8	25	76.2	82.8	15
Greece	73.0	77.8	15	77.5	82.7	17
Hungary	65.5	70.0	34	72.7	77.9	33
Iceland	73.7	79.7	1	79.7	83.3	11
Ireland	70.1	75.2*	28	75.6	82.5	22
Israel	72.1	79.7	1	75.7	83.5	8
Italy	70.6	79.1**	6	77.4	84.5**	4
Japan	73.3	79.6	3	78.8	86.4	1
Luxembourg	70.0	78.1	13	75.6	83.3	11
Mexico	64.1	72.9	30	70.2	77.6	34
Netherlands	72.5	78.5	11	79.2	82.7	17
New Zealand	70.1	78.8	8	76.2	82.7	17
Norway	72.4	78.7	9	79.3	83.2	13
Poland	66.0	71.5	31	74.4	80.0	30
Portugal	67.9	76.5	22	74.9	82.6	21
Republic of Korea	61.8	76.8	20	70.0	83.8	7
Russian Federation	61.4	59.0*	36	73.0	72.4*	36
Slovak Republic	66.8	71.3	33	74.3	78.7	32
Spain	72.3	78.6	10	78.5	84.9	2
Sweden	72.8	79.4	4	78.8	83.4	10

(Continues)

Table 7-3 Life Expectancy at Birth for Males and Females of Selected Countries *(continued)*

Country	Male			Female		
	1980	2009	Rank	1980	2009	Rank
Switzerland	72.3	78.9	7	79.0	84.6	3
Turkey	55.8	71.5	31	60.3	76.1	35
United Kingdom	70.2	78.3	12	76.2	82.5	22
United States	70.0	76.0	24	77.4	80.9	25

*2005 Data
**2008 Data

Source: Data from U.S. Centers for Disease Control and Prevention, *Health, United States*, 2011, Table 21.

Table 7-4 Years of Potential Life Lost (YPLL) Before Age 75 by Cause of Death and Rank, 2008

Cause of Death	YPLL	Rank by YPLL	Rank by No. of Deaths
Cancer	1437.9	1	2
Unintentional injuries	1094.9	2	5
Heart disease	1028.5	3	1
Suicide	367.3	4	10
Homicide	267.6	5	15
Chronic lower respiratory disease	181.8	6	3
Cerebrovascular disease	178.8	7	4
Diabetes	165.4	8	7
Chronic liver disease and cirrhosis	159.1	9	12
HIV disease	99.9	10	>15
Influenza and pneumonia	88.8	11	8

Sources: Reproduced from U.S. Centers for Disease Control and Prevention, *Health, United States*, 2011, Table 25 and *National Vital Statistics Report: Final Data for 2008*, Table 10.

Calculation of YPLL arbitrarily chooses 75 as the age before which a death is considered premature (age 65 was used before 1996). As an example, the death of a person 15 to 24 years of age counts as 55.5 YPLL before age 75. Unintentional injuries rank relatively high in YPLL because they are likely to kill young people, who have more years to lose. Table 7-4 shows a comparison of the leading causes of death in the United States with the leading causes of YPLL.

Risk Assessment and Risk Perception

While some statistical concepts may seem difficult and confusing, people have an intuitive understanding of statistics affecting their everyday lives. They understand that the future is full of uncertainties, and they intuitively try to minimize risks or at least weigh risks against expected benefits. Their intuitive judgment of risks, however, often does not coincide with the more scientific estimates of statisticians. It turns out that while judgments of risk by the average person include statistical estimates that are often fairly accurate, they are also influenced by psychological factors that should perhaps be taken into consideration by the public health professionals.

Public health's mission to protect the population from disease and injury requires governments to minimize risks or at least weigh risks against expected benefits, just as individuals do in their own lives. The formal process of risk assessment identifies events and exposures that may be harmful to humans and estimates the probabilities of their occurrence as well as the extent of harm they may cause.

Risk assessment is often done on the basis of historical data: for example, one may predict that the number of motor vehicle crashes next year will be similar to the number this year, increasing or decreasing according to the trend established over the past several years. Risks that certain chemicals cause cancer in humans are usually estimated by analogy with data obtained from animal studies. For many situations, however, there is little basis on which to make comparisons. In such cases, assessing risks involves making many assumptions, some of which may be little better than guesses. To estimate the probability of a mishap in a new technology, various possible chains of events are considered, and a risk for something going wrong is estimated for each step, perhaps by analogy with conventional technology. Risks of the individual steps are then added or multiplied to obtain a risk for the whole. This approach was used, for example, when nuclear power plants were first introduced, and it helped engineers to identify what kind of safety devices should be incorporated to reduce the probability of failure.[24] Still, the assessment appears to have underestimated the risk at Three Mile Island, as discussed later in this section.

Using such methods, scientists calculate probabilities that various injurious events will occur and rank them in order, as shown in Table 7-5. According to an analysis published in 1987, experts said that the most risky activities and technologies were motor vehicles, smoking, alcoholic beverages, handguns, and undergoing surgery. When the representatives of the general public were asked for their perceptions of risks, however, they headed their list with nuclear power, which was ranked 20th by the experts. Other risks that people tend to rank higher than the experts do are electromagnetic fields, genetic engineering, and radioactive waste.[25]

As a result of the apparent irrationality of the public in response to risks that the experts estimated to be small, a field of study has developed concerning risk perception. While experts

Table 7-5   Ordering of Perceived Risk for 30 Activities and Technologies

Activity or Technology	League of Women Voters	College Students	Experts
Nuclear power	1	1	20
Motor vehicles	2	5	1
Handguns	3	2	4
Smoking	4	3	2
Motorcycles	5	6	6
Alcoholic beverages	6	7	3
General (private) aviation	7	15	12
Police work	8	8	17
Pesticides	9	4	8
Surgery	10	11	5
Fire fighting	11	10	18
Large construction	12	14	13
Hunting	13	18	23
Spray cans	14	13	26
Mountain climbing	15	22	29
Bicycles	16	24	15
Commercial aviation	17	16	16
Electric power (nonnuclear)	18	19	9
Swimming	19	30	10
Contraceptives	20	9	11
Skiing	21	25	30
X-rays	22	17	7
High school and college football	23	26	27
Railroads	24	23	19
Food preservatives	25	12	14
Food coloring	26	20	21
Power mowers	27	28	28
Prescription antibiotics	28	21	24
Home appliances	29	27	22
Vaccinations	30	29	25

The ordering is based on the geometric mean risk ratings within each group. Rank 1 represents the most risky activity or technology.

Source: Reprinted with permission from P. Slovic, "Perception of Risk," *Science* 236:28. Copyright 1987, AAAS.

assess risk on the basis of expected mortality as predicted from historical data, the general public includes other considerations in its assessments. When these additional criteria are analyzed, it appears that the public's perception may not be so irrational after all.

Risk perception researchers have found that people's concern about a risk is affected by certain associated factors. For example, familiar risks are more acceptable than unfamiliar ones. Risks that people perceive they have control over are more acceptable than those that are uncontrollable. A risk with potentially catastrophic consequences is unacceptable, even if it is highly unlikely to occur. People are more likely to accept a risk from an activity that is perceived as beneficial, but they want the risks and benefits to be distributed equitably.

Risk perception researchers classify risks on two scales: dread and knowability. The more dreaded the risk, the less acceptable it is; similarly, unknown risks are less acceptable than known risks. **Figure 7-1** maps various risks according to the concern they evoke on the two scales. Thus although driving an automobile is, statistically, one of the most risky activities, it does not arouse great anxiety because it is neither dreaded nor unknown. Moreover, people perceive that they have control when they are driving, and the benefit is obvious to them. Conversely, a nuclear reactor accident is highly dreaded, and thus is perceived by the public as more risky than the experts believe it to be. People perceive that they lack control over nuclear reactors, and the benefits of nuclear power may not be clear to people who live in their vicinity.

The public's perception about nuclear power gained credibility after the 1979 accident at the Three Mile Island nuclear reactor in Pennsylvania. According to the experts, numerous safeguards were in place to prevent an accident, and the chance of a serious breakdown was remote. In fact, the safety systems worked to the extent that there was no disaster; no one was killed, and there was no significant radiation leak. Nevertheless, the fact that the breakdown occurred at all sent a signal that the experts may have underestimated the risks. Public opposition to nuclear power increased dramatically, and stricter requirements for reactor safety were imposed, raising construction and operating costs. The coup de grace for nuclear power came with the 1986 reactor meltdown at Chernobyl, in the Ukraine, which did cause lost lives and widespread radioactive contamination of the environment. Since then, no new nuclear reactors have opened in the United States.[25] With the recent concerns about fossil fuels' causing climate change, perceptions of the risk–benefit balance for nuclear power may change.

An interesting example of anomalous risk perception—one that is of great relevance to public health—is the paradox that adolescents so often engage in activities that they "know" to be dangerous, such as smoking, drunk driving, drug use, and unprotected sex. Studies aimed at understanding why teens engage in health-threatening behaviors can help to design interventions to prevent such behaviors. In the case of smoking, for example, surveys have

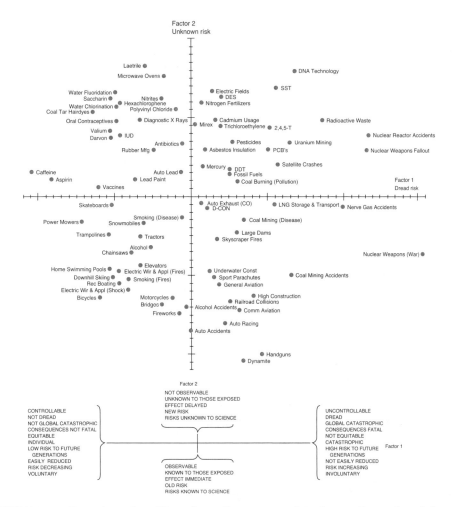

FIGURE 7-1   Location of 81 Hazards on Factors 1 and 2. *Source:* Reproduced from P. Slovic et al., in R. W. Kates et al., ed., *Perilous Progress: Managing the Hazards of Technology* (Boulder, CO: Westview Press, 1985), 108.

shown that teenagers can fairly accurately predict the probability that smokers will die of lung cancer and other diseases. However, the same surveys have found that teenage smokers perceive themselves to be at little or no risk. It turns out that they plan to quit smoking in the next few years, an inaccurate perception because they underestimate the addictive nature of nicotine and the difficulty of quitting once they are addicted.[26] Tobacco control programs, then, can be focused on convincing adolescents that tobacco companies are trying to lure them into addiction.

Cost–Benefit Analysis and Other Evaluation Methods

Other types of statistical calculations are frequently carried out as part of public health decision making. One of these is cost benefit analysis, discussed earlier in this text in relation to the controversy over setting occupational exposure limits to benzene.

Cost–benefit analysis weighs the estimated cost of implementing a policy against the estimated benefit, usually in monetary terms. In the benzene example discussed previously, the industry argued that setting a low exposure limit would be very expensive and that the benefit in lives saved would be small. Part of the difficulty in conducting such an analysis is the determination of what monetary value to place on a life saved. In other situations, the analysis provides a clearer justification for a program. For example, an analysis of the costs and benefits of immunizing children against measles, mumps, and rubella—comparing the costs of the immunization program with the costs of caring for the thousands of patients whose disease would not have been prevented if no immunizations had been done—yielded a 13 to 1 ratio of benefits to costs.[27]

Another evaluation technique is cost-effectiveness analysis, which compares the efficiency of different methods of attaining the same objective. For example, it may be so expensive to prevent heart attacks in healthy men by prescribing cholesterol-lowering drugs that a cost-effectiveness analysis would conclude that it is cheaper to skip the drugs and provide cardiac care for the men who do suffer an attack. Cost–benefit analysis and cost-effectiveness analysis "cannot serve as the sole or primary determinant of a health care decision," according to a congressional report, but the process of identifying and considering all the relevant costs and benefits can improve decision making.[28(p.211)]

Conclusion

The world is full of uncertainty. Science may not always be able to provide answers to people's questions. Statistics is a way to learn, at least, how certain people can be about what they think they know.

Statistics is a tool widely used in public health. Most epidemiologic studies and most studies in the other public health sciences depend on statistics to analyze data and interpret findings. Statistical analyses can establish the probability that what was observed occurred by chance alone. A measure commonly used to indicate the probability that a study finding is the result of chance is the p value. Even when a low p value indicates that a result is statistically significant, there is still a chance that the result is not valid, even if all sources of bias are ruled out. Studies with large numbers of subjects are more likely to be valid than small studies, although sources of error other than random variation are still possible in large studies.

Knowledge of statistics is also important in evaluating screening tests, used as a secondary prevention approach to detect diseases so that they can be treated at an early stage. Tests that are highly sensitive tend to yield false positives, while tests that are highly specific tend to yield false negatives. Most screening programs use sensitive tests and follow up positive results with more expensive tests that are both highly sensitive and highly specific. For conditions that are rare in the population being screened, the rate of false positives may be higher than the rate of true positives. Screening programs are also subject to biases, such as lead-time bias and overdiagnosis bias, which may make them less useful for saving lives than expected.

To put numbers into perspective, they are often converted into rates. Rates are useful in epidemiology and as a way of understanding the importance of the vast quantities of data used for assessment of the public's health and evaluation of public health programs. Rates commonly used as public health indicators are mortality (death) rates, birth rates, fertility rates, infant mortality rates, and maternal mortality rates. Rates may be statistically adjusted to make them comparable from one population to another. Age-specific rates can also be calculated. Other statistical concepts useful as public health indicators are life expectancy and years of potential life lost.

Public health's efforts to protect the population may require calculations of risk. Risk assessment is a formal process of calculating probabilities of various injurious events. The scientific assessment of risk sometimes conflicts with people's perception of risk.

Public health is based on science, including the science of statistics, which is the science of uncertainty. To paraphrase statistician and author Robert Hooke, scientific studies are often the only way to answer people's questions, but the studies do not produce "unassailable, universal truths that should be carved on stone tablets." Instead, they produce statistics, which must be interpreted.[11(p.64)]

References

1. R. Royce et al., "Sexual Transmission of HIV," *New England Journal of Medicine* 336 (1997): 1072–1078.
2. B. Fisher et al., "Reanalysis and Results After 12 Years of Follow-Up in a Randomized Clinical Trial Comparing Total Mastectomy with Lumpectomy with or Without Irradiation in the Treatment of Breast Cancer," *New England Journal of Medicine* 333 (1995): 1456–1467.
3. G. A. Colditz et al., "The Use of Estrogens and Progestins and the Risk of Breast Cancer in Postmenopausal Women," *New England Journal of Medicine* 332 (1995): 1589–1593.
4. J. L. Stanford et al., "Combined Estrogen and Progestin Hormone Replacement Therapy in Relation to Risk of Breast Cancer in Middle-Aged Women," *Journal of the American Medical Association* 274 (1995): 137–142.
5. G. Kolata, "Cancer Link Contradicted by New Hormone Study," *The New York Times*, July 12, 1995.

6. H. C. Sox, "Benefit and Harm Associated with Screening for Breast Cancer," *New England Journal of Medicine* 338 (1998): 1145–1146.
7. V. L. Ernster, "Mammography Screening for Women Aged 40 Through 49—A Guidelines Saga and a Clarion Call for Informed Decision Making," *American Journal of Public Health* 87 (1997): 1103–1106.
8. R. A. Smith, "Breast Cancer Screening Among Women Younger than 50: A Current Assessment of the Issues," *CA-A Cancer Journal for Clinicians* 50 (2000): 312–336.
9. K. Armstrong et al., "Screening Mammography in Women 40 to 49 Years of Age: A Systematic Review for the American College of Physicians," *Annals of Internal Medicine* 146 (2007): 516–526.
10. G. Kolata, "Get a Test. No Don't. Repeat," *The New York Times*, November 22, 2009.
11. V. Cohn and L. Cope, *News and Numbers: A Guide to Reporting Statistical Claims and Controversies in Health and Other Fields*, 2nd ed. (Ames, IA: Iowa State University Press, 2001), 11.
12. B. MacMahon et al., "Coffee and Cancer of the Pancreas," *New England Journal of Medicine* 304 (1981): 630–633.
13. G. Taubes, "Epidemiology Faces Its Limits," *Science* 269 (1995): 164–169.
14. P. Brodeur, *The Great Power-Line Cover-Up: How the Utilities and the Government Are Trying to Hide the Cancer Hazards Posed by Electromagnetic Fields* (Boston: Little, Brown, 1993).
15. C. Farquhar et al., "High-Dose Chemotherapy and Autologous Bone Marrow or Stem Cell Transplantation Versus Conventional Chemotherapy for Women with Early Poor Prognosis Breast Cancer," The Cochrane Library. http://onlinelibrary.wiley.com/doi/10.1002/14651858.CD003139/pub2/full, accessed May 25, 2012.
16. R. Bayer, *Private Acts, Social Consequences: AIDS and the Politics of Public Health* (New York: The Free Press, 1989).
17. International Early Lung Cancer Action Program Investigators, "Survival of Patients with Stage I Lung Cancer Detected on CT Screening," *New England Journal of Medicine* 355 (2006): 1763–1771.
18. P. B. Bach et al., "Computed Tomography Screening and Lung Cancer Outcomes," *Journal of the American Medical Association* 297 (2007): 953–961.
19. H. G. Welch et al., "How Two Studies on Cancer Screening Led to Two Results," *The New York Times*, March 13, 2007.
20. D. A. Berry et al., "Effect of Screening and Adjuvant Therapy on Mortality from Breast Cancer," *New England Journal of Medicine* 353 (2005): 1784–1792.
21. U.S. Centers for Disease Control and Prevention, "Deaths: Preliminary Data for 2010," *National Vital Statistics Report* 60, No. 4. http://www.cdc.gov/nchs/data/nvsr/nvsr60/nvsr60_04.pdf, accessed May 22, 2012.
22. U.S. Centers for Disease Control and Prevention, "Births: Final Data for 2009," *National Vital Statistics Report* 60, No. 1. http://www.cdc.gov/nchs/data/nvsr/nvsr60/nvsr60_01.pdf, accessed May 22, 2012.
23. U.S. Centers for Disease Control and Prevention, *Health, United States*, 2011. http://www.cdc.gov/nchs/data/hus/hus11.pdf, accessed May 22, 2012.

24. R. Wilson and E. A. C. Crouch, "Risk Assessment and Comparisons: An Introduction," *Science* 236 (1987): 267–270.
25. P. Slovic, "Perception of Risk," *Science* 236 (1987): 280–285.
26. P. Slovic, "Do Adolescent Smokers Know the Risks?" in P. Slovic, *The Perception of Risk* (London: Earthscan Publications Ltd., 2000), 363–371.
27. C. C. White et al., "Benefits, Risks and Costs of Immunization for Measles, Mumps and Rubella," *American Journal of Public Health* 75 (1995): 739.
28. G. Pickett and J. J. Hanlon, *Public Health: Administration and Practice* (St. Louis, MO: Times Mirror/Mosby, 1990), 211.

The Role of Data in Public Health

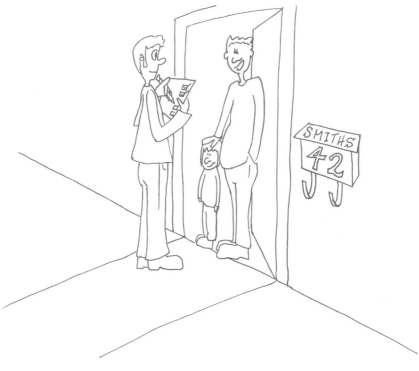

Collecting Data

Just as a doctor monitors the health of a patient by taking vital signs—blood pressure, heart rate, and so forth—public health workers monitor the health of a community by collecting and analyzing health data. These data are called health statistics. Statistics are a vital part of public health's assessment function, used to identify special risk groups, to detect new health threats, to plan public health programs and evaluate their success, and to prepare government budgets. The statistics collected by federal, state, and local government are the raw material for research on epidemiology, environmental health, social and behavioral factors in health, and for the medical care system.

At the federal level, the primary agency that collects, analyzes, and reports data on the health of Americans is the National Center for Health Statistics (NCHS), part of the Centers for Disease Control and Prevention (CDC). The NCHS collects its data in two main ways: First, states periodically transmit data they have compiled from local records; vital statistics, including virtually all births and deaths, are routinely collected this way. Second, the NCHS conducts periodic surveys of representative samples of the population, seeking information on certain characteristics such as health status, lifestyle and health-related behavior, onset and diagnosis of illness and disability, and the use of medical care. Some of these surveys are conducted on a state-by-state basis, and the data are thus useful to states and local communities. In addition, other federal agencies that collect data for their own purposes share it with the NCHS.

Vital Statistics

Births and deaths are the most basic, reliable, and complete data collected. Virtually every birth and death in the United States is recorded on a birth certificate or death certificate. Certificates are filed with the local registrar by the attending physician, midwife, undertaker, or other attendant. The state health department is generally responsible for collecting these reports and transmitting them periodically to the NCHS.

Birth certificates contain information supplied by the mother about the child's family, including names, addresses, ages, race and ethnicity, and education levels. Medical and health information is supplied by the hospital, doctor, or other birth attendant concerning prenatal care, birth weight, medical risk factors, complications of labor and delivery, obstetrical procedures, and abnormalities in the newborn. In the past decade many states have added a question on the mother's use of tobacco to the birth certificate. Much of the information on the certificate is confidential, withheld even from the person represented by the certificate. Its main use is for public health research, providing the data that can be used to relate features of the mother and her pregnancy to the health of the child.

The information on death certificates is subject to a number of uncertainties, depending on how well the informant knew the deceased and the circumstances of the death. For example, information on parents, education, and occupation may not be known if the decedent is an elderly person with no surviving relatives. There is often difficulty in the accuracy and consistency with which causes of death are specified. Incorrect diagnoses are common; in the absence of an autopsy, the exact cause of death may not be known. If a number of conditions contribute to the fatal process, underlying causes and immediate causes may be confused.

For some conditions such as AIDS or suicide, the cause of death may be misstated deliberately by the local official because of social stigma.

In addition to births and deaths, vital statistics include marriages and divorces, spontaneous fetal deaths, and abortions. Data on marriages and divorces are legal events that require universal reporting, but they are not very interesting from a public health point of view. Reporting of spontaneous fetal deaths is incomplete, especially for those that occur relatively early in a pregnancy; many may be unrecognized. Induced abortions are also probably somewhat underreported. In some states, the name of the woman who had the abortion is not included in the report for reasons of confidentiality.

Because infant mortality is an important public health issue, the NCHS has set up a special computer system that links vital records of infants born during a given year who died before their first birthday. The linkage allows researchers to compare information on the death certificates with that on the birth certificates, providing insight into factors that contribute to infant deaths.

The Census

The data collected through the vital statistics system and other methods must be converted into rates if they are to be useful for many public health purposes. The calculation requires information on the number of people in the population being referred to, the number that serves as the denominator when a vital statistic is used as the numerator. To calculate age-adjusted or age-specific rates, it is necessary to know how many people are in each age group. To determine sex-specific or race-specific rates, one needs to know how many males and females there are and how many blacks, whites, Hispanics, and people of other races in each sex and each age group. This information is collected by the U.S. Census Bureau, part of the Department of Commerce. Without an accurate count of the American population and all its characteristics, the government's health statistics would not be accurate.

As every schoolchild knows, the Constitution requires that the population of the United States be counted every 10 years to determine each state's representation in the House of Representatives. Based on that simple mandate, the Census Bureau has developed a national survey that provides data not only on the geographical distribution of the population and its sex, age, and ethnic characteristics, but also on a wide variety of social and economic characteristics, including education, housing, and health insurance status. Furthermore, because the population is always in flux and its circumstances tend to change fairly quickly, the Census Bureau tracks trends in the population between the decennial censuses, using polls and surveys and other sources of data such as birth and death records, immigration and emigration records, and school statistics. Census Bureau data are vital for the operation of the nation's social, political, economic, and industrial systems, and they are essential for the practice of public health.

Because census data can determine the political composition of the U.S. Congress and the distribution of federal funds to states and communities, various interest groups carefully monitor how the data are collected. An issue that was particularly controversial in preparing for the year 2000 census concerned how a person's race is determined. The broad categories previously used in the census were white, black, Hispanic, Asian and Pacific Islander, and American Indian and Alaska native. Individuals identify their own race and ethnic category. The issue has been further complicated by the fact that interracial marriage and parenthood has become increasingly common in the United States, and many of mixed racial parentage wanted an "interracial" category to be included on the year 2000 census. After considerable debate, the Census Bureau decided against such a category, but it allowed individuals to check more than one racial category for themselves.[1] This policy affects race-specific health statistics, but the effect is still small. Only 2.4 percent of the population chose to check more than one race in 2000. In 2010, 2.9 percent checked more than one race.[2] Among children, the increase in the multiracial population was dramatic between 2000 and 2010, reaching 4.2 million, with the most common combination being black and white.[3]

An even more politically controversial issue is the chronic problem of how to count every individual person in the United States. The census is mandated by the U.S. Constitution, and the Supreme Court has interpreted the mandate to mean that every person in the country must be enumerated; no statistical corrections are allowed.[4] The process for the 2010 census began in March 2010, when a short questionnaire was mailed or delivered to every household. The head of household was asked to complete the form, providing information on all the residents in the household, and return it to the Census Bureau. If the form was not returned, a second questionnaire was mailed. If there was still no response, the household was called or visited by a census worker to collect the information.

Inevitably, people are missed or counted twice. The missing ones are likely to be the poorest and most marginal members of the population—the homeless, illegal immigrants, fugitives from the law. Wealthy people who own more than one home might be counted twice. The Census Bureau estimates that the 2010 census missed about 10 million people and counted about 36,000 people twice.[5] Such errors can lead to systematic inaccuracies in health statistics. For example, blacks tend to be undercounted in the census, while black births and deaths are more accurately recorded, meaning that birth and death rates calculated for blacks tend to be higher than their true value would be if correct population numbers were used for the denominator.

Preparations for the 2010 census, according to *The New York Times*, were a shambles.[6] The agency's director and deputy director resigned in 2006 over the Bush administration's lack of support for the census, and it took over a year for a new director to be nominated and confirmed.[7] There were partisan battles in Congress about how much effort should be made to count racial and ethnic minorities: Republicans tend not to care that inaccurate counts affect congressional representation, because hard-to-count groups, like minorities, immigrants and the poor, tend to vote Democratic.[8] And because census numbers determine allocation of hundreds of billions of dollars in federal funds, cities and states whose populations are undercounted tend to suffer.

A major change in the way the 2010 census was conducted was that only the most basic data was collected from everyone, using what used to be called the short form, which asks for name, age, sex, race and ethnicity, and relationship of everyone living in the household. Previous censuses have sought to gain a fuller understanding of population characteristics by using a long form for about one in six addresses, asking questions about education, housing, employment, transportation, language, ancestry, and other issues useful for governments and businesses. In an attempt to make the collection of this detailed information more efficient and more timely, the Census Bureau in 2005 launched a new ongoing survey called the American Community Survey (ACS), which collects the same kind of information previously collected on the long form. The long form will no longer be used in the decennial census. The ACS is sent each year to about 3 million households selected to be representative of the populations of local jurisdictions. The ACS is designed to help communities plan transportation systems, zoning, schools, healthcare facilities, and housing, as well as the need for social services.[9]

Republican hostility to the census broke out again in May 2012, when the Republican-led House of Representatives voted to eliminate the ACS entirely on the grounds that it is too intrusive. A number of business groups, including the U.S. Chamber of Commerce and the National Association of Home Builders, have come out in favor of the ACS, which provides important economic data for business planning as well as government decision making. The Senate is unlikely to go along with the elimination proposal, but the outcome is still uncertain.[10]

NCHS Surveys and Other Sources of Health Data

As noted previously, the NCHS, in addition to collecting data from the states, actively conducts a number of surveys to gather additional information on the health of the American population. Follow-back surveys are a way to expand on the vital statistics data the NCHS has received. For example, in a survey conducted in 1988, NCHS chose a sample of birth certificates to investigate further, sending questionnaires to the mothers, doctors, and hospitals to learn more about family characteristics as well as the circumstances of the pregnancy and birth. Called the National Maternal and Infant Health Survey, the survey followed back a sample of fetal deaths and infant deaths, allowing researchers to study factors related to poor pregnancy outcomes.[11] Similar surveys are periodically conducted on a sampling of deaths; the person who filled out the death certificate is asked to provide more information on the lifestyle of the deceased as well as what medical care he or she received. The most recent mortality follow-back survey was conducted in 1993.

Two ongoing NCHS surveys aim to assess the health of the population as a whole, estimate the prevalence of selected diseases and risk factors, and look for trends. Every few years, interviewers for the National Health Interview Survey (NHIS) contact 35,000 to 40,000 households and ask questions about illnesses, injuries, impairments, chronic conditions, access to health care, utilization of medical resources, and other health topics.[12] The National Health and Nutrition Examination Survey (NHANES) is designed to obtain even more detailed and accurate information; doctors and nurses are sent in vans to conduct physical and dental examinations and laboratory tests on a carefully selected sample of the population. Each year, 15 counties are visited, and about 5000 individuals of all ages are selected to undergo the tests. Data are collected on the prevalence of chronic conditions, including cardiovascular disease, diabetes, kidney disease, respiratory disease, osteoporosis, and hearing loss, as well as risk factors for those conditions, such as smoking, alcohol consumption, sexual practices, physical fitness and activity, weight, and dietary intake.[13]

The NCHS is also collaborating with the National Institute on Aging on several follow-up studies of the population surveyed in previous NHIS surveys. In one follow-up study, over 7000 individuals who were 70 years of age or older in the 1984 NHIS survey were re-interviewed in 1986, 1988, and 1990. In a similar follow-up study, over 9000 individuals who were 70 years or older in 1994 were re-interviewed in 1997–1998 and 1999–2000. Since then, subjects have been re-interviewed at 2-year intervals. The interview data are linked to Medicare records and death certificates. The purpose of these studies is to describe the process by which older people progress from functioning in the community, becoming dependent, being institutionalized, and dying. Information is also collected on use of medical care and services. The second study looks for trends in healthy aging. The information provided by these follow-up studies is expected to be very valuable in relating the clinical, nutritional, and behavioral factors identified almost 3 decades ago to subsequent health status as people age, including their need for hospitalization or institutionalization in a nursing home.[14]

The Behavioral Risk Factor Surveillance Survey (BRFSS) conducted by the states, which report their findings to the CDC, is another way of obtaining information on health-related behavior. It asks questions about health, including high blood pressure, high blood cholesterol, diabetes, and weight, as well as about high-risk behaviors such as cigarette smoking, excessive alcohol consumption, drinking and driving, and physical inactivity. It also asks whether people get preventive medical care such as mammograms, Pap smears, colon-cancer screening, and immunizations.[15] The BRFSS gathers some of the same information as NHANES, but it has the advantage of surveying many more people, and it allows analysis of how the factors vary from one state to another. However, the information is self-reported and may be less reliable than that obtained in NHANES. For example, the BRFSS finds that, according to people's own reports, about 25 percent of adults are obese,[16] while the NHANES survey, using direct measurements, found a rate of about 34 percent.[17] This finding accords with previous observations that overweight people generally report that they weigh less than they do.

The NCHS conducts a variety of other surveys, including the National Youth Fitness Survey, the National Survey of Family Growth, the National Immunization Survey, and several surveys of hospitals, nursing homes, and other healthcare providers to gain information on healthcare utilization. Some surveys are done in collaboration with other agencies, such as the National Asthma Survey, in collaboration with the CDC's National Center for Environmental Health, the National Infant Feeding Practices Study, in collaboration with the Food and Drug Administration, and the National Health Interview Survey on Disability, in collaboration with several other agencies including the Social Security Administration.

Other governmental agencies collect health-related data according to the focus of their responsibilities. For example, the Environmental Protection Agency carries out surveillance for health hazards in the environment, including air pollutants and releases of toxic chemicals. The National Cancer Institute coordinates a program called Surveillance, Epidemiology, and End-Results (SEER), used to monitor long-term trends of cancer incidence and mortality. The Centers for Medicare and Medicaid Services has billing records for the Medicare program, which are useful for research on utilization and outcomes of medical care. The Food and Drug Administration collects reports of adverse reactions to drugs after they have been approved and are on the market, sometimes recommending recalls if a serious problem appears that was not noted during preapproval testing. Surveillance for product-related injuries is conducted by the Consumer Product Safety Commission.

Is So Much Data Really Necessary?

While it seems that the government collects enormous amounts of information on its citizens, there is never too much. These data are critically important in making up the surveillance systems that form the basis of effective public health practice as well as the planning and evaluation efforts that are increasingly being used in public health programming.

The statistics collected by federal, state, and local agencies are used in all areas of public health. Early notification of communicable disease cases is a classic use of public health information to protect the public's health. The need for public health intervention to control other problems may not be obvious without an analysis of data. This explains the Institute of Medicine committee's insistence on the importance of assessment as a core function of public health.[18]

Public health leaders are increasingly stressing the importance of planning, setting goals, and managing public health programs to meet these goals, a process that requires data at the local, state, and federal levels. For example, a community may not recognize that it has a problem with unintended pregnancy and low-birth weight unless it analyzes the data from birth certificates, comparing local data with statewide or national averages. Recognition of the problem might persuade local public health leaders to consider school-based birth control education and services.

Throughout this book, during discussions of public health issues (including biomedical, social and behavioral, environmental, and medical care issues), problems are defined according to the data that are available. In any area of public health, problems are identified in terms of statistics. The success of intervention programs to confront a problem is evaluated based on whether they improve the statistics.

In an era when people tend to frown on "big government" and yearn for lower taxes, there is always pressure to cut back fiscal support for data collection and analysis, activities that seem less urgent than fighting a known epidemic, for instance. Yet without data, experts cannot recognize that an epidemic is beginning. Inspired by the recommendations of *The Future of Pubic Health*,[18] the CDC has taken a lead in coordinating and encouraging the use of data in public health assessment. Recent events, including the emergence and resurgence of infectious diseases and the fear of bioterrorism, have stimulated the development of new surveillance systems within the United States and around the world.

With or without adequate data, decisions affecting public health policy and the allocation of scarce resources from government budgets must be made. It is increasingly important that these policy and fiscal decisions be made on the basis of timely and accurate information.

Accuracy and Availability of Data

British economist Sir Josiah Stamp (1880–1941) wrote in 1929, "The Government [is] very keen on amassing statistics. They collect them, add them, raise them to the nth power, take the cube root and prepare wonderful diagrams. But you must never forget that every one of those figures comes in the first instance from the village watchman, who just puts down what he damn well pleases."[19]

The process of data collection is always imperfect. Even data for births and deaths, the most accurately reported health events, may be flawed. The census produces errors, and there are political difficulties in trying to rectify them. Most other sources of health information, relying as they do on surveys or voluntary reports, are even more incomplete or subject to bias. For example, the Youth Behavioral Factor Risk Survey of high school students, conducted by states and reported to the CDC, misses adolescents who have the highest risks—those who have dropped out of school.

Errors in reporting cause of death on death certificates, a prime example of the errors about which Stamp warns, are especially worrisome for public health in that mortality data have such a strong influence on planning and priority setting for public health programs. Autopsies are being done with declining frequency, in part because of cost concerns, but also because doctors may believe that sophisticated diagnostic technology has rendered autopsies obsolete. In 1972, autopsies were performed in 19.3 percent of deaths; in 2007 that number had fallen to 8.5 percent.[20,21] Cause of death information is still subject to uncertainty in many cases, however, and several studies have found that evidence obtained from an autopsy contradicted the clinical judgment of doctors in 15 percent to 32 percent of cases. Information gained from an autopsy answers the question, did the patient receive the correct treatment for the correct disease? This information can improve the quality of medical care for future patients as well as improve the accuracy of vital statistics.

Because some of the inaccuracies on birth and death certificates may result from carelessness on the part of the busy health professionals who file them, new electronic methods of filing that are being introduced in some states are expected to improve the quality of the data. For example, maternal deaths are suspected of being underreported because doctors often fail to check off on a women's death certificate whether she was pregnant or gave birth in the time period prior to her death. If an electronic death certificate is used, the computer will refuse to accept the form—will not "send" it—until that question is answered.[22]

Computers are extensively used in the analysis of public health data, of course, and new applications are continually improving the timeliness and accessibility of the data. Weekly reports of notifiable diseases from state and local health agencies are transmitted electronically to the CDC, allowing prompt response to new outbreaks. Laboratory results are also reported electronically, facilitating the rapid identification of bacterial and viral strains that may be causing illness in scattered locations around the country. Databases that are kept up-to-date by electronic filings can provide rapid feedback on the effectiveness of new public health interventions as well as help detect emerging problems.

The new information technology—or public health informatics as it is sometimes called—has vastly improved the accessibility of public health information to public health workers and the general public. The CDC and most other federal and state public health agencies make information available over the Internet. For example, *Morbidity and Mortality Weekly Reports* is searchable online, and articles can be downloaded from the CDC's Web page. The National Cancer Institute provides the latest information on cancer therapies and prognoses tailored for doctors and for patients. Most of the information is freely available to all, although some data sets require users to have special passwords before they are allowed access; others are available to authorized users only on CDs or other media.

Confidentiality of Data

When anyone collects information on other people, questions always arise about how the information is going to be used and who is going to be allowed access to it. In general, all information collected from individuals by governments for whatever purpose is considered confidential and cannot be divulged without the consent of the individual. In most cases, the information is entered into a massive database from which individual names and addresses are removed. For research purposes, an identifying number may remain attached to the data to enable researchers to match information in one database with that in another. This technique is used, for example, in matching birth and death records as described above in order to learn more about the factors that contribute to infant mortality.

There is always concern that a determined snoop who works in an agency or knows an employee could obtain confidential information on an individual and use it to that individual's detriment. Agencies that handle confidential data impose stringent rules on access. Researchers must explain and justify their need for the data and promise to safeguard its confidentiality. Most agencies have an institutional review board or data protection committee, often including members from the community, which weighs the researchers' claims and decides whether to grant permission for access. Other than its use for research, the only exception made to the promise of confidentiality is when people must be notified that they have been exposed to a communicable disease.

The conflict between the need for confidentiality and the need for open access to information has been played out over various aspects of the AIDS epidemic. Because HIV-positive individuals feared, with good reason, that they might be discriminated against if employers, landlords, and others learned of their infection, public health practitioners were concerned that patients would refuse to be tested unless confidentiality was ensured. Hence, the rules for reporting HIV were handled differently from other communicable diseases: anonymous testing was allowed, and the system for reporting cases to many state health departments and the CDC was modified to maintain anonymity. More recently, however, with the advent of new drugs that can clearly help AIDS patients and slow the onset of AIDS in HIV-infected individuals, HIV's exempt status has, for the most part, been discontinued, and it is treated like other communicable diseases.

Conclusion

Statistics are the vital signs of public health. Local, state, and federal governments collect data on their citizens, starting with birth certificates and ending with death certificates. The U.S. census, conducted every 10 years, provides information on the age, sex, and ethnic composition of communities, information that allows the calculation of birth rates, death rates, infant mortality rates, life expectancies, and other data that form the basis for public health's assessment function.

The NCHS is the repository for the vital statistics data received from the states. The NCHS also conducts a number of periodic and ongoing surveys to collect additional information on Americans, including information on family structure, specific health conditions, behavioral risk factors, and other data useful in planning public health intervention programs.

Health statistics are used for all aspects of public health policy development and evaluation. Uses of the data include health needs identification, analysis of problems and trends, epidemiologic research, program evaluation, program planning, budget preparation and justification, administrative decision making, and health education.[23]

Increasingly, electronic means are being used to collect, transmit, store, and analyze data and to make the data available to public health workers and the general public. Strict precautions are taken to ensure confidentiality of information about individuals.

References

1. S. A. Holmes, "People Can Claim One or More Races on Federal Forms," *The New York Times*, October 30, 1997.
2. U.S. Census Bureau, "Overview of Race and Hispanic Origin: 2010," 2010 Census Briefs. http://www.census.gov/prod/cen2010/briefs/c2010br-02.pdf, accessed May 26, 2012.
3. S. Saulny, "Census Data Presents Rise in Multiracial Population of Youths," *The New York Times,* March 24, 2011.
4. L. Greenhouse, "In Blow to Democrats, Court Says Census Must Be by Actual Count," *The New York Times*, January 26, 1999.
5. U.S. Census Bureau, "Census Bureau Releases Estimates of Undercount and Overcount in the 2010 Census," News Release, May 22, 2012. http://www.census.gov/newsroom/releases/archives/2010_census/cb12-95.htm, accessed May 26, 2012.
6. Editorial, "Census Damage Control," *The New York Times*, June 23, 2008.
7. Editorial, "The Census at 'High Risk,'" *The New York Times*, March 25, 2008.
8. Editorial, "Rescue the Census," *The New York Times*, December 4, 2008.
9. C. Holden, "New Annual Survey Brings Census into the 21st Century," *Science* 295 (2002): 2202–2203.
10. C. Rampell, "The Beginning of the End of the Census," *The New York Times,* May 19, 2012.
11. National Center for Health Statistics, "National Maternal and Infant Health Survey." http://www.cdc.gov/nchs/nvss/nmihs.htm, accessed May 28, 2012.
12. National Center for Health Statistics, "National Health Interview Survey: The Principal Source of Information on the Health of the U.S. Population." http://www.cdc.gov/nchs/data/nhis/brochure2010january.pdf, accessed May 27, 2012.

13. National Center for Health Statistics, "National Health and Nutrition Survey, 2007–2008: Overview." http://www.cdc.gov/nchs/data/nhanes_07_08/overviewbrochure_0708.pdf, accessed May 27, 2012.

14. National Center for Health Statistics, "Longitudinal Studies of Aging." http://www.cdc.gov/nchs/lsoa/lsoa1.htm and http://www.cdc.gov/nchs/lsoa2.htm, accessed May 27, 2012.

15. U.S. Centers for Disease Control and Prevention, "About the BRFSS: Turning Information into Public Health." http://www.cdc.gov/brfss/about.htm, accessed May 28, 2012.

16. P. P. Chowdhury et al., "Surveillance of Certain Health Behaviors Among States and Selected Local Areas—United States, 2005," *Morbidity and Mortality Weekly Report* Surveillance Summary (2007) 56 (SS04): Table 25.

17. C. L. Ogden et al., "Obesity Among Adults in the United States—No Statistically Significant Change since 2003–2004. NCHS Data Brief No. 1 (2007). http://www.cdc.gov/nchs/data/databriefs/db01.pdf, accessed September 23, 2012.

18. U.S. Institute of Medicine, Committee for the Study of the Future of Public Health, *The Future of Public Health* (Washington, DC: National Academy Press, 1988).

19. J. Stamp, *Some Economic Factors in Modern Life* (London: P. S. King, 1929), 258–259, quoted in R. Goodman and R. Berkelman, "Physicians, Vital Statistics, and Disease Reporting," *New England Journal of Medicine* 258 (1987): 379.

20. National Center for Health Statistics, "The Changing Profile of Autopsied Deaths in the United States, 1972–2007," NCHS Data Brief No. 67. http://www.cdc.gov/nchs/data/databriefs/db67.pdf, accessed May 28, 2012.

21. National Center for Health Statistics, "The Autopsy, Medicine, and Mortality Statistics," *Vital and Health Statistics* Series 3, No. 32 (2001). http://www.cdc.gov/nchs/data/series/sr_03/sr03_032.pdf, accessed May 28, 2012.

22. Michael Zdeb and Mary Applegate, personal communication.

23. G. Pickett and J. J. Hanlon, *Public Health: Administration and Practice* (St. Louis, MO: Times Mirror/Mosby, 1990), 151–153.

Biomedical Basis of Public Health

The "Conquest" of Infectious Diseases

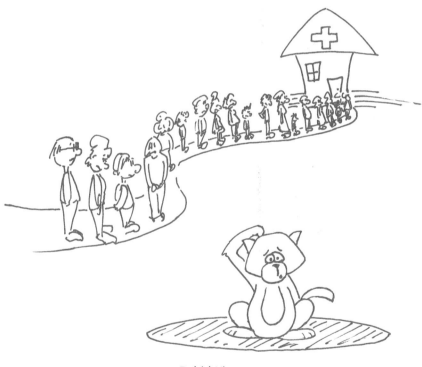

Rabid Kitten

Throughout history, until the beginning of the 20th century, infectious diseases were the major killers of humans. Bubonic plague, the "Black Death," is said to have wiped out as much as 75 percent of the population of Europe and Asia in the 14th century. Tuberculosis was the number one killer in England in the mid-19th century. An example of the toll of infectious diseases

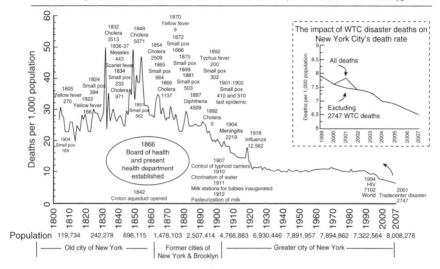

FIGURE 9-1   Death Rates in New York City, 1804–2007. *Source:* Courtesy of New York City Department of Health and Mental Hygiene.

is demonstrated in **Figure 9-1**, which provides death rates of the population of New York City over the period 1804 to 2000. Epidemics of smallpox and cholera swept through the city every few years, killing many people in each wave. In the mid-19th century, background mortality rates—largely from tuberculosis, typhoid, and miscellaneous respiratory and gastrointestinal diseases—were double what they became by 1930.

These infectious diseases were largely conquered through public health measures, including purification of water, proper disposal of sewage, pasteurization of milk, and immunization, as well as improved nutrition and personal hygiene. The discovery and introduction of antibiotics in the 1940s also played a role. In fact, by the 1960s, the threat of infectious diseases seemed to have been reduced to a minor nuisance.

In contrast to the fear, drama, and excitement that accompanied efforts to understand and control infectious diseases in the late 19th and early 20th centuries, public health in the 1960s and 1970s seemed to have become routine and boring. This period in the history of public health corresponds to the time when, according to the Institute of Medicine, public health was falling into disarray because of complacency.[1] This chapter will focus on the battles public health practitioners have won. It will discuss the causes of infectious diseases, how they are transmitted, and how classic public health measures have brought them under control.

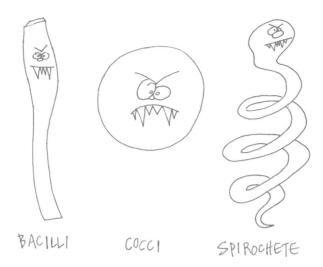

Bacilli, Cocci, Spirochete

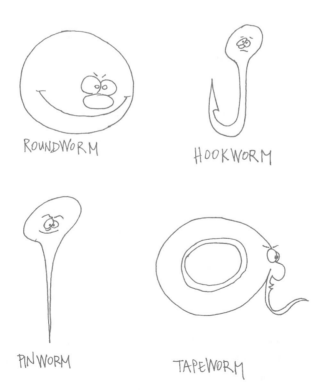

Roundworm, Hookworm, Pinworm, Tapeworm

Infectious Agents

The major epidemic diseases are caused by bacteria, viruses, or parasites. The fact that each of these diseases is caused by a specific microbe was established in the 1880s and 1890s, at a time of great scientific excitement, when almost every year marked a discovery of a new disease-causing bacterium.

Robert Koch, a German physician, developed techniques to classify bacteria by their shape and their propensity to be stained by various dyes. Since billions of bacteria—most of them harmless to humans—inhabit the skin, throat, mouth, nose, large intestine, and vagina, it was necessary to develop a set of rules that could be used to prove that a specific organism caused a specific disease. These rules, called "Koch's postulates," are (1) the organism must be present in every case of the disease; (2) the organism must be isolated and grown in the laboratory; (3) when injected with the laboratory-grown culture, susceptible test animals must develop the disease; and (4) the organism must be isolated from the newly infected animals and the process repeated.[2]

Koch applied these rules in his proof that tubercle bacilli were the cause of tuberculosis, the leading cause of death in Europe at that time. Bacilli are bacteria that appear rod-shaped when observed under the microscope. Koch identified another bacillus, *Vibrio cholera*, as the cause of cholera. Other disease-causing bacilli identified during that period were those that cause plague, typhoid, tetanus, diphtheria, and dysentery.

Round-shaped bacteria, called *cocci*, include *streptococci*, which cause strep throat and scarlet fever; *staphylococci*, which cause wound infections; and *pneumococci*, which cause pneumonia. Syphilis is caused by a corkscrew-shaped bacterium called a spirochete. All these bacteria were identified by the beginning of the 20th century.

For some infectious diseases, however, no bacterial agent could be found. Smallpox, for example, was known to be transmitted from a sick person to a healthy one by something in the pus of the patient's lesions. Yet attempts to isolate a microorganism were unsuccessful. The agent that caused the disease could pass through the finest available filters and could not be observed in any existing microscope. Smallpox was recognized to be one of a number of diseases caused by such "filterable agents" or viruses. It was not until 1935, when the American scientist W. M. Stanley crystallized tobacco mosaic virus, that the nature of viruses was demonstrated.

While bacteria are living, single-celled organisms can grow and reproduce outside the body if given the appropriate nutrients. Viruses are not complete cells, they are simply complexes of nucleic acid and protein that lack the machinery to reproduce themselves. Various kinds of viruses infect not only animal cells but also plant cells—as tobacco mosaic virus infects tobacco—and even bacteria. They can survive extreme conditions such as treatment with alcohol and drying in a vacuum and become active again when they are injected into a living cell.

They reproduce themselves by taking control of the cell's machinery, often killing the cell in the process. The human diseases caused by viruses include smallpox, yellow fever, polio, hepatitis, influenza, measles, rabies, and AIDS, as well as the common cold.

Human diseases can also be caused by protozoa, or single-celled animals that can live as parasites in the human body. Malaria, spread by mosquitoes; cryptospiridiosis, which caused the Milwaukee diarrhea epidemic described earlier in this text; and giardiasis, also known as "beaver fever" are examples of protozoal diseases. Other parasites, such as roundworms, tapeworms, hookworms, and pinworms, are the most common source of human infection in the world. Except for pinworms, they are not common in the United States today.

Means of Transmission

Infectious diseases are spread by a variety of routes, directly from one person to another or indirectly by way of water, food, or vectors such as insects and animals. Bacteria and viruses that cause respiratory infections, including colds, influenza, and tuberculosis, are transmitted through the air on aerosols, water droplets produced when an infected person coughs or sneezes. They can also be transmitted from an infected person to objects he or she touches, such as doorknobs, utensils, or towels, to be picked up by the next person to touch the contaminated object and transferred by hand to the nose. The early European settlers made use of this route of transmission to inflict a primitive form of germ warfare on the Native American people, giving them blankets that had been used by patients suffering from smallpox. The disease decimated Native American populations because they had no immunity to the virus.

Gastrointestinal infections such as cholera, cryptospiridiosis, and diphtheria, are generally spread by the fecal–oral route, by which fecal matter from an infected person reaches the mouth of an uninfected person. This may occur as a result of poor personal hygiene or by contamination of drinking water because of inadequate sanitary systems. Vector-born diseases, including malaria, yellow fever, and West Nile encephalitis, generally use a more complex route from one person to another, most often through an insect.

Each disease has its own pattern of development after a person is infected, and the time during which the patient is capable of transmitting the infection to others varies from one disease to another. Some diseases are most likely to be transmitted during the most symptomatic phase, for example, when a patient suffering from tuberculosis or the common cold is most actively coughing and sneezing. Others, such as measles and mumps, are most communicable during the day or two before noticeable symptoms develop. A few diseases can exist in a carrier state, in which the infected person can transmit the disease without having symptoms, as demonstrated by the infamous case of Typhoid Mary.[3]

Mary Mallon worked as a cook in a series of wealthy New York homes at the beginning of the 20th century. After an increasing number of family members in these homes became sick with typhoid fever, some of them fatally, suspicion fell on the cook. Because she was healthy, and because cooking was the only way she knew to support herself, Mary resisted medical tests and, when finally proven to be a carrier of the bacteria, refused to accept the results. Eventually she had to be incarcerated to prevent her from taking jobs where she spread the disease by the fecal-oral route. She remained in the custody of the New York City Health Department for the rest of her life. It was Mary's occupation, of course, that made her such a threat to the public health. The discovery of antibiotics, too late to help Mary, made it possible to eliminate the bacteria in typhoid carriers. However some viruses, such as herpes and hepatitis B, can persist in carrier states, and no treatment is known to eliminate them.

Chain of Infection

Control of infectious diseases is still an important component of public health. The public health approach to controlling infectious diseases is to interrupt the chain of infection. Many methods used to accomplish this interruption have now become routine, but vigilance is always required.

The chain of infection, a term used to describe the pattern by which an infectious disease is transmitted from person to person, is composed of several links, as illustrated in **Figure 9-2**. These are listed here:

1. Pathogen. The pathogen is a virus, bacterium, or parasite that causes the disease in humans.
2. Reservoir. The reservoir is a place where the pathogen lives and multiplies. Some pathogens spread directly from one human to another and have no other reservoir. Others, however, may infect nonhuman species, spreading from them to humans only occasionally. Plague, for example, is a disease of rodents that is transmitted to humans by the bite of a flea. Rats are the reservoir of plague. Raccoons and bats are reservoirs for rabies, which spreads to humans only through the bite of a rabid animal. Contaminated water or food may also serve as reservoirs for some human diseases.
3. Method of transmission. The pathogen must have a way to travel from one host to another, or from a reservoir to a new host. The flea is a vector for plague, transferring the plague bacillus from rat to human by sucking it up when it bites the rat and then injecting it into a human host with a second bite. Food-borne diseases are transmitted when a person eats contaminated food; water-borne diseases are transmitted when someone drinks contaminated water. Many respiratory diseases are transmitted by aerosol. AIDS, syphilis, gonorrhea, and a number of other diseases are transmitted by sexual contact.

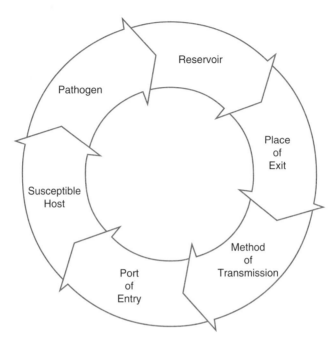

FIGURE 9-2   Chain of Infection. *Source:* Courtesy of Henry Schneider.

4. Susceptible host. Even if the pathogen gains entry, a new potential host may not be susceptible because the host has immunity to the pathogen. Immunity may develop as a result of previous exposure to the pathogen, or the host may naturally lack susceptibility for a variety of reasons. Most microorganisms are specifically adapted to infect certain species. Canine distemper virus, for example, does not infect humans. Even within species, susceptibility to specific viruses varies among individuals. Scientists have been puzzled why a very few people who have been repeatedly exposed to the human immunodeficiency virus (HIV) do not become infected; recent studies have found a genetic mutation that makes them resistant to the virus.

Public health measures to control the spread of disease are aimed at interrupting the chain of infection at whichever links are most vulnerable. At link 1, the pathogen could be killed, for example, by using an antibiotic to destroy the disease-causing bacteria. At link 2, one could eliminate a reservoir that harbors the pathogen. For example, controlling rat populations in cities by picking up garbage is a way of preventing the spread of plague to humans. Adequate water and sewage treatment prevents the spread of water-borne diseases, and proper food-handling methods eliminate reservoirs of food-borne pathogens.

At link 3, transmission from one host to another could be prevented by quarantining infected individuals, for example, or by warning people to boil their water if the water supply becomes contaminated. Hand washing is an important way to prevent the spread of disease: it prevents restaurant workers from contaminating food, hospital workers from carrying pathogens from one patient to another, and allows all individuals to protect themselves against pathogens they may pick up from the environment and put in their mouth. The spread of sexually transmitted diseases can be prevented by use of a condom, a simple matter of blocking the movement of the pathogens to the uninfected person.

At link 4, the resistance of hosts can be increased by immunization, which stimulates the body's immune system to recognize the pathogen and to attack it during any future exposure. Vaccination not only keeps the individual from contracting a disease but also makes it harder for the pathogen to find susceptible hosts. In some cases, it may even be possible to completely eliminate a pathogen from the earth by eliminating the susceptibility of its potential hosts. This was accomplished in the case of smallpox, as discussed below.

Other links are often included separately as part of the chain of infection when it is useful to consider them as sites for public health intervention. For example, the port of entry into the host for a mosquito-borne disease would be the skin, a link that could be interrupted if the potential host wears long sleeves and gloves. Similarly, the place of exit is the route by which the pathogen leaves the host.

Public health measures to control the spread of infectious disease include both routine prevention measures and emergency measures to control an outbreak once it has begun. Many of the measures referred to above—especially those concerning links 2 and 3—come under the category of "environmental health." Immunization—link 4—is a major weapon that has had great success against the dread diseases that created the epidemics of the past. However, vaccines do not exist for all diseases—notably, a vaccine has not yet been developed against AIDS. Even when vaccines do exist, some diseases are too rare to justify the trouble and expense of vaccinating everyone. This is where surveillance is especially important.

Epidemiologic surveillance is the system by which public health practitioners watch for disease threats so that they may step in and break the chain of infection, halting the spread of disease. In the early history of public health, the solution was often quarantine—isolation of the patient to prevent him or her from infecting others. Quarantine is still used occasionally, when the disease is serious and there is no effective vaccine. For example, a patient diagnosed with tuberculosis—which is slow to respond to medication—might be ordered to stay home for 2 to 4 weeks after treatment is started until the disease is no longer infectious.

More often, the public health response when an outbreak is detected by surveillance is to locate people who have had contact with the infected individual and to immunize them or give them medical treatment, as appropriate. For tuberculosis, contact tracing is used in addition to quarantine: people who have been exposed to the patient are given prophylactic doses of antibiotics. Tuberculosis has presented new and more difficult problems to the public health system in recent years because of the development of drug-resistant strains of the bacteria.

Contact tracing is also routinely used for controlling sexually transmitted diseases, such as syphilis and gonorrhea. Syphilis, which tends to affect the poor, the homeless, drug users, and prostitutes, can be diagnosed by a blood test. Because it has few symptoms in the early stages, it may go untreated and is easily spread. The challenge for public health is to identify those with the disease through screening programs carried out, for example, in a city jail. Once a case is identified, public health workers try to discreetly alert those who have been exposed. The public health worker asks the person who has been diagnosed to identify sexual contacts; the worker then notifies the contacts that they have been exposed without identifying the source of the exposure. Syphilis is readily cured by penicillin. If untreated, it may cause long-term damage to the heart and brain; congenital syphilis in infants born to infected mothers can be lethal.

The classic public health measures of surveillance and quarantine were key components in combating severe acute respiratory syndrome (SARS), a highly infectious new disease that first broke out in southern China in November 2002. Because China did not at first report the disease, it was not recognized as a major threat until March 2003, when the World Health Organization (WHO) issued a global alert and a travel advisory. WHO had been alerted by Dr. Carlo Urbani, an infectious disease specialist working in Vietnam, who noticed that a patient who had recently arrived in Saigon from Hong Kong was suffering from an atypical form of pneumonia. Dr. Urbani himself soon contracted the disease and died. Epidemiologic detective work found that the patient in Saigon, as well as patients soon identified in Toronto and Singapore, had all stayed in the same hotel in Hong Kong where a traveler from southern China had spent 1 night before falling ill with the syndrome. More than a dozen guests at the hotel had been infected by that one traveler, and they carried the disease to several other countries.[4]

By July 5, 2003, when WHO declared that SARS had been contained, the disease had infected 8439 people in 30 countries and had killed 812 people.[5] Although a virus was identified, lab tests could not diagnose the disease until weeks after a patient had developed symptoms. No drug has been found effective against the virus, and treatment requires intensive respiratory therapy during extended hospital stays. SARS was contained by old-fashioned measures: quickly isolating patients who were suspected to have the disease—because of fever, cough, and previous contact with a known SARS patient—and quarantining anyone who had come in contact with them. The epidemic had severe economic impact wherever it broke out, keeping business and vacation travelers from affected areas and even scaring away visitors from Chinatowns in American cities.

There was concern that the disease would be seasonal and would break out again in 2004, but this did not occur. A few small outbreaks in 2004 stemmed from inadequate safety measures in research laboratories, but alert health workers kept the disease from spreading. Since 2004 there have not been any known cases of SARS anywhere in the world.[6]

Rabies

Rabies, a fatal disease of the nervous system caused by a virus, kills an estimated 55,000 people around the world each year, usually contracted through a dog bite. In the United States, transmission of the disease to humans is very effectively prevented by routine public health measures, including epidemiologic surveillance. Although there is an effective vaccine against rabies, routine immunization of everyone is not recommended. Human exposure to the rabies virus in this country is relatively rare, and the vaccine is expensive and inconvenient to deliver, requiring several injections over a period of approximately a month.

The rabies virus infects only mammals, and it is almost always transmitted when a rabid animal bites another animal or a human. Since the animal most likely to bite a human is the dog, mandatory immunization of dogs against rabies is the first line of defense in the protection of people. Wild animals serve as the reservoir of rabies, and dogs are most likely to be exposed by being bitten by a rabid wild animal. Domestic cats are also at risk for exposure to rabies from wildlife, and immunization is recommended for them as well.

The public health system has defined clear guidelines for responding to a report of a person's being bitten by a domestic or wild animal, depending on the likelihood that the animal is rabid. Because immunization of dogs is widespread in the United States, less than 100 cases of rabies occur annually in the 60 million dogs in this country, and a dog bite is considered unlikely to transmit the disease. If the biting dog (or cat) appears to be healthy, it need only be observed for 10 days to ensure that it remains healthy. Rabies virus affects the brain and from there travels to the salivary glands and is secreted in saliva. An animal capable of transmitting the virus in its saliva will already have brain involvement, exhibit symptoms, and be dead within a few days. That is sufficient time for the bitten person to be given the series of vaccinations that will protect him or her from the disease.

If the biting animal is wild, or if there is other reason to suspect that it is rabid, it must be killed and its brain tested for signs of rabies virus infection. There is no way to determine definitively whether a living animal has rabies. If the test shows the animal to be rabid, the bite victim receives the vaccinations. If no sign of rabies is found, no vaccinations are given. There is no room for error in these tests, because once symptoms of rabies appear, it is too late to save the victim. Public health laboratories take this responsibility very seriously. Generally, immunizations are given to anyone who is bitten by a wild animal that cannot be captured and tested.

To control rabies, public health practitioners conduct surveillance for rabies in wildlife. When raccoons, skunks, and foxes in a geographic area are infected with the virus, they are likely to be a threat to humans and domestic animals. In Europe and in some parts of the United States, public health officials are attempting to control rabies in wildlife by distributing bait containing an oral rabies vaccine.

Bats are the most dangerous rabies threat to humans. Even in parts of the country where the disease is not endemic among most wildlife, rabid bats are likely to be found. Because the animals are nocturnal and elusive, contact with bats may go unnoticed. During the period between 2000 and 2011, 24 of the 36 cases of human rabies in the United States were caused by a strain of the virus that is associated with bats. Many of these victims were not aware of having been bitten by a bat and did not realize that any exposure to bats might constitute a rabies risk. Of the 12 cases not attributable to bats, all except three were caused by dog bites outside of the United States; one was from a raccoon in an Eastern state, one from a fox bite in Mexico, and one suspected to be caused by a feral cat in California.[7] Remarkably, three people have survived rabies infection; all were young healthy people who received intensive medical treatment.[8]

The rabies surveillance system has been remarkably successful. The cost of rabies control is significant, however. Testing the brain of an animal for rabies costs about $100, and the price of a series of vaccinations for a person suspected of being exposed may amount to $1500. In 1994, after a kitten in a New Hampshire pet store tested positive for rabies, 665 people received post-exposure treatment at a cost of over $1 million for the vaccines alone.[9] In 2008, a rabid puppy was among a group of 24 dogs and 2 cats that were brought to the United States in a rescue mission aimed at reuniting American soldiers with pets they had adopted in Iraq. By the time the puppy was diagnosed, the animals had been dispersed to 16 states around the country. Concerned that the puppy might have bitten other animals in the group, federal and state public health workers tracked them all down, vaccinated them and placed them in quarantine for 6 months.[10] This incident spotlights the risks in the importation of animals to the United States. According to its report on the incident, the Centers for Disease Control and Prevention (CDC) is working to update current regulations.

Smallpox, Measles, and Polio

While constant vigilance is required to protect people from rabies because wild animals serve as a reservoir of the disease, some pathogenic viruses, including measles and polio, have no nonhuman reservoir. It is a possibility, therefore, that universal immunization against these diseases could eliminate the measles and polio viruses from the earth. This has been achieved with smallpox, one of public health's greatest victories.

Smallpox was a particularly feared disease that is believed to have first emerged in Asia about the time of Christ and tended to spread in major epidemics that claimed millions of lives in China, Japan, the Roman Empire, Europe, and the Americas.[2] It was highly contagious, spread by aerosol or by touch. The concept of vaccination originated with smallpox: the observation that survivors of the disease were immune to future infection inspired the idea that people could be protected against serious illness by inoculating them with small amounts of infected matter from a person suffering a mild case. While the procedure was not entirely safe, the practice became widespread in the American colonies, and George Washington ordered his entire army to be inoculated. In 1796, the practice of immunization became less risky when the British physician Edward Jenner—inspired by the observation that milkmaids appeared to be immune to smallpox—proved that inoculation with cowpox matter, which was harmless to humans, provided immunity against smallpox.[11]

By 1958, routine immunization had eliminated smallpox in the United States and other industrialized countries. However, it was still widespread in 33 underdeveloped countries, killing two million people per year. With support from both the United States and the Soviet Union, WHO developed plans for a program to eliminate smallpox. Between 1967 and 1977, medical teams traveled all over the world in search of outbreaks of the disease. Local governments were mobilized to vaccinate residents of areas where an outbreak was occurring. Because the lesions of smallpox were so conspicuous, it was possible for the investigators to track outbreaks by showing pictures of victims and asking people if they knew of anyone with this disease. Once a patient was located, he or she could be quarantined and everyone in the vicinity vaccinated, sometimes by force. The last case was found in Somalia in October 1977.[2]

Now the smallpox virus officially remains in only two places, stored in laboratories at the CDC and in a Russian laboratory in Siberia. By international agreement, genetic studies were being conducted, after which both stocks of the virus were scheduled to be destroyed in 1999.[12] The decision to destroy the virus was controversial, with some scientists believing that valuable information might be gained in future studies using techniques that are not yet known. In 1999, WHO decided to defer the destruction for a few more years.[13]

Meanwhile, word was leaking out of the former Soviet Union that the Soviets had been working on smallpox as a bioweapon. There were fears that they had shared their stocks of the virus with rogue states such as Iraq and North Korea. The anthrax attacks of 2001 further raised fears about bioterrorism. Plans for destruction of the smallpox virus have been put on hold, and research priorities have focused on developing an improved vaccine and finding drugs that would be effective against the virus.

Poliovirus, like smallpox virus, infects human beings only, and polio similarly has the potential to be eradicated. In 1988, at a time when 350,000 children were being paralyzed each year, WHO set a goal of eradicating polio by the year 2000.[14] This goal was not met, but substantial progress has been made against this crippling disease: polio has been essentially eliminated from the Western Hemisphere, Europe, and the Western Pacific, and by 1999, annual polio cases were reduced by 99 percent worldwide. Many countries hold National Immunization Days each year, distributing doses of oral polio vaccine to millions of children.

Only Southern Asia and Sub-Saharan Africa still have a significant incidence of polio. An important reason that eradication did not succeed in these countries is that rumors spread in 2003 among Muslims, especially in Nigeria, that the polio vaccine had been deliberately contaminated to cause AIDS or infertility.[14] Several Nigerian states halted vaccinations, the number of cases in Nigeria jumped to 800 in 2004, and the virus spread to several other African countries that had previously been polio free. Under pressure from WHO, Nigeria resumed polio immunizations the following year. Now, only three countries continue to have endemic polio—Nigeria, Pakistan, and Afghanistan but eradication from these countries has proven extremely difficult. As long as the disease exists in these countries, it tends to spread to neighboring countries; several African countries have reestablished transmission.[15]

There are several reasons why polio is proving more difficult to eradicate than smallpox.[16] Unlike smallpox, there are many "invisible" cases of polio, in which children may be infected, able to spread the virus by the fecal-oral route but not show symptoms. Thus it is not possible to focus on small outbreaks as was done with smallpox. The vaccine is imperfect and must be administered several times to become effective. India has made major effort to vaccinate children with repeated rounds of National Immunization Days each year, but in poverty-stricken areas of the country children suffering from other intestinal infections tend not to develop immunity even after multiple doses of the vaccine. Political upheaval in parts of Pakistan and Afghanistan has interfered with immunization campaigns in those countries. Some experts have argued that the goal of eradicating polio is unrealistic and that efforts should be focused on "control" rather than eradication.[16] They say that other vaccine-preventable diseases are being neglected because of the intensive effort on polio, that the campaign has been going on too long and has become too expensive. However, India was removed from the list of endemic countries in 2012, giving hope that success can be achieved elsewhere, and the effort continues.[15]

Measles, another viral disease that could in theory be eradicated, offers an example of what happens when public health relaxes its vigilance. Before a vaccine was available, almost all children contracted measles, causing 400 to 500 deaths a year in the United States and 1000 cases of chronic disability from measles encephalitis.[17] Worldwide, an estimated 750,000 children died of measles as recently as 2000.[18] A vaccine became available in 1963, and the number of cases in the United States dropped precipitously. In 1978, the U.S. Department of Health and Human Services set a goal to eradicate measles from this country by 1982. That ambition proved overly optimistic. Two problems interfered.[19]

First, outbreaks of measles began to occur among high school and college students who had been vaccinated as babies. It became clear that the immunity conferred by vaccination in infancy wears off and that a booster vaccination is necessary in older children, a practice that is now recommended at the age of 4 to 6. The booster should be given to adolescents if they did not receive it earlier.

The greater problem was that too many children were not being immunized until it was required for entry into school. This was particularly true in large cities among poor African-American and Hispanic children. Immunization rates in the United States were worse than those of some third-world countries. More than 27,000 American children contracted measles in 1990, and 89 died.[20] Even the surveillance system was doing poorly: a study in New York City during 1991 found that up to 50 percent of cases were not reported.[21] The public health system was shaken by this evidence of failure, and a better job is now being done on measles immunization. In fact, measles was declared eliminated from the United States in 2000, meaning that all cases can be traced to individuals who contracted the disease outside the country and brought it here. However, in 2011, 222 measles cases were reported to the CDC, compared to a median of 60 per year during 2001 to 2010.[22] Of the 2011 cases, 196 were American residents, the majority of them children, and 86 percent of them were unvaccinated or had unknown vaccination status. Of the 66 children who were unvaccinated but should have been, 50 were unvaccinated because of philosophical or religious beliefs, discussed later in this chapter.

Public health leaders had hoped that when and if polio is eradicated, the organizational and medical resources that had been mobilized in that campaign could then be used in a vaccination campaign against measles. Given the uncertainties with polio eradication and the difficulties with achieving universal immunization in the United States, the prospect for measles eradication worldwide is doubtful. Measles is still endemic in some European countries as well as at higher levels in Africa and Southeast Asia. However, some progress has been made. The number of estimated deaths from measles has been reduced from 750,000 in 2000 to 164,000 in 2008.[23] The WHO has set a goal of 90 percent reduction in measles mortality by 2010.[18]

An attempt to eradicate an eradicable disease can backfire if it is not conducted with sufficient political will, knowledge, and resources. This was the case with malaria, which was the target of an international eradication campaign in the 1950s and 1960s. There is no nonhuman reservoir for the malaria-causing parasites, but the route of transmission is a vector, certain species of mosquito. The primary weapon in the eradication effort was the pesticide DDT. While the campaign produced dramatic results, funding ran out before the objective was achieved, and there was a resurgence of the disease with greater impact than ever. A combination of factors contributed to the calamity: DDT-resistant mosquitoes emerged; the pathogen developed resistance to the main antimalarial drug, chloroquine; and populations in former malarial areas lost their immunity to the disease because of lack of exposure.[24] Now, malaria is one of the most widespread potentially fatal infectious diseases in the world, killing an estimated one million people annually, mainly children.[25] The disease occurs mainly in tropical and subtropical areas and has been largely eliminated in the United States, but global climate change and international travel could contribute to the re-emergence of malaria as a public health problem in the South.

Fear of Vaccines

The benefits of vaccination are obvious to public health and medical professionals. However, just as Muslim leaders in Nigeria resisted polio vaccination with the rumor of infertility, so suspicion has spread in the United States that measles immunization causes autism. Autism often becomes apparent at about the age when the vaccine is given. Consequently, some parents refused to allow their children to be vaccinated against measles. Similarly, unfounded stories about side effects of the pertussis (whooping cough) vaccine—that it might cause sudden infant death syndrome (SIDS)—led many parents to resist the vaccine.[26]

Because parental concerns became so widespread, the Institute of Medicine has conducted periodic reviews of the latest evidence on vaccine safety. In 2003, it published a review on SIDS and concluded that "the evidence favors rejection of a relationship between some vaccines and SIDS."[27] In 2004, the Institute of Medicine reviewed evidence on a possible link between the measles-mumps-rubella vaccine (MMR) and autism and again concluded that "the body of epidemiological evidence favors rejection of a causal relationship between the MMR vaccine and autism."[28] In both cases, the review committees acknowledged that the concern about the vaccines was understandable because the diseases are poorly understood, and they recommended more research on the causes of SIDS and autism.

The evidence cited in the autism report included a major study done in Denmark, in which records of a half million children were analyzed. About one in five children had not received the vaccine, and the researchers found that these children developed autism at the same rate as children who had received the vaccine.[29] Some vaccines do have real risks, including fever and seizures that occur in a small number of infants after they are vaccinated for pertussis and rare cases of polio caused by the oral polio vaccine, which contains the live, weakened virus. These risks are much smaller than the risks of the diseases in an unvaccinated population. However, many American parents are too young to remember the fears aroused by polio in the past, and they may be unaware that formerly common childhood diseases such as measles and chicken pox sometimes have serious complications. Whooping cough can be fatal in infants exposed to unvaccinated older siblings who contract the disease. Because of the success of vaccinations, people have never seen these diseases and thus no longer fear them.

The measles outbreaks in 2011, discussed above, illustrate the dangers of leaving children unvaccinated. That year, 222 cases of measles were reported in the United States, more than three times the average number reported in previous years. Most of the cases were linked to people who traveled abroad or visited from another country and spread the virus to unvaccinated children in this country. Seventy of the patients required hospitalization.[22]

It is often in wealthy communities that parents refuse to subject their children to the small risk of immunization. They count on the fact that most other children are vaccinated to protect their own children from being exposed. However, much of the protection afforded by a high rate of immunization in a population comes from "herd immunity," the phenomenon by which even infants too young to be vaccinated, old people with weakened immune systems, and those who refuse to be immunized are unlikely to be exposed to a disease because the majority of the population is immune. If the percentage of immunity in the population falls too low, however, outbreaks are likely. Then even vaccinated people are at risk, because no vaccine is perfect.

Another drawback of people's fear of vaccines is that pharmaceutical companies have become reluctant to invest in developing them. Parents' tendency to blame a recent immunization for any serious health problem suffered by their children leads them to sue the company that made the vaccine. This experience, together with the fact that prices that can be charged for vaccines tend to be low, has caused many companies to drop vaccine production altogether. While immunization is considered the most effective intervention for preventing disease and promoting health, it is not clear that even the current vaccines will continue to be available.[29] The example of the former Soviet Union stands as a warning to us. Diphtheria is virtually unknown in the West now, but in the 1980s, when the public health system in Russia was in chaos and immunizations stopped, the disease surged, with 200,000 cases and 5000 deaths there.[30]

Public health in the United States can celebrate success in the fight against many common diseases. In 2007, the CDC reported that death rates for 13 infectious diseases were at all-time lows; for nine of them, including whooping cough, polio, and diphtheria, deaths and hospitalizations declined by more than 90 percent since vaccines against them were approved.[31] However, it has become clear that infectious diseases are far from being conquered. The development of resistance to the chemical arsenal for combating disease is discussed elsewhere together with other new and emerging problems in infectious diseases.

Conclusion

Public health has had great success in controlling infectious diseases. Classic public health measures prevent transmission of disease-causing bacteria, viruses, and parasites by interrupting the chain of infection. Measures employed at various links in the chain include killing the pathogen, eliminating the reservoir that harbors the pathogen, preventing transmission from one host to another or from reservoir to host, and increasing the resistance of hosts by immunization.

Rabies is an example of a disease that has been successfully controlled in the United States by public health measures. Immunization of dogs is the primary barrier protecting humans from the reservoir of the virus, which is wild animals. By maintaining surveillance and intervening with vaccination when a person has been exposed to a possibly rabid animal, public health has kept the number of human deaths from rabies very low. SARS, a new, highly communicable disease first recognized in Asia in 2003, was successfully controlled by the classic public health measures of surveillance, isolation, and quarantine.

Smallpox, measles, and polio are viral diseases against which effective vaccines have been developed and which have no nonhuman reservoir. In theory, therefore, they could be eliminated from the earth. This has been accomplished with smallpox, with only two known stocks of the virus remaining. Polio has been eliminated from the United States and many other parts of the world, and a campaign is underway to eradicate it, although progress has been erratic and some experts doubt that the goal is realistic. The prospects for measles eradication are even less clear. The United States has had epidemics of measles as recently as the early 1990s, and cases of measles still occur when infected people enter this country from endemic areas. Reluctance by some parents to vaccinate their children weakens herd immunity and threatens to cause outbreaks of infectious diseases that could have been controlled.

Success in controlling infectious diseases requires adequate resources and political will to maintain effective immunization programs and ongoing epidemiologic surveillance.

References

1. U.S. Institute of Medicine, Committee for the Study of the Future of Public Health, *The Future of Public Health* (Washington, DC: National Academy Press, 1988), 19.
2. L. Garrett, *The Coming Plague: Newly Emerging Diseases in a World out of Balance* (New York: Farrar, Straus & Giroux, 1994), 403.
3. G. Pickett and J. J. Hanlon, *Public Health: Administration and Practice* (St. Louis, MO: Times Mirror/Mosby, 1990).
4. J. M. Hughes, "The SARS Response—Building and Assessing an Evidence-Based Approach to Future Global Microbial Threats," *Journal of the American Medical Association* 290 (2003): 3251–3253.
5. K. Bradsher, "SARS Declared Contained, with No Cases in Past 20 Days," *The New York Times*, July 6, 2003.
6. U.S. Centers for Disease Control and Prevention, "Severe Acute Respiratory Syndrome (SARS). http://www.cdc.gov/SARS/index.html, accessed June 2, 2012.
7. U.S. Centers for Disease Control and Prevention, "Human Rabies." http://www.cdc.gov/rabies/location/usa/surveillance/human_rabies.html, accessed June 2, 2012.
8. U.S. Centers for Disease Control and Prevention, "Recovery of a Patient from Clinical Rabies—California, 2011," *Morbidity and Mortality Weekly Report* 61 (2012): 61–65.
9. D. L. Noah et al., "Mass Human Exposure to Rabies in New Hampshire: Exposures, Treatment, and Cost," *American Journal of Public Health* 86 (1996): 1149–1151.
10. U.S. Centers for Disease Control and Prevention, "Rabies in a Dog Imported from Iraq—New Jersey, June 2008," *Morbidity and Mortality Weekly Report* 57 (2008): 1076–1078.

11. G. Rosen, *A History of Public Health* (Baltimore, MD: Johns Hopkins University Press, 1993).

12. E. Marshall, "Bioterror Defense Initiative Injects Shot of Cash," *Science* 283 (1999): 1234–1235.

13. L. Altman, "Killer Smallpox Gets a New Lease on Life," *The New York Times*, May 25, 1999.

14. L. Roberts, "Polio Eradication: Is It Time to Give Up?" *Science* 312 (2006): 832–835.

15. Global Polio Eradication Initiative, "Polio Eradication Shifts into Emergency Mode." http://www.polioeradication.org/Mediaroom/Newsstories.aspx, accessed October 30, 2012.

16. I. Arita et al., "Is Polio Eradication Realistic?" *Science* 312 (2006): 852–854.

17. U.S. Centers for Disease Control and Prevention, "Measles—United States, January 1–April 25, 2008," *Morbidity and Mortality Weekly Report* 57 (2008): 494–498.

18. U.S. Centers for Disease Control and Prevention, "Progress in Global Measles Control and Mortality Reduction, 2000–2007," *Morbidity and Mortality Weekly Report* 57 (2008): 1303–1308.

19. U.S. Centers for Disease Control and Prevention, "Measles Prevention: Recommendations of the Immunization Practices Advisory Committee," *Morbidity and Mortality Weekly Report* 38, No. S-9 (1989): 1–11.

20. U.S. Centers for Disease Control and Prevention, "Measles—United States, 1990," *Morbidity and Mortality Weekly Report* 40 (1991): 369–372.

21. S. F. Davis et al., "Reporting Efficiency During a Measles Outbreak in New York City, 1991," *American Journal of Public Health* 83 (1993): 1011–1015.

22. U.S. Centers for Disease Control and Prevention, "Measles—United States, 2011," *Morbidity and Mortality Weekly Report* 61 (2012): 253–257.

23. U.S. Centers for Disease Control and Prevention, "Global Vaccines and Immunization." http://www.cdc.gov/globalhealth/immunization, accessed October 30, 2012.

24. U.S. Centers for Disease Control and Prevention, "The History of Malaria, an Ancient Disease." http://www.cdc.gov/malaria/about/history/index.html, accessed June 2, 2012.

25. U.S. Centers for Disease Control and Prevention, "Impact of Malaria." http://www.cdc.gov/malaria/malaria_worldwide/impact/.html, accessed June 2, 2012.

26. E. W. Campion, "Suspicions About the Safety of Vaccines," *New England Journal of Medicine* 347 (2002): 1474–1475.

27. U.S. Institute of Medicine, Immunization Safety Review Committee, *Vaccinations and Sudden Unexpected Death in Infancy* (Washington, DC: National Academies Press, 2003).

28. U.S. Institute of Medicine, Immunization Safety Review Committee, *Vaccines and Autism* (Washington, DC: National Academies Press, 2004).

29. K. M. Madsen et al., "A Population-Based Study of Measles, Mumps, and Rubella Vaccination and Autism," *New England Journal of Medicine* 347 (2002): 1477–1482.

30. R. Rappuoli et al., "The Intangible Value of Vaccination," *Science* 297 (2002): 937–939.

31. D. G. McNeil, Jr., "Sharp Drop Seen in Deaths from Ills Fought by Vaccine," *The New York Times*, November 14, 2007.

The Resurgence of Infectious Diseases

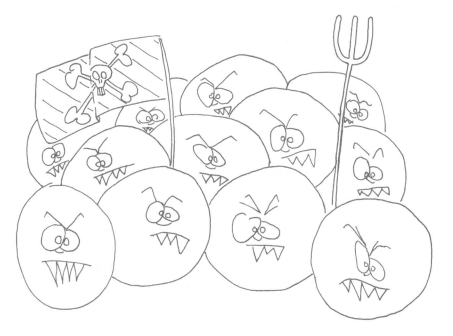

Bacterial Resistance

The appearance of AIDS in the early 1980s challenged the widely held belief that infectious diseases were under control. However, there had been intimations during the previous 2 or 3 decades that the microbes were not as controllable as generally believed. The influenza virus was proving stubbornly unpredictable, deadly new variants of known bacteria were beginning to crop up, and the familiar old bacteria were becoming strangely resistant to antibiotics. That trend has continued, and the importance of public health in combating these growing problems has become increasingly apparent.

The Biomedical Basis of AIDS

By the turn of the 21st century, the exotic disease that seemed to strike only gay men has turned into a world-wide scourge: the human immunodeficiency virus (HIV) now infects over 33 million individuals and kills almost 2 million a year.[1] In the United States as of 2009, some 619,400 people had died of AIDS.[2] Since the outbreak was first recognized, a great deal has been learned about HIV, how it causes AIDS, and how it is spread.

HIV is a retrovirus, a virus that uses RNA as its genetic material instead of the more usual DNA. Retroviruses have long been known to cause cancer in animals, and they were extensively studied for clues to the causes of human cancer, research that proved helpful for understanding the immunodeficiency virus when it was identified. Two human retroviruses—causing two types of leukemia—were known before HIV was discovered. Retroviruses infect cells by copying their RNA into the DNA of the cell, penetrating the genetic material like a "mole" in a spy agency. This DNA may sit silently in the cell, being copied normally along with the cell's genetic material for an indefinite number of generations. Or it may take over control of the cell's machinery, causing the uncontrolled reproduction typical of cancer.

The target of HIV is a specific type of white blood cell called the CD4-T lymphocyte, or T4 cell. T4 cells are just one of many components of the complicated immune machinery that is activated when the body recognizes a foreign invader such as a bacterium or a virus. The T4 cell's role is to divide and reproduce itself in response to such an invasion and to attack the invader. In a T4 cell that is infected with HIV, activation of the cell activates the virus also, which then produces thousands of copies of itself in a process that kills the T4 cell. The T4 cells are a key component of the immune system because, in addition to attacking foreign microbes, they also regulate other components of the immune system, including the cells that produce antibodies, the proteins in the blood that recognize foreign substances. Thus destruction of the T4 cells disrupts the entire immune system.[3]

The course of infection with HIV takes place over a number of years. After being exposed to HIV, a person may or may not notice mild, flu-like symptoms for a few weeks, during which time the virus is present in the blood and body fluids and may be easily transmitted to others by sex or other risky behaviors. The body's immune system responds as it would to any viral infection, producing specific antibodies that eliminate most of the circulating viruses. The infection then enters a latent period, with the viruses mostly hidden in the DNA of the T4 cells, although a constant battle is taking place between the virus and the immune system. Billions of viruses are made, and millions of T4 cells are destroyed daily.[4] During this time, the person is quite healthy and is less likely to transmit the virus than during the early stage of infection (although transmission is still possible). Eventually however, after several years, the immune system begins to lose the struggle, and so many of the T4 cells begin to die that they cannot be replaced rapidly enough. When the number of T4 cells drops below 200 per cubic millimeter of blood, about 20 percent of the normal level, symptoms are likely to begin appearing, and the person is vulnerable to opportunistic infections and certain tumors. At the same time, the number of circulating viruses increases, and the person again becomes more capable of transmitting the infection to others.[5] At this stage, the person meets the criteria for AIDS, which is defined by the T4 cell count and/or the presence of opportunistic infections.

The development and licensing of a screening test in 1985 was a major step forward in the fight against HIV. The test measures antibodies to the virus, which begin to appear 3 to 6 weeks after the original infection. This test is relatively fast and inexpensive; it is a sensitive screening test, giving the first indication that the individual may be HIV positive. The test is used for three purposes: diagnosing individuals at risk to determine whether they are infected so that they may be appropriately counseled and, if necessary, treated; monitoring the spread of HIV in various populations via epidemiologic studies; and screening donated blood or organs to ensure that they do not transmit HIV to a recipient of a transfusion or transplant. A major drawback of the antibody screening test is the absence of antibodies in the blood during the initial 3- to 6-week period after infection. This "window" of nondetectability may give newly infected people a false sense of security. More accurate tests that look for the virus itself in the blood are now available. These tests are used to confirm infection in people who have tested positive in the screening test. In the United States, they are also done on all donated blood to ensure that no virus-infected blood is used for transfusions.

Tests that directly measure a virus in the blood have contributed a great deal to understanding the biomedical basis of HIV infection. Measurement of "viral load"—the concentration of viruses in the blood—is a valuable tool for evaluating the effectiveness of therapeutic drugs. Viral load has also been found to influence the individual's chances of transmitting the virus by sexual and other means. Thus a therapy that is effective in reducing viral load can help to control the spread of HIV.

The major pathways of HIV transmission vary in different populations. Homosexual relations between men are still the leading route of exposure for men in the United States. Injection drug use accounts for 9 percent of new HIV infections in Americans.[2] Transmission by heterosexual relations, especially male to female, is becoming increasingly common in this country; it is the leading route of infection for females. In the developing countries of Asia and Africa, where HIV infection is spreading rapidly, heterosexual relations are the most common means of transmission. Several studies have found that circumcision protects men against contracting HIV from infected women; there is also evidence that circumcision reduces male-to-female transmission, but the effect is smaller.[6]

The sharing of needles is a common route of transmission in developing countries because of insufficient supplies of sterile equipment for medical use. In poor countries, including Russia and some nations in Eastern Europe, medical personnel often use one syringe repeatedly for giving immunizations or injections of therapeutic drugs. If one of the patients is HIV positive, this practice may transmit the infection to everyone who later receives an injection with the same needle. According to the World Health Organization (WHO), 40 percent of injections worldwide are given with unsterile needles.[7] Transfusion with HIV-contaminated blood is no longer a significant source of HIV infection in the United States, but it still occurs in countries too poor to screen donated blood.

A special case of HIV transmission occurs from mother to infant, *in utero* or during delivery, in 25 to 33 percent of births unless antiretroviral drugs are given. The virus can also be transmitted to breast-fed babies in their mother's milk. All infants of HIV-positive women will test positive during the first few months after birth. This is because fetuses in the womb receive a selection of their mothers' antibodies, providing natural protection against disease (though not HIV) during their first months of life. Testing a baby's blood for HIV antibodies provides evidence of the mother's HIV status. Many states in the United States routinely perform HIV screening tests on newborns' blood as part of their newborn screening programs. The special issues raised by maternal–fetal transmission of the virus have been the subject of ethical, legal, and political controversy at the national and state levels. Drug therapies are now capable of preventing transmission of the virus from mother to infant in 99 percent of cases.[8] Similar drug treatment of mothers and/or infants can prevent transmission in breast milk.

HIV/AIDS has become a disease of minorities. Although African Americans make up only 14 percent of the U.S. population, almost half of new cases being diagnosed in recent years are among blacks. According to the Centers for Disease Control and Prevention (CDC), in 2009, the rate of infection was almost seven times higher in black men than in white men and 15 times higher in black women than white women.[9] Hispanics are diagnosed at three times the rate of whites.[10] Among the factors that contribute to the higher rates among minorities are the fact that people tend to have sex with partners of the same race and ethnicity; minorities tend to experience higher rates of other sexually transmitted diseases, which increase the risk of transmission of HIV; socioeconomic issues associated with poverty; lack of awareness of HIV status; and negative perceptions about HIV testing.[9]

Progress in treating HIV/AIDS over the past 2 decades has been dramatic. Early therapy focused on treating opportunistic infections, which were often the immediate cause of death in AIDS patients. The first antiretroviral therapy, zidovudine (AZT), was approved by the Food and Drug Administration (FDA) in 1987.[11] The drug interfered with the replication of HIV by inhibiting the enzyme that copies the viral RNA into the cell's DNA. However, the virus's tendency to mutate rapidly leads to the development of resistance to the drug, meaning that its effectiveness can wear off.

As scientists gained a better understanding of the virus, they developed drugs that target different stages of viral replication. Protease inhibitors, which interfere with the ability of newly formed viruses to mature and become infectious, were introduced in 1995.[11] At the same time, scientists recognized that treating patients with a combination of drugs that attack the virus in different ways reduces the opportunity for HIV to mutate and develop resistance. The introduction of these drug combinations, called highly active antiretroviral therapy (HAART), led to dramatic improvements in the survival of HIV-infected patients. As a result, the number of AIDS deaths fell by more than half between 1996 and 1998 and has continued to decline since then.[12]

The development of effective treatments for HIV/AIDS has had many beneficial consequences. HAART can reduce viral load to undetectable levels in the blood and body fluids of many patients, which greatly reduces the likelihood that the virus will be transmitted to others through sexual contact and other means. The availability of effective therapy also encourages at-risk people to be tested and counseled on ways to protect themselves and to prevent transmission of the virus to others. Scientists hoped that HAART would be able to completely eradicate HIV from the body, but this hope has not been realized. The virus manages to survive in protected reservoirs of the body, rebounding into active replication when the drugs are withdrawn.[10] For some patients, side effects of the drugs can be severe and even fatal; about 40 percent of patients treated with protease inhibitors develop lipodystrophy, characterized by abnormal distributions of fat in the body, sometimes accompanied by other metabolic abnormalities.[13] Moreover, the virus can develop resistance to these drugs if used improperly. A survey of blood samples taken between 1999 and 2003 found that 15 percent were resistant to at least one drug.[14]

New drugs continue to be developed, including a new class called "fusion inhibitors," introduced in 2003, which interfere with HIV's ability to enter a host cell, and a class called integrase inhibitors, introduced in 2002, which prevents the virus from integrating into the genetic material of human cells.[15] Thus for many patients, HIV infection has become a chronic disease, necessitating life-long therapy but enabling them to live a relatively normal life. The drugs are expensive however, costing an average of $13,000 per year per patient.[16] Even in the United States, only half of those in need of therapy are on continuous treatment.

The greatest hope for controlling AIDS, especially in the developing world where the new drugs are unaffordable, is to develop an effective vaccine. Prevention through immunization has been the most effective approach for the viral scourges of the past, including smallpox, measles, and polio. Early hopes for the rapid availability of a vaccine against AIDS have faded, however. In fact, after several promising vaccine candidates failed in clinical trials, the NIH held a meeting of vaccine researchers in March, 2008, to reassess whether a vaccine will ever be possible and what new approaches could be tried.[17] It should perhaps not be surprising that a virus so well adapted to disabling the immune system should be so effective at eluding attempts to employ that same immune system against it. Part of the difficulty in developing an effective vaccine is that the virus itself is constantly changing its appearance, making it unrecognizable to the immune mechanisms that are mobilized against it by a vaccine. This quality is common to RNA viruses. Another difficulty is that there is no good animal model for studying HIV/AIDS.[18]

At present, the most effective way to fight AIDS is to prevent transmission (step 3 in the chain of transmission). This requires education and efforts at motivating people to change their high-risk behavior, an exceedingly difficult task.

HIV seems to have appeared from nowhere and to have spread over the entire world within a decade. Where did the virus come from? Genetic studies of HIV show that it is related to viruses that commonly infect African monkeys and apes, and it seems likely that a mutation allowed one of these viruses to infect humans. There is evidence that this type of event—cross-species transmission of viruses—may occur fairly frequently. Monkeys and chimpanzees are killed for food in parts of Africa, which could explain how humans were exposed.[11] HIV is remarkable, however, for the speed with which it has spread into the human population worldwide.

Scientists conjecture that the human form of the virus may have existed in isolated pockets of Africa for some time, but that its rapid spread was the result of social conditions in Africa and the United States in the late 1970s. Because symptomatic AIDS does not appear until several years after the original infection, the first victims of the 1980s were probably infected in the early and mid-1970s. Investigators trying to track the early spread of the epidemic have gone back to test stored blood samples drawn in earlier times, and they have found HIV-infected samples from as early as 1966, in the blood of a widely traveled Norwegian sailor who died of immune deficiency. The sailor's wife and one of his three children later died of the same illness, and their stored blood, when tested, was also found to be infected with HIV.[19] An even older blood sample drawn from a West African man in 1959 has been found to contain fragments of the virus, but it is not known whether the man developed AIDS.[20] This evidence implies that sporadic early outbreaks of the disease occurred in isolated African villages, going undetected for decades.

The reasons for the recent emergence of HIV disease as a significant problem include the disruption of traditional lifestyles by the movement of rural Africans to urban areas, trends magnified by population growth, waves of civil war, and revolution. The apparent worldwide explosion of AIDS then occurred because of changing patterns of sexual behavior and the use of addictive drugs in developed and developing countries, together with the ease of international air travel.

Other Emerging Viruses

In 1976, before the AIDS epidemic was recognized but while, as scientists now believe, the virus was spreading silently into African cities, another viral illness broke out with much more dramatic effect in Zaire and Sudan. Symptoms caused by the previously unidentified Ebola virus include fever and severe bleeding from various bodily orifices. Several hundred people became ill from the disease, and up to 90 percent of its victims died. The disease spread rapidly from person to person, affecting especially family members and hospital workers who had cared for patients. Investigators from the CDC and WHO identified the virus and helped devise measures, including quarantine, to limit the spread of the disease, which eventually disappeared. The Ebola virus broke out again in Zaire in the summer of 1995, killing 244 people before it again seemed to vanish.[21] Since then, there have been repeated outbreaks in West and Central Africa.[22] According to CDC data, almost 800 Africans have died of Ebola since 1995.[23]

The Ebola virus infects monkeys as well as humans, and on a number of occasions infected monkeys have been imported into the United States. In 1989, a large number of monkeys imported from the Philippines died of the viral infection at a primate quarantine facility in Reston, Virginia. In that episode, which served as the basis for Richard Preston's book, *The Hot Zone*, several laboratory workers were exposed to the virus, which fortunately turned out to be a strain that did not cause illness in humans.[24] Scientists have been searching for an animal species that serves as a reservoir for the virus between outbreaks in the human population. There are indications that, like HIV, Ebola may spread to humans when they handle the carcasses of apes used for food. Unlike HIV, the Ebola virus kills the apes it infects, leading to significant declines in populations of gorillas and chimpanzees; outbreaks in humans have been preceded by the discovery of dead animals near villages where the outbreaks occur.[22] There is now concern that Ebola may be pushing West African gorillas to extinction. Attempts to develop a vaccine for humans have had success in protecting monkeys in laboratory studies; whether such a vaccine could be delivered safely to wild gorillas is uncertain.[25]

Other new or resurgent viruses have appeared in various parts of the world, including the United States, in the recent past. In May and June 2003, for example, public health authorities in Illinois and Wisconsin received reports of a disease similar to smallpox among people who had had direct contact with prairie dogs. Prompt investigation by state officials and the CDC identified the cause as monkeypox virus, which was known from outbreaks in Africa. Although known to infect monkeys, the primary hosts for monkeypox are rodents.[26]

The outbreak in the United States spread to 72 people in 6 Midwestern states. Fortunately, monkeypox is not highly contagious in humans, and it is a less severe disease than smallpox. No one died in the outbreak. However, the incident raised alarms about exotic pets. The illness in the prairie dogs was traced back through pet stores and animal distributors to an Illinois distributor, who in April had imported several African rodents, including a Gambian giant rat that had died of an unidentified illness. In June 2003, the U.S. government banned the import of all rodents from Africa. Careful surveillance and isolation of exposed people and animals halted the outbreak by the end of July, and no further cases of monkeypox have been reported since then.[26]

In 1993, the CDC was called in when two healthy young New Mexico residents living in the same household died suddenly within a few days of each other of acute respiratory distress, their lungs filled with fluid. Within 3 weeks, biomedical scientists had recognized that the illness, which had claimed several other victims in the Four Corners area of the Southwest, was caused by hantavirus. Named after the Hantaan River in Korea, the hantavirus had been responsible for kidney disease among thousands of American soldiers in Korea during the 1950s. In New Mexico, the virus was found to be carried by deer mice, which had been unusually plentiful in the Four Corners area because of an unusually wet winter. All of the human victims of hantavirus had had significant exposure to mouse droppings, either in their homes or in their places of work.[27]

The CDC declared hantavirus pulmonary syndrome (HPS) a notifiable disease in 1995, and as of the end of 2011, 587 cases had been reported in 34 states.[28] Over one-third of the victims have died, often in a matter of hours. It is hoped that adding HPS to the list of notifiable diseases will help medical workers to recognize it more readily. In the case of a Rhode Island college student who may have contracted the disease in 1994 from exposure to mouse droppings while making a film at his father's warehouse, the hospital did not recognize that he was seriously ill and sent him home from the emergency room the first time he appeared there; 2 days later he returned much sicker, and he died 5 hours after being hospitalized.[29]

Rodents are suspected as carriers of several hemorrhagic fevers with symptoms similar to those caused by hantavirus or the Ebola virus: Bolivian hemorrhagic fever (caused by the Machupo virus), Argentine hemorrhagic fever (caused by the Junin virus), and Lassa fever in Sierra Leone are all carried by rats. Well-known, insect-borne viruses, such as yellow fever and equine encephalitis, are resurgent in areas of South and Central America where they had been thought to be vanquished. Dengue fever, also spread by mosquitoes, has taken on the new, deadly form of a hemorrhagic fever and is spreading north through Central America, threatening people along the southern border of the United States.[21]

In the summer of 1999, the United States first experienced the effects of West Nile virus, which spread rapidly across the country over the next few years. The first sign of the new disease was a report to the New York City Health Department by an infectious disease specialist in Queens, New York that an unusual number of patients had been hospitalized with encephalitis, an inflammation of the brain. The disease was suspected to be St. Louis encephalitis, a mosquito-borne disease that is endemic in the southern United States, and the diagnosis was supported by the patients' reports that they had been outdoors in the evenings during peak mosquito hours. Soon, however, it became obvious that a great number of dead crows were being found in the New York area, and a veterinarian at the Bronx Zoo reported that there had been unprecedented deaths among the zoo's exotic birds. Lab tests confirmed that the virus causing the human disease was the same as the one that was killing the birds, but St. Louis encephalitis virus was not known to infect birds. West Nile virus was well known in Africa,

West Asia, and the Middle East. It is known to be fatal to crows and several other species of birds. It also infects horses. Fifty-six patients were hospitalized in the New York epidemic, seven of whom died.[30,31]

How the West Nile virus came to New York is not known. The most likely explanation is that it came in an infected bird, perhaps a tropical bird that was smuggled into the country. The virus is easily spread among birds by several species of mosquitoes, some of which also bite humans. Although the threat disappeared with the mosquitoes after the first frost in the fall, the next summer saw a spread of the disease to upstate New York and surrounding states. Carried by migratory birds, the virus has now arrived in all 48 contiguous states.[32] It appears that West Nile virus is here to stay. In 2011 it caused illness in 486 people.[33] While the infection proves fatal to a small percentage of human victims, it often leaves patients with long-term impairments, including fatigue, weakness, depression, personality changes, gait problems, and memory deficits.[34]

Public health professionals fight the virus by educating the public about eliminating standing water where mosquitoes breed, wearing long sleeves, and using repellant. A vaccine is available for horses, and scientists are working on developing a vaccine that will be effective for humans.

A variety of environmental factors are responsible for the recent emergence of so many new pathogens. Human activities that cause ecological changes, such as deforestation and dam building, bring people into closer contact with disease-carrying animals. Modern agricultural practices, such as extreme crowding of livestock, intensify the risk that previously unknown viruses will incubate in crowded herds and be widely dispersed to human consumers. International distribution of meat and poultry may help to spread new pathogens. The popularity of exotic pets in the United States also can lead to the spread of pathogens, like monkeypox and perhaps West Nile virus, from animals or birds to people. A breakdown of public health efforts such as mosquito control programs because of complacency or insufficient funding has resulted in the reappearance of insect-borne diseases. Spread of the viruses in developing countries is facilitated by urbanization, crowding, war, and the breakdown of social restraints on sexual behavior and intravenous drug use. U.S. residents will not be able to escape the effects of these new pathogens. The ease and speed of international travel means that a new infection first appearing anywhere in the world could traverse entire continents within days or weeks. This was dramatically illustrated by the emergence and rapid spread of SARS. The SARS virus is believed to have been transmitted to humans from an animal species used for food in China, possibly the civet cat.

Influenza

Influenza—the "flu"—may seem like an old familiar infectious disease. However, it can be a different disease from 1 year to the next and has the capacity to turn into a major killer. This happened in the winter of 1918–1919, when the flu killed 20 million to 40 million people worldwide, including 196,000 people who died in the United States in October.[35] Even in the average year, influenza kills 250,000 to 500,000 people worldwide.[36] Although normally most deaths from flu occur in people above age 65, the 1918 epidemic preferentially struck young people.

Influenza virus has been studied extensively, and vaccination can be effective, but constant vigilance is necessary to protect people from the disease. Like HIV, influenza is an RNA virus, constantly changing its appearance and adept at eluding recognition by the human immune system. Because of the year-to-year variability of the flu virus, flu vaccines must be changed annually to be effective against the newest strain. Each winter, viral samples are collected from around the world and sent to WHO, where biomedical scientists conduct experiments designed to predict how the virus will mutate into next year's strain. These educated guesses form the basis for next year's vaccine.

At unpredictable intervals, however, a lethal new strain of the flu virus can come along, as it did in 1918. A strain that caused the Asian flu emerged in 1957, and a third, called Hong Kong flu, arrived in 1968. Neither of the latter outbreaks was as deadly as the 1918 epidemic, although a not insignificant 70,000 Americans died from the Asian flu. In 1976, CDC scientists thought they had evidence that another deadly strain—swine flu—was emerging, and the country mobilized for a massive immunization campaign. That time, the scientists had made a mistake; the anticipated epidemic never occurred. Infectious disease experts have for decades been expecting a new epidemic, which did occur in 2009, as discussed later in this section.

New strains of influenza virus, especially those that have undergone major changes, tend to arise in Asia, particularly China, and then spread around the world from there. One of the reasons China is an especially fertile source of new flu strains is that animal reservoirs for influenza—pigs and birds—are common there, living in close proximity to humans. Human and animal influenza viruses incubate in a pig's digestive system, forming new genetic combinations, and are then spread by ducks as they migrate. While such hybrid viruses, containing human and animal genes, are only rarely capable of infecting humans, those that are able to do so are the most likely to be deadly.

Until recently, little was known about what made the 1918 strain of influenza so deadly, or how to predict the lethality of new strains that come along. Recently, however, genetic studies have been possible using samples of the 1918 virus. Tissue taken from soldiers who died in 1918 had been stored at the Armed Forces Institute of Pathology in Washington, D.C. and from victims in an Alaskan village who were buried in permanently frozen ground. Scientists have found that the 1918 virus has features in common with avian flu viruses that make them especially dangerous to humans, and they also resemble the human virus enough that they can spread easily among people.[37] Similar avian features were found in the viruses that caused epidemics in 1957 and 1968.

Thus influenza experts were alarmed in 1997, when a 3-year-old Hong Kong boy died from a strain of influenza virus that normally infected chickens. There had been an epidemic of the disease in the birds a few months earlier. Antibodies to the virus were found in the blood of the boy's doctor, although he did not become ill, and public health authorities watched for more cases with great concern. Two dozen other people became sick by December, and six died. To prevent further transmission from chickens to humans, the Hong Kong government ordered that all 1.5 million chickens in the territory be killed. That action seems to have been effective in halting the epidemic in humans.[38]

Bird flu emerged again in 2003 and has become widespread in Asia, sub-Saharan Africa, and some European countries, despite efforts to eliminate it by killing millions of birds.[39] More than 600 human cases in 15 countries have been reported since 2003 and more than half have died.[40] Thus far it appears that most of the human victims of the bird flu caught the virus from chickens, not from other humans. There is great concern that mixing of the viral genes could occur in a person infected with both the bird virus and a human flu virus, resulting in a much more virulent strain capable of spreading among humans. The new virus could start a global pandemic of a lethal form of the disease, as in 1918. The U.S. government has developed a vaccine against bird flu and has stockpiled some doses in the event that the virus were to begin spreading easily from person to person.[40]

In late 2011, controversy arose over research funded by the National Institutes of Health that created a highly transmissible form of the avian flu virus. The work was done in ferrets, which are a good model of how flu viruses behave in humans. Two groups of researchers, at the University of Wisconsin and a Dutch university, created mutations in the virus that enabled it to spread by aerosol. The National Science Advisory Board for Biosecurity asked that details of the experiments be withheld from publication to prevent terrorists from replicating them.[41] However, a meeting of the WHO in February 2012 concluded that the risk of its use by bioterrorists was outweighed by the danger that changes might occur naturally in the wild that would give the virus the ability to cause a pandemic.[42] Full publication will allow scientists to recognize warning signals that the virus is becoming more dangerous, which also might lead to better treatments.

While avian flu is still a cause for concern, another strain of influenza emerged in spring 2009, which was quickly declared a pandemic by the WHO, making it the first pandemic since 1968. The virus, which originated in pigs and is known as swine flu or, more accurately, H1N1, spread rapidly around the world. The term "pandemic" refers to its worldwide spread rather than its severity, and in most patients the symptoms are mild. In August 2010, the WHO declared an end to the pandemic, but the H1N1 virus is expected to circulate in many parts of the world, like seasonal flu viruses, and the annual flu vaccines will provide protection against it.[43]

The public health approach to influenza control can serve as a model for how to predict and possibly prevent the spread of other new viral threats. As the AIDS epidemic has shown, a new virus can come from "nowhere" and wreak havoc all over the world within a few years. Complacency over the "conquest" of infectious diseases has led governments to cut budgets and reduce efforts at monitoring disease. That should not happen again. The public health information-gathering network is more important than ever.

New Bacterial Threats

Bacteria, which a few decades ago seemed easily controllable because of the power of antibiotics to wipe them out, have, like viruses, emerged in more deadly forms. Previously unknown bacterial diseases such as Legionnaires' disease and Lyme disease have appeared. More baffling is the fact that some ordinary bacterial infections have turned unexpectedly lethal. A great cause for concern is the development of resistance to drugs. Resistance can spread among pathogens of the same species and even from one bacterial species to another.

Legionnaires' disease and Lyme disease are not new, but only recently have they become common enough to be recognized as distinct entities and for their bacterial causes to be identified. *Legionella* bacteria were able to flourish in water towers used for air conditioning. Regulations requiring antimicrobial agents in the water have been effective in limiting the spread of Legionnaires' disease. The conditions that promote the spread of Lyme disease, however, are more difficult to change. The pathogen that causes Lyme disease was identified in 1982 as a spirochete that is spread by the bite of an infected deer tick.[44] The reservoir for Lyme disease is the white-footed mouse, on which the deer tick feeds and becomes infected. Deer, on which the ticks grow and reproduce, are an important step in the chain of infection, and it is because of the recent explosion in the deer population in suburban areas that Lyme disease has now become such a problem for humans.

Infection with *streptococci*, the bacteria that cause strep throat, had normally been easily cured with penicillin. However, for reasons that are not well understood, a more lethal strain of the bacteria, called *group A streptococci*, has become increasingly common. The sudden death of Muppets puppeteer Jim Henson in 1990 from fulminating pneumonia and toxic shock was caused by this new, virulent strain. The headline-grabbing "flesh-eating bacteria" that infect wounds to the extent of necessitating amputations and even causing death are also *group A streptococci*. The group A strain, which produces a potent toxin, was prevalent in the early part of the 20th century, when it caused scarlet fever, frequently fatal in children, and rheumatic fever, which often caused damage to the heart. For decades, the group A strain was superseded by strains B and C, which were much milder in their pathogenic effects. But now, for reasons that are not clear, the group A strain has become much more prevalent.[45,46]

Another bacterium that has recently become more deadly is *Escherichia coli*, which is normally present without ill effect in the human digestive tract. In 1993, the new threat gained national attention when a number of people became severely ill after eating hamburgers at a Jack in the Box restaurant in Seattle, and four children died of kidney failure. The culprit was found to be a new strain of *E. coli*, which had acquired a gene for shiga toxin from a dysentery-causing bacterium. The toxin, against which there is no treatment, causes kidney failure, especially in children and the elderly. The shiga toxin gene had "jumped" from one species of bacteria to another while they were both present in human intestines. The resulting strain, called *E. coli* serotype O157:H7, is now quite common in ground beef, leading public health authorities to recommend or require thorough cooking of hamburgers.[19(p.427)] The "jumping gene" phenomenon has also been found in cholera and diphtheria bacteria, bacterial strains that can be benign or virulent depending on the presence or absence of genes that produce toxins.

Since the finding that *E. coli* O157:H7 is common in hamburger, it has been discovered to cause illness by a number of other exposures, including unpasteurized apple cider and alfalfa sprouts.[47(p.160–161)] In 1999, there was an outbreak in upstate New York among people who had attended a county fair. The bacteria were found in the water supplied to food and drink vendors. It turns out that *E. coli* O157:H7 is widespread in the intestines of cattle, especially calves, which excrete large quantities of the bacteria in manure. The manure may contaminate apples fallen from trees or other produce, which if not thoroughly washed before being consumed, may spread the disease to people. At the New York State county fair, the water was contaminated because heavy rain washed manure from the nearby cattle barn into a well.[48] A vaccine against the toxic bacteria has been approved for cattle in the hope of reducing the risk of human exposure.[49]

Perhaps the most disturbing development in infectious diseases is the antibiotic resistance among many species of bacteria, a development that leaves physicians powerless against many diseases they thought to be conquered. The process by which bacteria become resistant to an antibiotic is a splendid example of evolution in action. In the presence of an antibiotic drug, any mutation that allows a single bacterium to survive confers on it a tremendous selective advantage. That bacterium can then reproduce without competition from other microbes, transmitting the mutation to its offspring. The result is a strain of the bacteria that is resistant to that particular antibiotic. The mutated gene can also "jump" to other bacteria of the same or different species by the exchange of plasmids, small pieces of DNA that can move from one bacterial organism to another. Different mutations may be necessary to confer resistance to different antibiotics. Some bacteria become resistant to many different antibiotics, making it very difficult to treat patients infected with those bacteria.

Improper use of antibiotics favors the development of resistance, and the current widespread existence of resistant bacteria testifies to the carelessness with which these lifesaving drugs have been used. For example, since antibiotics are powerless against viruses, the common practice of prescribing these drugs for a viral infection merely affords stray bacteria the opportunity to develop resistance. Another example of improper use is the common tendency of patients to stop taking an antibiotic when they feel better instead of continuing for the full prescribed course. The first few days' dose may have killed off all but a few bacteria, the most resistant, which may then survive and multiply, becoming much more difficult to control. In some countries, antibiotics are available without a prescription, increasing the likelihood that they will be used improperly.

A practice that significantly contributes to antibiotic resistance is the widespread use in animal feeds of low doses of antibiotics for the purpose of making livestock grow bigger and healthier. More antibiotics are used in this manner than in medical applications, and the practice has clearly led to the survival of resistant strains of bacteria that may not only contaminate the meat but that may also spread the antibiotic resistance genes to other bacteria.[50] Studies have shown that these "superbugs" can be transmitted to humans.[51] Because the agricultural industry benefits from the practice and has fought restrictions, the government has found it difficult to impose regulations on it. In 2012, the FDA took a step in the direction of restricting the practice by requiring a veterinarian's prescription for use of antibiotics in farm animals.[52]

The bacteria *salmonella* and *campylobacter* are estimated to cause 3.8 million cases of foodborne illness in the United States each year. In a 1999 study, 26 percent of the salmonella cases and 54 percent of the campylobacter cases were found to be resistant to at least one antibiotic, probably because of antibiotic use in animal feed.[53] Resistance to erythromycin and other common antibiotics is increasingly found in *group A streptococci*, the lethal strain discussed previously.[54] Infection with *methicillin-resistant Staphylococcus aureus (MRSA)* is a major problem in hospitals, burn centers, and nursing homes, where hospital staff may carry the bacteria from one vulnerable patient to another. Intensive efforts have succeeded in reducing the rates of MRSA infections in hospitalized patients by nearly 50 percent between 1997 and 2007.[55] Healthcare-associated infections, many of them caused by drug-resistant bacteria, are estimated to cost $20 billion and contribute to some 99,000 deaths annually in the United States.[56]

Multidrug-Resistant Tuberculosis (MDR TB)

Tuberculosis, which is spread by aerosol, used to be a major killer in the United States. Between 1800 and 1870, it accounted for one out of every five deaths in this country. Worldwide, it is still the leading cause of death among infectious diseases. It is a disease associated with poverty, thought to be conquered in the affluent United States, where the incidence of tuberculosis steadily declined between 1882 and 1985. Much of the success came from the early public health movement, which emphasized improvement of slum housing, sanitation, and pasteurization of cows' milk, which harbored a bovine form of the bacillus that was pathogenic to humans. Patients were isolated in sanatoriums, where they were required to rest and breathe fresh air and, incidentally, were prevented from infecting others. With the introduction of antibiotics in 1947, mortality from tuberculosis was dramatically reduced, sanatoriums were closed, and tuberculosis seemed vanquished.

In 1985, however, the trend reversed. There were several reasons for the increase in the incidence of tuberculosis, which was particularly concentrated in cities and among minority populations. The HIV epidemic was certainly a major factor. People with defective immune systems are more susceptible to any infection, but HIV-positive people are especially vulnerable to tuberculosis. An increasing homeless population and the rise in intravenous drug use, both of which are associated with HIV infection, were also factors in increasing tuberculosis rates. Homeless shelters, prisons, and urban hospitals are prime sites for the transmission of tuberculosis.

But tuberculosis is not limited to the "down and out" or those who participate in high-risk behavior. "The principal risk behavior for acquiring TB infection is breathing," as one expert says.[57(p.1058)] People have been infected with tuberculosis bacilli in the course of a variety of everyday activities: a long airplane trip sitting within a few rows of a person with active tuberculosis,[58] hanging out in a Minneapolis bar frequented by a homeless man with active tuberculosis,[59] and, most frighteningly, attending a suburban school with a girl whose tuberculosis went undiagnosed for 13 months.[60]

When tuberculosis bacilli are inhaled by a healthy person, they do not usually cause illness in the short term. Most often, the immune system responds by killing off most of the bacilli and walling off the rest into small, calcified lesions in the lungs called tubercles, which remain dormant indefinitely. Evidence that a person has been exposed shows up in tuberculin skin tests, which cause a conspicuous immune response when a small extract from the bacillus is injected under the exposed person's skin. For reasons that are not well understood, probably having to do with individual immune system variations, a small percentage of people develop active disease soon after exposure; others may harbor the latent infection for years before it becomes active, if ever. Infected people have a 10 percent lifetime risk of developing an active case. The risk for people who are HIV positive is much higher: up to 50 percent.[47] Most cases of active tuberculosis are characterized by growth of the bacilli in the lungs, causing breakdown of the tissue and the major symptom—coughing—which releases the infectious agents into the air.

Before the introduction of antibiotics, about 50 percent of the patients with active tuberculosis died. Antibiotics dramatically reduced not only the mortality rate, but the incidence rate as well, since the medication relieved coughing and therefore inhibited the spread of disease. However, the development of multidrug resistance (MDR), in some strains of the bacilli, has meant that the disease is much more difficult and expensive to treat, and the mortality rate is much higher.

The increased prevalence of the antibiotic resistant strains in all parts of this country during the 1980s is thought to be due to the fact that many patients did not take their medications regularly. The tuberculosis bacillus is a particularly difficult pathogen to deal with because it grows slowly and because diagnostic testing can take several weeks. Once the disease is diagnosed, even the most potent antibiotic must be taken for several months to wipe out the pathogens. Patients commonly begin to feel better after 2 to 4 weeks of taking an effective prescribed drug and, if they stop taking the medication at that point, they may relapse with a drug-resistant strain.

That MDR TB can be a threat to all strata of society was made clear by an epidemic that was finally recognized in a suburban California school in 1993. The source of the outbreak was a 16-year-old immigrant student who had contracted the disease in her native Vietnam.[60] She had developed a persistent cough in January 1991, but her doctors had failed to diagnose the cause as tuberculosis until 13 months later. Even then, they did not report the case to the county health department, as required by law, and when the case was reported by the laboratory that had analyzed her sputum, the doctors refused to cooperate with the health department. By the time the county authorities took over her case in 1993, the girl had developed a drug-resistant strain. In accordance with standard public health practice, the health department then began screening all the girl's contacts for tuberculosis infection. Some 23 percent of the 1263 students given the tuberculin skin test were found to be positive for exposure to the infection. Of those, 13 students had active cases of the drug-resistant strain of the disease. Fortunately, no one died.[61]

It is clearly in the community interest to ensure that all tuberculosis patients be properly diagnosed and provided a full course of medications, whether or not they can afford to pay, to prevent them from spreading the disease. New York City has proven that, by applying public health measures, it is possible to reverse the trend of increasing MDR TB, a trend that had been worse in that city than anywhere else in the nation. In 1992, the number of tuberculosis cases diagnosed in the city had nearly tripled over the previous 15 years, and 23 percent of new cases were resistant to drugs. The city and state began intensive public health measures, which included screening high-risk populations and providing therapy to everyone diagnosed with active tuberculosis. A program of directly observed therapy (DOT) was instituted for patients who were judged unlikely to take their medications regularly. Outreach workers traveled to patients' homes, workplaces, street corners, park benches, or wherever necessary to observe that each patient took each dose of his or her medicine. As a result of these measures, the number of new cases of tuberculosis fell in 1993, 1994, and 1995, and the percentage of new cases that were MDR also fell by 30 percent in a 2-year period.[62] New York's success has been echoed by national trends, as shown in Figure 10-1, giving hope that concerted public health efforts can eliminate tuberculosis as a serious public health threat in the United States. DOT is recognized all over the world as the most effective approach to dealing with tuberculosis.

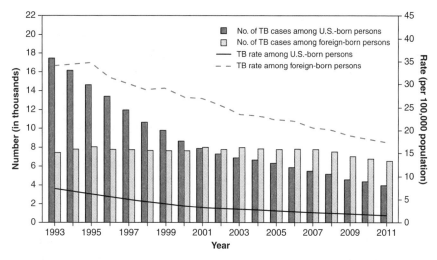

FIGURE 10-1   Number and rate of tuberculosis (TB) cases among U.S.-born and foreign-born persons, by year reported—United States, 1993–2011. Data are updated as of February 22, 2012. Data for 2011 are provisional. *Source:* Reproduced from U.S. Centers for Disease Control and Prevention, *Morbidity and Mortality Weekly Report* 61 (2012): 181–185, Figure 2.

As Figure 10-1 shows, the majority of tuberculosis cases reported in the United States are found among foreign-born persons. This reflects the fact that tuberculosis infection is widespread throughout the world, especially in developing countries and in countries with high rates of HIV infection. The prevalence of MDR TB strains is a major concern; the proportion of TB cases that are MDR can reach 20 percent in some countries of the former Soviet Union and parts of China.[63] In the United States, the proportion of multidrug-resistant cases is only about 1 percent, mainly occurring among foreign-born persons. Because of immigration and international travel, the United States will need to continue tuberculosis control programs at home and to actively participate in global efforts to control the disease around the world to avoid future outbreaks in this country.

The CDC in 2007 revised its requirements for overseas medical screening of applicants for immigration to the United States.[64] Federal agencies also developed measures to prevent individuals with certain communicable diseases, including active tuberculosis, from traveling on commercial aircraft. Names of these individuals are placed on a Do Not Board list by federal, state, or local public health agencies and distributed to international airlines. A similar list is distributed to border patrol authorities in order to prevent individuals deemed dangerous to the public health from entering the country through a seaport, airport, or land border. These lists are managed by the CDC and the Department of Homeland Security.[65]

In the 1990s, even more threatening strains of tuberculosis began to appear around the world—extensively drug-resistant, or XDR TB. While strains of MDR TB are resistant to the most common anti-TB drugs, there are still some drugs that are effective against them, although they are more expensive and are difficult to administer. XDR TB is resistant to virtually all antituberculosis drugs, leading to a mortality rate of 50 percent or more. According to one expert, this raises "concerns about a return to the pre-antibiotic era in TB control."[66]

In May 2007, an American lawyer, Andrew Speaker, caused an international health scare when, after being tested for tuberculosis in Atlanta, he flew to Paris to be married in Greece and spend his honeymoon in Europe. When the test results came in a few days later, showing that he had XDR TB, the CDC contacted him in Rome and recommended that he make arrangements for medical treatment there. Instead, he traveled to the Czech Republic, took a flight from Prague to Montreal, and then drove to New York City where he turned himself in at a hospital. He later explained that he preferred to be treated at home and was afraid he would not be allowed to board a plane bound for the United States. The incident inspired headlines around the world as U.S. authorities tried to locate Mr. Speaker and to track down passengers and crew members on the two trans-Atlantic flights so that they could be tested for the infection. Back in the United States, Mr. Speaker was held in isolation and eventually had surgery to remove the infected portions of his lung. Further tests showed that he did not have XDR TB after all, although his infection was MDR TB.[67] The incident presumably inspired the development of Do Not Board lists, as described above.

It is clear that in the struggle between microbes' ability to evolve new variations and human ingenuity in devising new defenses against them, the microbes are gaining. In a special issue of *Science* magazine devoted to emerging infections, a CDC scientist says that a "post-antimicrobial era may be rapidly approaching," when effective antibiotics will no longer be available to treat bacterial infections.[68(p.1055)] If so, that era will force public health professionals back to more emphasis on prevention of disease transmission with classical public health measures such as surveillance, immunization, sanitation, and infection control procedures.

Prions

As if new viruses and drug-resistant bacteria were not worrisome enough, a novel form of infectious disease grabbed headlines in the 1990s. Creutzfeldt-Jakob disease (CJD) is a rare and devastating disorder in which the patient becomes demented and ultimately dies, and the brain appears spongy on autopsy because many brain cells have died. Similar diseases in animals can be transmitted by injecting brain tissue from an infected animal into the brain of a previously healthy one. However, no virus or bacteria has been found responsible for causing the condition. In 1997, Stanley Prusiner, a scientist at the University of California Medical School in San Francisco, won the Nobel Prize for his controversial theory that this type of disease is caused by particles called prions, which contain protein but no nucleic acid and thus no traditional genetic material.

In 1996, a paper appeared in a British medical journal reporting that 10 persons in the United Kingdom younger than 45 years of age had been diagnosed with a CJD-like condition, an unusually high incidence in a group much younger than those usual struck by the disease.[69] The authors suggested a link with an epidemic of bovine spongiform encephalopathy (BSE), known as "mad cow disease," which had killed over 160,000 cattle in Britain over the previous decade. The disease was spread by the practice, now discontinued, of grinding up discarded animal parts and adding them to feed for other cattle. A flurry of alarm and a European ban on British beef led the British government in 1996 to order the mass slaughter of all at-risk cattle to prevent the possibility of human exposure to infected beef.[70]

The evidence is strong that consumption of contaminated beef is the cause of new variant CJD (vCJD). As of October 2009, 217 cases had been reported worldwide, of which 170 were in the United Kingdom. Most of them had lived there during the years of the BSE outbreak among cattle. Three cases have been reported in the United States, two of them who probably contracted the disease in the United Kingdom and one who probably contracted the disease in Saudi Arabia.[71] Americans have little chance of being exposed to BSE in the United States. Regulations on cattle feed have been tightened, and restrictions have been introduced that prohibit importation of live ruminants, such as cattle, sheep, and goats. Certain ruminant parts are prohibited from entering the food supply. Although there was controversy about whether enough is being done to protect American cattle from BSE, only three cases have been identified in American cows between 2003 and 2006.[72] No cases of vCJD have been attributed to consumption of American beef.

Public Health Response to Emerging Infections

The American public health system, criticized in 1988 for being in disarray, has taken many steps toward responding to the emerging threats of infectious diseases. While still underfunded and challenged from all sides, American public health agencies have devoted significant resources to developing plans and priorities for confronting the threats.

The Institute of Medicine has undertaken several studies to address the environmental, demographic, social, and other factors leading to the emergence or re-emergence of infectious diseases. One of its conclusions is that most of the emerging infectious disease events have been caused by zoonotic disease pathogens—those infectious agents that are transmitted from animals to humans. Factors that contribute to the risk of this animal to human transmission include human population growth, changing patterns of human–animal contact, increased demand for animal protein, increased wealth and mobility, environmental changes, and human encroachment on farmland and previously undisturbed wildlife habitat. Clearly, these diseases are an international problem, and dealing with them requires an international response.[73]

Global surveillance for infectious diseases is critically important for identifying potential epidemics early enough to bring them under control. Diseases that went unnoticed in animals but have spread to humans include AIDS, Ebola, avian influenza, and SARS. Effective control of emerging infectious diseases requires worldwide disease surveillance focusing not only on human populations, but also on domestic animals and wildlife. Thus, the CDC is collaborating with, in addition to the World Health Organization, the World Organization for Animal Health, and the Food and Agricultural Organization of the United Nations. In addition, the CDC has established the International Emerging Infections Program, which has laboratories in China, Egypt, Guatemala, Kenya, and Thailand.

Other priorities that the Institute of Medicine has identified for controlling emerging infections include reducing inappropriate use of antibiotics by banning their use for growth promotion in animals and by developing improved diagnostic tests for infectious diseases so that antibiotics are not used for viral diseases. The Institute of Medicine also recommends developing new vaccines, new antimicrobial drugs, and measures aimed at vector-borne diseases.[74]

Public Health and the Threat of Bioterrorism

In the late 1990s, concern increased in the United States about the possibility that biological organisms could be used as agents of warfare and terrorism. The anthrax attacks of 2001 demonstrated that the concern was well founded. Earlier incidents had raised awareness of the possible threat, including revelations by a Russian defector that the Soviets had developed systems for loading smallpox virus on ballistic missiles.[75] Concern was heightened by evidence that Iraq had produced missile warheads and bombs containing anthrax spores and botulinum toxin. The Aum Shinrikyo cult that released sarin gas in a Tokyo subway was found later to have experimented with releases of aerosolized anthrax and botulinum toxin throughout the city.[76] Closer to home, a 1984 outbreak of salmonellosis that sickened 751 people in The Dalles, Oregon was eventually traced to intentional contamination of salad bars in several restaurants, details of which were revealed much later in a criminal prosecution of the Baghwan religious cult that was responsible for the incident.[77]

Even before the anthrax attacks of 2001, the CDC had developed plans for dealing with biological terrorism. Since then, awareness of the possibility of biological attacks has increased, and planning has continued. It is clear that, in contrast with bombings or chemical attacks, dissemination of biological agents is likely to be done in a covert way. Thus, the first signs of an attack are likely to be seen by physicians and hospital emergency rooms. Local health departments will carry out the initial investigations of unusual disease outbreaks, and good surveillance is vital for recognizing outbreaks as early as possible. In sum, the approach to bioterrorism preparedness is much the same as the response to an epidemic of any other origin.

Conclusion

Infectious diseases have increasingly threatened the health of Americans over the past 2 decades, in a challenge to the earlier view that infectious diseases were under control. The appearance of AIDS in the early 1980s was an early sign that a new disease could appear out of "nowhere" and rapidly become a lethal, worldwide epidemic. Other viruses such as Ebola and other hemorrhagic fevers have emerged in tropical areas and could be brought to the United States if conditions were right. A deadly hantavirus appeared in the United States in 1993 and has been reported in 34 states. West Nile virus was first recognized in New York City in 1999 and has spread across the country to almost all states. Monkeypox, a virus similar to smallpox that primarily infects rodents, was brought to the United States in exotic pets imported from Africa and sickened a number of people in 2003. Influenza is a highly infectious disease that can spread rapidly all over the world. While the public health system has worked internationally, adapting vaccines to keep up with the rapidly mutating viruses, everyone is frightened by the prospect of another worldwide flu epidemic like the one in 1918 that killed 20 to 40 million people.

New bacterial diseases have also been appearing in the United States as ecological and cultural conditions change. Lyme disease and Legionnaires' disease have been significant problems in the past 2 decades. *Streptococci* and *E. coli* have become much more deadly in recent years. Many bacteria, including *M. tuberculosis*, have developed resistance to antibiotics, making them much less vulnerable to treatment.

To combat today's emerging infectious threats, public health professionals must update measures successful in the early part of the 20th century. Plans are in place to fortify the public health system to improve surveillance and response to the new threats. As with many other aspects of public health, however, political controversy and economic concerns tend to impede the implementation of effective measures, such as those needed to deal with antibiotic resistance stimulated by agricultural practices. New concerns about the threat of biological terrorism have added urgency to the call for strengthening the public health system in the United States.

References

1. UNAIDS. "Global Report: UNAIDS Report on the Global AIDS Epidemic," 2010. http://www.unaids.org/globalreport/Global_report/htm. 2010, accessed October 30, 2012.
2. U.S. Centers for Disease Control and Prevention, "HIV/AIDS in the United States: At a Glance." http://www.cdc.gov/hiv/resources/factsheets/us.htm, accessed June 3, 2012.

3. W. C. Greene, "AIDS and the Immune System," *Scientific American* (September 1993): 99–103.

4. M. Pope and A. T. Haase, "Transmission, Acute HIV-1 Infection and the Quest for Strategies to Prevent Infection," *Nature Medicine* 9 (2003): 847–852.

5. M. A. Nowak and A. J. McMichael, "How HIV Defeats the Immune System," *Scientific American* (August 1995): 58–65.

6. U.S. Centers for Disease Control and Prevention, "Male Circumcision and Risk for HIV Transmission and Other Health Conditions: Implications for the United States." http://www.cdc.gov/hiv/resources/factsheets/circumcision.htm, accessed June 3, 2012.

7. R. O. Valdiserri et al., "Accomplishments in HIV Prevention Science: Implications for Stemming the Epidemic," *Nature Medicine* 9 (2003): 881–886.

8. U.S. Centers for Disease Control and Prevention, "Mother-to-Child (Perinatal) HIV Transmission and Prevention." http://www.cdc.gov/hiv/topics/perinatal/resources/factsheets/perinatal.htm, accessed June 3, 2012.

9. U.S. Centers for Disease Control and Prevention, "HIV Among African Americans." http://www.cdc.gov/hiv/topics/aa/index.htm, accessed June 3, 2012.

10. U.S. Centers for Disease Control and Prevention, "HIV Among Latinos." http://www.cdc.gov/hiv/latinos/index.htm, accessed June 3, 2012.

11. A. S. Fauci, "HIV and AIDS: 20 Years of Science," *Nature Medicine* 9 (2003): 839–843.

12. U.S. Centers for Disease Control and Prevention, "HIV Mortality (Through 2008)," http://www.cdc.gov/hiv/topics/surveillance/resources/slides/mortality/index.htm, accessed June 4, 2012.

13. A. Garg, "Acquired and Inherited Lipodystrophies," *New England Journal of Medicine* 350 (2004): 1220.

14. B. Masquelier et al., "Prevalence of Transmitted HIV-1 Drug Resistance and the Role of Resistance Algorithms," *Journal of Acquired Immune Deficiency Syndrome* 40 (2005): 505–511.

15. National Institute of Allergy and Infectious Diseases, "Drugs That Fight HIV." http://www.niaid.nih.gov/topics/HIVAIDS/Documents/HIVPillBrochure.pdf, accessed June 4, 2012.

16. K. A. Gebo et al, "Contemporary Costs of HIV Healthcare in the HAART Era," AIDS 24 (2010): 2705.

17. L. A. Altman, "Rethinking is Urged on a Vaccine for AIDS," *The New York Times*, March 26, 2008.

18. K. O. Kallings, "The First Postmodern Pandemic: 25 Years of HIV/AIDS," *Journal of Internal Medicine* 263 (2007): 218–243.

19. L. Garrett, *The Coming Plague: Newly Emerging Diseases in a World Out of Balance* (New York: Farrar, Straus and Giroux, 1994).

20. T. Zhu et al., "An African HIV Sequence from 1959 and Implications for the Origin of the Epidemic," *Nature* 391 (1998): 594–597.

21. B. Le Guenno, "Emerging Viruses," *Scientific American* (October 1995): 56–64.

22. E. M. Leroy et al., "Multiple Ebola Virus Transmission Events and Rapid Decline of Central African Wildlife," *Science* 303 (2004): 387–390.

23. S. Centers for Disease Control and Prevention, "Known Cases and Outbreaks of Ebola Hemorrhagic Fever, in Chronological Order." http://www.cdc.gov/ncidod/dvrd/spb/mnpages/ebola/ebolatable.htm, accessed June 4, 2012.

24. R. Preston, *The Hot Zone* (New York: Random House, 1994).

25. G. Vogel, "Scientists Say Ebola Has Pushed Western Gorillas to the Brink," *Science* 317 (2007): 1484.

26. K. D. Reed et al., "The Detection of Monkeypox in Humans in the Western Hemisphere," *New England Journal of Medicine* 350 (2004): 342–350.

27. U.S. Centers for Disease Control and Prevention, "Outbreak of Acute Illness—Southwestern United States, 1993," *Morbidity and Mortality Weekly Report* 42 (1993): 421–424.

28. U.S. Centers for Disease Control and Prevention, "Annual U.S. HPS Cases and Case-fatality, 1993–2011." http://www.cdc.gov/hantavirus/surveillance/annual-cases.html, accessed June 6, 2012.

29. U.S. Centers for Disease Control and Prevention, "Hantavirus Pulmonary Syndrome—Northeastern United States, 1994," *Morbidity and Mortality Weekly Report* 43 (1994): 548–549, 555–556.

30. U.S. Centers for Disease Control and Prevention, "Outbreak of West Nile-Like Viral Encephalitis—New York, 1999," *Morbidity and Mortality Weekly Report* 48 (1999): 845–849.

31. U.S. Centers for Disease Control and Prevention, "Update: West Nile Virus Encephalitis—New York, 1999," *Morbidity and Mortality Weekly Report* 48 (1999): 944–946.

32. U.S. Centers for Disease Control and Prevention, "Summary of Notifiable Diseases—United States, 2006," *Morbidity and Mortality Weekly Report* 55 (2006): 8.

33. U.S. Centers for Disease Control and Prevention, "Final 2011 West Nile Virus Infections in the United States." http://www.cdc.gov/ncidod/dvbid/westnile/surv&controlCaseCount11_detailed.htm, accessed June 6, 2012.

34. R. Voelker, "Effects of West Nile Virus May Persist," *Journal of American Medical Association* 299 (2008): 2135–2136.

35. J. M. Barry, *The Great Influenza: The Story of the Deadliest Pandemic in History* (London: Penguin Books, 2004).

36. World Health Organization, "Spreading the Word About Seasonal Influenza." http://www.who.int/bulletin/volumes/90/4/12-030412/en/index.html, accessed June 6, 2012.

37. E. C. Holmes, "1918 and All That," *Science* 303 (2004): 1787–1788.

38. E. C. J. Claas et al., "Human Influenza A H5N1 Virus Related to a Highly Pathogenic Avian Influenza Virus," *The Lancet* 351 (1998): 472–477.

39. U.S. Centers for Disease Control and Prevention, "Avian Influenza A Virus Infections of Humans." http://www.cdc.gov/flu/avian/gen-info/avian-flu-humans.htm, accessed June 6, 2012.

40. U.S. Centers for Disease Control and Prevention, "Highly Pathogenic Avian Influenza A (H5N1) in People." http://www.cdc.gov/flu/avianflu/h5n1-people.htm, accessed June 6, 2012.

41. D. Grady and W. J. Broad, "Seeing Terror Risk, U.S. Asks Journals to Cut Flu Study Facts," *The New York Times*, December 20, 2011.

42. D. Grady, "Despite Safety Worries, Work on Deadly Flu to Be Released, *The New York Times,* February 17, 2012.

43. U.S. Centers for Disease Control and Prevention, "2009 H1N1 Flu." http://www.cdc.gov/h1n1flu/, accessed June 6, 2012.

44. F. S. Kantor, "Disarming Lyme Disease," *Scientific American* (September 1994): 34–39.
45. R. M. Krause, "The Origin of Plagues: Old and New," *Science* 257 (1992): 1073–1078.
46. R. K. Aziz and M. Kotb, "Rise and Persistence of Global M1T1 Clone of Streptococcus pyogenes," *Emerging Infectious Diseases* 14 (2008): 1511–1517.
47. D. L. Heymann, *Control of Communicable Diseases Manual* (Washington, DC: American Public Health Association, 2004), 160–161.
48. U.S. Centers for Disease Control and Prevention, "Public Health Dispatch: Outbreak of *Escherichia coli* O157:H7 and Campylobacter Among Attendees of the Washington County Fair—New York 1999," *Morbidity and Mortality Weekly Report* 48 (1999): 803.
49. U.S. Department of Agriculture, "Vilsack Issues Conditional License for Vaccine to Reduce E. coli in Feedlot Cattle." http://www.usda.gov/wps/portal/usda/usdahome?contentidonly=true&contented=2009/03/0058.xml, accessed June 5, 2012.
50. W. Witte, "Medical Consequences of Antibiotic Use in Agriculture," *Science* 279 (1998): 996–997.
51. B. M. Kuehn, "Antibiotic-Resistant 'Superbugs' May Be Transmitted from Animals to Humans," *Journal of the American Medical Association* 298 (2007): 2125–2126.
52. G. Harris, "U.S. Tightens Rules on Antibiotics Use for Livestock," *The New York Times,* April 11, 2012.
53. S. L. Gorbach, "Antimicrobial Use in Animal Feed—Time to Stop," *New England Journal of Medicine* 345 (2001): 1202–1203.
54. P. Hudvinen, "Macrolide-Resistant Group A Streptococcus—Now in the United States," *New England Journal of Medicine* 346 (2002): 1243–1245.
55. U.S. Centers for Disease Control and Prevention, "MRSA Statistics." http://www.cdc.gov/mrsa/statistics/index.html, accessed June 6, 2012.
56. K. S. Sack, "Guidelines Set for Preventing Hospital Infections," *The New York Times,* October 9, 2008.
57. B. R. Bloom and C. J. L. Murray, "Tuberculosis: Commentary on a Reemergent Killer," *Science* 257 (1992): 1055–1064.
58. T. A. Kenyon, "Transmission of Multidrug-Resistant Mycobacterium Tuberculosis During a Long Airplane Flight," *New England Journal of Medicine* 334 (1996): 935–938.
59. S. Kline et al., "Outbreak of Tuberculosis Among Regular Patrons of a Neighborhood Bar," *New England Journal of Medicine* 333 (1995): 222–227.
60. "California School Becomes Notorious for Epidemic of TB," *The New York Times,* July 18, 1994.
61. R. Ridzon et al., "Outbreak of Drug-Resistant Tuberculosis with Second-Generation Transmission in a High School in California," *Journal of Pediatrics* 131 (1997): 863–868.
62. T. R. Frieden et al., "Tuberculosis in New York City—Turning the Tide," *New England Journal of Medicine* 333 (1995): 229–233.
63. World Health Organization, *Anti-Tuberculosis Drug Resistance in the World. Report No. 4* (Geneva, Switzerland: World Health Organization; 2008). http://whqlibdoc.who.int/hq/2008/WHO_HTM_TB_2008.394_eng.pdf, accessed June 6, 2012.
64. U.S. Centers for Disease Control and Prevention, "Trends in Tuberculosis—United States, 2007," *Morbidity and Mortality Weekly Report* 57 (2008): 281–285.

65. U.S. Centers for Disease Control and Prevention, "Federal Air Travel Restrictions for Public Health Purposes—United States, June 2007–May 2008," *Morbidity and Mortality Weekly Report* 57 (2008): 1009–1012.

66. N. S. Shah et al., "Extensively Drug-Resistant Tuberculosis in the United States, 1993–2007," *Journal of the American Medical Association* 300 (2008): 2153–2160.

67. L. K. Altman, "Traveler's TB Not as Severe as Officials Thought," *The New York Times*, July 4, 2007.

68. M. I. Cohen, "Epidemiology of Drug Resistance: Implications for a Post-Antimicrobial Era," *Science* 257 (1992): 1050–1055.

69. R. G. Will et al., "A New Variant of Creutzfeldt-Jakob Disease in the U.K.," *The Lancet* 347 (1996): 921–925.

70. P. G. Smith and S. N. Cousens, "Is the New Variant of Creutzfeldt-Jakob Disease from Mad Cows?" *Science* 273 (1996): 748.

71. U.S. Centers for Disease Control and Prevention, "Fact Sheet: Variant Creutzfeldt-Jakob Disease." http://www.cdc.gov/ncidod/dvrd/vcjd/factsheet_nvcjd.htm, August 23, 2010, accessed June 6, 2012.

72. U.S. Centers for Disease Control and Prevention, "BSE (Bovine Spongiform Encephalopathy, or Mad Cow Disease)." http://www.cdc.gov/ncidod/dvrd/bse/index.htm, accessed June 6, 2012.

73. U.S. Institute of Medicine, *Achieving Sustainable Global Capacity for Surveillance and Response to Emerging Diseases of Zoonotic Origin: Workshop Report* (Washington, DC: National Academies Press, 2008).

74. U.S. Institute of Medicine, *Microbial Threats to Health: Emergence, Detection, and Response* (Washington, DC: National Academies Press, 2003).

75. C. J. Davis, "Nuclear Blindness: An Overview of the Biological Weapons Programs of the Former Soviet Union and Iraq," *Emerging Infectious Diseases* 5 (2000): 509–512.

76. K. B. Olson, "Aum Shinrikyo: Once and Future Threat?" *Emerging Infectious Diseases* 5 (2000): 513–516.

77. T. J. Torok, "A Large Community Outbreak of Salmonellosis Caused by Intentional Contamination of Restaurant Salad Bars," *Journal of the American Medical Association* 278 (1997): 389–395.

The Biomedical Basis
of Chronic Diseases

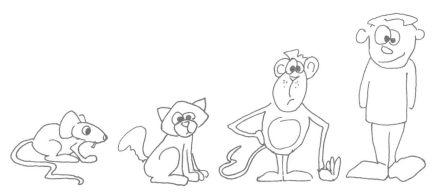

Evolution of the Research Study

The early successes of public health against infectious diseases led to a change in the major causes of illness and death beginning in the 1920s. Chronic degenerative diseases, especially heart disease and cancer, are now the leading causes of death in the United States. While they are primarily diseases of old age—when everyone must die of something—they also strike people in their prime, robbing them of productive years of life. Cancer is the leading cause of death among Americans aged 45 to 65, and cardiovascular disease runs a close second. Cardiovascular disease kills the most people overall. Other significant diseases of current public health concern include diabetes, arthritis, and Alzheimer's disease, which may not be as deadly in the short run but have severe impacts on the quality of life. It is the mission of public health to prevent such premature death and disability.

Prevention of disease usually requires some understanding of the cause, a requirement that is generally much more difficult to fulfill for chronic diseases than for infectious ones. There is no single pathogen that causes cancer or heart disease, nor is there one for arthritis, diabetes, or Alzheimer's disease. In most cases, chronic diseases have multiple causes, making it more difficult for scientists to recognize significant risk factors and establish preventive measures. Moreover, these diseases tend to develop over long periods of time, further complicating the task of pinning down causes. In some cases, however, the gradual onset provides the advantage of early detection, permitting secondary prevention—interventions early in the disease process that can mitigate its impact.

As chronic degenerative diseases became a growing problem during the 20th century, scientists began to focus on efforts to understand their causes. The growth of the National Institutes of Health (NIH), which sponsors most biomedical research in the United States, has reflected the growth of concern about these diseases. In its early days as a one-room Laboratory of Hygiene that opened in 1887, the NIH conducted research primarily on infectious diseases. Congress created the National Cancer Institute in 1937 and the Heart Institute—now called the National Heart, Lung, and Blood Institute (NHLBI)—in 1948. Now there are 27 different institutes and centers, each of them focused on a different organ or problem, mostly chronic diseases. One institute, for example, is concerned with arthritis, one with diabetes, and one with neurological disorders and stroke.

Research into the causes of chronic disease, like research into the causes of infectious disease, relies on epidemiologic methods and laboratory research, which usually includes studies of animals as models, or stand-ins for human patients. The importance of research on animal models to the understanding of human disease cannot be overemphasized. Epidemiology is generally limited to observation and analysis of events that occur spontaneously. Ethical concerns severely limit the experiments that can be done on humans. In experiments on laboratory animals, scientists can carefully control the conditions so that cause-and-effect relationships can be clearly proven. Mice and rats are the most commonly used laboratory animals; as mammals, they share the majority of biochemical and physiological processes with humans. Because of their short life spans, the effects of various exposures and interventions can be studied over the lifetime of the animals. However, mammals can differ in unpredictable ways in their susceptibility to infectious or toxic agents. Different experimental animals have proven useful for studying different diseases, and extrapolation of results from any particular mammal to humans is not always valid.

The identification of an animal model can significantly improve progress toward understanding a disease. It is not always easy to find an experimental animal that is susceptible to the disease one wishes to study. For instance, there is no good animal model for AIDS, a fact that has hampered progress in developing drug therapies or vaccines. Asian macaque monkeys, which can be made sick by simian immunodeficiency virus, a relative of human immunodeficiency virus (HIV), are the closest substitute. Only chimpanzees can be infected with HIV, and chimps are no longer used for research for ethical reasons and cost.[1] Animals also differ in how they metabolize some chemicals; a dose of dioxin that would kill a guinea pig has no effect on a mouse or rat, and it is difficult from this evidence to predict the chemical's toxicity to humans.

Scientists have been increasingly successful in devising methods of growing cells and tissues in laboratory glassware for studying biomedical processes. Such laboratory cultures are commonly used to investigate the cancer-causing potential of various chemicals. Much of the research on HIV has been done using cultured human cells, and a great deal has been learned. However, such experiments provide oversimplified conditions that may lead to invalid conclusions about the complex interactions that occur in intact animals. In the case of HIV, for example, a number of drugs that appeared to inactivate the virus in test tube experiments have proved to be ineffective in human patients.

Cardiovascular Disease

Cardiovascular disease encompasses two of the three leading causes of death in the United States: heart disease and stroke. Risk for dying from cardiovascular disease increases with age, is higher in men than in women, and is higher in African Americans than in whites.

The causes of cardiovascular disease have been relatively well established through epidemiologic studies, including the Framingham Study, which identified high blood cholesterol, high blood pressure, and smoking as major risk factors. Animal experiments and examination of the bodies of people who have died of the disease have also contributed to an understanding of how it develops. Knowledge about cardiovascular disease has been facilitated by its prevalence in the United States and the fact that it follows a similar progression in many of its victims. The important role of blood components in determining individual risk was readily established because blood is easy to study; it can be drawn from patients and experimental subjects without major discomfort or ethical objections.

It has been known for decades that atherosclerosis—hardening of the arteries—is part of the development of cardiovascular disease. Pathologists performing autopsies on people who died of heart attacks found, within the inner-wall lining of the deceased's arteries, a buildup of plaque composed of fat and cholesterol, blood cells, and clotting materials. The formation of plaque begins at an early age in the United States. Fatty streaks, the first stage in the development of plaque, have been found on autopsy in half the children aged 10 to 14 who died of accidental causes.[2] A classic study, published in 1955, examined the arteries of American soldiers killed in the Korean War and found that 77 percent of the men, whose average age was 22, showed some signs of atherosclerosis.[3] More recent studies have confirmed these findings and have shown that plaque was more likely to be found in adolescents and young adults with risk factors such as smoking, hypertension, obesity, and high levels of low-density lipoprotein cholesterol.[4]

Animal studies showed that diet plays a role in the formation of plaque. Rabbits fed milk, meat, and eggs instead of their normal vegetarian diet were found to develop atherosclerotic plaque very similar to that found in humans.[5] It was easy to deduce that the American diet was responsible for the high rate of cardiovascular disease in the United States.

Experiments on rats, rabbits, and monkeys have clarified the process by which high cholesterol and fat in the blood interact with other risk factors such as smoking, high blood pressure, and diabetes to form plaque in the arteries. These factors cause chronic injury of the artery's inner wall, which the body attempts to repair, leading to a "healing" process that runs wild, becoming a disease in itself. The higher the levels of cholesterol and other fats in the blood, the more they are incorporated into the scab-like buildup, and the faster the plaque forms. A heart attack or stroke results when the plaque ruptures, releasing clots that may block an artery in the heart or brain, cutting off the blood supply.[6]

Recent evidence suggests that atherosclerosis may also have an infectious component caused by bacteria that are often found in plaque.[7] The blood cells in plaque are characteristic of an immune response, and a number of chemicals in the blood suggest that atherosclerosis is an inflammatory condition like arthritis. These findings may lead to new approaches to prevention, diagnosis, and treatment of atherosclerosis.[6]

With the major risk factors for cardiovascular disease well established, much of the recent epidemiologic and biomedical research has focused on trying to understand what determines the relative presence or absence of these risk factors. A great deal has been learned about the various lipids (fats) in the blood, each of which plays a role in the individual's risk of cardiovascular disease, and how their concentrations may be increased or decreased. Factors that affect blood pressure have also been extensively studied. Diabetes, which has its own research institute at NIH, greatly increases the risk of cardiovascular disease (see later in the chapter for a discussion of the biomedical basis of diabetes). All of these risk factors are determined in part by genetics, but they can be significantly modified by individual behavior and are thus susceptible to public health intervention.

High blood cholesterol is a well-known risk factor for atherosclerosis and heart disease. Cholesterol levels of 200 mg/dL (milligrams per deciliter of blood) or below are considered desirable: persons with that level of cholesterol have less than one-half the heart attack risk of those with levels above 240 mg/dL.[8] Most of the cholesterol in the blood is bound up with protein in various forms, and some forms are more harmful than others. For example, if a high percentage of a person's cholesterol is in the form of high-density lipoprotein (HDL), sometimes called "good cholesterol," the person's risk of heart disease is much lower than that of someone with a high percentage of cholesterol in the form of low-density lipoprotein (LDL), "bad cholesterol." Many current studies try to identify factors that affect not only total cholesterol, but also the relative concentrations of HDL and LDL.

The main sources of cholesterol in the American diet are eggs, meat, and milk. In humans, as in rabbits, vegetarians have lower cholesterol levels than meat eaters. Vigorous exercise lowers total cholesterol and increases HDL. Moderate consumption of alcoholic beverages has a similar effect, although heavy drinking damages the heart. Other dietary substances such as fish, olive oil, and oat bran also appear to have favorable effects on blood lipids. Smoking lowers HDL levels. Genes play an important role in the HDL-LDL balance. Some people can eat lots of fat with very little effect on their blood cholesterol, while others must work much harder to maintain favorable levels.

In the past decade, the use of cholesterol-lowering drugs called statins has increased dramatically. The number of Americans who took the drugs grew from about 2 million in 1998 to 30 million in 2005.[9,10] Epidemiologic studies have clearly shown that statins can prevent heart attacks, even in people with cholesterol levels previously considered normal and, for the most part, they appear to be safe for long-term use. However, from a public health perspective, the trend toward prescribing drugs for healthy people to take for the rest of their lives is troubling. Moreover, statins can be expensive. As a spokesman for the American Heart Association is quoted as saying, "If you're going to increase my health insurance because my next door neighbor has borderline high cholesterol, and if he's sitting around and watching TV and eating and getting fat, do you want me to pay for that?"[11]

While the availability of statins appears to be good news for secondary prevention in people who already have atherosclerosis or who have risk factors that put them at high risk, the preferable public health approach to preventing heart disease is primary prevention. This means promoting healthy behavior, including exercise, not smoking, and eating a healthy diet. Eating a healthy diet is not easy in American society.

High blood pressure—hypertension—is a major risk factor for cardiovascular disease, especially stroke, contributing to the injury in the artery walls that is part of atherosclerosis. It also increases the risk of kidney disease. While some medical conditions are known to cause high blood pressure, most cases occur without known cause, and these people are said to have "essential hypertension." Factors that have been linked with essential hypertension are obesity, smoking, lack of exercise, and stress. In the United States, 140/90 is generally considered the borderline above which blood pressure is considered too high. In this reading, 140 is the systolic pressure, that pressure exerted by the blood on the artery walls during the heart's contraction when the pressure is greatest. The diastolic pressure—90 in this case—occurs between contractions, when the heart is relaxed. New evidence prompted the NHLBI to issue guidelines in 2003 that classified blood pressure as "normal" only if it is below 120/80. Pressures between this level and 140/90 are classified as "prehypertension," meaning that individuals with these readings are at risk of developing hypertension. Since the risk of stroke rises continuously as blood pressure rises, people are advised to take medication if necessary to maintain a healthy blood pressure. For those with other risk factors, such as diabetes or kidney disease, it is even more important to keep blood pressure under control.[12]

The U.S. government launched a major blood pressure awareness program in 1972; since then, the annual rate of fatal strokes has been cut by more than half. Many people can keep their blood pressure under control by eating a healthy diet, exercising, and abstaining from smoking, the same behaviors that promotes healthy cholesterol levels. Secondary prevention is important: people should know their own blood pressure and take appropriate measures if it is too high.

Dietary salt (sodium chloride) is believed to be a factor in causing some cases of essential hypertension, but sensitivity to salt is variable and is probably determined by genetics. Laboratory studies have found that some strains of rats get high blood pressure when fed large amounts of salt, while rats of other strains do not seem to react to salt. Rats of one sensitive strain tend to have strokes when subjected to salt and stress, while rats of some other strains are unaffected.[13] The NHLBI recommends that everyone limit their salt intake to about a teaspoon a day, but the question of whether this measure would reduce blood pressure in the average person is controversial. Some researchers have argued that high dietary salt damages the heart and kidneys even in people with normal blood pressure.[14]

At a population level, it is clear that hypertension has a higher prevalence in groups that consume greater amounts of sodium, and that sodium intake is higher in the United States than in many other countries. The prevalence of hypertension in the United States is high; one in three adults have high blood pressure; about 65 percent of those age 60 or older have it.[15] Therefore public health experts have noted that reducing the amount of salt in the American diet would be expected to reduce the prevalence of hypertension. They estimate that, for example, if the average systolic blood pressure could be reduced by five points, mortality due to stroke would be reduced by 14 percent. Because Americans tend to get most of their salt from packaged foods and restaurant meals, the American Public Health Association together with an interagency committee coordinated by NHLBI, has recommended that the food industry, including manufacturers and restaurants, reduce sodium in the food supply by 50 percent over the next decade.[12]

Smoking is believed to increase the risk of cardiovascular disease through the actions of two components of tobacco smoke: nicotine and carbon monoxide. Nicotine, the addictive component of tobacco, is a stimulant that raises blood pressure, increases the pulse rate, stimulates release of stress hormones, and increases irritability of the heart and blood vessels. Carbon monoxide, a poisonous gas, binds to hemoglobin in the blood, blocking the hemoglobin's ability to carry oxygen throughout the body. Both nicotine and carbon monoxide place stress on the heart and blood vessels, with the long-term effect of contributing to atherosclerosis. In the short term, the effects of nicotine and carbon monoxide can provoke irregularities in heartbeat, which may result in sudden death.

Tobacco is especially significant as a cause of heart attack in younger adults. While heart attacks are relatively rare among people in their 30s and 40s, those that do occur are likely to be caused by smoking. One epidemiologic study found that smokers in this age group have a five times greater rate of heart attacks than nonsmokers.[16]

Cancer

Cancer has proven much more difficult to understand than cardiovascular disease, in part because it has so many different manifestations. It is sometimes said that cancer is not one disease, but 100 diseases. In many ways, breast cancer is different from lung cancer, which is different from leukemia. They typically differ in terms of risk factors, appearance under a microscope, response to various forms of treatment, and so forth. For the biomedical scientist and the public health professional trying to understand the cause and prevention of cancer, each kind of cancer must be studied separately. What all cancers have in common is that they arise when the activities of a cell are transformed and the cell begins to grow out of control. Understanding cancer, therefore, requires understanding normal cell function, so that it is possible to recognize what goes wrong in a cancer cell. In general, a normal cell turns cancerous through a mutation in the genetic material, DNA—usually a mutation in one of the genes that regulate cell growth and differentiation. When that cell divides, the mutation is transmitted to the daughter cells, which, because of the disruption in control caused by the mutation, tend to divide more rapidly than normal. As the cells continue to divide abnormally, errors tend to occur as the DNA is copied, leading to additional mutations and more abnormalities in the cells that are becoming a tumor.[17,18] Other changes that may accompany the formation of a tumor are the stimulation of the growth of blood vessels that feed the tumor and the tendency to metastasize—a process by which cancer cells detach from the main tumor and spread to distant parts of the body. Understanding the molecular mechanisms through which tumors form and grow can lead to the development of effective therapies, specific approaches to halting the process or killing the cancerous cells.

To achieve the public health goal of preventing disease, it is important to know what causes the mutations that initiate the cancer. It turns out that mutations in DNA can be caused by many different types of agents, including chemicals, viruses, and radiation. Other factors, such as hormones and diet, play a role in determining whether a mutation progresses to the development of a tumor. Hormones, which function in the body to stimulate or inhibit cell growth, may have an enhanced effect on a mutated cell. The mechanisms by which dietary factors influence the development of cancer—in addition to the fact that some foods may contain carcinogens, or cancer-causing chemicals—are less well understood. There is some evidence that dietary fiber protects against some cancers, perhaps because it speeds the passage of possible carcinogens through the digestive tract, lessening the likelihood that they will be absorbed. High fat in the diet increases the risk of many forms of cancer, but it is not clear why. Diets high in fruits and vegetables seem to be protective.

Exposure to certain kinds of radiation has long been known to cause cancer in humans. Many of the early scientists who unsuspectingly worked with radioactive materials died of the disease, including Marie Curie, the Nobel Prize winner who discovered radium. Curie died of leukemia in 1934 at age 66.[19] Laboratory studies demonstrated clearly that ionizing radiation was capable of damaging DNA and causing mutations in all forms of life, from bacteria to plants to mammals. Later, exposure to certain chemicals was observed to cause some of the same kinds of genetic damage as did radiation, and many of these same chemicals could be demonstrated to cause cancer in laboratory animals.

Viruses have long been known to cause some cancers in plants and animals, but only recently have some human cancers, including liver cancer and cervical cancer, been shown to be of viral origin. Cancer viruses transform cells by integrating themselves into the DNA of the host cell; the viral genes may override the host's genes, for example, by turning on inappropriate cell division. In fact, viruses that cause cancer in humans have been found to carry altered forms of human genes.

The knowledge gained by studying cancer viruses has helped scientists to understand more generally how mutation of the cell's own genes can turn a normal cell into a cancer cell by inappropriately turning on cell division. Some of the genes that, when mutated, lead to cancer—known as oncogenes—stimulate cell division; others, known as tumor suppressor genes, normally function to keep cell division turned off. The new genetic understanding of cancer causation also helps to explain why some families are more susceptible to some kinds of cancer. Since in most cases more than a single mutation is required before a cell is fully malignant, a member of a family that carries one mutation in a gene might need only one additional event to develop a tumor.

The public health approach to primary prevention of cancer is to prevent human exposure to the agents that cause mutation. In the case of ionizing radiation, the danger of which was recognized early, government standards have been developed to protect the population against exposure from various sources such as nuclear power plants, medical and dental x-rays, and radon gas. Sunlight, another proven cause of cancer, cannot be regulated: education in the importance of sunscreen and hats is the favored approach. Because viruses have only recently been recognized to cause cancer in humans, the public health response to these agents is evolving. Immunization is one approach: Hepatitis B vaccination is now recommended for all children, not only to prevent acute hepatitis infection but because chronic infection with hepatitis B virus has been shown to lead to liver cancer. A recently developed vaccine against human papilloma virus has been shown to be effective for the prevention of cervical cancer. It is controversial, however, because it must be given to young girls before they become sexually active.

The extent to which chemicals in the environment cause cancer is one of the most difficult and controversial questions in public health. The tars in tobacco smoke are clearly a major cause, and the American Cancer Society estimates that almost one-third of cancer deaths in the United States are due to tobacco use.[20] In addition to being the major cause of lung cancer, smoking increases the risk of cancer in many other organs, including the mouth, nasal cavities, larynx, pharynx, esophagus, stomach, liver, pancreas, kidney, bladder, and cervix. Although Americans are greatly concerned about the possibility of cancer-causing chemicals in their food, water, or air, little is known about whether these sources contribute significantly to the number of cases diagnosed each year. Most industrial chemicals have not been tested for carcinogenicity. Chemicals added to food, however, must be tested.

The testing of chemicals for carcinogenicity in humans is fraught with difficulties. The standard, most definitive approach is a controlled experiment in which a large group of rats, mice, or guinea pigs is fed a diet containing the suspect chemical over their whole lifetime— about 2 years for these animals—and the incidence of tumors in this group is compared with that in an equivalent group of animals that did not receive the chemical. If the exposed animals have more tumors than the unexposed, the chemical is labeled a carcinogen. Aside from the potential frustration of the experiment by some unpredictable factor—for example, an outbreak of mouse flu that kills off all the animals after the first year, necessitating a new start—there are many reasons why this approach may not accurately predict carcinogenicity in humans. Differences in metabolism between mouse and human sometimes mean differences in carcinogenicity of a chemical in the two species; or the dose of the chemical necessary to produce a detectable increase in tumors may be so high that it disrupts the animals' metabolism, making the results meaningless.

Another approach to determining carcinogenicity—one that is much faster, simpler, and cheaper—is to test whether the chemical can cause mutations in a colony of cells growing in a laboratory dish. This test has its own drawbacks. While mutation is necessary for the development of cancer, not all chemicals that cause mutations are carcinogens. These test-tube experiments ignore the role of hormones and other secondary influences that determine whether a mutated cell will actually grow into a tumor.

Diabetes

The number of Americans diagnosed with diabetes is rising rapidly, having more than tripled in the past 20 years.[21] Officially, diabetes ranks seventh overall as a cause of death in the United States; it is fifth among blacks, Hispanics, and Asians, and fourth among American Indians.[22] However, there are reasons to believe that diabetes contributes to premature death more often than reported by death certificates. Examination of death certificates of people known to have diabetes have found that only 35 percent to 40 percent of them had diabetes listed anywhere on the certificate. Many deaths listed as caused by heart disease may be linked with diabetes. Heart disease death rates are two to four times higher for people with diabetes than for those without it. Overall, the risk of death for people with diabetes is double the risk for people of the same age who do not have diabetes.[23]

Diabetes is a major cause of disability. Although it is usually treatable and can be controlled over long periods of time, there has been little that public health could do to prevent the disease except to make unpopular recommendations for changes in lifestyle. The Centers for Disease Control and Prevention (CDC) refers to twin epidemics of diabetes and obesity,[24] because obesity greatly increases the risk of diabetes, and the number of Americans who are obese has been increasing rapidly.

Diabetes is a deficiency in the body's ability to metabolize sugar, a function that is normally controlled by the hormone insulin. There are two major forms of diabetes: type 1 diabetes, which usually has its onset in childhood, is caused by a failure of the insulin-producing cells of the pancreas; type 2 diabetes, more common with increasing age, is a more complex mix of impaired insulin production and resistance to the hormone's action. Both forms of diabetes are significantly affected by genetics. Research on the causes of diabetes has thus far yielded very little information on how type 1 diabetes could be prevented. Type 2 is closely correlated with obesity, and is largely preventable with proper diet and exercise. However, public health has not been very successful in persuading most people to adopt such healthy behaviors, which could prevent a number of other chronic diseases as well.

While public health may not be able to prevent diabetes, it is concerned with preventing the disability that is inevitable when the disease is not well controlled. An estimated one out of four people with diabetes are unaware that they have it.[23] This is a major public health problem because the high blood sugar that is typical of uncontrolled diabetes causes damage to blood vessels throughout the body, especially the eyes and kidneys. Complications of diabetes include blindness, kidney failure, cardiovascular disease, poor wound healing, and amputations of the extremities. Secondary prevention requires early diagnosis of the disease so that treatment can begin at an early stage. Lack of access to routine medical care—a common problem in the United States—contributes to the seriousness of diabetes as a public health problem. The necessary long-term monitoring and treatment required to manage a case of diabetes can be complicated and expensive, and those who need it the most may have the greatest difficulty in receiving care.

Other Chronic Diseases

There is much more to learn about other diseases that have a major impact on the health of the population. Mental illness is a major cause of disability in this country, and yet very little is known about its causes and prevention. Alzheimer's disease and other forms of dementia in older people cause anguish to their families and force affected people into nursing homes at a tremendous cost to society. The NIH and other funding sources are supporting a great deal of research on understanding genetic and other factors that affect people's risk of developing dementia as they age, but not much is known yet on how people can protect themselves. Arthritis, while not a major killer, can severely impact the quality of life for many older people, causing great pain and suffering in their last years.

Conclusion

Chronic diseases are the leading causes of death and disability in the United States, with cardiovascular diseases and cancer leading the list. Diabetes is becoming increasing prevalent and is a major cause of disability. Preventing these diseases—an important public health priority—is based on understanding their causes. The success of biomedical science and epidemiology in understanding causes of cardiovascular disease and how to prevent or delay its onset serves as a model for what society would hope to achieve for all the diseases that cause premature death or disability. Progress in understanding the functioning of normal cells and what goes wrong when they turn malignant gives researchers hope that they will eventually learn to prevent many kinds of cancer.

Despite the tremendous progress made by biomedical science in the understanding of the bases of chronic diseases, a great deal is left to learn about what can go wrong with the human body and how to prevent it. People cannot expect, and maybe would not wish, to live forever, but biomedical research holds the key to preventing many premature deaths, as well as much of the pain and anguish that many people suffer toward the end of their lives. Because it offers such hope, NIH's work is generally well supported by Congress and the American people.

References

1. J. Cohen, "Monkey Puzzles," *Science* 296 (2002): 2325–2326.
2. R. Ross, "The Pathogenesis of Atherosclerosis: A Perspective for the 1990s," *Nature* 362 (1993): 801–809.
3. W. F. Enos, Jr. et al., "Pathogenesis of Coronary Disease in American Soldiers Killed in Korea," *Journal of the American Medical Association* 158 (1955): 912–914.
4. H. C. McGill and C. A. McMahan, "Starting Earlier to Prevent Heart Disease," *Journal of the American Medical Association* 290 (2003): 2320–2322.
5. S. J. Dudrick et al., "Experimental and Clinical Atherosclerosis: Their Experimental Reversal," in R. C. Maulitz, ed., *Unnatural Causes: The Three Leading Killer Diseases in America* (New Brunswick, NJ: Rutgers University Press, 1989), 35–61.
6. D. J. Rader and A. Daugherty, "Translating Molecular Discoveries into New Therapies for Atherosclerosis," *Nature* 451 (2008): 904–913.

7. S. O'Connor et al., "Potential Infectious Etiologies of Atherosclerosis: A Multifactorial Perspective," *Emerging Infectious Diseases* 7 (2001): 780–788.

8. National Heart Lung and Blood Institute, "What Is Cholesterol?" http://www.nhlbi.nih .gov/health/health-topics/topics/hbc/, accessed June 16, 2012.

9. E. J. Topol, "Intensive Statin Therapy—A Sea Change in Cardiovascular Prevention," *New England Journal of Medicine* 350 (2004): 1562–1564.

10. Agency for Healthcare Quality and Research, "Trends in Statins Utilization and Expenditures for the U.S. Civilian Noninstitutionalized Population, 2000 and 2005." http://www.meps .ahrq.gov/mepsweb/data_files/publications/st205/stat205.pdf, accessed October 31, 2012.

11. G. Kolata, "A Broader Benefit Is Found in a Drug Against Cholesterol," *The New York Times*, May 27, 1998.

12. A. V. Chobanian et al., "Seventh Report of the Joint Commission on Prevention, Detection, Evaluation, and Treatment of High Blood Pressure," *Hypertension* 42 (2003): 1206–1252.

13. J. J. Nora et al., *Cardiovascular Diseases: Genetics, Epidemiology, and Prevention* (New York: Oxford University Press, 1991).

14. E. D. Frohlich, "The Salt Conundrum: A Hypothesis," *Hypertension* 50 (2007): 161–166.

15. National Heart, Lung and Blood Institute, "Who Is at Risk for High Blood Pressure?" http://www.nhlbi.nih.gov/health/health-topics/topics/hbp/atrisk.html, accessed September 23, 2012.

16. R. Collins et al., "Cigarette Smoking, Tar Yields, and Non-Fatal Myocardial Infarction," *British Medical Journal* 311 (1995): 471–477.

17. W. K. Cavenee and R. L. White, "The Genetic Basis of Cancer," *Scientific American* (March 1995): 50–57.

18. H. J. Burstein and R. S. Schwartz, "Molecular Origins of Cancer," *New England Journal of Medicine* 358 (2008): 527.

19. *The New Encyclopedia Britannica*, Vol. 3 (Chicago: Encyclopaedia Britannica, 1995), 799.

20. American Cancer Society, "Tobacco-Related Cancer Fact Sheet." http://www.cancer .org/docroot/PED/content/PED_10_2x_Tobacco-Related_Cancers_Fact_Sheet.asp?site, accessed September 23, 2012.

21. U.S. Centers for Disease Control and Prevention, "Long-Term Trends in Diagnosis of Diabetes." http://www.cdc.gov/diabetes/statistics/slides/long_term_trends.pdf, accessed June 16, 2012.

22. U.S. Centers for Disease Control and Prevention, "Health, United States, 2011," Table 26. http://www.cdc.gov/nchs/data/hus/hus11.pdf, accessed June 16, 2012.

23. U.S. Centers for Disease Control and Prevention, "National Diabetes Fact Sheet, 2011." http://www.cdc.gov/diabetes/pubs/pdf/ndfs_2011.pdf, accessed June 16, 2012.

24. U.S. Centers for Disease Control and Prevention, "Twin Epidemics of Diabetes and Obesity Continue to Threaten the Health of Americans CDC Says," press release. http://www.cdc .gov/media/pressrel/r010911.htm, accessed June 16, 2012.

Genetic Diseases and Other Inborn Errors

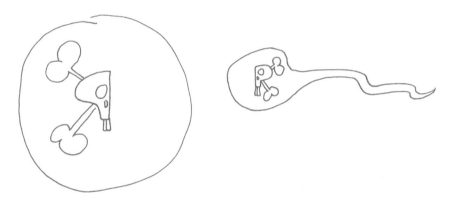

Bad Genes

Congenital defects are a major cause of death and disability in infants and children. Some 3 percent to 4 percent of newborns have a major abnormality apparent at birth. Other problems show up later; up to 7.5 percent of children are diagnosed with a congenital defect in their first 5 years.[1] Such abnormalities may be inherited in the child's genes, or they may be caused by birth injury or by the mother's exposure to an infectious agent or toxic substance during pregnancy. Genes also play a role in many diseases of later life.

Because the birth of healthy children has been a high priority traditionally for public health, education and prenatal care for pregnant women have been encouraged. As more has been learned about how certain infectious agents, drugs, and chemicals can cause birth defects, greater public health efforts have been directed toward preventing women's exposure to these substances. Until the past few decades, little could be done to prevent genetic abnormalities.

Now, however, technological developments have opened up vast possibilities in the detection of defective genes. These discoveries have had many clear benefits, but they have also raised many difficult ethical questions.

Environmental Teratogens

Birth defects may be caused by a variety of environmental agents, called teratogens, which include some bacteria and viruses, various drugs and chemicals, and radiation. Many teratogens are also carcinogens, capable of causing cancer. In some cases, the teratogenic effect, like the carcinogenic effect, is known to be the result of mutation in the DNA. However, much less is known about the disruptions of fetal development that lead to birth defects than is known about carcinogenesis.

Infectious diseases known to damage the fetus include syphilis, rubella (German measles), and toxoplasmosis. Congenital syphilis, caused by bacteria passed from a mother to her fetus through the placenta, was a devastating disease of newborns before penicillin was discovered. The disease damaged the infants' nerves, bones, and skin and often resulted in blindness and mental retardation. Beginning in the 1930s, many states required blood tests for syphilis—the Wasserman test—for all couples about to be married in an effort to identify and treat infected people before they could transmit the disease to a child.[2] Most states have discontinued that requirement.

Rubella, ordinarily a mild disease of childhood, causes profound deafness in children whose mothers were infected by the virus while pregnant. Routine vaccination of children against rubella accomplishes the longer-term purpose of immunizing childbearing women, and the incidence of congenital deafness has been dramatically reduced. Toxoplasmosis, a parasitic disease that may go unnoticed in adults, can cause major neurological damage in the fetus. Since cats are a reservoir for the parasite and the route of transmission is most commonly through cat feces, toxoplasmosis is best prevented by education—warning pregnant women about the risks of contracting the disease through gardening and contact with litter boxes.

A pregnant woman's exposure to teratogenic drugs and environmental chemicals can have very obvious results because the effects become apparent within 9 months, dramatically altering a young life. One memorable tragedy occurred in the 1950s at Minamata, Japan, where a plastics factory contaminated the bay with high levels of mercury. A highly toxic form of the mercury accumulated in the fish, the staple of the community's diet. While adults were relatively unaffected, many children were born with severe neurological deformities, including profound brain damage.[3] The tragedy of Minamata, captured by the famous photographs of W. Eugene Smith and Aileen M. Smith, accessible on the Internet, alerted the world to the dangers of environmental pollution.[4] Laws controlling air and water pollution and disposal of toxic wastes have been effective in preventing such disasters in the United States, but they continue to occur in other parts of the world, including the former Soviet Union.

Another famous teratogenic event was the epidemic of limb deformities that occurred in Europe and Australia in the early 1960s that was caused by the sedative thalidomide. Women who took the drug to relieve morning sickness gave birth to babies whose arms and legs were drastically shortened into flipper-like appendages.[3] The United States escaped the epidemic because one skeptical Food and Drug Administration (FDA) official, Dr. Frances Kelsey, was suspicious of the drug and resisted great pressure from the manufacturer before the dangers became apparent. In 1998, in a controversial decision, thalidomide was approved by the FDA as an effective treatment for leprosy and some forms of cancer. However, it can be used only under very strict regulations that require women taking it to undergo monthly pregnancy tests and to use two forms of birth control.[5]

One of the FDA's most important missions is to protect American citizens against such tragic side effects of drugs by prohibiting them entirely if their value is not judged to be worth the associated risks or by mandating clear communications about risks when there are also clear benefits. The antibiotic tetracycline, the anti-epilepsy drug Dilantin, the hormone diethylstilbestrol, and the acne medication Accutane are among the common prescription drugs that have been found by painful experience to cause birth defects. Pregnant women are now advised to refrain from taking any medication that is not absolutely necessary.

Alcohol was recognized to be a teratogen only in the 1970s. Although most cases of fetal alcohol syndrome have been identified in children of heavy drinkers, no level of alcohol has been judged safe for the fetus, and pregnant women are advised not to drink at all. Tobacco smoke increases the risk of premature birth and low birth weight, as well as sudden infant death syndrome. Cocaine and heroin use by pregnant women causes addiction in the fetus, bringing about painful withdrawal symptoms in the newborn and sometimes leaving permanent neurological damage.

Genetic Diseases

Essentially all the information required for the development of a new human being is contained in the genetic material located in the 46 chromosomes, half of which come from the mother's egg and half of which come from the father's sperm. Mistakes are common in the reproductive process. The most visible are chromosomal abnormalities, which can be seen under a microscope. Such defects cause a variety of malformations in the developing fetus, many of which are incompatible with survival. More than half of pregnancies in healthy women end in spontaneous abortion, and chromosomal abnormalities are obvious in many of these aborted fetuses.[1] When the affected fetus does survive, the disability is usually profound, almost always including mental retardation and often leading to early death. Down syndrome, caused by an extra copy of chromosome 21, is the best-known disorder of this type, largely because its effects are less lethal than those of other chromosomal defects, and most affected infants survive.

The majority of genetic diseases are caused by defects that are not visible under a microscope. Those that are best known and understood are caused by a defect in a single gene inherited more or less according to classical Mendelian genetics (see Figure 12-1). In the first part of the figure, the pattern of inheritance of a dominant gene is shown. The father carries the gene

Pattern of Inheritance of a Dominant Gene: Huntington's Disease

Father

	H	**h**
h	Hh	hh
h	Hh	hh

(Mother)

H = dominant gene for Huntington's disease
h = normal gene

The father carries the gene for Huntington's on one of a pair of chromosomes. The mother carries two normal genes. Half of the children will inherit the disease from the father.

Pattern of Inheritance of a Recessive Gene: Sickle-Cell Disease

Father

	S	**S**
S	*SS*	*S*S
S	*S*S	SS

(Mother)

S = recessive gene for sickle-cell disease
S = normal gene

Father and mother both carry one recessive gene. Neither parent has symptoms and they may be unaware they are carriers. One-quarter of the children will inherit two recessive genes and have the disease. One-half the children will be carriers.

FIGURE 12-1   Mendelian Genetics.

for Huntington's disease on one of a pair of chromosomes. The mother carries two normal genes. Half of the children will inherit the disease from the father. In the second part of the figure, the pattern of inheritance of a recessive gene is shown. Both parents carry one recessive gene, but neither parent has symptoms, and the parents may be unaware that they are carriers. One-quarter of the children will inherit two recessive genes and will have the disease. One-half the children will be carriers.

In sum, of the two copies of each gene that an individual inherits, one from each parent, the gene for a disease may be dominant or recessive. When the presence of a single copy is sufficient to cause the disease—an autosomal dominant disorder—the affected person will transmit that gene on average to half of his or her children. (Autosomal genes are on a nonsex chromosome.) Examples of autosomal dominant disorders are Huntington's disease, a midlife deterioration of the brain whose best-known victim was the folk singer Woody Guthrie; achondroplasia, a type of dwarfism made famous by the French painter Toulouse-Lautrec; and Marfan's syndrome, characterized by extreme height and cardiovascular abnormalities, which occasionally makes the news after the sudden death of an unsuspecting basketball player.[1]

Autosomal recessive disorders do not become obvious unless the individual inherits two copies of the gene. The disease may appear unexpectedly in a child of two parents who were unaware that they each carried one copy of the gene. The best-known autosomal recessive disorders tend to predominate in certain ethnic groups: Tay-Sachs disease in Jews of Eastern European descent, sickle-cell disease in Africans and African Americans, cystic fibrosis in people of northern European ancestry, and thalassemia in populations of Mediterranean or Asian descent.[1]

X-linked disorders, such as hemophilia and Duchenne's muscular dystrophy, are caused by a defective gene on the female sex chromosome, called the X chromosome. These diseases occur predominantly in males. Since females have two X chromosomes, inheritance of the defective gene has minimal impact on them because of the second, normal gene's presence. Males, who inherit an X chromosome from the mother and a Y chromosome from the father, can inherit the disease only from the mother.

While the patterns of inheritance are well established for many genetic diseases, new mutations may sometimes occur, affecting a child whose family has no history of the disease. Many autosomal dominant conditions cause such severe handicaps that the affected individuals are unable or unlikely to reproduce; for these conditions, the majority of cases arise from mutations. With recessive and X-linked genetic defects, birth of an affected infant into a family that lacks a history of the condition may or may not indicate that a new mutation has occurred. A recessive gene would not be apparent unless someone who carried it married another carrier. X-linked genes might not appear for several generations in small families or those in which most of the children happened to be girls.

Some genetic conditions vary in their impact depending on environmental factors. For example, anencephaly—the absence of a brain—and the related spinal-cord defect, spina bifida, appear to be the result of a combination of genetic and environmental factors. The incidence of these disorders has been found to vary by geographical area, a hint that further research will provide evidence that environmental factors are involved. One important finding is that if a woman takes dietary supplements of folic acid before conception and during early pregnancy, her infant's risk of these devastating conditions is substantially reduced.

Genetic makeup also influences people's susceptibility to most of the common diseases of adulthood; most of these diseases involve complex interactions between genes and the environment. Genes for cholesterol and other blood lipids affect an individual's risk of cardiovascular disease. High blood pressure has a genetic component. A variety of genes affect people's risk for various forms of cancer, including breast cancer and colorectal cancer. Susceptibility to diabetes is strongly influenced by genes. Knowing individuals' family health history can help determine whether they need more intensive screening for these diseases.

Mental disorders including schizophrenia, manic depression, and Alzheimer's disease are also believed to be affected by genetics, although the evidence is fragmentary. While it is well known that people with high cholesterol can lower their risk of heart disease or diabetes by exercising, eating a healthier diet and, if necessary, taking appropriate medications, current knowledge offers little guidance about how to counteract a family history of Alzheimer's disease or other mental disorders. One can only hope that, with advances in biomedical research, prevention will someday be possible.

Genetic and Newborn Screening Programs

Short of performing surgery on the genetic material, the public health mandate of preventing death and disability from many genetic diseases can be fulfilled only by predicting and preventing the birth of affected children. The process involves various methods of prenatal diagnosis and, when an affected fetus is identified, termination of the pregnancy. One of the most common genetic abnormalities, Down syndrome, is caused by an extra copy of chromosome 21. Affected individuals have a distinctive appearance and are likely to have heart defects and mild to moderate mental retardation. The risk of bearing an infant with the syndrome is well known to increase with the mother's age and, in the past, women age 35 and older were advised to undergo prenatal testing by amniocentesis, using a needle to sample fetal cells from the uterus. With the option of abortion available, this practice reduced the number of Down syndrome births by about 25 percent.[1] However, even though younger women have a lower risk, the number of infants born to them is much higher overall, and they bear most of the affected infants. The American College of Obstetricians and Gynecologists now recommends that all women be screened.[6] In the United States, about 90 percent of women who are found to be carrying an infant with Down syndrome choose to have an abortion.[7]

There is a more significant role for public health in the prevention of disorders that are caused by recessive genes. When the gene is known, members of populations that have a high incidence of a disease, such as Jews of Eastern European descent, can be screened for carrier status, allowing young people to make informed decisions about marriage and child bearing. In the 1970s, after the gene for Tay-Sachs disease was identified, a major voluntary program offered screening to Jewish people. The response was enthusiastic because the horror of the disease was well known: apparently healthy infants begin to deteriorate soon after birth, developing paralysis, dementia, and blindness, and die by age 3 or 4. Couples who are both Tay-Sachs carriers can choose to undergo prenatal testing by amniocentesis, allowing for termination of an affected pregnancy.[8]

However, religious Jews are opposed to abortion. An alternative approach is offered by an organization called Dor Yeshorim, established in the 1980s by a rabbi who had lost four children to Tay-Sachs. The organization offers Jewish high school students in the United States, Israel, and other countries blood tests to determine if they are carriers. To maintain anonymity, and to avoid the stigma of being labeled a carrier, each student is given an identification number and a telephone number that couples can call to learn whether they are genetically "compatible." In ultra-orthodox communities that practice arranged marriage, a confidential registry was established that allows matchmakers to avoid arranging marriages between carriers of Tay-Sachs and several other debilitating or lethal genetic diseases.[9] As a result of the availability of screening, the incidence of Tay-Sachs has been reduced by more than 90 percent in the United States and Canada.[8]

Another public health approach to preventing the death and disability caused by genetic diseases is provided by newborn screening for metabolic disorders that can be treated if diagnosed soon after birth. An estimated 5000 of the 4.1 million infants born in the United States each year have a potentially severe or lethal condition for which screening and treatment could prevent many or all of the complications.[10] The first such condition to be recognized was phenylketonuria (PKU), which was identified as the cause of mental retardation in a significant number of institutionalized adults. Biomedical scientists found that the problem was a genetic inability to metabolize the amino acid phenylalanine, which therefore accumulates in the blood with toxic effects on the brain. They recognized that if affected infants could be identified early they could be put on a special diet low in phenylalanine, and the damage would be prevented.

Dr. Robert Guthrie, a pediatrician from Buffalo, New York, who is considered the "father of newborn screening," developed a simple, inexpensive test that could diagnose PKU from a drop of a baby's blood placed on a piece of filter paper. Routine newborn screening for PKU began in the 1960s and is now mandated in all states and most developed countries. Before each baby is discharged from the hospital, the blood sample is obtained by a prick of the baby's heel. Filter paper specimens bearing the dried blood spots are sent to state public health laboratories for testing.[11]

A number of other inborn metabolic errors can be identified from testing the same dried drop of blood, and tests for these conditions are mandated by various states depending on the characteristics of their populations. In addition to PKU, all states screen for congenital hypothyroidism, a deficiency of thyroid hormone leading to mental retardation and dwarfism that can be easily treated with regular doses of the hormone. Many states screen for sickle-cell disease, prevalent in African-American populations, a program that raised ethical issues when first implemented, as discussed below. The newborn blood samples are used in some states to identify infants who may have been exposed to the human immunodeficiency virus (HIV) prenatally.

Laboratory tests used for newborn screening have become increasingly sophisticated. A method called tandem mass spectrometry searches for more than 20 metabolic disorders in one process, using the dried blood-spot specimen.[12] However, the technical ability to detect these disorders has confronted states with dilemmas of how extensively to implement screening for them. Resources are needed to follow up on an abnormal test result, including further testing to confirm the presence of a disease and counseling of parents and pediatricians about a condition that may be extremely rare. There are concerns about who is responsible for treating a disease that has been identified through screening. For example, the special diet required for infants with PKU may be considered a food rather than a drug and thus not be covered by a family's health insurance. For some conditions, no treatment exists. States differ not only on which conditions they screen for, but also on whether parental consent is required before screening, whether a fee is charged, and the extent of services provided for follow-up.[13]

The information gained from a genetic test or the screening of a newborn is not always so unambiguous as a fatal diagnosis of Tay-Sachs disease or a clear need for a special diet, as in PKU. With many conditions, uncertainties in the test results as well as in the prognosis complicate decision making. For example, cystic fibrosis (CF), which causes abnormal secretions of the lungs, pancreas, and sweat glands, is the second most common potentially lethal genetic diseases in the United States.[14] About 1 in 25 Caucasian Americans, the group at highest risk, carries the recessive gene, which has been identified. The screening test, which measures an enzyme in the blood, yields many false positives. Scientists learned that the accuracy of the diagnosis could be improved by following up the enzyme test with a test on the DNA. As scientists studied the gene, however, they found hundreds of different mutations that could cause CF, and there seemed to be little correlation between the mutation and the symptoms. While many patients with CF die young of breathing problems associated with thick mucus in the lungs, some individuals identified by genetic tests have much milder symptoms. Although only a few states now include CF in their newborn screening programs, a major clinical trial found that early identification of affected infants helped to prevent some of the nutritional deficits and deterioration of lung function suffered by children who were identified only when they developed symptoms at an older age.[14] The CDC now recommends screening for CF.

The identification of the CF gene allows prospective parents to be tested for carrier status, as in Tay-Sachs disease. However, in the case of CF, test results are not as clear. Each of the many possible mutations must be tested for individually, and it is not feasible for laboratories to test for all of them. Currently, the accepted approach for white Americans is to test for the 25 most common mutations. About 78 percent of carrier couples can be identified this way, but one in five couples with a normal test result is still at risk to bear a child with CF. The frequencies of mutations are different in other ethnic groups, and identification of carriers is even less reliable.[15]

In addition to the conditions that can be identified using the blood spot, the CDC recommends screening for hearing loss using computerized equipment now available in many hospitals. Profound and permanent congenital hearing loss is estimated to occur in approximately one in 1000 births. About half of these cases are thought to be due to genetic mutations, and about half are due to environmental factors, including prenatal drug exposures and infections such as rubella.[16]

Because of the variation from state to state in the number of disorders included in newborn screening programs, a federal advisory committee in 2006 recommended a panel of 29 disorders that all states should include in their newborn screening programs.[17] As of 2009, all the states had implemented the full screening panel.[18] A list of the metabolic conditions for which the CDC recommends screening is shown in Table 12-1. An additional two conditions have been added since then: severe combined immunodeficiency and critical congenital heart disease.

Table 12-1   Recommended Newborn Screening Panel and Estimated Number of U.S. Children Who Would Have Been Identified with Disorders in 2006

Disorder	Est. no. cases, 2006
Amino acid disorders	
Phenylketonuria (PKU)	215
Maple syrup urine disease	26
Homocystinuria	11
Citrullinemia 1	24
Argininosuccinic acidemia	7
Organic acid metabolism disorders	
Isovaleric acidemia	32
Glutaric acidemia type 1	38
Hydroxymethylglutaric aciduria	3
Multiple carboxylase deficiency	3

(Continued)

Table 12-1   Recommended Newborn Screening Panel and Estimated Number of U.S. Children Who Would Have Been Identified with Disorders in 2006 (*Continued*)

Disorder	Est. no. cases, 2006
Methylmalonic acidemia	62
3-Methylcrotonyl-CoA carboxylase deficiency	100
Proprionic acidemia	15
Beta-ketothiolase deficiency	7
Hemoglobinopathies	
Hb SS	1128
Hb SC	484
Hb S/beta thalassemia	163
Fatty Acid Oxidation Disorders	
Medium chain acyl-CoA dehydrogenase deficiency	239
Very long-chain acyl-CoA dehydrogenase deficiency	69
Long-chain 3-hydroxyacyl-CoA dehydrogenase deficiency	13
Trifunctional protein deficiency	2
Carnitine uptake defect	85
Other Disorders	
Primary congenital hypothyroidism	2156
Biotinidase deficiency	62
Congenital adrenal hyperplasia	202
Classical galactosemia	224
Cystic fibrosis	1248
Hearing loss	5073 (2009)
Total (all disorders, 2006)	**6439**

Source: Reproduced from U.S. Centers for Disease Control and Prevention, *Morbidity and Mortality Weekly Report* 61(2012): 390–393.

Genomic Medicine

The science underlying human genetics has made great advances over the past decade, facilitated by the federally sponsored Human Genome Project, which aims to analyze the whole of human DNA and make a map of all human genes. The successful identification of key genes has enabled many couples cursed with a family heritage of crippling disease to bear a healthy child. Most diseases of later life are more complex, not single-gene defects, and thus the presence or absence of a specific gene does not provide any definite predictions. Nevertheless, an individual's risks of developing some cancers, heart disease, diabetes, Alzheimer's disease, and other major afflictions of adulthood are closely tied to his or her genetic makeup. Knowledge of the genes can potentially provide benefits in preventing the diseases as well as better treatments when the individual becomes sick with one of these diseases later in life. The study of how genes act in the body, and how they interact with environmental influences to cause disease is called genomics, a science that promises to transform the prospects of medical practice and has major implications for public health.

There are many potential benefits of identifying genetic risks early in life. For example, scientists are investigating ways to prevent the onset of type 1 diabetes in children whose genes put them at high risk. Antibodies detectable in the blood of these children attack and ultimately destroy the insulin-producing cells of the pancreas, but there is hope of disrupting this process with appropriate drugs or immune modifiers. If these experiments are successful, diabetes risk could be included in newborn screening programs, and treatment could avert the need for lifelong insulin therapy and lifestyle modifications.[19]

Genes have been identified that significantly increase a woman's risk of breast cancer. The BRCA1 and BRCA2 genes can be screened for, but they account for a relatively small percentage of breast cancer; these genes also increase the risk of ovarian cancer. Genetic screening may benefit women who have a family history of breast cancer, especially when the cancer occurs at an early age, as tends to happen with inherited BRCA mutations. Women who inherit these mutations are advised to undergo more intensive and frequent breast exams than average and to begin this screening when they are younger. The most effective intervention currently available for BRCA carriers is the surgical removal of a woman's breasts and ovaries. Scientists hope that, in the future, a better understanding of the genes' actions may lead to less drastic therapy.[20]

Scientists have mapped more than 3 million places along the human genome where individuals or populations may differ in a base pair. These places are known as single-nucleotide polymorphisms (SNPs), and the chart of where they are located is called the HapMap. Numerous studies are underway attempting to find links between specific SNPs and risks of various diseases. In most cases, the difference in risk is relatively small. This has not stopped companies from patenting and commercializing the tests. Several companies are now offering "gene profiles," promising that if a customer sends a cheek swab and a fee, he or she will receive a readout of his or her risk of diseases such as diabetes, heart disease, and various forms of cancer. Most knowledgeable scientists believe that these promises are overblown, for several reasons.[21]

First, because these tests are not regulated, their validity and accuracy are unreliable. Second, the science of predicting susceptibility to these complex diseases based on the presence of specific genes is still at an early stage. The risk detected by the tests does a poor job of distinguishing people who will develop the disease from those who will not. Third is the question of what can be done for a person who has been found at increased risk. There is an argument that knowledge of an increased susceptibility to a disease might motivate people to practice a healthier lifestyle. For example, a person with a genetic susceptibility to lung cancer might be more likely to quit smoking, or individuals at risk of diabetes might increase their physical activity. However, there is little evidence that people do respond in this way. Certainly, a concerned individual would be better off spending his money on a gym membership than a genetic profile. From a public health perspective, it makes more sense to promote healthy behaviors for everyone.[22]

Findings from the Human Genome Project are expected to have major implications for the use of drugs in the treatment of diseases. A great deal is being learned about how genes affect the metabolism of various drugs. It has been known for some time that different individuals may respond to some drugs in different ways. Medicines that are dramatically effective in some patients may be ineffective in others with the same disease and may cause major side effects in still others. It is becoming possible to predict which patients will respond to a drug and even to determine that some patients may require higher or lower doses of the drug than others. Scientists are also able to design drugs for specific patients depending on their genetic makeup. Cancer therapy is especially suitable for targeted drug therapy: already there have been successes in blocking tumor growth using specially designed drugs that attack cellular mechanisms specific to certain mutations. Lives of patients with leukemia, gastric cancer, melanoma, and colon cancer have been extended with such drugs.[23]

Ethical Issues and Genetic Diseases

There has been great excitement about the potential uses of genetics and genomics in preventing and treating disease. However, the discoveries have opened a Pandora's box of ethical, legal, social, and scientific questions.

There are lessons to be learned from the mistakes made in early attempts to screen for sickle-cell disease, a disorder of hemoglobin, the oxygen-carrying protein in the blood. In this disease, painful crises of impaired blood circulation occur in individuals who have inherited two copies of the recessive gene, which was identified in the 1970s. However, well-meaning attempts to initiate screening programs for sickle-cell disease, inspired by the success of Tay-Sachs screening in Jews, caused widespread confusion and ill feeling among African Americans, the group at highest risk for carrying the sickle-cell gene. The meaning of the tests was not understood, and many people who were healthy carriers of one gene were discriminated against in school and in employment and were denied health insurance. Many African Americans became suspicious that the intent of the program was genocidal.[24] Considerable time, effort, and money were required to overcome the early mistakes. Now, most states include sickle-cell disease in their newborn screening programs. While there is no cure for sickle-cell disease, infant and childhood mortality is reduced by prophylactic treatment with penicillin, which prevents infections associated with the crises.[25]

Difficult questions always arise when a serious disorder is diagnosed in a fetus or the genetic potential for such a problem is recognized in the parents. Aborting a fetus with a genetic or teratogenic abnormality is often the only alternative to the birth of a child with a handicap. Many Americans are uncomfortable with, if not morally opposed to, abortion. However, attitudes vary with the severity of the abnormality: most people would support the parents' decision to abort a fetus with anencephaly, the absence of a brain, a condition that is rapidly and inevitably lethal. The acceptability of a Down syndrome child varies significantly among prospective parents; some couples choose abortion, while others are happy to have the child.

Matters become even more complicated when the genes being identified are those that are known to cause diseases of later life. One of the cruelest of these is Huntington's disease, a single-gene defect in which symptoms first appear between the ages of 30 and 50. During the next 10 to 20 years, the disease progresses toward death, with symptoms that include extreme involuntary movements, intellectual deterioration, and psychiatric disturbances. Because Huntington's disease is inherited in an autosomal dominant fashion, each child of an affected individual has a 50 percent chance of developing the disease. Although a test is now available that allows individuals to learn whether they carry the gene and are thus destined to develop the symptoms, many people who are at risk have decided they would prefer not to know. The psychological impact of such knowledge can be devastating, and the potential for being denied insurance or employment is significant. On the other hand, individuals with a family history of Huntington's disease may wish to know whether they carry the gene before deciding whether to beget children.[26]

There is a fine line between the worthy goal of preventing disease and disability and the use of genetic screening and abortion to select desirable traits and eliminate undesirable ones from the gene pool. The former is part of the mission of public health, but the latter comes dangerously close to the kind of eugenics practiced by Nazi Germany. The Human Genome Project set aside 3 percent to 5 percent of its funding to study the many social, ethical, and legal dilemmas that result from better understanding of human heredity. Since genetic screening first became possible in the 1960s, various groups have proposed guidelines for how screening should be done and who should be screened. Most of the principles are consistent with the recommendations proposed by an Institute of Medicine committee, which include the following:

- Newborn screening should be done only when there is a clear indication of benefit to the newborn, when a system is in place to confirm the diagnosis, and when treatment and follow-up are available for affected infants.
- Carrier identification programs should be voluntary and confidential, and they should include counseling about all choices available to the identified carriers.

- Prenatal diagnosis should include education and counseling before and after the test, informing the parents about risks and benefits of the testing procedure and the alternatives available to them.
- All tests should be of high quality, because life and death decisions are based on the results. New tests should be evaluated by the FDA, and there should be more government oversight of laboratory proficiency.
- There should be more education for the general public about genetics.[27]

With the increasing availability of genetic tests, there is great concern about how the information will be used. The knowledge can help individuals and their doctors make informed decisions about their lifestyle and medical care. However, there has been great concern about harmful consequences, for example if insurance companies use the information to deny coverage or prospective employers deny employment to individuals who may be more vulnerable in the work environment or who may potentially be more expensive to insure. According to some estimates, every individual carries at least 5 to 10 genes that could make him or her sick under the wrong circumstances or could adversely affect his/her children.[9] All people have an interest in ensuring that any knowledge about their genetic makeup will be used to do them good and not harm. In 2008, Congress passed and President Bush signed the Genetic Information Nondiscrimination Act, which prohibits discrimination by health insurers or employers on the basis of DNA. Part of the justification for the law was that some people might otherwise avoid getting genetic tests that could benefit their health. Another benefit is that the law would encourage people to be more willing to participate in research studies without fear that their genetic information might be used against them.[28]

From a public health perspective, there is danger that the enthusiasm for genomics may deflect attention and resources from the important mission of preventing disease in the population. Although individuals differ in their genetic susceptibility to the most common diseases, these diseases are associated with well-known environmental and behavioral risks that are traditional targets of public health intervention. Smoking, for example, increases risk for heart disease, several kinds of cancer, and a number of other diseases. To reduce smoking in the whole population is a far more efficient and effective approach to improving the population's health than attempts to identify risk genes in individual smokers. There is a place for genomics in understanding the biological basis of diseases that cannot be prevented with existing knowledge, such as breast cancer, type 1 diabetes, and Alzheimer's disease. However, many public health advocates believe that resources would be better spent on research and interventions aimed at modifying health-related behaviors, including smoking, diet and physical activity patterns, and sexual behavior.[29]

According to one skeptical epidemiologist, the benefits of genomics are likely to be greatest for treatment rather than prevention, and "our resources allocated to treatment already massively outweigh those spent for disease prevention."[30]

Conclusion

People's health is determined significantly by their genes, and sometimes by prenatal exposure to infectious agents and toxic substances. Public health measures can sometimes prevent unfortunate health outcomes caused by genes or by exposures before birth.

A number of bacteria, viruses, and parasites are known to damage a developing fetus. Immunization of children against some of these infectious agents prevents infections from affecting future generations. Some chemical substances, including several well-known prescription drugs as well as alcohol and illegal drugs, can also cause birth defects. Public health efforts to prevent these exposures include environmental protection and regulation by the FDA.

With increasing knowledge about the genetic basis of some diseases, public health is able to take some actions to minimize their impact. Some conditions, such as Down syndrome, can be easily detected during pregnancy, permitting parents to choose whether to bear an affected child. For a few notorious diseases in children who receive a defective gene from each parent, such as Tay-Sachs and sickle-cell disease, prevention involves screening at-risk populations, allowing potential parents to choose whether to conceive an affected child. A major public health effort is focused on diagnosing severe metabolic disorders that can be treated if detected soon after birth. All states have newborn screening programs that test dried spots of blood taken from each infant soon after birth.

The increasing knowledge about the role of genetics in health and the growing capacity to test for individuals' genetic makeup raise many ethical issues concerning how the information should be used and whether application of this knowledge will divert resources from public health's mission of preventing disease in the whole population.

References

1. P. A. Baird and C. R. Scriver, "Genetics and the Public Health," in J. M. Last and R. B. Wallace, eds., *Maxcy-Rosenau Public Health and Preventive Medicine* (Norwalk, CT: Appleton and Lange, 1992), 983–994.
2. R. R. Faden et al., *AIDS, Women, and the Next Generation* (New York: Oxford University Press, 1991), 62.
3. A. Nadakavukaren, *Our Global Environment: A Health Perspective*, 6th ed. (Long Grove, IL: Waveland Press, 2006).

4. W. E. Smith and A. M. Smith, "Minamata," slides. aileenarchive.or.jp/minamata_en/slides/swf.html, accessed June 16, 2012.

5. National Library of Medicine, "Thalidomide: Warning." http://www.ncbi.nlm.nih.gov/pubmedhealth/PMH0001053/, accessed June 17, 2012.

6. American College of Obstetricians and Gynecologists, "New Recommendations for Down Syndrome Call for Offering Screening to All Pregnant Women." http://www.acog.org/About_ACOG/News_Room/News_Releases/2006/New_Recommendations_for_Down_Syndrome, accessed June 17, 2012.

7. C. Mansfield et al., "Termination Rates After Prenatal Diagnosis of Down Syndrome, Spina Bifida, Anencephaly, and Turner and Klinefelter Sydromes: A Systematic Literature Review," *Prenatal Diagnosis* 19 (1999): 808–812.

8. M. M. Kaback, "Population-Based Genetic Screening for Reproductive Counseling: The Tay-Sachs Model," *European Journal of Pediatrics* 159 (Suppl. 3) (2000): S102–S195.

9. A. George, "The Rabbi's Dilemma," *New Scientist*. http://www.newscientist.com/article/mg18124345.400-the-rabbis-dilemma/html, accessed June 17, 2012.

10. M. Mitka, "Newborn Screening Bill," *Journal of the American Medical Association* 299 (2008): 2141.

11. R. Guthrie, "Newborn Screening: Past, Present, and Future," in T. Carter and A. M. Willey, eds., *Genetic Disease Screening and Management* (New York: Alan R. Liss, 1986), 318–339.

12. U.S. Centers for Disease Control and Prevention, "Using Tandem Mass Spectrometry for Metabolic Disease Screening Among Newborns," *Morbidity and Mortality Weekly Report* 50 (RR03) (2001): 1–22.

13. American Academy of Pediatrics Newborn Screening Task Force, "Serving the Family from Birth to the Medical Home," *Pediatrics* 106 (2000): 389–422.

14. U.S. Centers for Disease Control and Prevention, "Newborn Screening for Cystic Fibrosis: Evaluation of Benefits and Risks and Recommendations for State Newborn Screening Programs," *Morbidity and Mortality Weekly Report* 53 (RR-13) (2004).

15. L. A. Bradley and I. Lubin, "Carrier Testing for Cystic Fibrosis: Transition from Research to Clinical Practice," in Centers for Disease Control and Prevention, Office of Genomics and Disease Prevention, *Genomics and Population Health: United States 2003* (Atlanta, GA: 2004).

16. American Academy of Pediatrics, "Newborn Screening Fact Sheets," *Pediatrics* 118 (2006): e940–e942.

17. U.S. Centers for Disease Control and Prevention, "Impact of Expanded Newborn Screening—United States, 2006," *Morbidity and Mortality Weekly Report* 57 (2008): 1012–1015.

18. U.S. Centers for Disease Control and Prevention, "C.D.C. Grand Rounds: Newborn Screening and Improved Outcomes," *Morbidity and Mortality Weekly Report* 61 (2012): 390–393.

19. E. A. M. Gale, "Can We Change the Course of Beta-Cell Destruction in Type 1 Diabetes?" *New England Journal of Medicine* 346 (2002): 1740–1741.

20. J. Couzin, "Choices—and Uncertainties—for Women with BRCA Mutations," *Science* 302 (2003): 592.

21. E. Pennisi, "Breakthrough of the Year: Human Genetic Variation," *Science* 318 (2007): 1842–1843.

22. D. J. Hunter et al., "Letting the Genome out of the Bottle—Will We Get Our Wish?" *New England Journal of Medicine* 358 (2008): 105–107.

23. A. Pollack, "Drugs May Turn Cancer into Manageable Disease," *The New York Times*, June 6, 2004.

24. J. Rennie, "Grading the Gene Tests," *Scientific American* (June 1994): 89–97.

25. U.S. Centers for Disease Control and Prevention, "Mortality Among Children with Sickle Cell Disease Identified by Newborn Screening During 1990–1994—California, Illinois, and New York," *Morbidity and Mortality Weekly Report* 47 (1998): 169–172.

26. National Institute of Neurological of Neurological Disorders and Stroke, "Huntington's Disease: Hope Through Research." http://www.ninds.nih.gov/disorders/huntington/detail_huntington.htm#160513137, accessed June 17, 2012.

27. U.S. Institute of Medicine, Committee on Assessing Genetic Risks, *Assessing Genetic Risks: Implications for Health and Social Policy* (Washington, DC: National Academies Press, 1994).

28. National Institutes of Health, National Human Genome Research Institute, "Genetic Information Nondiscrimination Act of 2008." http://www.genome.gov/10002328, accessed June 17, 2012.

29. K. R. Merikangas and N. Rich, "Genomic Priorities and Public Health," *Science* 302 (2003): 599–601.

30. W. C. Willett, "Balancing Life-Style and Genomics Research for Disease Prevention," *Science* 296 (2002): 695–598.

Social and Behavioral Factors in Health

Do People Choose Their Own Health?

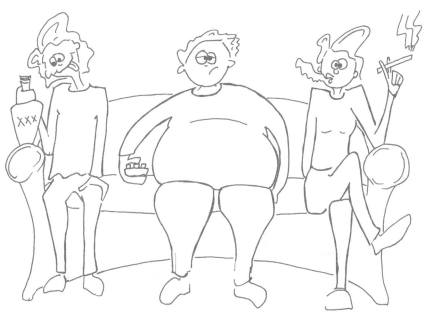

The Leading Causes of Death

Early successes of public health, in its mission to prevent death and disability, often came from focusing on specific diseases or groups of diseases, seeking particular causes, and finding ways to interrupt the cause-and-effect relationships. This approach was validated in the early 20th century by victories over infectious diseases. Public health professionals learned to break the chains of infection, most often by removing etiologic agents (bacteria, viruses, parasites) from the environment (water, food) or by developing vaccines to immunize potential hosts.

As infectious diseases were brought under control and as chronic diseases became more significant as causes of death and disability, it became increasingly apparent that the challenges faced by public health regarding chronic diseases would be more complex. Compare the leading causes of death in the United States in 1900 with those in 2008, as shown in Table 13-1 and Table 13-2. The top three killers of 1900, which were of infectious origin, have moved down or disappeared from the 2008 list, while heart disease has moved from fourth to first and cancer from eighth to second. The diseases at the top of the 2008 list have complex causes and most have no clear etiologic agent. Despite decades of biomedical research, there are no vaccines or environmental solutions to the problems of cancer and heart disease.

Table 13-1   Leading Causes of Death in the United States, 1900

Cause	% of All Deaths
Pneumonia and influenza	11.8
Tuberculosis (all forms)	11.3
Diarrhea, enteritis, ulceration of intestines	8.3
Diseases of the heart	8.0
Intracranial lesions of vascular origin	6.2
Nephritis	5.2
All accidents	4.2
Cancer and other malignant tumors	3.7
Senility	2.9
Diphtheria	2.3

Source: Reproduced from National Center for Health Statistics, "Leading Causes of Death, 1900–1998," page 67. www.cdc.gov/nchs/data/dvs/lead1900_98.pdf, accessed October 1, 2012.

Table 13-2   Leading Causes of Death in the United States, 2008

Cause	Number of Deaths	% of All Deaths
Diseases of heart	616,828	25.0
Malignant neoplasms (cancer)	565,469	22.9
Chronic lower respiratory diseases	141,090	5.7
Cerebrovascular diseases	134,148	5.4
Unintentional injuries	121,902	4.9
Alzheimer's disease	82,435	3.3
Diabetes	70,553	2.9
Influenza and pneumonia	56,284	2.3
Kidney diseases	48,237	2.0
Suicide	36,035	1.5

Source: Reproduced from National Center for Health Statistics. *Health, United States, 2011.* www.cdc.gov/nchs/data/hus/hus11.pdf, Table 26, May 2012, accessed October 1, 2012.

In 1990, a group of public health experts from the Centers for Disease Control and Prevention (CDC) decided that they should look at the data in a different way. They observed that the leading causes were not, in fact, root causes but were merely the diagnoses identified at the time of death. These diseases result from a combination of inborn (largely genetic) and external factors. The panel of experts undertook to identify, where possible, the underlying causes of death from each of the leading diseases. They came up with a list of nongenetic factors that they called the leading actual causes of death.[1] While the mortality figures are only estimates, they are based on the best data available. These factors are highly significant for public health because they are preventable causes of death and disability and because they provide targets for public health intervention. In 2000, CDC scientists repeated the analysis with new data and found some changes, although the order of importance is almost the same.[2] Table 13-3 shows the leading actual causes of death in 2000.

Tobacco was found to be the leading actual cause of death in the United States. According to the study, tobacco accounts for 30 percent of all cancer deaths and 21 percent of cardiovascular disease deaths. In addition, it causes chronic obstructive lung disease, infant deaths due to low birth weight, and burns due to accidental fires. Of the 435,000 deaths attributed to tobacco smoking, 35,000 were caused by second-hand smoke.

Poor diet and physical inactivity are listed as the second most important actual cause of death. These two factors are closely related to each other, with overeating and inactivity combining to lead to obesity. Dietary fat, sedentary behavior, and obesity have all been associated with

Table 13-3 Actual Causes of Death in the United States, 2000

Cause	Number of Deaths	% of All Deaths
Tobacco	435,000	18.1
Poor diet and physical inactivity	365,000	15.2
Alcohol consumption*	85,000	3.5
Microbial agents	75,000	3.1
Toxic agents	55,000	2.3
Motor vehicle	43,000	1.8
Firearms	29,000	1.2
Sexual behavior	20,000	0.8
Illicit drug use	17,000	0.7

*16,653 deaths from alcohol-related crashes are included in both alcohol consumption and motor vehicle death categories.

Source: Reproduced from A.H. Mokdad, J.S. Marks, D.F. Stroup, and J.L. Gerberding, "Actual Causes of Death in the United States, 2000," *Journal of the American Medical Association* 291 (2004): 1238–1245; 298, Table 1.

heart disease, stroke, several forms of cancer, and diabetes. The number of deaths attributed to this factor increased by 22 percent from the 1990 estimates, the largest change among all actual causes of death. The prevalence of overweight and obesity among Americans increased dramatically during the 1990s and continues to increase.

In 2005, an analysis by scientists from the CDC and the National Cancer Institute found fault with the calculations of obesity as a leading cause of death.[3] The new calculations, using different statistical methods, led to the conclusion that being moderately overweight was actually protective, especially in older people, although obesity still caused premature deaths. The publication of this study prompted great glee among critics of the "health police" and libertarians who object to being told what to do by the government. It is not clear why this analysis produced such different conclusions from the previous ones. The evidence is still strong that excess weight increases risks for heart disease, diabetes, high blood pressure, and some kinds of cancer. One possible explanation for the new findings is that medical care has become increasingly effective in preventing deaths from these diseases. Despite the controversy, public health professionals continue to regard excess weight and obesity as a major threat to people's health.

Misuse of alcohol was listed as the third actual cause of death, causing 35 percent to 40 percent of motor vehicle fatalities, as well as chronic liver disease and cirrhosis, home injuries, drowning, fire fatalities, job injuries, and 3 percent to 5 percent of cancer deaths.[2] Alcohol consumption by people under 21, the legal drinking age, is associated with many health and social problems, including alcohol-impaired driving, physical fighting, poor school performance, sexual activity, and smoking. Underage drinking to excess contributes to more than 4600 deaths in the United States each year.[4]

Number four on the list—microbial agents—encompasses the top three killers of 1900. The fact that mortality from infectious diseases has become so much less significant is testimony to public health's successes. As discussed previously, however, infectious diseases have by no means been conquered, and they could move to a higher position on the list in the future.

The fact that toxic agents are listed fifth as an actual cause of death is evidence of successes in environmental health. The list's authors call this figure the most uncertain; environmental threats may actually belong farther up the list. Certainly, environmental pollution is much more significant as a cause of death in the former Soviet Union, where environmental health has not been given the priority it has in the United States.

Firearms, sexual behavior, motor vehicles, and the illicit use of drugs round out the list. The authors, recognizing that some deaths may have multiple causes, choose what they believe to be the most significant. For example, they attribute most AIDS deaths to sexual behavior or drug use, although they recognize of course that a microbial agent is involved. The number of deaths attributed to these actual causes has declined since 1990 because of improved treatments for human immunodeficiency virus (HIV). Deaths from alcohol-related motor vehicle crashes have also declined since 1990, largely due to better enforcement of drunk-driving laws.[2]

These nine actual causes of death account for approximately 50 percent of all deaths in the United States. The other half includes genetic factors, which were specifically excluded from the analysis, and other less clearly identifiable causes. Lack of access to health care was cited as a significant factor. Presumably, many deaths could legitimately be attributed to old age. The nine identified factors are of particular public health significance because they cause premature deaths; they are often preceded by impaired quality of life; and many could be prevented by public health measures.

In trying to prevent premature death and disability, public health must focus on these nine factors. Two of them—microbial agents and toxic agents—have traditionally been public health issues. The other seven are rooted in the behavioral choices of individuals. This is the biggest challenge now faced by public health. How can people be persuaded to behave in healthier ways in a democratic society, where every step is fraught with political, economic, and moral controversy?

There are two obvious approaches that the government has traditionally taken to promote healthy behavior: education and regulation. Both of these approaches have had successes and both have had failures. Both continue to be important components of public health's struggle to accomplish its mission.

Education

Most simply, education informs the public about healthy and unhealthy behavior. Many people who are concerned about their health and that of their families do in fact adjust their behavior in accordance with new information. For example, the 1964 surgeon general's report called *Smoking and Health*,[5] the first authoritative statement from the federal government that smoking caused cancer and other life-threatening diseases, had a significant impact on the prevalence of smoking in the United States. Many people quit the habit after learning the information, and the prevalence of smoking began to decline for the first time after 1964.

Information on healthful eating habits has traditionally been provided by the federal government. In the early 20th century, concern focused on nutritional deficiencies, and the government conducted research on requirements for various vitamins and minerals, leading to listings of recommended dietary allowances or daily values. The educational process was furthered by Food and Drug Administration (FDA) requirements for labeling of prepared foods, which must accurately identify the percentage of the daily value provided by each serving.

While the prevention of nutritional deficiencies is still a valid concern, especially among the poor, the focus of government educational programs on nutrition has shifted to the prevention of the major killers—cancer, cardiovascular disease, and diabetes, which tend to be associated with nutritional excesses. Research over the past several decades has led to a greater understanding of the importance of overall dietary pattern in the onset of these diseases. The government's educational efforts have stressed the importance of eating less fat (especially saturated fat), less salt, and more fruits, vegetables, and grains. The FDA has revised its labeling requirements to provide consumers with the information that will allow them to follow its guidelines. There is evidence that Americans have responded to the message that they should cut down on fat in their diet and that this behavior may have helped bring down the high rates of heart disease over the past 30 years.

Results of efforts to modify dietary and smoking behaviors, while showing some success, also illustrate the limitations of the educational approach. The impact of both messages has been limited. While the percentage of Americans who smoke has declined, almost one in five adults maintains the habit despite widespread knowledge about the dangers of tobacco.[6] Evidence of dietary improvement is difficult to verify, since surveys of people's eating habits are notoriously unreliable. While the decline in heart disease is encouraging, the prevalence of obesity has increased, casting doubt on the extent to which Americans have really improved their eating habits.

Educational efforts to modify health-related behavior can be controversial, even when the messages seem benign and obvious. For decades the tobacco industry used all its political and economic power to dispute the evidence that smoking was harmful. Even the government's policy on diet has generated opposition, for example, from the meat industry, which has fought to delay the release of proposed recommendations that people eat less meat and more fruits, vegetables, and grains—recommendations that, if widely followed, would financially harm the industry.[7] Similarly, the sugar industry has fought government recommendations that people should reduce sugar in the diet.[8]

The educational messages most guaranteed to generate controversy, however, are those concerning sexual behavior. American attitudes about sex are notoriously ambivalent. Though movies and television shows frankly depict sexual activity, many people are puritanically reluctant to talk about how people can protect themselves against the natural consequences of that activity: unintended pregnancy and sexually transmitted diseases. For example, the tenure of Joycelyn Elders as President Clinton's surgeon general was extremely controversial because she spoke out openly on these issues, recommending condom use and masturbation, until she was forced by political pressures to resign her office.

Schools are naturally a prime site for health education programs. The goal is to teach children from an early age how to live healthy lives, providing information, for example, on diet, exercise, and the dangers of smoking, alcohol use, and drug abuse. Studies have shown that school education programs are effective in teaching children the facts about health and safety. It is less clear, however, that they actually influence young people to behave in healthier ways.

Sex education in the schools is highly controversial. Opponents have argued for years that teaching young people about sex encourages them to indulge in immoral behavior. When AIDS came along, the controversy became more intense because it meant that sexual behavior could be a matter of life and death. Many proponents of explicit education about safe sex argue that young people have sex no matter what they are taught and that they should be informed about how to protect themselves. Opponents argue that condoms are only partially effective in preventing pregnancy and sexually transmitted diseases and that young people should be taught that they can protect themselves only by abstinence. This was the policy of the Bush administration, which allocated hundreds of millions of dollars of federal funds for abstinence-only education. Many of these programs commonly contained multiple scientific and medical inaccuracies. According to Richard Daines, the New York State Commissioner of Health, "the Bush administration's abstinence-only program is an example of a failed national health-care policy directive, based on ideology rather than on sound scientific evidence that must be the cornerstone of good public health-care policy."[9]

In fact, a number of studies have shown that students who have received comprehensive sex education in school delay initiation of sex, reduce the number of partners, and are more likely to use contraception when they do have sex.[8] And while the use of condoms cannot guarantee protection against pregnancy and HIV transmission, condoms do reduce risk. Nevertheless, the controversy continues in many communities. The decision on what students should be taught about sex is made by local school boards and depends on "community standards."

An extension of the educational approach to changing behavior is the use of advertising to reinforce the public health message. Most people are subjected to large doses of media messages promoting unhealthy behavior, including cigarette ads in magazines, beer commercials on television, and movie portrayals of unsafe sex. The occasional public service announcements meant to convey countervailing messages are feeble weapons in the battle for public health, although there is evidence that counter advertising about the dangers of smoking helped to reduce smoking rates in the 1960s. The "Just Say No" antidrug campaign during the Reagan administration was strong enough to make an impression; whether it persuaded people to change their behavior is doubtful. Recently there have been efforts to develop more effective approaches to conveying public health messages in the media. One of these was the successful Harvard School of Public Health campaign to persuade several television producers to write "designated drivers" into their sitcom scripts as a way of advocating an alternative to drinking and driving.[10]

Another variation on health education that has become popular with college administrators to curb high-risk student drinking is the social norms approach. This approach is based on an influential study from the 1980s, which surveyed students about their perception of the frequency and amount of drinking among their peers. It turned out that students generally believed that other students drank more than they actually did. The remedy to the misperception that "everyone is doing it" is to advertise the actual norms on campus. Institutions could reduce high-risk drinking by up to 20 percent over a relatively short period of time by conducting surveys on campus and advertising the results.[11] Although use of the social norms approach is in an early stage, its proponents believe it can be used for a variety of other issues, such as tobacco prevention, seat-belt use, and prevention of high-risk sexual activity.

Health education messages may also be delivered by a medical professional during an office visit. Doctors who care for people with chronic diseases such as diabetes and asthma know that they can keep their patients healthier if they include a health education component in their treatment plans. Studies have shown that, while patients do not always follow the doctor's orders, a physician's recommendation can increase the likelihood that people will change their behavior.[12]

Public health's mission is to prevent disease, while medicine traditionally focuses more on treatment and cure. However, the fact that the medical profession can—and often does—play an important role in communicating public health messages about healthy behavior means that public health has a role to play in educating medical providers about health risks and health-related behaviors.

Regulation

Governments have always regulated people's behavior by passing and enforcing laws. The regulatory approach is clearly warranted when its intent is to restrain people from harming others. Laws against murder and assault are in effect public health laws, and there is no question about their legitimacy. Traffic laws—also aimed at protecting public health—are clearly accepted as necessary. Though not scrupulously obedient, everyone recognizes the importance of stopping at red lights, keeping to the right side of the road (in the United States), and driving at speeds appropriate to the conditions.

Most states have laws concerning alcohol and tobacco use aimed at protecting the public's health. Laws against drunk driving are clearly justified as a means of protecting others. Laws that regulate smoking in indoor public places are also justified on the basis that smokers create a health hazard by polluting the air that others must breathe. Most adults agree with laws aimed at preventing children and teenagers from behaving in ways that may harm their health, such as restrictions on access to alcohol and tobacco. The greatest controversy about governmental attempts to regulate behavior arises when these efforts are perceived as interfering with a mature individual's freedom to take risks with his or her own health. Laws requiring seat-belt use or motorcycle helmets, accordingly, are less well accepted than speed limits.

Controversy over public health laws is not new. In the 19th century, major controversies raged in Britain and the United States over laws requiring immunization against smallpox. In the United States the matter was decided in the 1905 Supreme Court decision *Jacobson v. Commonwealth of Massachusetts*, which upheld that state's right to require vaccination "for the common good."[13]

Another hot issue in the 19th century, both in Britain and the United States, was the control of venereal diseases, a campaign fraught with moral and social implications that presaged more recent controversies over AIDS. In Britain, a series of Contagious Diseases Acts were passed in the 1860s and 1870s, providing for compulsory medical examinations of known and suspected prostitutes and detention of those found to carry disease. Such laws were justified by arguing that venereal diseases were a national defense issue: military recruits affected by syphilis and gonorrhea would be unfit for service. Proponents also argued that irresponsible men, infected by prostitutes, carried diseases home to their innocent wives. It was especially urgent to prevent the spread of syphilis, which can be transmitted from an infected woman to her fetus during pregnancy, causing severe damage to the child. In the United States, most states adopted laws that required couples to be certified free of disease before they could obtain a marriage license.[14]

Many of the themes that occurred in the debates over venereal disease control have recurred today in debates about AIDS prevention. In fact, two states passed laws in the 1980s requiring premarital screening for HIV infection—similar to the old requirement for syphilis testing. However, these laws were soon repealed, as the syphilis laws have been. Changes in social norms mean that premarital screening occurs too late to protect women— or men—against sexually transmitted diseases. The conflict between, on the one hand, the protection of the privacy and freedom of the infected individual and, on the other hand, the protection of the health of potential "innocent" victims is the same with AIDS as it was with syphilis. However, the political power of gay men, the group most affected by AIDS in the early days of the epidemic, was much stronger than was the power of prostitutes in the 19th century. The gay community fought against many proposals designed to prevent the spread of the virus. For example, legal battles were fought in San Francisco and New York over the closing of gay bathhouses, which were the site of many unsafe sexual practices. New York State's 1985 decision to close the bathhouses in New York City was upheld by the courts. In San Francisco, legal action by the gay community forced an overturn of the city's order to close the bathhouses. However, the court ordered bathhouse owners to hire monitors to prevent high-risk sexual activity.[15]

Does Prohibition Work?

The most ambitious attempt by the U.S. government to regulate the behavior of its citizens was Prohibition, passed by a constitutional amendment in 1919 that was repealed 14 years later. Common wisdom holds that Prohibition was a failure, but today's society treats "recreational" drugs—marijuana, heroin, cocaine—in much the same way that the Eighteenth Amendment treated alcohol, and few public health leaders are willing to call for an end to the "war on drugs." In fact, the Prohibition approach to regulating behavior appears to have mixed results, combining success and failure in a complex way.

The movement to legally ban alcohol became a moral crusade in the late 19th century, with prohibitionists blaming alcohol for all the ills of society. According to the rhetoric, drinking drove men to violence, especially against their wives and children; drunkards were a threat to public safety; and drunkenness itself was looked on as a sin and a crime. In fact, public disapproval had convinced many people to cut down on or quit their use of alcohol, and consumption had declined even before the Eighteenth Amendment was approved.[16] During Prohibition, the rate of cirrhosis of the liver declined to half that of 1910. Despite the image of the Roaring Twenties—with speakeasies, flappers, and bathtub gin—consumption of alcohol fell by two-thirds.[17] However, it was also true that flouting of the law became socially acceptable, and organized crime flourished.

The debate about Prohibition resurfaces occasionally in the context of illegal drugs. In an exchange of letters published in the *Wall Street Journal* in 1989, two prominent conservatives debated whether the war on drugs was doing more harm than good.[18,19] The economist Milton Friedman argued that while drugs are "tearing asunder our social fabric, ruining the lives of many young people, and imposing heavy costs on some of the most disadvantaged among us," much of the harm results from the fact that the drugs are illegal.[18] The illegality drives up the price of the drugs, providing a financial incentive to drug dealers, causing desperate addicts to commit crimes to pay for their addiction, and corrupting law enforcement officials tempted by bribery. Removing the "obscene profits" from the drug market, Friedman wrote, would reduce the motivation of drug pushers to recruit future addicts among vulnerable young people.

Opposing this view was William Bennett, who was the leader of the first President Bush's drug-control efforts. Bennett admitted that the war on drugs is costly, but argued that the cost of not enforcing laws against drugs would be higher. He claimed that after repeal of Prohibition, the consumption of alcohol soared by 350 percent and asked if the country could afford such a dramatic increase in drug use. He blamed current levels of drug use for lost productivity, rising health insurance costs, flooding of hospitals with drug overdose emergencies, and drug-related accidents. He disputed the argument that addicts turn to crime to support their habit, claiming that many addicts were criminals before they turned to drugs.[19]

The argument has not been resolved. In 2001, the National Academy of Sciences published a report suggesting that the Prohibition-like approach may not be working. The report stated that, although the federal government spends some $17 billion each year on drug enforcement programs, there is little information on the effectiveness of these programs. The number of people arrested and incarcerated for drug offenses increased throughout the 1980s and 1990s, despite a lack of evidence that this approach helped to deter illegal drug use. "It is unconscionable for the country to continue to carry out a public policy of this magnitude and cost without any way of knowing whether and to what extent it is having the desired effect," the report concluded.[20(p.279)]

Other arguments against the war on drugs were put forward by Nicholas Kristof in a 2009 *New York Times* column entitled "Drugs Won the War." Kristof notes that the United States incarcerates people at a rate nearly five times the world average, adding up to 500,000 people in 2009. The prohibition approach is expensive, costing federal, state, and local governments some $44.1 billion annually. Drug prohibition also raises prices, empowering criminals at home and terrorists abroad. The Mexican government is engaged in a vicious war against the drug cartels, which supply drugs mainly to the American market. And the Taliban in Afghanistan support themselves largely by the opium trade.[21]

Although it seems unlikely that the United States will abandon the war on drugs completely, President Obama's drug czar, Gil Kerlikowske, has declared an intention to shift the emphasis more toward treatment rather than imprisonment, more consistent with the public health approach. Evidence on the effectiveness of treatment and prevention programs is also thin, however. The most widespread prevention program used in the United States, the school-based D.A.R.E. (Drug Abuse Resistance Education) program, which has a "zero-tolerance strategy," has been found to have little impact on drug use.[20]

Later in this text, we undertake a more theoretical discussion of what influences people to behave in the ways that they do. It is clear that, to be effective, public health must expand beyond the traditional approaches of education and regulation in its attempt to change people's unhealthy behaviors. Elsewhere, we discuss ways in which a combination of education and regulation is being used to change people's behavior in relation to the substance that tops the list of hazards to health: tobacco smoking.

Conclusion

As infectious diseases have become less predominant causes of death in the United States, a major focus of public health programs has shifted to people's behavior. An analysis conducted by a group of public health leaders has concluded that the top three actual causes of death are smoking, poor diet and physical inactivity, and alcohol consumption. Other behavioral factors that are among the top nine causes of death are firearms, sexual behavior, motor vehicles, and the illicit use of drugs. For public health to significantly reduce the death rates beyond what it can achieve in controlling infectious diseases, it must find ways to promote behavioral change.

Two approaches that government has traditionally taken to persuade people to change their behavior are education and regulation. Education about health includes simply informing people about risks, which can be an effective strategy when new knowledge becomes available, as occurred with the 1964 surgeon general's report called *Smoking and Health*. Food labeling is also part of an educational effort to encourage Americans to eat a healthier diet. Regulation is another effective approach to promoting behavioral change, although it is often unpopular. Historically, the most ambitious attempt to regulate Americans' behavior was Prohibition, which did in fact improve their health by reducing the rate of cirrhosis of the liver. Whether the Prohibition-like approach currently used for control of illegal drugs is effective has not been demonstrated.

Research in the social and behavioral sciences has led to the development of theories of why people behave as they do and how they can be influenced to change their behavior. The evidence indicates that health promotion programs are most effective when they target individuals at many different levels of influence.

References

1. J. M. McGinnis and W. H. Foege, "Actual Causes of Death in the United States," *Journal of the American Medical Association* 270 (1993): 2207–2212.
2. A. H. Mokdad, J. S. Marks, D. F. Stroup, and J. L. Gerberding, "Actual Causes of Death in the United States, 2000," *Journal of the American Medical Association* 291 (2004): 1238–1245.
3. K. M. Flegal et al., "Excess Deaths Associated with Underweight, Overweight, and Obesity," *Journal of the American Medical Association* 293 (2005): 1861–1867.
4. U.S. Centers for Disease Control and Prevention, "Fact Sheet: Alcohol and Public Health." http//:www.cdc.gov/alcohol/fact-sheets.htm, accessed September 15, 2012.
5. *Smoking and Health: Report of the Advisory Committee to the Surgeon General of the Public Health Service* (Washington, DC: U.S. Department of Health, Education and Welfare, 1964).
6. U.S. Centers for Disease Control and Prevention, *Health United States*, 2011. http://www.cdc.gov/nchs/data/hus/hus11.pdf, Table 62, accessed September 15, 2012.
7. M. Nestle, *Food Politics* (Berkeley, CA: University of California Press, 2002).
8. Editorial. "The Food Pyramid Scheme." *The New York Times*, September 1, 2004.
9. T. Hampton, "Abstinence-Only Programs Under Fire," *Journal of the American Medical Association* 299 (2008): 2013–2015.
10. K. C. Montgomery, "Promoting Health Through Entertainment Television," in C. Atkin and L. Wallack, eds., *Mass Communication and Public Health: Complexities and Conflicts* (Newbury Park, CA: Sage Publications, 1990), 114–128.

11. University of Virginia, National Social Norms Institute, "Social Norms: An Introduction." http://www.socialnorms.org/FAQ/FAQ.php, accessed June 19, 2012.

12. U.S. Public Health Service. *Healthy People 2000: National Health Promotion and Disease Prevention Objectives*, Publication No. (PHS) 91-50212 (Washington, DC: Department of Health and Human Services, 1990), 153–154.

13. T. Christoffel, *Health and the Law: A Handbook for Health Professionals* (New York: Free Press, 1982).

14. H. M. Leichter, *Free to Be Foolish: Politics and Health Promotion in the United States and Great Britain* (Princeton, NJ: Princeton University Press, 1991).

15. R. Bayer, *Private Acts, Social Consequences: AIDS and the Politics of Public Health* (New York: Free Press, 1989).

16. G. Pickett and J. J. Hanlon, *Public Health: Administration and Practice* (St. Louis, MO: Times Mirror/Mosby, 1990).

17. D. Beauchamp, *The Health of the Republic: Epidemics, Medicine, and Moralism as Challenges to Democracy* (Philadelphia: Temple University Press, 1988).

18. M. Friedman, "An Open Letter to Bill Bennett," *The Wall Street Journal,* September 7, 1989: A14.

19. W. Bennett, "A Response to Milton Friedman," *The Wall Street Journal,* September 19, 1989: A30.

20. Committee on Data and Research for Policy on Illegal Drugs, *Informing America's Policy on Illegal Drugs: What We Don't Know Keeps Hurting Us* (Washington, DC: National Academies Press, 2001).

21. N. Kristof, "Drugs Won the War," *The New York Times,* June 14, 2009.

How Psychosocial Factors Affect Health Behavior

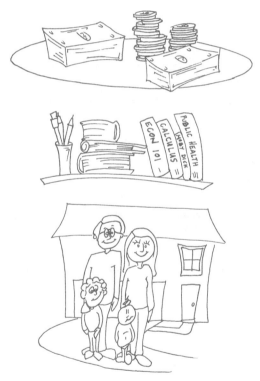

Healthy, Wealthy, and Wise

While individual behavior plays a major role in determining a person's health, many factors influence individual behavior. Humans are social creatures, and their behavior is strongly affected by their social environment. This accounts, at least in part, for the fact that diseases tend to be distributed in the population according to certain patterns: certain groups have characteristic disease patterns that remain constant over time even when individuals in the group change. From a public health perspective, it may be more efficient to try to change the social environment that influences people to behave in unhealthy ways than to try to change people's behavior one individual at a time.

Another reason to consider the social environment in studying health behavior is that when the focus is on the individual, the conclusion is likely to be that the person is to blame for his or her illness. Unhealthy behaviors may be maintained and reinforced by aspects of the social environment that are beyond the individual's control. It may be more appropriate for public health intervention programs to focus on these social aspects or at least consider them in designing programs aimed at promoting healthy behavior.

Demographic factors—including race, gender, and marital status—are consistently found to influence health. Statistics show that most ethnic minorities in the United States have significantly higher mortality rates from most diseases than whites. Males have higher mortality rates than females at all ages, although females tend to suffer more from chronic illness. Married people are in general healthier than people who are not married, whether single, separated, widowed, or divorced. The reasons for these differences are believed to be primarily social.

The most important predictor of health is *socioeconomic status* (SES), a concept that includes income, education, and occupational status, factors that tend to be strongly associated with each other. SES accounts in part, though not entirely, for the health differences by race, sex, and marital status. For example, blacks tend to be less healthy than whites, and they generally have lower SES than whites. However, even wealthy, educated blacks have higher mortality rates than whites of comparable SES.[1]

Groups with the lowest SES have the highest mortality rates, a fact that is true in many different countries and has been true for centuries, for reasons known and unknown.[2] In London in 1665, the poor were more likely to die in the plague epidemic because of poor nutrition and sanitation and because they could not flee the city to escape infection as the wealthy did. In the United States today, the health of the poor is threatened by the adverse environmental conditions of the inner cities, such as lead paint and air pollution, crime, and violence. Poor people also have poorer nutrition, less access to medical care, and more psychological stress.

It is not only the effects of poverty that account for socioeconomic variations in health, however. The association is seen at all levels of the socioeconomic scale, the very rich being healthier than the rich, who are healthier than the middle class, and so on. In a study of British civil servants called the Whitehall Study, mortality rates over a 10-year period were compared across four employment grades. Top administrators were compared with executives and professionals, the clerical staff, and unskilled laborers.[3] As seen in Figure 14-1, higher employment status was associated with a lower risk of dying.

Part of the reason that people with higher SES are healthier seems to be that people with more education behave in healthier ways. For example, in 2010, 26.9 percent of Americans without a high school diploma smoked, while of those with a bachelor's degree or higher, only 8.3 percent smoked. Those with more education were also more physically active.[4(Table 61,73)] Similarly, the Whitehall Study questioned subjects about their habits and found that those in higher employment grades were less likely to smoke, more likely to exercise, and more likely to eat a healthful diet that included skim milk, whole grains, and fresh fruits and vegetables.[3]

Variable access to medical care is another factor that has been blamed for some of the socioeconomic differences in health. In the United States, where 15 percent to 20 percent of the population—mostly those in low socioeconomic groups—lacks health insurance, it is often argued that universal health insurance could reduce health inequalities. However, the SES differences in mortality are also seen in Britain, Scandinavian nations, and other countries that have national health programs. The British civil servants in the Whitehall Study all had the same medical coverage by the National Health Service; yet the mortality

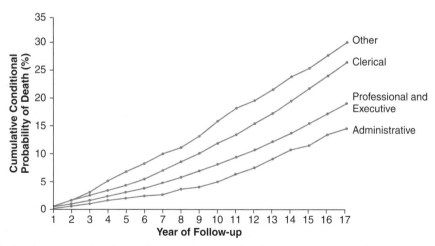

FIGURE 14-1   Mortality from All Causes by Year of Follow-Up and Grade of Employment, in Whitehall (U.K.) Male Civil Servants, Initially Aged 40–64. *Source:* Reproduced from M. G. Marmot, M. J. Shipley, and G. Rose, "Inequalities in Death—Specific Explanations of a General Pattern?" *The Lancet*, 323:1003–1006, 1984, with permission from Elsevier.

risks were still higher at lower employment grades, even when behavioral factors were taken into consideration.

Health of Minority Populations

Race and ethnicity have been seen to profoundly affect health in the United States. Most data on health status of different population groups show that the health of African Americans, the largest racial minority, constituting about 13 percent of the population, is poorer than that of white Americans. Hispanics are a heterogeneous group, and their health status varies among different subgroups. American Indians generally have poorer health indicators than whites, while Asian Americans have better health status.

While the overall health of the U.S. population has improved over the past decades, health disparities among racial and ethnic groups have persisted. Life expectancy at birth in 2009 was 78.8 for whites and 74.5 for blacks.[4(Table 22)] The infant mortality rate of blacks was 2.4 times higher, and the rate for American Indians/Alaska Natives was 1.5 times higher than that of whites.[4(Table 17)] Mortality from diabetes is 1.7 times as high in American Indians as in whites, and more than twice as high in blacks as in whites.[4(Table 26)] Black men die of prostate cancer at 2.3 times the rate of white men.[5] The death rate from HIV/AIDS is 9 times higher among blacks than whites, way out of proportion to their percentage of the population.[4(Table 24)]

The health disparities may be accounted for in part by the lower SES of blacks, who live in households with median incomes $17,000 less than the average for the nation.[6] Over 27 percent of blacks were living in poverty in 2010, as compared with 1 out of 10 white non-Hispanics.[6] Blacks have less education on average than whites, and they have higher unemployment rates. The reasons for the socioeconomic disparities are complex and somewhat inaccessible to public health interventions. Moreover, the relationship between socioeconomic status and health is not entirely understood. Nevertheless, public health must find ways to improve the health of groups that have historically been disadvantaged economically, educationally, and politically. The federal government predicts that by 2050, nearly half of Americans will belong to racial and ethnic minorities. If the health disparities are not remedied, the overall health of the U.S. population is likely to decline.[7]

Public health interventions aimed at improving the health of minority groups include efforts to influence their health behaviors. These efforts begin with attempts to understand what factors influence health and health behavior, how these factors may affect people of various ethnic and racial groups differently, and what kind of interventions can be effective in modifying these factors. This chapter and later chapters that consider specific health behaviors will examine how minority groups differ from the majority white population and how those differences may be related to the observed disparities in health.

Stress and Social Support

A number of psychological factors have been found to influence health, some of which may have a role in the health effects of SES. One of these factors is stress, which is due to the adverse physical and social conditions associated with lower SES, which may act both directly, by affecting physiological processes, and indirectly, by influencing individual behavior. Early evidence of the health effects of stress came from observations that widows and widowers seemed to have an unusually high risk of dying soon after the death of their spouses. Several studies in the 1960s and 1970s found that mortality rates of survivors are 40 percent to 50 percent higher during the 6 months after the death of a spouse compared to the mortality of married people of the same age. These studies were expanded to include the effects of other stressful life events such as death of other family members, divorce, and loss of a job, all of which were found to increase the risk of illness or death.[8]

Stress is well established as a contributor to heart disease, a relationship that has been demonstrated in a variety of epidemiologic studies. A particularly convincing example is a study of the male employees of two banks. At first, the two groups were similar, but one bank changed its management policies to become commercial. The employees of the commercial bank had to deal with considerable competition, risk, and responsibility for investing funds; employees of the other bank, a semipublic savings bank, had less competition and fewer responsibilities. Over a 10-year period, the employees of the commercial bank were found to have 50 percent higher rates of heart attacks and sudden death.[9]

Experiments on animals ranging from rats to baboons have found that various psychosocial stresses induce physiological changes such as decreased immune response and increased atherosclerosis. A 1991 experiment on humans demonstrated that stress suppresses the immune response in humans also. In that experiment, investigators measured levels of psychological stress in 420 healthy volunteers, then administered nasal drops containing cold viruses to all but a small control group. They found that the subjects whose stress levels were higher were more likely to be infected with cold viruses and more likely to develop colds, with symptoms including sneezing, coughing, eye watering, nasal discharge, sore throat, and increased use of tissues.[10] A whole new field of research called psychoneuroimmunology has arisen to study the impact of stress on health.

There are many reasons why lower SES exposes people to greater life stress. Daily hassles are greater at lower levels on the SES hierarchy: cars break down, landlords complain about late rent checks, child care is unreliable, officials are rude. Members of racial and ethnic minorities may be exposed to incidents of racial prejudice. These minor but constant stresses may be as debilitating as such major life events as deaths in the family. Higher income and education provide resources that help to buffer the impact of life's hassles, thereby protecting health.

A number of factors can help people cope with life's stresses. Money, of course, can solve a multitude of problems. Education is important because it provides the information and skills to solve problems. Family and friends can also help by providing both emotional and instrumental assistance. In fact, social support has proven to be surprisingly significant in determining an individual's health.

Early evidence for the influence of social support on health came from an epidemiologic cohort study conducted on residents of Alameda County in California. Persons aged 30 to 69 were surveyed in 1965 on their physical, mental, and social well-being as well as their health-related habits such as exercise and the use of cigarettes and alcohol. They were also asked about their social networks, such as marital status, number of close friends and relatives, church membership, and affiliation with other organizations. Death certificates were then monitored over the next 9 years to assess mortality rates and, in 1974, a follow-up survey was conducted on survivors to assess their health status.[11]

The study, as expected, found a strong association between certain unhealthy behaviors and higher mortality rates. More surprising, the study also found that an individual's health status and risk of dying were strongly associated with the extent and nature of his or her social network. This was true for both men and women and for individuals of high SES and low SES. The association remained true even after unhealthy behaviors were taken into consideration. Throughout the socioeconomic spectrum, men and women with few social contacts had mortality rates two to three times higher than those with many social connections.

Many more recent studies have supported the conclusions of the Alameda County study. Absence of social support has been related to an increase in coronary heart disease, complications in pregnancy and delivery, suicide, and other unhealthy outcomes.[12] Why social support should have such a broad and consistent effect on health is very poorly understood. It probably acts in part through its ability to buffer stress. A better understanding of the relationship between social support and health may come from research in the field of psychoneuroimmunology.

Psychological Models of Health Behavior

While public health does not have much power to change people's SES, stressful life events, or social networks, it is hoped that understanding how these factors affect health may permit more effective interventions to promote healthier behavior. With this goal, social and behavioral scientists have proposed various theories and models attempting to explain how psychosocial factors affect health-related behavior. Some of these theories focus on individual psychology, while others attempt to explain the effect of the social environment on individual behavior. The goal of these analyses is to understand the most effective ways to promote healthier behavior.

The classic frame of reference for understanding health behavior, and especially behavior change, is the health belief model. Assuming that people act in rational ways, the health belief model specifies several factors that determine whether a person is likely to change behavior when faced with a health threat. These factors are (1) the extent to which the individual feels vulnerable to the threat, (2) the perceived severity of the threat, (3) perceived barriers to taking action to reduce the risk, and (4) the perceived effectiveness of taking an action to prevent or minimize the problem.

Based on the health belief model, the public health approach to changing behavior would be to convince people that they are vulnerable, that the threat is severe, and that certain actions are effective preventive measures. For example, surveys of low-income minority women who had not had mammograms found that many had misperceptions about the disease. Some women underestimated their susceptibility to breast cancer (factor 1); others were embarrassed or afraid of the pain or radiation involved in a mammogram (factor 3); and others felt that cancer was not curable and therefore there would be no point in diagnosing it early (factor 4). Screening rates among these women could be improved by counseling that included personally tailored messages that addressed the women's beliefs and concerns.[13]

Another important concept in understanding health behavior is self-efficacy, the sense of having control over one's life. People who are confident that they can control their lives are said to have high self-efficacy. People who believe their lives are subject to chance or external forces are said to have low self-efficacy. Self-efficacy is often added as a fifth factor in the health belief model. People are more likely to adopt healthy behavior if they are confident that they have the ability to do so.[13]

A sense of control is beneficial for health in a number of ways. Clearly, it reduces stress. A number of studies in both humans and animals have shown that an individual's perception of the stressfulness of an adverse event can be reduced by two factors: knowledge of when the stressful event will occur and the ability to regulate the timing and intensity of the event. This knowledge and ability give the individual a sense of control, or self-efficacy. The lowest self-efficacy is seen in people (or animals) who have experience of being unable to avoid noxious events, especially if they have repeatedly tried and failed. They may develop a pattern of "learned helplessness," a pattern described as a "numbed acceptance of a negative situation, so that an individual no longer tries to change that situation for the better because he or she does not expect those efforts to make any difference."[14(p.44)]

A number of studies have shown that people with high self-efficacy are more likely to engage in health-promoting behavior than those with low self-efficacy. An attitude of learned helplessness is common in people who have repeatedly tried and failed to quit smoking or lose weight.

A great deal of research has been focused on how to increase people's self-efficacy, thereby helping to motivate them to practice healthy behaviors. An individual's self-efficacy is increased by previous successful performance of the behavior in question. It may also be increased by seeing others successfully perform the behavior, especially if the observed behavior is being performed by someone similar to themselves. For example, the most successful school drug prevention programs include role-modeling, small group exercises, and skills practice to teach students how to identify and resist internal and external pressures to use drugs. These programs have been found to be much more effective in enhancing students' self-efficacy to resist drugs if they are led by older teens, with whom they can identify, rather than by adult health educators.[15]

A theory that has proved widely useful in health education is the transtheoretical model, which envisions change—for example smoking cessation or adopting a healthy diet—as a process involving progress through a series of five stages: precontemplation, contemplation, preparation, action, and maintenance. People in the *precontemplation* stage have no intention to change their behavior; the first step in getting them to change involves consciousness-raising to increase their awareness that their behavior is unhealthy and should be changed. In the second, *contemplation* stage, the person is more aware of the benefits of change, but is also very aware of the difficulties and barriers to change and still is not ready to take action. The third step is *preparation*, when a person has decided to make the change and has planned concrete actions he or she could take, such as signing up for a class, discussing the plan with their physician, or buying a self-help book. The fourth step, *action*, requires that individuals actually modify their behavior by abstaining from smoking or adhering to a healthier diet. Finally, *maintenance* is the stage in which people have achieved the healthier behavior but must strive to prevent relapse.[16] Knowing which stage an individual has reached can help a physician or health educator move him or her along to the next stage.

The health belief model and the transtheoretical model are not contradictory; they are merely alternative ways of looking at what may be the same psychological factors. Both models can be useful in designing public health messages aimed at changing behavior.

Ecological Model of Health Behavior

In accordance with the recognition that individual beliefs and behaviors occur in a social context and that health promotion may be more effectively achieved through changing the social environment, so-called ecological models have been proposed for understanding health behavior.[17] An ecological model looks at how the social environment, including interpersonal, organizational, community, and public policy factors, supports and maintains unhealthy behaviors. The model proposes that changes in these factors will produce changes in individual behavior.

The ecological model, illustrated in **Figure 14-2**, describes five levels of influence that determine health-related behaviors; each level is a potential target for health promotion intervention. The first level—*intrapersonal* factors—encompasses the knowledge, attitudes, and skills of the individual. This is the level that has been explored by the psychological theories discussed

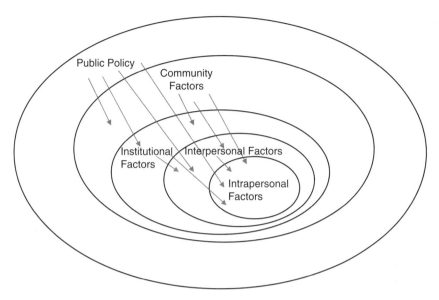

FIGURE 14-2   Ecological Model

earlier in this chapter. The second through fifth levels—interpersonal relations, institutional factors, community factors, and public policy—each have an impact on individual behavior both directly and indirectly, by interaction with the factors at other levels of influence.

The second level of influence, *interpersonal* relations—including family, friends, and coworkers—has very important effects on health-related behavior. Families, of course, are the origin of many health behaviors, especially habits learned early in life such as tooth brushing, exercising, and eating patterns. In the teen years, pressure from peers becomes more significant in influencing individual behaviors, such as smoking, using alcohol and drugs, and engaging in other risk-taking behavior. On the positive side, family and peer relationships provide the social support discussed earlier in this chapter.

Application of the ecological model at the interpersonal level would lead to different strategies in a teen drug prevention program depending on the nature of the teens' social relationships. A teen who belongs to a dense, homogeneous network will be more influenced by the norms and values of that group than a teen who relates individually to a number of separate individuals. In the close-knit group, drug prevention programs would have to focus on changing the norms about drug use within the existing network. When social networks are more loosely organized, the program might focus on creating drug-free networks, encouraging teens to associate with those networks, and reducing the desirability of membership in drug-using networks.

The third level of influence is significant because people spend one-third to one-half of their waking lives in *institutional* settings, especially schools and workplaces, which may have profound effects on their health and health-related behavior. In the workplace, employees may encounter hazardous chemicals or risks from injuries and accidents. Stress may be a problem. Alternatively, organizations may provide a corporate culture that supports positive behavior change. Workplace or school cafeterias may provide health-conscious menus; exercise facilities may be available and their use encouraged; smoking restrictions may prevail. Schools and work-places provide ideal settings for public health intervention.

The larger *community*—the fourth level—can be a significant influence on behavior. Organizations can work together in a community to jointly promote healthy goals. An under-standing of community organization and networks can offer insight into promising avenues for health promotion. For example, churches are the social centers for many black and rural communities and may provide a focal point for health-related interventions. Conversely, com-munity factors may sabotage public health efforts to promote healthy behavior. In the South, where tobacco is a pillar of local economies, public health advocates may find it difficult to even raise the issue of the health consequences of smoking.

At the fifth level, *public policy* encompasses the regulations and limitations on behavior that have been discussed previously. These are the most explicit and controversial measures that local, state, and national governments take to promote healthy behaviors. Such measures include smoking restrictions, age limits on alcohol sales, seat-belt laws, and so forth.

Health Promotion Programs

As social and behavioral scientists gain a better understanding of how people's behavior is affected by their own beliefs and by the various levels of influence in their social environment, theories such as the health belief model and the ecological model are being used to design more effective public health and disease prevention programs. A good example is provided by an AIDS prevention program targeted at gay men in San Francisco in the mid-1980s.[18] Prevention of infection through behavior change was and is still the most effective approach to AIDS control because there is as yet no biomedical solution to the problem—no vaccine and no proven cure.

In the 1980s, San Francisco was the city with the second highest number of AIDS cases in the United States. Most of the cases occurred in gay men, and the primary means by which the virus was transmitted was by sexual intercourse between men. Almost as soon as this was under-stood, a prevention campaign was launched by the city health department in collaboration with community-based AIDS organizations and a research group from the University of California. They mounted an intensive media effort to inform at-risk individuals about the practice of safer sex. However, researchers understood that merely providing knowledge was not sufficient to change people's behavior. By interviewing small groups of gay men, they identified key beliefs that must be addressed if the messages were to be acted on by the target population.

This approach combines elements of three theories discussed above: the health belief model, self-efficacy, and the ecological model. The campaign's goals were to promote the following beliefs among high-risk individuals:

1. Belief in personal threat (i.e., "I am susceptible to infection").
2. Belief in response efficacy (i.e., "There is something I can do that will lessen the threat of infection").
3. Belief in personal efficacy (i.e., "I am capable of making these changes").
4. Belief that new behaviors are consistent with group norms (i.e., "My peers support new behaviors").[18]

The first belief was relatively easy to achieve because of the extensive publicity about AIDS in the general media. News and entertainment media aimed at gay men, including gay newspapers, comic books and leaflets, and telephone hot lines could be used to focus more on the second and third beliefs. Gay organizations held small group training sessions to teach skills in the use of condoms as well as interpersonal communication skills such as the ability to negotiate safer sex practices with prospective sex partners; this helped to enhance perceptions of self-efficacy among those at risk. To achieve the fourth belief, messages sought to encourage the perception that low-risk behaviors could be pleasurable and satisfying.

The first three elements of the campaign targeted individual health beliefs and self-efficacy. The fourth element addressed interpersonal and community influences. The campaign targeted community influences by providing educational programs for bartenders in establishments frequented by gay men. Condoms were made widely available in bars and small group meetings and were distributed by volunteers on street corners. The public policy, government level of influence was brought in through provision by the city of free, confidential testing for the human immunodeficiency virus (HIV) antibody. Because public bathhouses were a frequent site of high-risk behavior, there was pressure on the city government to close them, as was done in New York City. However, the campaign as a whole was so successful in changing the behavior of gay men that business at the bathhouses fell off, and public health officers were satisfied with merely posting warnings to the clientele about safe sex.[19]

The San Francisco AIDS prevention program was highly successful. Surveys done between 1984 and 1988 found that gay men had dramatically reduced their high-risk sexual behaviors during that period. For example, the percentage of men who reported engaging in unprotected receptive anal intercourse—the behavior most likely to transmit HIV—fell from 44 percent to 3 percent over the 4 years of the study.[20] When rates of seroconversion among gay men from HIV-negative to HIV-positive were analyzed, the researchers found that the behavior changes had paid off: between 1982 and 1986, seroconversion rates fell from 13 percent to only 1 percent.

The early success of AIDS prevention programs among gay men, in the rest of the country as well as in San Francisco, was attributable largely to the fact that the gay community was in general well educated and politically astute. The epidemic's potential victims tended to be of high SES, motivated to preserve their health and able to mobilize resources to cope with the impending threat. Thus, they were more receptive to the health promotion campaign than other groups at risk for HIV. However, the success at reducing high-risk behavior has not been maintained. Ongoing studies of gay men in San Francisco found that the prevalence of unprotected anal intercourse had increased from 31 percent in 1998 to 46 percent in 2007. Despite continuing HIV prevention programs, the prevalence of HIV-positive status among gay men in San Francisco has stabilized at about 24 percent.[21]

Public health workers attribute the resurgence of sexual risk behaviors to the advent of highly active antiretroviral therapy in 1995. Because of the remarkable effectiveness of the new drug treatments, many younger gay men saw HIV infection as a less severe threat (a factor in the Health Belief Model) than did older gay men. The growing number of infected individuals, who are living longer because of therapy, and the persistence of unsafe sexual behaviors have led to a high rate of new infections, which more than replace the number of gay men who die from AIDS, which remains stable.[21]

Researchers in San Francisco believe that high rates of infection will persist in that community and stress the need for intensification of effective prevention strategies. In other parts of the country, different approaches may be necessary to reach high-risk groups. For example, among blacks—the population with the highest prevalence of HIV—men who have sex with men (MSM) often do not identify as gay. Thus prevention messages targeted at them might need to be different from those used in San Francisco.[22] A large number of studies have been done on behavioral interventions for HIV prevention and their effectiveness at reducing risky sexual behaviors. Evidence has shown effectiveness for individual person-to-person counseling, group-level programs that include a skill-building component delivered by other MSM, and to a lesser extent, community-level programs that can motivate and reinforce behavior change. There is little evidence, however, on how to reach minority MSM who do not regard themselves as part of the gay community. Other high-risk groups that need targeted programs include black women, who may be at risk of infection because of heterosexual intercourse with bisexual black men, and intravenous drug users.

Unfortunately, health promotion and disease prevention programs cannot be done once and for all. They must be repeated for every generation and every new at-risk group.

Changing the Environment

As more is being learned about what influences people to behave the way they do, many advocates believe that public health programs, to be effective, must concentrate less on individual behavior and more on changing the environment—both the social environment and the physical environment—to make it easier for people to behave in healthy ways. For example, there are many fewer deaths from motor vehicle crashes now than there were 2 decades ago. This public health success comes less from educational programs about safe driving than it does from safer design of highways and automobiles.

Similarly, the San Francisco HIV researchers suggest that social biases against homosexuality may contribute to the AIDS epidemic. They propose that recognition of same-sex marriage might encourage more stable relationships among gays, reduce the number of sexual partners by each individual, and thereby reduce the individual's risk of being infected. Public policy affects risk of HIV infection among intravenous drug users by providing access to needle exchange programs, which are illegal in some communities.

Environmental factors influence people's diet and activity patterns, which are the second most important factor in Americans' poor health. The government recommends that people eat five servings daily of fresh fruit and vegetables, but educating people who live in poor areas of the inner city will not help improve their diets if they do not have access to supermarkets or produce stands. Similarly, federal policies that since World War II have favored a suburban lifestyle must bear much of the blame for Americans' lack of exercise: people live in their cars because most places are not within walking distance.

The environmental perspective forces people to think of public health problems as social and political issues that require collective action. Instead of blaming smokers for lack of will power, public opinion has shifted its focus to the tobacco industry and the enormous resources the industry has put into making their product attractive to young people, a way of thinking that has led to a remarkable change in public attitudes toward smoking. People take action, as black activists did against the alcoholic beverage industry when it began aggressively marketing high-powered malt liquors to young black males.[23] This approach may lead to confrontations with very powerful economic interests, and it will not always be successful. However, when whole communities become involved, it has the potential of being the most effective way to bring about major changes in health and behavior.

Conclusion

Because health is so strongly affected by behavior, it is important for public health advocates to understand what influences people to behave in healthy or unhealthy ways. The social and behavioral sciences offer insights into why people behave as they do, and they provide a basis for developing interventions aimed at persuading people to change their behavior.

There is evidence that factors such as race, gender, marital status, and especially SES influence health, and the reasons for these differences are likely to be social. Life expectancy, infant mortality, and mortality rates from a variety of diseases vary profoundly among different racial and ethnic groups. Stress, which may be brought on by social factors, has an adverse effect on health for a number of reasons. Social support has been found to have a positive effect on health, probably in part by providing a buffer against stress. The health of black Americans tends to be poorer than that of the white majority. Health data on the population is usually analyzed by race and ethnicity, and public health efforts focus on understanding the disparities and trying to eliminate them.

Theories of health behavior include the health belief model and the theory of self-efficacy. Both theories focus on the individuals' attitudes and beliefs as determinants of their behavior. The transtheoretical model of stages of change can be used in health education programs to promote behavior change. A broader perspective is provided by the ecological model of health behavior. This model considers all the levels of influence that may affect the individual's attitudes and beliefs, including interpersonal relationships such as family and friends, institutional influence such as school and work, the larger community and its values and beliefs, and public policy including laws and regulations.

The most effective public health intervention programs influence people's beliefs at several levels with the goal of creating a social environment favorable to healthy behavior. The San Francisco AIDS prevention program is an example of an effective program that succeeded in significantly reducing the transmission of HIV early in the epidemic. Evidence shows, however, that in order to maintain the success of such a program, intensive public health efforts must be maintained, both to prevent relapses into unhealthy behavior and to educate new generations of at-risk people.

Increasingly, public health advocates realize that the most effective ways of improving health-related behavior of individuals is to focus on involving whole communities in improving the social and physical environment to be more conducive to healthy behavior.

References

1. P. D. Sorlie, E. Backlund, and J. B. Keller, "U.S. Mortality by Economic, Demographic, and Social Characteristics: The National Longitudinal Mortality Study," *American Journal of Public Health* 269 (1995): 949–956.

2. N. Adler, T. Boyce, M. A. Chesney, S. Folkman, and S. L. Syme, "Socioeconomic Inequalities in Health: No Easy Solution," *Journal of the American Medical Association* 269 (1993): 3140–3145.

3. M. G. Marmot et al., "Health Inequalities Among British Civil Servants: The Whitehall II Study," *Lancet* 337 (1991): 1387–1393.

4. National Center for Health Statistics, *Health, United States, 2011.* http://www.cdc.gov/nchs/data/hus/hus11.pdf, May 2012, accessed June 21, 2012.

5. National Cancer Institute, "SEER Stat Fact Sheets: Prostate." http://seer.cancer.gov/statfacts/html/prost.html#incidence-mortality, accessed June 21, 2012.

6. C. DeNavas-Walt, B. D. Proctor, and J. C. Smith, U.S. Census Bureau, *Income, Poverty, and Health Insurance Coverage in the United States: 2010.* http://www.census.gov/prod/2011pubs/p60-239.pdf, accessed June 21, 2012.

7. U.S. Centers for Disease Control and Prevention, "Health Disparities Experienced by Racial/Ethnic Minority Populations," *Morbidity and Mortality Weekly Report* 53 (2004): 755.

8. K. J. Helsing and M. Szklo, "Mortality After Bereavement," *American Journal of Epidemiology* 114 (1981): 41–52.

9. F. Kittel, M. Kornitzer, and M. Dramaik, "Coronary Heart Disease and Job Stress in Two Cohorts of Bank Clerks," *Psychotherapy and Psychosomatics* 34 (1980): 110–123.

10. S. Cohen, D. A. J. Tyrrell, and A. P. Smith, "Psychological Stress and Susceptibility to the Common Cold," *New England Journal of Medicine* 325 (1991): 606–612.

11. L. F. Berkman and L. Breslow, *Health and Ways of Living: The Alameda County Study* (New York: Oxford University Press, 1983), 31–54.

12. J. S. House, K. R. Landis, and D. Umberson, "Social Relationships and Health," *Science* 241 (1988): 540–545.

13. N. K. Janz, V. L. Champion, and V. J. Strecher, "The Health Belief Model," in K. Glanz, B. K. Rimer, and F. M. Lewis, eds., *Health Behavior and Health Education: Theory, Research, and Practice*, 3rd ed. (San Francisco: Jossey-Bass, 2002), 45–66.

14. R. R. Lau, "Beliefs about Control and Health Behavior," in D. S. Gochman, ed., *Health Behavior: Emerging Research Perspectives* (New York: Plenum Press, 1983), 43–63.

15. C. A. Marlatt, J. S. Baer, and L. A. Quigley, "Self-Efficacy and Addictive Behavior," in A. Bandura, ed., *Self Efficacy in Changing Societies* (Cambridge, UK: Cambridge University Press, 1995), 289–315.

16. J. O. Prochaska, "The Transtheoretical Model and Stages of Change," in K. Glanz, B. K. Rimer, and F. M. Lewis, eds., *Health Behavior and Health Education: Theory, Research, and Practice*, 3rd ed. (San Francisco: Jossey-Bass, 2002), 99–120.

17. K. R. McLeroy, D. Bibeau, A. Steckler, and K. Glanz, "An Ecological Perspective on Health Promotion Programs," *Health Education Quarterly* 15 (1988): 351–377.

18. A. L. McAlister, P. Puska, M. Orlandi, L. L. Bye, and P. L. Zbylot, "Behaviour Modification: Principles and Illustrations," in W. Holland, R. Detels, and G. Knox, eds., *Oxford Textbook of Public Health*, 2nd ed., vol. 3. (Oxford, England: Oxford University Press, 1991), 3–16.

19. R. Bayer, *Private Acts, Social Consequences: AIDS and the Politics of Public Health* (New York: Free Press, 1989).

20. L. McKusick, T. J. Coates, S. F. Morin, L. Pollack, and C. Hoff, "Longitudinal Predictors of Reductions in Unprotected Anal Intercourse Among Gay Men in San Francisco: The AIDS Behavioral Research Project," *American Journal of Public Health* 80 (1990): 978–983.

21. S. Scheer et al., "HIV Is Hyperendemic Among Men Who Have Sex with Men in San Francisco: 10-Year Trends in HIV Incidence, HIV Prevalence, Sexually Transmitted Infections and Sexual Risk Behaviour," *Sexually Transmitted Infections* 84 (2008): 493–498.

22. J. H. Herbst et al., "The Effectiveness of Individual-, Group-, and Community-Level HIV Behavioral Risk-Reduction Interventions for Adult Men Who Have Sex with Men: A Systematic Review," *American Journal of Preventive Medicine* 32 (2007), (Supplement 1): 38–67.

23. L. Wallack, L. Dorfman, D. Jernigan, and M. Themba, *Media Advocacy and Public Health: Power for Prevention* (Newbury Park, CA: Sage Publications, 1993).

Public Health Enemy Number One: Tobacco

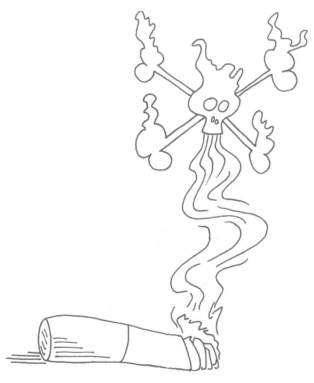

Deadly Habit

Cigarette smoking—the leading actual cause of death in the United States—is clearly the nation's most significant public health issue. The problem of tobacco-caused disease embodies the complex interactions by which psychological, social, cultural, economic, and political factors influence individual behavior to cause over 400,000 deaths each year. Table 15-1 lists the major diseases caused by smoking and estimates the annual number of deaths from each disease.

Table 15-1   Major Diseases Caused by Smoking and Estimated Annual Number of Deaths, 2000–2004

Disease	Number of Deaths
Cardiovascular disease	128,497
Cancer of the lung, trachea, bronchus	125,522
Respiratory disease, including bronchitis, emphysema and chronic airway obstruction	103,339
Other cancers, including laryngeal, oral, stomach, esophageal, pancreatic, urinary	35,326
Diseases among infants	776
Fire-related	736

Source: Data from U.S. Centers for Disease Control and Prevention, "Smoking-Attributable Mortality, Years of Potential Life Lost, and Productivity Losses—United States, 2000–2004," *Morbidity and Mortality Weekly Report* 57 (2008): 1226–1228.

The struggle to understand and deal with tobacco-caused illness involves all areas of public health. Epidemiology provided the first solid evidence that smoking caused cancer and heart disease and has continued to yield information on the health effects of this very human habit. Biomedical studies were slow to provide evidence because laboratory animals could not be persuaded or forced to smoke cigarettes, but eventually they yielded valuable information on the role of tobacco in the causation of cancer and heart disease. In recent years, smoking has increasingly been seen as an environmental health threat, producing indoor air pollution that has been shown to cause adverse health effects in nonsmokers. Ultimately, however, smoking is a behavior, and it is the social and behavioral sciences that must provide insights into why people smoke and how they can be persuaded to quit.

Public health faces a fundamental dilemma in confronting the current epidemic of tobacco-caused disease: What should be the role of a democratic government in confronting a behavior that is practiced by one out of five adults and will kill up to half of them? Political and economic forces that favored tobacco have opposed strong government measures against cigarettes. Public health efforts involving education and health promotion campaigns have persuaded many people to stop smoking but seem to have reached the limit of their effectiveness in bringing smoking prevalence down to about 20 percent among adults.

However, the 1990s saw a major shift in federal and state governments' attitudes toward smoking. Recognition that the nicotine in tobacco is addictive, together with evidence that cigarette companies have purposely manipulated nicotine levels in cigarettes to keep people hooked, have forced politicians to look with suspicion on what was previously considered a freely chosen behavior. Moreover, evidence of the high economic costs paid by government-financed programs, including Medicare and Medicaid, for the treatment of tobacco-caused disease has forced governments to question their previous assumptions about the economic advantages of supporting the tobacco industry.

Biomedical Basis of Smoking's Harmful Effects

The basic fact underlying the popular success of cigarettes is that they deliver nicotine, an addictive drug. Nicotine is absorbed by the linings of the mouth and the respiratory tract and travels rapidly to the heart and then to the brain. The drug produces a sense of enhanced energy and alertness, while also having a calming effect on addicted smokers. When people try to quit smoking, they experience withdrawal reactions with unpleasant physical and psychological symptoms. In 2010, 44 percent of smokers reported that during the past year they had tried to quit; only 4 to 7 percent of them succeeded.[1]

In addition to nicotine, an important component of tobacco smoke is tar, the residue from burning tobacco that condenses in the lungs of smokers. Tars provide the flavor in cigarette smoke; they are also a major source of its carcinogenicity. As early as the 1930s, experiments were done in which these tars were painted on the ear linings of rabbits or the shaved backs of mice and found to cause tumors. Decades of studies by biomedical researchers—and clandestinely by tobacco companies, which did not wish to publicize their results—have confirmed the carcinogenicity of the tars as well as other ingredients of the smoke, including arsenic and benzene. When filters were added to cigarettes with the ostensible purpose of removing tars and other harmful ingredients, it turned out that they tended also to remove the taste and "satisfaction" from smoking. Thus filter cigarettes, to be acceptable to smokers, had to deliver significant levels of tar and nicotine, meaning that there were limits to how "safe" a cigarette could be.

Tars not only cause cancer but also contribute to other lung diseases through their tendency to damage cilia, the tiny hairs on the linings of the respiratory tract that sweep the lungs and bronchi clear of microbes, irritants, and toxic substances. Damage to cilia and irritation of respiratory tract linings by components of smoke increase susceptibility to infectious diseases like bronchitis, influenza, and pneumonia as well as to diseases brought on by chronic irritation such as emphysema and asthma.

In contrast to the long-term processes leading to cancer and emphysema, the effect of smoking on the cardiovascular system can be very rapid. The nicotine in cigarette smoke raises blood pressure and heart rate. It may also cause spasms in the blood vessels of the heart, especially if damage already exists, increasing the risk of sudden cardiac death. Carbon monoxide in cigarette smoke interferes with the oxygen-carrying capacity of red blood cells, leading to oxygen shortages in the hearts of patients suffering from coronary artery disease. Smoking increases the risk of stroke and heart attacks by altering the clotting properties of blood. Components of cigarette smoke also have been shown to raise total blood cholesterol levels and reduce levels of HDL, the "good" cholesterol.

Historical Trends in Smoking and Health

Although it has been smoked and chewed for hundreds of years, tobacco was not used intensively enough to cause widespread illness until the 20th century. Before then, almost all tobacco was smoked in pipes and cigars or used as chewing tobacco and snuff. Cigarette-rolling machines and safety matches were invented in the 1880s, but cigarette smoking began to increase dramatically only after 1913, when Camel, followed by other brands, began mass marketing campaigns.[2] The distribution of free cigarettes to soldiers during the two world wars further stimulated smoking among men. Smoking among women was frowned on early in the century, but women began to take up the habit during and after World War II, and by 1960 about 34 percent of American women smoked.[2] While estimates of the percentage of men and women who smoked during the early part of the century are imprecise [they were done before the Centers for Disease Control and Prevention (CDC) began systematic surveys of the population in 1965], a general idea of the trends in much of the century can be seen in **Figure 15-1**. The percentage of Americans who smoke has continued to decline since 1980. A better sense of the extent of smoking in this country, and the circumstances influencing it comes from U.S. Department of Agriculture data on total manufactured cigarette consumption, as shown in **Figure 15-2**.

The first disease clearly linked to smoking was lung cancer, which is caused predominately by smoking and is relatively rare in nonsmokers. Lung cancer was virtually nonexistent in the United States and Britain in 1900. In the 1930s, the increase in deaths from lung cancer began to attract attention, and a link to cigarette smoking began to be suspected. This link was confirmed in the epidemiologic studies published in the 1950s. Cigarette consumption dropped as a result of these reports (as shown in Figure 15-2) but began to climb again when tobacco companies promoted filter cigarettes as a safer alternative.

In 1964, the U.S. surgeon general released a report, *Smoking and Health*, a summary of the evidence to date, the result of an exhaustive deliberation by a panel of 10 renowned scientists.[3] The panel unanimously agreed and wrote that cigarette smoking caused lung cancer and chronic bronchitis and was strongly associated with cancer of the mouth and larynx. It also

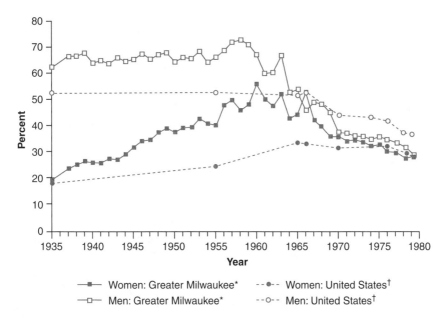

*Adapted from Howe 1984: *Milwaukee Journal*, Consumer analysis of the Greater Milwaukee market, 1924–1979. Before 1941, the wording of questions eliciting information on cigarette use and type of respondent are not recorded. In 1941–1954, men were asked, "Do you smoke cigarettes?" In 1955–1959, respondents were asked, "Do any men [women] in your household smoke cigarettes with [without] a filter tip?" In 1960–1965 and 1967, women and men were asked, "Have you bought, for your own use, cigarettes with [without] a filter tip in the past 30 days?" In 1966 and 1968–1979, women and men were asked, "Have you bought, for your own use, cigarettes with [without] a filter tip in the past 7 days?" Data since 1955 are based on the sum of the percentage of smokers who bought filter-tipped cigarettes and the percentage who bought nonfilter-tipped cigarettes in the past 30 days. Results overestimate smoking prevalence because respondents could answer "yes" to both questions. Data for women in 1976–1979 include only the percentage buying filter-tipped cigarettes; the question on the use of nonfilter-tipped cigarettes was dropped because of low response.

†Absence of data points from national surveys from 1935–1965 means these lines should not be interpreted as trends. The 1935 data are from the 1935 *Fortune* Survey III (*Fortune Magazine,* 1935), the 1955 data are from the 1955 Current Population Survey (Haenszel et al., 1956), and the 1965–1979 data are from the National Health Interview Survey (Giovino et al., 1994).

FIGURE 15-1   Prevalence (%) of Current Smoking Among Adults Aged 18 Years or Older in the Greater Milwaukee Area and in the General U.S. Population, by Gender 1935–1979. *Source:* Reproduced from the Centers for Disease Control and Prevention (2001). "Women and Smoking: A Report of the Surgeon General, 2001," Figure 2.1. www.cdc.gov/tobacco/data_statistics/sgr/2001/complete_report/pdfs/chp2.pdf, accessed October 1, 2012.

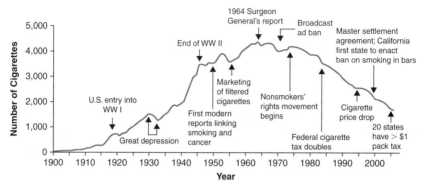

FIGURE 15-2   Annual Adult per Capita Cigarette Consumption, U.S., 1900–2005.
Source: Reproduced from U.S. Centers for Disease Control and Prevention. http://
smokingcessationleadership.ucsf.edu/Downloads/ppt_June_172009.pdf, accessed October 1, 2012.

reported that smoking increased the risk of heart disease. The surgeon general's report was very influential, convincing many smokers to quit and providing ammunition for advocates wishing to impose controls on the tobacco industry.

Women were hardly mentioned in the 1964 surgeon general's report. Lung cancer was rare in women, and all the studies had been done on men. However, women soon began to catch up. In 1980, the surgeon general issued another report that focused entirely on women. *Health Consequences of Smoking for Women* addressed "the fallacy of women's immunity."[4] The report points out that the first signs of an epidemic of smoking-related diseases among women were just beginning to appear, because women had only begun smoking intensively 25 years after men had. Indeed, lung cancer was about to surpass breast cancer and become the leading cause of cancer death in women, as it is today.[5] The report noted that, in addition to suffering the same ill health effects as men, female smokers are at increased risk for complications of pregnancy and that infants of female smokers are more likely to be premature or lagging in physical growth.

Historically, the prevalence of smoking among black men was higher than that for white men; accordingly, lung cancer mortality rates have been higher among black men. Rates of smoking among blacks have declined and are now slightly lower than those among whites. American Indians and Alaskan Natives smoke at much higher rates than other ethnic groups, averaging 36.4 percent overall. Very large differences in smoking rates are seen among groups of different socioeconomic status, and there is a particularly strong association with lack of education. Prevalence of smoking is only about 8.3 percent among male and female college graduates, while 27 percent of those without high school diploma are smokers.[6]

Regulatory Restrictions on Smoking—New Focus on Environmental Tobacco Smoke

Public health efforts at discouraging smoking have had to contend with the enormous economic and political power of the tobacco industry. Congress, which still provides subsidies to tobacco growers, has been very reluctant to pass legislation opposed by the industry. However, the 1964 surgeon general's report carried great credibility, and its publication led to a number of government actions aimed at restricting cigarette marketing. These included Federal Trade Commission requirements that cigarette packages contain warning labels and a Federal Communications Commission mandate in 1968 that radio and television advertisements for cigarettes be balanced by public service announcements about their harmful effects. The latter requirement, called the Fairness Doctrine, was so effective in countering the tobacco companies' ads, as seen in the drop in cigarette consumption shown in Figure 15-2, that in 1971 the industry submitted to a total ban on cigarette advertising on radio and television. In return, the public service announcements ceased. The tobacco companies shifted their advertising efforts to magazines, newspapers, billboards, product giveaways, and sponsorship of sporting and cultural events.[2]

Over the past 3 decades, new awareness of the harm caused by "second-hand smoke" has led to some of the most effective actions against smoking. Studies began to show that exposure to environmental tobacco smoke caused some of the same health problems as active smoking. For example, the nonsmoking spouses of smokers have an increased risk of lung cancer and heart disease, and children of parents who smoke are more likely to suffer from asthma, respiratory infections, and sudden infant death syndrome. In 1992, the Environmental Protection Agency issued a report that declared environmental tobacco smoke to be a carcinogen, causing 3000 lung cancer deaths a year.[7] Evidence of the harm caused by passive smoking inspired the nonsmokers rights movement, which largely bypassed the Congress and focused political pressure on state and local governments.

In 1974, Connecticut was the first state to enact restrictions on smoking in restaurants. Minnesota passed a comprehensive statewide clean indoor air law in 1975. In 1983, San Francisco passed a restrictive law against smoking in the workplace, including private workplaces. The clean indoor air movement blossomed. At the state level, laws were passed that restricted smoking on public transit and in elevators, cultural and recreational facilities, schools, and libraries. Over the objections of the tobacco industry, a ban on smoking on all domestic airline flights was passed by Congress in 1989.[2] Restrictions on indoor smoking became more widespread in the 1990s. By January 1, 2012, 24 states and the District of Columbia had banned or severely restricted smoking in all public places, including work sites, restaurants, and most bars. All but one other state—Wyoming—had enacted some limitations on indoor smoking, and many counties and municipalities have passed legislation to promote clean indoor air.[8]

The effectiveness of the nonsmokers' rights movement stems from its success in transforming smoking into a socially unacceptable activity. Bans in so many public places force smokers to refrain for extended periods and to segregate themselves when they wish to smoke, often by going outdoors. By making smoking inconvenient, bans encourage people to quit. As Figure 15-2 shows, cigarette consumption has declined steadily since the nonsmokers rights movement began.

Advertising—Emphasis on Youth

While smoking rates among adults have fallen, public health advocates have become increasingly concerned about smoking among youth. Teenagers tend to be less worried about their health in the distant future than they are with their image and social status among their peers. Tobacco companies exploit those concerns in their attempts to win over young people to smoking.

In order to maintain a constant number of customers over time, the tobacco industry must persuade 2 million people to take up the habit each year to balance the number of smokers who die or quit.[9] Cigarette advertising and promotional expenditures amounted to $12.4 billion in 2006, almost double the amount spent in 1997.[10] Because the teen years are the critical period for smoking initiation—90 percent of adult smokers started when they were teenagers, and the average age at which they took up the habit is 14.5—tobacco companies have targeted their advertising toward children and young people.[2] For example, Joe Camel ads were strongly appealing to children. A 1991 study found that 91 percent of 6-year-olds recognized the cartoon character, the same percentage that recognized the Mickey Mouse logo of the Disney channel. Some 98 percent of high school students recognized Joe Camel, compared with only 72 percent of adults.[11] Between 1988, when the Joe Camel ad campaign was introduced, and 1990, it is estimated that Camel cigarette sales to minors went from $6 million to $476 million.[2] In response to an outburst of negative publicity and public anger at the tobacco companies, Joe Camel was retired in 1997.

Tobacco companies also targeted youth with promotional items, such as T-shirts, caps, and sporting goods bearing a brand's logo. They managed to evade the ban on broadcast advertising by sponsoring sporting events, at which brand names were displayed in the background, ensuring that they would be visible on television throughout the event.

As part of the 1998 Master Settlement Agreement (MSA), discussed later in this chapter, major tobacco companies agreed to stop advertisements targeted at children, including some promotional activities. Although the most blatant appeals to youth are gone, the companies began running ads that, while ostensibly antitobacco public service ads, were actually more sophisticated messages designed to encourage youth smoking.[12] The messages were that smoking is for adults only, and that parents should talk to their children about not smoking. Analyses of their impact on teens have shown that these ads were ineffective in discouraging young people from smoking and may have increased their intention to smoke. This may have been the intention when the ads were designed. Nevertheless, a combination of public health efforts, including the MSA, have contributed to a decline in the number of teens who smoke. The CDC's biannual survey of high school students found in 2011 that 18.1 percent had smoked in the previous month, down from 36.4 percent in 1997, the year when the highest number of students reported having smoked.[13]

All states have laws prohibiting the sale of tobacco to minors, but enforcement of the laws varies. The CDC's 2011 survey found that 14 percent of the student smokers bought cigarettes from stores or gas station. There is evidence that increasingly, youths are buying cigarettes via the Internet, making age laws difficult to enforce. A 2007 Institute of Medicine committee has recommended that Congress pass legislation to prohibit all online tobacco sales and shipment of tobacco products directly to consumers.[14]

As advertising to children and teens has become increasingly restricted, tobacco companies have focused their efforts on young adults, who are still receptive to social pressures, may smoke occasionally, and may be vulnerable to advertising. The companies use promotional activities in bars and nightclubs, such as distributing free cigarette samples or brand-labeled articles of clothing, with the goal of turning occasional smokers into addicts. Social events at college campuses are other occasions where companies can gain access to young adults. A study in 2000–2001 of 119 colleges found that events at which free cigarettes were distributed occurred at all but one of them. Many of the events took place at bars and nightclubs, but fraternities and sororities were also popular sites for the events.[15] Indoor smoking bans, which have become more widespread in the last few years, have blocked the effectiveness of this kind of marketing. Portrayal of smoking in movies and on television has been shown to exert a powerful influence in inspiring adolescents to smoke, and the Institute of Medicine has recommended that the movie rating system take this into consideration when G, PG, PG-13, or R ratings are assigned.[14]

The tobacco industry has targeted advertising at women and minorities, groups identified as promising sources of new smokers. Young women have been attracted by suggestions that smoking will help them lose weight, beginning with the Lucky Strike ads of the 1920s that advised, "Reach for a Lucky instead of a sweet." More recently, Virginia Slims ads have taken a similar approach. Shortly after the Virginia Slims advertising campaign began in the 1960s, the proportion of 14- to 17-year-old girls who started smoking nearly doubled.[2] African Americans historically had higher rates of smoking—and of lung cancer—than whites, though the difference has shrunk over the past decade.[6] Tobacco companies try to win over black leaders by donating to black causes, such as the National Association for the Advancement of Colored

People and the United Negro College Fund, and by sponsoring black cultural events such as jazz festivals. They advertise heavily in African-American publications and, before the MSA, blanketed neighborhoods with billboards.

Taxes as a Public Health Measure

Antismoking activists, supported by economics research, have concluded that one of the most effective measures to discourage young people from smoking is to raise the tax on cigarettes. One reason is that a pack of cigarettes represents a more significant proportion of a teenager's disposable income than it does for adults, and the higher price is likely to have more impact on someone who is not yet addicted. Low income and minority smokers are also sensitive to price.[16]

Recent research on teenage smoking suggests that teenagers are indeed sensitive to price. For example, after Philip Morris cut the price of Marlboro cigarettes, a brand favored by young people, by 40 percent in April 1993, the proportion of teenagers in 8th, 10th, and 12th grades who smoked rose from 23.5 percent to 28 percent in 1996. Other studies have shown that a 10 percent increase in price reduces the number of teenagers who smoke by approximately 7 percent to 12 percent.[17] "Raising tobacco taxes is our number one strategy to damage the tobacco industry," an American Cancer Society executive was quoted as saying. "The industry has found ways around everything else we have done, but they can't repeal the laws of economics."[17(p.293)]

Raising taxes on cigarettes is effective in reducing smoking among adults as well. In 1989, California increased cigarette taxes from 10 cents to 35 cents per pack. The law specified that 20 percent of the proceeds were to be designated for programs designed to prevent and reduce tobacco use, especially among children. Surveys conducted before and after implementation of the tax increase found that the prevalence of cigarette smoking among adults in California was reduced from 22.7 percent in 1988 to 20.0 percent in 1992 to 15.9 percent in 1995.[18] It is difficult to determine the share of the decline that can be attributed to the price increase as compared with other antismoking measures, including indoor smoking bans and the antismoking campaign funded by the tax.

In recent years, state and local governments have found that raising taxes on cigarettes is a painless way of closing budget shortfalls, and many states have followed this policy.[19] In 2012, for example, New York had the highest rate, with a tax of $4.35 per pack. By contrast, tobacco-producing states have low cigarette taxes: Virginia's rate was 30 cents per pack, and Missouri's rate, the lowest, was 17 cents.[8] California, a leader in raising cigarette taxes for public health goals, had fallen to a rank of 33rd among states, with a tax of 87 cents per pack. In June 2012, California voters rejected a proposed $1 a pack increase, the proceeds of which would have been used to finance cancer research. The tobacco industry spent nearly $50 million to defeat the measure.[20] The federal tax on cigarettes, last raised in 2009, is $1.01.per pack.[8]

California's Tobacco Control Program

Despite California's failure in recent years to maintain its leadership in tobacco control efforts, its voter-initiated program begun in 1989 with a 25-cent tax increase on cigarettes, has proved successful in maintaining low smoking rates statewide. The initiative mandated mass media antitobacco advertising as well as school and community education and intervention activities. It also mandated that the effectiveness of the program be evaluated after a decade. Thus, the California experience has provided evidence on what methods are effective in reducing smoking.

The tax increase itself contributed to the success of the program, as discussed in the previous section. Immediately after the increase was implemented, the rate of decline in cigarette consumption increased significantly in California compared with the rest of the nation. The rate of decline then leveled off until the media campaign was launched in 1990 and 1991, when there was a further 12 percent decline.[21] In 1994, the California legislature passed a law prohibiting smoking statewide in all workplaces except bars, taverns, and casinos. The law has since been strengthened to include these workplaces as well.

Overall, per capita cigarette consumption in California fell by 59 percent between 1988 and 2004.[22] This reduction was achieved by a combination of a reduction in the number of smokers and reduction of the number of cigarettes each smoker consumed per day. In California, according to the CDC's Behavioral Risk Factor Survey, the prevalence of smoking was 12.1 percent in 2010, compared to 19.3 percent in the nation as a whole.[23] California's antitobacco campaign suffered budget cuts after the first few years, and tobacco companies stepped up their political efforts to oppose the state's control measures, as well as their advertising and promotion of cigarettes; but the permanent changes in policy, as well as additional tax increases, have helped California to maintain its lead over all other states except Utah in keeping smoking levels relatively low.[23]

California's campaign included an aggressive advertising component, which contributed significantly to the campaign's overall success. Studies of the effectiveness of antismoking messages have shown that some messages are much more effective than others. In fact, some programs sponsored by the tobacco industry, which are presented as smoking prevention efforts, have been shown to make smoking more attractive to youths. For example, these advertisements often present the messages that smoking is an "adult" choice, that parents have a responsibility to help their kids fight peer pressure for smoking, and that "it's the law" that retailers not sell cigarettes to youth. Examination of industry documents, discussed in the next section, has found that the industry has purposely used these "forbidden fruit" messages to generate good public relations and fight restrictive legislation without actually discouraging youth smoking.[24]

The evaluation component of California's media campaign identified which antismoking messages were most effective in reaching youth. Researchers found that the message most effective in reaching both youths and adults is that "Tobacco industry executives use deceitful, manipulative, dishonest practices to hook new users, sell more cigarettes and make more money."[25(p.774)] One such successful ad, called "Nicotine Soundbites," showed the actual footage of tobacco executives testifying before Congress in 1994, raising their right hands and swearing that nicotine is not addictive. Ads with this message made both adults and teenagers angry, because no one likes to learn that they are being manipulated.

Another message that was found to be effective among both adults and teens was that second-hand smoke harms others. One ad portrayed a boy smoking, sitting with his little sister watching television. The little girl begins coughing and smoke comes out of her mouth. In the early 1990s, California also ran ads that encouraged quitting and provided information on smoking cessation programs, including toll-free quit lines; calls to the quit lines dramatically increased. Ads with some other messages, including those that focused on health effects, were found to be ineffective.[25]

Researchers concluded that, to be effective, antitobacco advertisements need to be "ambitious, hard-hitting, explicit, and in-your-face."[25(p.776)] The industry recognized the effectiveness of the ads and worked hard to limit them. R. J. Reynolds threatened to sue the California Department of Health and the television stations that ran the Nicotine Soundbites ad; the lawsuit was not filed, but the ad was later dropped. During the state campaign, the tobacco industry tried to counter the antitobacco efforts by increasing spending in California on advertising, incentives to merchants, and promotional items. One study calculated that after 1993, the industry spent nearly $10 for every $1 spent by the state.[21]

The Master Settlement Agreement (MSA)

The 1990s saw dramatic developments in the battle against smoking, and suddenly it seemed possible that effective tobacco control measures would be enacted at the federal level. The changes resulted from several separate political and legal events, as well as public revelations that have discredited the tobacco industry.

In February 1994, David Kessler, then Commissioner of the Food and Drug Administration (FDA), launched an offensive against the tobacco industry by asserting that his agency had the authority to regulate tobacco. Kessler, who was appointed by the first President Bush but now had the support of an antismoking president, Bill Clinton, based his claim on thoroughly documented evidence that nicotine is an addictive drug and cigarettes are drug delivery systems. He proposed a series of measures aimed to protect children and teenagers against tobacco company efforts to get them hooked.

Coincidentally, in March 1994, a class-action lawsuit was filed against American tobacco companies in federal district court in Louisiana on behalf of "all nicotine-dependent persons in the U.S." and their families and heirs, seeking compensatory and punitive damages, attorneys fees, an admission of wrongdoing, and other remedies. Although this suit was dismissed, it was followed by other major lawsuits, including one in May 1994 by Michael Moore, the attorney general of Mississippi, who sought to recover the medical costs that the state had incurred treating smoking-related illnesses. Attorneys general from most of the other states followed suit over the next 3 years.[26]

Also in 1994, an anonymous informant from the Brown & Williamson tobacco company, who called himself "Mr. Butts" after the Doonesbury comic strip character, sent a box of top-secret tobacco industry internal documents to Stanton Glantz, a professor of medicine at the University of California at San Francisco and a well-known critic of the tobacco industry. The papers provided a wealth of information on discrepancies between what the industry knew about the ill effects of tobacco and what they were telling the public. For example, a lawyer for Brown & Williamson had written in a 1963 internal memo, "Nicotine is addictive. We are, then, in the business of selling nicotine, an addictive drug effective in the release of stress mechanisms."[27(p.58)] Glantz, with the support of University of California lawyers and librarians, published the papers on the Internet.

The tobacco companies, of course, challenged the FDA's authority to regulate tobacco, and they also vigorously defended against the lawsuits by attorneys general and injured smokers. However, the documents released by Glantz, together with other internal industry documents that were leaked, seriously undermined the industry's ability to defend itself in court. In April 1997, a North Carolina court affirmed the FDA's authority over tobacco as a drug, although it struck down some of the advertising restrictions proposed by the agency. However, in August 1998, an appeals court ruled the other way, stating that only Congress has authority to regulate the tobacco industry. The Supreme Court agreed to take up the issue, and in 2000 it supported the appeals court decision that the FDA did not have the authority to regulate tobacco.[28]

In early 1997, when the tobacco industry was on the defensive, it began negotiations with the attorneys general, hoping to reach a settlement that would protect them against unlimited lawsuits and possible financial ruin. A historic settlement was announced in June, in which the companies agreed to pay $368.5 billion over a 25-year period to compensate states for treating smoking-related illnesses and to set up a fund to pay damage claims for ill smokers, as well as for other purposes including financing of nationwide antismoking programs. The industry also agreed to a number of restrictions on advertising and promotion and to allow the FDA to regulate the nicotine in cigarettes. However, the settlement required Congressional approval, which did not materialize. In 1998, the tobacco industry reached a more limited settlement with the attorneys general, agreeing to pay 46 states $206 billion over 25 years and accepting some restrictions on advertising, including a ban on billboard ads. The settlement also provided $1.7 billion over a 5-year period to create the American Legacy Foundation, which used the funds for public education and other tobacco control activities.[29]

The MSA has been something of a disappointment for public health advocates. It was hoped that the states would use some of the settlement dollars for tobacco control programs. Smoking-cessation programs that include counseling and nicotine-replacement therapy, such as nicotine gum or patches, can double or even triple a smoker's chance of quitting.[29] Telephone quit lines, sponsored by some states and sometimes by voluntary organizations, can be effective at motivating people to quit. However, most states have used little of the MSA funds for such programs, using the windfall to close state budget gaps. On the other hand, tobacco companies have had to increase the price of cigarettes by 45 cents a pack to pay for the settlement. As discussed previously, higher prices discourage people from smoking, especially young people.

The American Legacy Foundation has used its part of the settlement to run aggressive ad campaigns against smoking targeted at youth, called the "truth" campaign. Drawing on findings from evaluations of the California and other tobacco control programs, the ads convey the message that tobacco companies manipulate the truth, deny adverse health effects and the addictive nature of tobacco, and try to make smoking appear attractive. The "truth" ads featured statements such as: "In 1984, one tobacco company referred to new customers as 'replacement smokers'" and "In 1990 tobacco companies put together a plan to stop coroners from listing tobacco as a cause of death on a death certificate." Another ad features a young man trying to ship a box of cigarettes at the post office, saying, "I'd like to ship this arsenic and cyanide spreading mechanism," insisting that it's perfectly legal and being met with skepticism by the clerk.[30] The "truth" ads were placed in youth-oriented magazines and television programs. Two national youth surveys, used to evaluate the effect of the "truth" campaign, found that young people who had seen the ads were significantly more likely than those who had not seen them to hold negative attitudes toward tobacco.[31] The "truth" campaign, together with the increased tobacco prices, has contributed to reducing youth smoking to a 27-year low of 20 percent in 2003 and 18.1 percent in 2011.[12,29] Smoking rates among young African Americans are lower than those among white youths.

The American Legacy Foundation's funding from the MSA expired in 2003. However, the foundation has succeeded in finding funds to continue the truth campaign and to launch the "EX" campaign, designed to help smokers quit by "re-learning to live their lives without cigarettes."[32] It also collaborates with the University of California at San Francisco in maintaining an on-line library of previously secret tobacco industry documents, which can be searched through a user-friendly interface. Ads for the truth campaign can be seen on the Foundation's website at http://www.thetruth.com. The digital library is found at http://legacy .library.ucsf.edu/.

FDA Regulation

The original agreement negotiated by the state attorneys general and the tobacco companies contained a provision allowing the FDA to regulate tobacco. Because that agreement was not approved by Congress, the MSA did not contain such a provision. There are many advantages to giving regulatory authority over tobacco to the FDA. Until 2009, there were no legal restrictions concerning ingredients in tobacco smoke or on labeling or advertising concerning health claims by the companies. There is evidence, for example, that companies manipulated nicotine levels in tobacco to promote addiction, and they added ammonia to increase the effect of the nicotine. Tobacco smoke contains toxic chemicals such as nitrosamines and arsenic in addition to the tars known to be carcinogenic.[27] It also contains radioactive polonium, which is not widely recognized.[33] In fact, the American Legacy Foundation has focused on some of these toxic ingredients in their antismoking ads.

Finally in 2009, after previous attempts had failed, Congress passed and President Obama signed the Family Smoking Prevention and Tobacco Control Act.[34] The law gives the FDA authority to regulate tobacco products and to restrict advertising and promotion. It requires larger and more graphic warning labels on cigarette packages, and it forbids tobacco companies from sponsoring sporting events. The law requires the disclosure of ingredients of cigarettes, as is done with food. It gives the FDA authority to require the removal of harmful ingredients, and to regulate health-related claims made by the companies, insisting that such claims be proven. The truth-in-advertising provision makes it possible for cigarettes to be made safer, so that smokers who cannot or will not quit would suffer less harm. Unless the government has the authority to verify claims, tobacco companies could continue to label their products "light" or "safer" without needing to actually reduce the hazards of smoking. One proposed advantage of giving the FDA regulatory authority would be to allow the agency to gradually reduce the amount of nicotine allowed in cigarettes to make them less addictive and to taper smokers off the addictive drug.[14]

The new law bans candy-flavored cigarettes, designed to appeal to young people. However, menthol was not included in the banned flavorings. Menthol masks the harshness of inhaled smoke and appears to ease the initiation of smoking among youths. It is also popular among African-American smokers, three-quarters of whom smoke menthol cigarettes, while only 25 percent of white smokers choose the menthol flavoring.[35,36]

"The key to public health action on the tobacco front seems to lie in combining strategies to discourage children from smoking and in producing a safer and less addictive cigarette for those who cannot, or will not, resist the temptation to smoke," wrote the ethicist George Annas in January 1997,[37(p.307)] when the possibility of a negotiated settlement was first being considered. Whether Congress or the courts or both will finally make possible the demotion of tobacco as public health enemy number one remains to be seen.

Conclusion

Cigarette smoking is the leading actual cause of death in the United States. The fact that smoking causes lung cancer has been known since the 1950s, and the behavior has been responsible for an epidemic of lung cancer, the leading cause of cancer death among both men and women. Smoking also causes cardiovascular disease, chronic lung disease, low birth weight in infants, and a number of other unhealthy conditions.

Since the surgeon general's *Smoking and Health* report was published in 1964, summarizing the evidence about the harm caused by smoking, public health advocates have been attacking the habit in as many ways as possible. Cigarette consumption in the United States peaked in the early 1960s and has declined since then, demonstrating significant success from the public health efforts. In the 1990s, however, there was a leveling off of the percentage of adults who smoke. Currently about 20 percent of the adult population smoke cigarettes, down from over 42 percent in 1965.

Public health has fought the tobacco industry on many fronts. In the 1960s, Congress passed legislation that required that cigarette ads on radio and television be balanced by counter-advertising about the harmful effects of smoking. This publicity, together with warning labels on cigarette packages, helped to persuade many people to quit. Tobacco companies have become increasingly sophisticated about marketing their products, especially to children, and public health has had to work hard to oppose them. Since nicotine in tobacco is addictive, it has become clear that the most effective approach to reducing smoking is to prevent young people from taking up the habit.

Public health interventions that have demonstrated some success in preventing the onset of smoking and in reducing its prevalence include the enactment and enforcement of laws prohibiting the sale of tobacco to minors, restrictions on indoor smoking, and—most effectively—increases in cigarette prices through imposition of taxes.

California was a leader among states in imposing a tax on cigarettes to be used for tobacco control programs. Evaluation of its mass media advertising campaign has helped antismoking activists to understand what messages are most effective in persuading youths not to smoke. California was also a leader in legislation to ban smoking in public places.

In the mid- and late-1990s, legal and regulatory attacks on the tobacco industry were launched by the Clinton administration and a number of states. The MSA between the attorneys general of 46 states and the tobacco industry contained restrictions on tobacco advertising aimed at young people and provided billions of dollars to the states to compensate them for medical costs they incurred for treating smoking related illnesses. It also provided funds to establish the American Legacy Foundation, which has run an effective media campaign to discourage young people from smoking.

In 2009, Congress passed and President Obama signed a law authorizing the FDA to regulate tobacco products. It is hoped that the agency will devise ways to rein in the industry's deceptive practices, wean smokers off their addiction to nicotine, and reduce demand for cigarettes.

The battle continues. It seems that progress is being made, but prospects for victory in public health's battle against the powerful tobacco industry are uncertain.

References

1. U.S. Centers for Disease Control and Prevention, "Tobacco Use Screening and Counseling During Physician Office Visits Among Adults," *Morbidity and Mortality Weekly Report* 57 (2008): 1221–1226.
2. C. E. Bartecchi, T. D. MacKenzie, and R. W. Schrier, "The Global Tobacco Epidemic," *Scientific American* (May 1995): 44–51.
3. U.S. Public Health Service, *Smoking and Health: Report of the Advisory Committee to the Surgeon General* (Washington, DC: 1964).
4. U.S. Public Health Service, *Health Consequences of Smoking for Women, Report of the Surgeon General* (Rockville, MD: 1980).
5. American Cancer Society, *Cancer Facts & Figures—2012*, p. 3. http://www.cancer.org/acs/groups/content/@epidemiologysurveillance/documents/document/aspc-031941.pdf, accessed October 31, 2012.
6. National Center for Health Statistics, *Health, United States, 2011.* http://www.cdc.gov/nchs/data/hus/hus11.pdf, May 2012, accessed June 25, 2012.
7. Environmental Protection Agency, *Respiratory Health Effects of Passive Smoking, 1992.* http://cfpub2.epa.gov/ncea/cfm/recordisplay.cfm?deid=2835, accessed June 27, 2012.
8. American Lung Association, "State of Tobacco Control, 2012." http://www.stateoftobaccocontrol.org/SOTC_2012.pdf, accessed June 27, 2012.
9. R. Kluger, "A Peace Plan for the Cigarette Wars," *New York Times Magazine*, April 7, 1996: 28–30, 35, 50, 54.
10. U.S. Centers for Disease Control and Prevention, "Tobacco Industry Marketing." http://www.cdc.gov/tobacco/data_statistics/fact_sheets/tobacco_industry/marketing/, accessed September 23, 2012.
11. P. M. Fischer, M. P. Schwartz, J. W. Richards, Jr., A. O. Goldstein, and T. H. Rojas, "Brand Logo Recognition by Children Aged 3 to 6 Years: Mickey Mouse and Old Joe the Camel," *Journal of the American Medical Association* 266 (1991): 3145–3148.

12. M. Wakefield et al., "Effect of Televised, Tobacco Company-Funded Smoking Prevention Advertising on Youth Smoking-Related Beliefs, Intentions, and Behavior," *American Journal of Public Health* 96 (2006): 2154–2160.

13. U.S. Centers for Disease Control and Prevention, "Youth Risk Behavior Surveillance—United States, 2011," *Morbidity and Mortality Weekly Report* 61 (SS04) (2012): 1–62.

14. Institute of Medicine (U.S.), *Ending the Tobacco Problem: A Blueprint for the Nation* (Washington, DC: National Academies Press, 2007).

15. N. A. Rigotti, S. E. Moran, and H. Wechsler, "US College Students' Exposure to Tobacco Promotions: Prevalence and Association with Tobacco Use," *American Journal of Public Health* 95 (2005): 138–144.

16. U.S. Centers for Disease Control and Prevention, "Response to Increases in Cigarette Prices by Race/Ethnicity, Income, and Age Groups—United States, 1976–1993," *Morbidity and Mortality Weekly Report* 47 (1998): 605–609.

17. M. Grossman and F. J. Chaloupka, "Cigarette Taxes: The Straw to Break the Camel's Back," *Public Health Reports* 112 (1997): 291–297.

18. California Department of Public Health, "Adult Smoking Prevalence." http://www.cdph.ca .gov/Programs/tobacco/Documents/CTCPAdultSmoking06.pdf, accessed June 29, 2012.

19. S. Dewan, "States Look at Tobacco to Balance the Budget," *The New York Times*, March 20, 2009.

20. I. Lovett, "California: Cigarette Tax Defeated," *The New York Times,* June 22, 2012.

21. J. P. Pierce et al., "Has the California Tobacco Control Program Reduced Smoking?" *Journal of the American Medical Association* 280 (1998): 893–899.

22. California Department of Health Services, "Cigarette Consumption." http://www.cdph.ca .gov/programs/tobacco/Documents/CTCPConsumption05.pdf, accessed June 29, 2012.

23. U.S. Centers for Disease Control and Prevention, "Vital Signs: Current Cigarette Smoking Among Adults Aged > 18 Years—United States," *Morbidity and Mortality Weekly Report* 60 (2011): 1207–1212.

24. A. Landman, P. M. Ling, and S. A. Glantz, "Tobacco Industry Youth Smoking Prevention Programs: Protecting the Industry and Hurting Tobacco Control," *American Journal of Public Health* 92 (2002): 917–930.

25. L. K. Goldman, and S. A. Glantz, "Evaluation of Antismoking Advertising Campaigns," *Journal of the American Medical Association* 279 (1998): 772–777.

26. J. M. Broder, "Cigarette Makers in a $368 Billion Accord to Curb Lawsuits and Curtail Marketing," *The New York Times*, June 21, 1997.

27. S. A. Glantz et al., *The Cigarette Papers* (Berkeley, CA: University of California Press, 1996).

28. M. L. Myers, "Protecting the Public Health by Strengthening the Food and Drug Administration's Authority over Tobacco Products," *New England Journal of Medicine* 343 (2000): 1806–1809.

29. S. A. Schroeder, "Tobacco Control in the Wake of the 1998 Master Settlement Agreement," *New England Journal of Medicine* 350 (2004): 203–301.

30. American Legacy Foundation. www.thetruth.com/, accessed June 29, 2012.

31. M. C. Farrelly et al., "Getting to the Truth: Evaluating National Tobacco Countermarketing Campaigns," *American Journal of Public Health* 92 (2002): 901–907.

32. American Legacy Foundation. www.legacyforhealth.org/, accessed June 29, 2012.
33. M. E. Muggli et al., "Waking a Sleeping Giant: The Tobacco Industry's Response to the Polonium-210 Issue," *American Journal of Public Health* 98 (2008): 1543–1650.
34. G. D. Curfman, S. Morrisey, and J. M. Drazen, "Tobacco, Public Health, and the FDA," *New England Journal of Medicine* 361 (2009): 402–403.
35. Centers for Disease Control and Prevention, "Highlights: African Americans and Tobacco." http://www.cdc.gov/tobacco/data_statistics/sgr/1998/highlights/african_americans/index.htm, accessed June 30, 2012.
36. L. W. Green, "New Anti-Smoking Ads a Smart Move," CNN Opinion. http://www.cnn.com/2012/03/16/opinion/green-tobacco-education/index.html?iref=allsearch, accessed June 30, 2012.
37. G. Annas, "Tobacco Litigation as Cancer Prevention: Dealing with the Devil," *New England Journal of Medicine* 336 (1997): 304–308.

Public Health Enemy Number Two and Growing: Poor Diet and Physical Inactivity

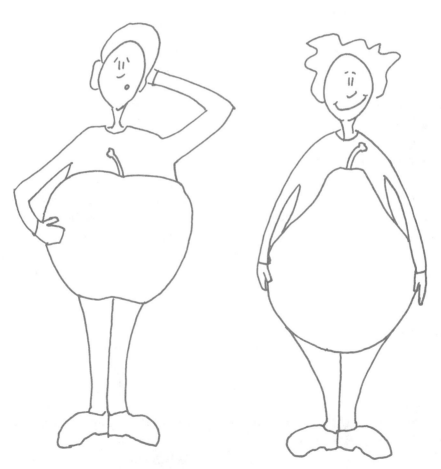

Pear-Shaped is Healthier

Throughout evolutionary history, humans had to exert a great deal of physical activity to obtain their food. Only over the past century has a substantial and increasing percentage of the population had access to an excess of food with no need to exercise. The consequence of this imbalance has been that Americans are becoming fatter, an exceedingly unhealthy trend. Today, poor diet and physical inactivity have been ranked second among the factors identified as leading actual causes of death in the United States, although the analysis is controversial.

Many studies have shown that weighing too much increases people's risk of cardiovascular disease, diabetes, most kinds of cancer, and a variety of other diseases. Thus, it is in the interest of public health to reduce the prevalence of overweight and obesity, which in 2007–2010 affected 68.5 percent of the adult population.[1] Getting people to lose weight, however, seems to be even more difficult than getting them to quit smoking, although many of them want to be thinner. According to the 2005–2006 National Health and Nutrition Examination Survey, 57 percent of women and 37 percent of men are trying to lose weight, most of them unsuccessfully.[2] An Institute of Medicine report on the problem states, "It is paradoxical that obesity is increasing in the United States while more people are dieting than ever before, spending, by one estimate, more than $33 billion per year on weight-reduction products (including diet foods and soft drinks, artificial sweeteners, and diet books) and services (e.g., fitness clubs and weight-loss programs)."[3(p.27)]

The association of obesity with certain health risks is easy to measure, but the relationship may not be a simple one of cause and effect. Obesity is a complex condition, influenced by genes as well as by many individual and social factors that include eating and exercise patterns. While being overweight has a health impact in itself, a person's disease risk may also be affected independently by dietary patterns and the amount of physical activity, whether or not he or she is overweight. Public health advocates, therefore, seek to promote healthier eating patterns among Americans, to encourage them to exercise more, and to reduce the percentage of people who are overweight.

Epidemiology of Obesity

Obesity is, to an extent, in the eyes of the beholder—often the beholder who is looking in the mirror. In the public health perspective, obesity is usually defined more precisely in terms of body-mass index (BMI). BMI is calculated by dividing a person's weight in kilograms by the square of his or her height in meters. Table 16-1 presents BMIs in terms of inches and pounds for a range that includes most Americans.

Most studies show that weight-associated health risks begin to appear at a BMI of about 25, and rise more significantly above 30, with the risks increasing in proportion to the severity of an

Table 16-1   Body Mass Index Table

BMI	19	20	21	22	23	24	25	26	27	28	29	30	31	32	33	34	35
Height (inches)							Body Weight (pounds)										
58	91	96	100	105	110	115	119	124	129	134	138	143	148	153	158	162	167
59	94	99	104	109	114	119	124	128	133	138	143	148	153	158	163	168	173
60	97	102	107	112	118	123	128	133	138	143	148	153	158	163	168	174	179
61	100	106	111	116	122	127	132	137	143	148	153	158	164	169	174	180	185
62	104	109	115	120	126	131	136	142	147	153	158	164	169	175	180	186	191
63	107	113	118	124	130	135	141	146	152	158	163	169	175	180	186	191	197
64	110	116	122	128	134	140	145	151	157	163	169	174	180	186	192	197	204
65	114	120	126	132	138	144	150	156	162	168	174	180	186	192	198	204	210
66	118	124	130	136	142	148	155	161	167	173	179	186	192	198	204	210	216
67	121	127	134	140	146	153	159	166	172	178	185	191	198	204	211	217	223
68	125	131	138	144	151	158	164	171	177	184	190	197	203	210	216	223	230
69	128	135	142	149	155	162	169	176	182	189	196	203	209	216	223	230	236
70	132	139	146	153	160	167	174	181	188	195	202	209	216	222	229	236	243
71	136	143	150	157	165	172	179	186	193	200	208	215	222	229	236	243	250
72	140	147	154	162	169	177	184	191	199	206	213	221	228	235	242	250	258
73	144	151	159	166	174	182	189	197	204	212	219	227	235	242	250	257	265
74	148	155	163	171	179	186	194	202	210	218	225	233	241	249	256	264	272
75	152	160	168	176	184	192	200	208	216	224	232	240	248	256	264	272	279
76	156	164	172	180	189	197	205	213	221	230	238	246	254	263	271	279	287

Source: Reproduced from National Institutes of Health, "Body Mass Index Table." www.nhlbi.nih.gov/guidelines/obesity/bmi_tbl.pdf, accessed September 27, 2012.

individual's obesity. The National Institutes of Health and the Centers for Disease Control and Prevention (CDC) have agreed on a definition of overweight as a BMI between 25 and 29.9 and obesity as a BMI of 30 or greater.[4] Using this definition, 73.3 percent of men and 63.9 percent of women 20 years of age and older were found to be overweight or obese in the National Health and Nutrition Examination Survey (NHANES) conducted between 2007 and 2010.[1] The prevalence of obesity was 34.4 percent in men and 36.1 percent in women.

The prevalence of overweight and obesity has increased dramatically over the past 3 decades, as shown in **Figures 16-1** and **16-2**. There are significant racial differences in the prevalence of overweight among women: 80.3 percent of nonpregnant black women are overweight, compared with 60.2 percent of white women. Black men and white men are more equally likely to be overweight: 70.2 percent of black men compared with 73.5 percent of white men.[1] The health effects of overweight and obesity are less marked among blacks. The optimal BMI has been calculated to be 23 to 25 for whites, while it is 23 to 30 for blacks.[5] The risks of excess weight are known to be higher for Asian populations; so the BMI cutoffs recommended by the World Health Organization are lower for them.[6] Due to insufficient data, it has not been possible to calculate ideal weights in other ethnic groups, including Mexican Americans, who are known to have a high prevalence of obesity. Overweight increases with age, as seen in Figures 16-1 and 16-2, but declines in the age group 75 years and older.

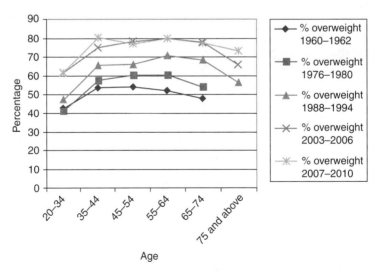

FIGURE 16-1   Percentage of Overweight Males. *Source:* Data from *Health, United States*, 2011, Table 74. http://www.cdc.gov/nchs/data/hus/hus11.pdf, accessed March 16, 2012.

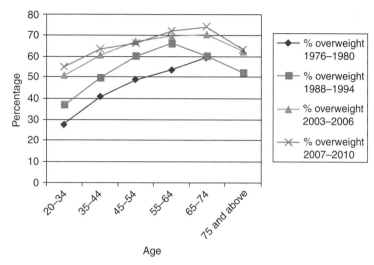

FIGURE 16-2   Percentage of Overweight Females. *Source:* Data from *Health, United States,* 2011, Table 74. http://www.cdc.gov/nchs/data/hus/hus11.pdf, accessed March 16, 2012.

Socioeconomic status has a significant influence on the prevalence of obesity. College graduates of both sexes are thinner than men and women with fewer years of education. The difference is especially significant among females: those with less than 12 years of education are nearly twice as likely to be overweight than female college graduates. Among men, the relationship of obesity with education is less clear.[1]

The greater prevalence of obesity in black women compared to white women doubtless contributes to poorer health among blacks. Rates of cardiovascular disease and diabetes are higher in blacks than in whites, and an unhealthy diet is likely to be part of the problem. Many Hispanics and American Indians are also overweight, accounting for high rates of diabetes among these groups.

While being fat is bad for people's health, the distribution of fat on the body makes a difference. Obesity researchers distinguish between apple-shaped people and pear-shaped people, and they have found health risks to be greater for those shaped like apples. People who gain weight in the abdominal area, as men usually do, have a higher risk of cardiovascular disease and diabetes than people who gain weight in the hips and buttocks—a pattern more common in females. Fat distribution is measured as a waist-to-hip ratio (WHR), with the waist measured at the smallest point and the hips at the widest point around the buttocks. Health risks in men who have a WHR more than 1.0 and women whose WHR is more than 0.8 are greater than the risks due to excess weight alone.[3]

In an alarming trend, overweight among children has been increasing steadily since the 1960s. Definitions of overweight and obesity in children are complex calculations, based on growth curves of BMI for age. The CDC identifies children as overweight if they are at or above the 85th percentile on growth curves established before 1980 and as obese if they are above the 95th percentile.[7,8] The prevalence of obesity among children and adolescents 6 to 19 years old increased from under 5 percent in the earliest surveys to more than 18 percent in the 2007–2010 NHANES. The prevalence of obesity is higher in some ethnic groups: among Mexican American teenage boys, almost 28 percent are obese, while the prevalence is over 27 percent among black teenage girls.[9]

Children who are fat are likely to become fat adults and suffer the concomitant risks of chronic disease. For example, a study that tracked 679 school children for 16 years found that weight during childhood was a good predictor of whether an adult would exhibit risk factors for cardiovascular disease and diabetes.[10] Obese children are for the first time being diagnosed with type 2 diabetes, which is sometimes called "adult-onset diabetes" because until recently it was believed to occur almost exclusively in adults.[11] This is especially likely to occur in American Indian adolescents, who have a high prevalence of obesity, but blacks and Hispanics are also affected. Complications of childhood obesity involve virtually every organ, including the cardiovascular system, the respiratory system, the kidneys, the gastrointestinal system, and the musculoskeletal system.[12] Evidence suggests that the harmful effects of excess weight increase with longer duration of obesity, implying that obese children are especially likely to suffer excess morbidity and mortality when they grow up.[5] One study found that the obese adolescent girls are two or three times as likely to die by middle age as girls of normal weight.[12]

Obesity in children also tends to cause psychological problems such as depression, anxiety, social isolation, and low self-esteem. Children who are worried about their weight may undertake diets that affect their physical as well as their psychological health, and they are at increased risk for eating disorders such as anorexia and bulimia. Obese children are less likely than thinner ones to complete college and are more likely to live in poverty.[12]

Diet and Nutrition

Obesity is caused by unhealthy eating patterns combined with inadequate physical activity, each a factor that influences people's health whether or not they weigh too much. The public health aspects of physical activity will be discussed later in this chapter. This section and the next explore the role of diet in the prevention of chronic diseases, including obesity, and describe public health efforts to encourage people to eat a healthier diet.

Most analyses find that Americans eat too much protein and fat and too few fruits and vegetables. This pattern contributes to high levels of cholesterol and other blood lipids and to high blood pressure—risk factors for cardiovascular disease. The evidence is less clear on how the American diet increases cancer risk, but epidemiologic studies show that breast and colon cancer risks are greater in populations that eat diets high in meat and low in fruits and vegetables. Diet is a major factor in type 2 diabetes, which is often brought on by obesity and which can usually be controlled by careful eating. Osteoporosis, a debilitating disease of the elderly, especially white women, is likely to become increasingly common because young women are not getting enough calcium, best obtained in low-fat dairy products.

The federal government, in a number of reports over the years by various advisory committees, has developed recommendations on how Americans should eat to maintain health and prevent chronic disease. Since 1980, the U.S. Department of Agriculture and the Department of Health and Human Services have reviewed the recommendations every 5 years and have released reports called Dietary Guidelines for Americans.[13] Agreeing on recommendations has often proved controversial, because the food industry tends to oppose any recommendation that calls for eating less of any food substance.[14] However, evidence clearly supports the recommendations included in the 2010 guidelines that people's diets should emphasize fruits, vegetables, whole grains, and fat-free or low-fat milk and milk products; they should include lean meats, poultry, fish, beans, eggs, and nuts but less saturated fats, transfats, cholesterol, salt, and added sugar.[13]

While the 2010 food guidelines did not change significantly from those issued earlier, the image used to illustrate the recommendations changed from the familiar food guide pyramid to a place setting for a meal, shown in **Figure 16-3**. MyPlate.gov recommends, for example, that half the plate should consist of fruits and vegetables, and at least half the grains should be whole grains. The website includes an option for an individual to create a personal profile with a calorie limit, affected by his or her physical activity, and a recommended food plan.[13]

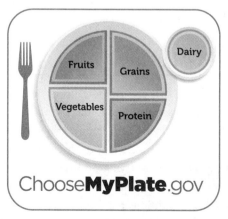

FIGURE 16-3   ChooseMyPlate.gov. *Source:* Courtesy of USDA.

Dietary surveys conducted by the Department of Agriculture have shown that while the diet of Americans has improved over the past several decades, people fall far short of the federal recommendations. One-third of the population eats at least some food from all food groups, but only 1 percent to 3 percent eat the recommended number of servings from all food groups on a given day. Fruits are the most commonly omitted item. Intake of fat and added sugars continues to be too high. While people appear to eat close to the recommended number of vegetable servings, half of these servings are iceberg lettuce, potatoes (including chips and fries), and canned tomatoes.[14] One unfortunate trend is that African Americans of low socioeconomic status, who used to eat a more healthful diet than wealthy whites, have now adopted eating patterns that have traditionally been associated with higher incomes. It is as if, as one commentator suggests, they feel they are now "able to afford steak instead of having to 'fill up' on bread or peas or beans."[15(p.739)]

Federal surveys suggest that, among the causes of increasing obesity, especially in children, is the increased intake of sweetened beverages. The proportion of calories that the average American obtained from soft drinks and fruit drinks more than doubled between 1977 and 2001.[16] The trend was similar for all age groups, but the numbers were highest in the younger age groups, rising from 4.8 percent to 10.3 percent of calories in the 2- to 18-year-old group and from 5.1 percent to 12.3 percent among those between the ages of 19 and 39. Meanwhile, consumption of milk decreased by 38 percent overall, including among children age 2 to 18, the group for whom milk consumption is most important for future health. Consumption of other beverages has not changed significantly over the period studied. These trends are unhealthy, not only because soft drinks and sweetened juice drinks contain "empty calories" that contribute to weight gain, but also because consuming milk products appears to help people control their weight in addition to providing calcium for their bones. According to the researchers, reducing soft drink and fruit drink intake "would seem to be one of the simpler ways to reduce obesity in the United States."[16(p.209)]

Promoting Healthy Eating

It might seem that what each individual eats is under his or her individual control. But many social, cultural, and economic factors contribute to dietary patterns. Eating habits and dietary preferences develop over a lifetime, influenced by family, ethnicity, the media, and other factors in the social environment. The high prevalence of overweight in the United States combined with the large numbers of people who are trying unsuccessfully to lose weight makes it clear that changing eating patterns is very difficult, even for highly motivated people. Studies of patients with a variety of medical conditions requiring special diets have found that even they have difficulty sticking to the prescribed diet. The rate of adherence to a diet by people with diabetes ranged from 20 percent to 53 percent to 73 percent in three different studies. People with kidney failure who were on dialysis were found to have a rate of adherence to the recommended diet of 39 percent and 42 percent in two separate studies. Another study found that the ability of people with high cholesterol to adhere to a low-cholesterol diet was only 30 percent.[17]

Several major public health campaigns conducted in entire communities and aimed at reducing cardiovascular risks found that obesity was the most difficult risk factor to control. The Stanford Three-Community Study, the Stanford Five-City Study, the Minnesota Heart Health Program, and the North Karelia (Finland) Project all had reasonable success in reducing risk factors such as smoking, hypertension, and blood cholesterol, but none of them interrupted the increase in the prevalence of obesity in the communities studied.[3]

Nevertheless, public health advocates have attempted to apply the ecological model of health behavior to create a social environment that favors healthier eating. For example, making nutritious foods more readily available—intervention at the community and institutional levels—should encourage people to choose their foods more wisely. The food industry is responding to many consumers' concerns about weight and health by providing a greater choice of low-fat and low-calorie foods. Many restaurants offer "heart healthy" selections on the menu and label them thus. Worksite and school cafeterias provide healthy food choices including salad bars. While such measures do not guarantee that people will eat a healthier diet, they remove barriers that make it hard for people to do so.

Enhancing self-efficacy and providing social support are ways of promoting healthy eating at the level of the individual and his or her family and friends.[17] Social support is provided when a whole family is willing to adopt a diet together, or by group programs such as Weight Watchers. Self-efficacy can be improved by "point of choice" postings of nutritional information, which can help shoppers who are concerned about the nutritional content of food but do not know how to make wise choices. Several major campaigns using point of choice postings have been conducted by supermarket chains in collaboration with health advocacy organizations such as the American Heart Association, but the results have been mixed. Other approaches to enhancing self-efficacy and adherence to diets include demonstrations of healthy cooking methods and practice in calculating portion sizes.

Public health advocates look at evidence from antismoking campaigns for ideas on how to improve the social environment to affect the American diet. The success of the public service announcements of the 1960s, together with later bans on cigarette advertising in the broadcast media, in reducing smoking prevalence inspired a number of media campaigns to promote more healthful eating. One such campaign was California's "5-A-Day" Campaign for Better Health, which attempted to increase fruit and vegetable consumption among state residents to five servings per day.[14] The assumption is that eating more fruits and vegetables leads to eating less of nonnutritious foods. The program proved to be successful in increasing consumption of fruits and vegetables in the state. Later, the National Cancer Institute launched the program nationwide, although funding was never adequate to maintain the early successes of the California program. As in the case of antismoking campaigns, public health advocates must compete with well-financed advertising campaigns by food manufacturers promoting highly attractive but nonnutritious foods.

Another problem with the "5-A-Day" approach is that fresh fruits and vegetables are relatively expensive and are often unavailable in poor neighborhoods. Fast food restaurants, on the other hand, are inexpensive and are often concentrated in low-income neighborhoods. Moreover, U.S. government policy subsidizes industrial agriculture, which produces high-calorie commodities at the expense of more nutritious produce.[18] Food advertising focuses predominately on processed foods, which are more profitable for the industry.[3]

The food and beverage industries use some of the same approaches to increasing their sales as the tobacco companies have used. As documented in Marion Nestle's book, *Food Politics: How the Food Industry Influences Nutrition and Health*,[14] companies do everything they can to encourage Americans to eat more. They do this by processing foods to make them taste good, which often means sweet, fatty, or salty. They push larger portions, often by promoting them as good buys; for example, a large serving of fries might cost only pennies more than a small serving while it might have twice as many calories. The companies also advertise extensively, especially to children. They take advantage of the fact that, with most women working outside the home, convenience and efficiency are major factors in food choice and fewer family meals than in the past are home cooked. As Nestle describes, food companies "conduct systematic, pervasive, and unrelenting . . . campaigns to convince government officials, health organizations, and nutrition professionals that their products are healthful or harmless, to undermine any suggestion to the contrary, and to ensure that federal dietary guidelines and food guides will help promote sales."[14(p.26)] Like tobacco companies, food companies argue that diet is a matter of individual choice, and they use science to sow confusion about the harm their products can do.

The Institute of Medicine, after a thorough study aimed at developing criteria for evaluating the outcomes of programs to prevent and treat obesity, concluded in a report called *Weighing the Options* that prospects were dim for people seeking to lose weight. "The fact is that despite the billions of dollars spent, few people reduce their body weight to a desirable or healthy level and even fewer maintain the weight lost beyond two or three years."[3(p.158)] The report noted that for most people, weight is not lost once and for all but that its control demands continuing effort. Accordingly, the Institute of Medicine recommends thinking in terms of lifelong weight management, encouraging overweight people to try at least to avoid gaining additional weight. According to the report, even small weight losses can raise self-esteem and improve the health of people suffering from obesity-related chronic conditions.

Public health advocates believe that tackling the obesity epidemic will require community-based efforts to increase the availability of healthy foods, changes in national agricultural policy to encourage the availability of nutritious food at a reasonable cost, and regulation of food industry advertising to promote ethical marketing standards.[19] A number of proposals have been made to tackle the obesity epidemic with tools similar to those that proved successful in the "tobacco wars." In addition to the educational campaigns such as the one for "5-A-Day" fruits and vegetables, they include requirements for food labeling and advertising to carry information on calorie, fat, and sugar content and prohibitions on making misleading health claims. Fast food restaurants should be required to provide nutritional information on packages and wrappers. The nutritionist Nestle proposes taxes on soft drinks and other junk foods to fund "eat less, move more" campaigns and perhaps to subsidize the costs of fruits and vegetables.[14(p.367)]

Some of these proposals are beginning to be implemented in some places, but they have proved controversial. New York City requires calorie counts to be posted on the menus of fast food restaurants. The New York State governor, David Paterson, proposed a tax on sugar-sweetened soft drinks and juice drinks as part of his 2009 budget proposal, but the idea met vigorous opposition. When the Maine legislature passed a similar tax, the law was repealed by voters.[20]

Because the impact of lawsuits against tobacco companies was so successful, forcing the companies to raise prices, limiting their advertising and marketing, and publicizing their fraudulent claims, public health advocates are beginning to think about similar lawsuits against fast food companies. Although a lawsuit against McDonald's by obese teenagers was laughed out of court, some lawyers see potential for challenging food companies on deceptive advertising and marketing practices, using consumer protection laws. In 2006, the Center for Science in the Public Interest announced a lawsuit against the Kellogg Company and the makers of the television show SpongeBob SquarePants for using the cartoon character to sell sweetened cereals, Pop Tarts, and cookies to children under 8.[21] One lawyer who was involved in tobacco cases and is now reportedly preparing suits against food companies is quoted as saying, "The issue is what goes on with the kids, the advertising, what's in schools. That's an issue that has some oomph to it."[22]

In fact, many public health advocates believe that the best hope of preventing obesity in adulthood is to influence children's habits. Thus a great deal of attention is being paid to preventing overweight in children. One proven approach is to encourage breastfeeding, which has many other health advantages as well, for both mother and infant. A number of studies have shown that breastfeeding has a long-term protective effect against obesity in children. It also helps the mother to lose weight she gained during pregnancy.[23]

It is also important to increase parents' awareness that their children are at risk. In a follow-up to the 1988–1994 NHANES survey, after children were weighed and measured, mothers were asked whether their child was overweight, underweight, or about the right weight. Nearly one-third of mothers of overweight children reported that their child was about the right weight.[24] The state of Arkansas addressed this problem by mandating that schools send home a weight report card, and a number of other states and school districts have followed suit, although the practice is controversial because of concerns about stigma.[25] It is clear, however, that efforts to prevent and treat childhood obesity must involve parents. The American Academy of Pediatrics recommends that doctors should measure and chart children's BMI at least once a year.[26] However, a 2002 study found that fewer than 10 percent of practitioners follow all the guidelines.[27] Many pediatricians feel unprepared to educate the parents on what to do if their child is overweight.

In 2005, the Institute of Medicine published a report called *Preventing Childhood Obesity: Health in the Balance*.[28] Calling childhood obesity a "critical public health threat,"[28(p.2)] the report recommends steps that federal, state, and local governments should take to make prevention of obesity in children and youth a national priority. Recommendations include developing guidelines for advertising and marketing of foods and beverages to children and giving the Federal Trade Commission authority and resources to monitor compliance. The report notes that "more than 50 percent of television advertisements directed at children promote foods and beverages such as candy, fast food, snack foods, soft drinks, and sweetened breakfast cereals that are high in calories and fat, low in fiber, and low in nutrient density."[28(p.172)] It also recommends that governments should develop and implement nutritional standards for all foods and beverages sold or served in schools. Food and beverage companies have invaded schools with vending machines selling unhealthy drinks and snacks, fast food in school cafeterias, and special educational programs and materials accompanied by advertisements for fast food and junk food.

As discussed later in this chapter, obesity and chronic disease are as much a result of lack of physical activity as they are of unhealthy diets. Weight-loss programs are most successful, in adults as well as in children, when they combine diet and exercise. "Exercise is today's best buy in public health," one commentator notes. "It is positive and acceptable, has insignificant side effects, and can be inexpensive."[29(p.252)]

Physical Activity and Health

Most studies on how to lose weight have found that the most effective approach combines dieting and physical activity. Dieters who are physically active are more likely to lose fat while preserving lean mass. This combination not only promotes a healthier distribution of body weight (a lower WHR), but it also helps people avoid the weight loss plateaus that can result from dieting. Since lean mass burns more calories than fat burns, a dieter who loses muscle mass will end up with a higher proportion of his or her weight consisting of fat, and thus fewer calories will be needed to maintain the new weight, making it more difficult to lose additional pounds. Exercising when dieting helps to ensure that the weight lost will be fat. Raising the amount of physical activity without reducing calorie intake, while a relatively inefficient way to lose pounds, is likely to reduce the waist-to-hip ratio and thus improve health.[30]

A number of epidemiologic studies have demonstrated that people who are more physically active live longer. For example, a study of almost 17,000 male Harvard alumni found that those who engaged in vigorous activities for 3 or more hours per week were less than half as likely to die within the 12- to 16-year follow-up period than those who had the lowest activity levels.[31] Among Harvard graduates who were sedentary at the beginning of the study, those who took up moderate sports activity at some time during the follow-up period had a 23 percent lower death rate than those who remained sedentary.[32]

Exercise clearly protects against cardiovascular disease, as demonstrated by epidemiologic studies and through biomedical evidence. The Framingham Study found, as early as the 1970s, that the risk for both men and women of dying from cardiovascular disease was highest among those who were the least physically active and that more activity was associated with lower risk.[33] Exercise offers protection against both heart disease and stroke. Several studies have indicated that inactive men and women are more likely to develop high blood pressure than those who are active and that moderate intensity exercise may help reduce blood pressure in people whose pressure is elevated.[34]

There is some biomedical evidence for how physical activity protects against cardiovascular disease. One major factor is the effect on blood cholesterol, especially the tendency for exercise training to increase levels of high-density lipoprotein, "the good cholesterol." Even a single episode of physical activity has been found to improve the balance of blood lipids, an effect persisting for several days.[35] By lowering cholesterol levels in the blood, exercise protects against atherosclerosis. Studies on monkeys have demonstrated that exercise has a protective effect even when the animals are fed a diet high in cholesterol and fats.[36] Other favorable effects of physical activity on the cardiovascular system include a lowering of blood pressure, an increase in circulation to the heart muscle, and a reduced tendency of blood to form clots. Moreover, physical activity reduces the risk of diabetes, which is an important risk factor for cardiovascular disease.

Type 2, or adult-onset diabetes is related to weight gain in adults, especially weight gain distributed in an "apple" shape, a consequence of insufficient physical activity. The high prevalence of obesity among Americans contributes to the ranking of diabetes as the seventh leading cause of death, probably an underestimate because many cardiovascular deaths have diabetes as an underlying cause.

Early suspicions that physical inactivity contributed to diabetes were raised by observations that prevalence of the disease was higher in societies or groups that moved from a traditional lifestyle to a more technologically advanced environment. This transition has been extensively studied in certain American Indian and Pacific Islander communities. While the increased risk stems in part from changes in diet and increased prevalence of obesity, physical activity may be an independent risk factor.[37] The Nurses' Health Study and the Physicians' Health Study have both found that regular physical exercise reduces the incidence of type 2 diabetes.[38,39] The protective effect of exercise against the development of diabetes seems to work largely by increasing the sensitivity of muscle and other tissues to insulin.

There is also evidence that physical activity protects against cancer, especially colon cancer and breast cancer. Some studies suggest a protective effect against cancer of the lung, prostate, and uterine lining. Exercise also improves survival and quality of life among individuals who have been diagnosed with several kinds of cancer.[40]

How Much Exercise Is Enough, and How Much Do People Get?

There is some controversy over how much exercise is enough to provide a health benefit. Part of the problem is that it is difficult to obtain reliable measures of study subjects' degree of activity. Most studies use self-reported information given in response to questionnaires, and many measure activity at a single point in time. Since the studies suffer from weaknesses in measurements of exposure (to exercise), most do not yield a clear dose–response effect. However, most researchers agree that the amount of benefit increases with the intensity, frequency, and duration of the physical activity, and that the activity must be regular and ongoing to provide an ongoing benefit.[30]

To send a clear message to Americans about the importance of increasing their physical activity, a panel of researchers convened by the CDC and the American College of Sports Medicine (ACSM) developed recommendations for how much and what kind of exercise people should aim for.[30] They arrived at a minimum standard of about 150 kilocalories of energy per day of light to moderate activity, which could be broken up over the course of the day. People can achieve the expenditure of 150 kilocalories each day by walking briskly for about 30 minutes or by running at 10 minutes per mile for about 15 minutes, or by performing other activities shown in Table 16-2. This recommendation, endorsed in a surgeon general's report, is supported, for example, by a study of almost 74,000 women aged 50 to 79, which found that those who did the recommended amount of exercise for 30 minutes a day, 5 days a week had 30 percent less heart disease than those who were less active.[30] More exercise was better, but the greatest benefit was gained in going from being sedentary to 30 minutes of walking.[41]

Table 16-2   Examples of Moderate Amounts of Activity

Washing and waxing a car for 45–60 minutes	**Less Vigorous, More Time**
Washing windows or floors for 45–60 minutes	↑
Playing volleyball for 45 minutes	
Playing touch football for 30–45 minutes	
Gardening for 30–45 minutes	
Wheeling self in wheelchair for 30–40 minutes	
Walking 1¾ miles in 35 minutes (20 min/mile)	
Basketball (shooting baskets) for 30 minutes	
Bicycling 5 miles in 30 minutes	
Dancing fast (social) for 30 minutes	
Pushing a stroller 1½ miles in 30 minutes	
Raking leaves for 30 minutes	
Walking 2 miles in 30 minutes (15 min/mile)	
Water aerobics for 30 minutes	
Swimming laps for 20 minutes	
Wheelchair basketball for 20 minutes	
Basketball (playing a game) for 15–20 minutes	
Bicycling 4 miles in 15 minutes	
Jumping rope for 15 minutes	
Running 1½ miles in 15 minutes (10 min/mile)	↓
Shoveling snow for 15 minutes	
Stairwalking for 15 minutes	**More Vigorous, Less Time**

*A moderate amount of physical activity is roughly equivalent to physical activity that uses approximately 150 Calories (kcal) of energy per day, or 1000 Calories per week.

†Some activities can be performed at various intensities; the suggested durations correspond to expected intensity of effort.

Source: Reproduced from U.S. Department of Health and Human Services, *A Report of the Surgeon General: Physical Activity and Health at a Glance* (1996). www.cdc.gov/nccdphp/sgr/pdf/sgraag.pdf, accessed September 24, 2012.

Some scientists have disputed the validity of the CDC/ACSM recommendation, arguing that more vigorous, sustained exercise is necessary to achieve a significant benefit.[42] This view is supported by an Institute of Medicine report issued in 2002 that calls for 60 minutes a day of moderate exercise. The report concluded that 30 minutes a day is not adequate to maintain normal weight.[43] The 2005 Dietary Guidelines for Americans follow the Institute of Medicine recommendations for exercise. Others argue, however, that it is preferable to set realistic goals for modest improvement, given that a very small percentage of the population gets even the minimal amount of exercise recommended by the CDC/ACSM panel.

In fact, 39 percent of American adults report that they engage in no physical activity at all during their leisure time, according to the 2007 National Health Interview Survey.[44] Lack of activity is more common in females than males and more common in African Americans and Hispanics than whites. People with less education and lower incomes are more likely to be inactive than those of higher socioeconomic status, and older adults tend to be more inactive than younger ones.[1]

Lack of physical activity is a major factor in the trend toward increasing prevalence of obesity in children. The federal government recommends that children and adolescents should be physically active at least 60 minutes every day.[45] While most younger children report having engaged in exercise that makes them "sweat and breathe hard," surveys show that activity falls off dramatically during the high school years. Only 29 percent of high school students reported in 2011 that they got the recommended amount of exercise, while 14 percent did not participate in 60 minutes of physical activity on any day during the week before they were surveyed.[46] Only 24 percent of students were enrolled in daily physical education classes when they were in 12th grade.

There is evidence that television and computers may be important factors in children's physical inactivity. American children spend more time watching television and videotapes and playing video games than doing anything else except sleeping.[47] A national study of children and adolescents from diverse socioeconomic backgrounds found that obesity was directly associated with the amount of time spent watching television.[48] In fact, children with a television in their bedroom are especially likely to be overweight, in part because their parents underestimate the amount of time they spend watching.[49] Black and Hispanic children are more likely than white children to have a television in their bedroom. A trial conducted among third and fourth grade students in a California school found that reducing the hours they spent watching television by half to a third over a period of 6 months reduced their BMI significantly compared with a control group.[47] Television encourages not only physical inactivity, but also snack consumption; children are bombarded with television commercials for nonnutritious food products.

Promoting Physical Activity

As with most attempts to change people's behavior, the most effective approach to promoting physical activity is likely to employ the ecological model, intervening at a number of levels of influence. Efforts to motivate individuals to be more active must be combined with interventions that make the physical and social environment more conducive to physical activity. In part because research on the effectiveness of these interventions is difficult to do, most studies have focused on short-term changes in exercise behavior. There is very little evidence that any program has had long-term success in increasing physical activity among significant numbers of people.

Many organizations and federal agencies recommend that healthcare providers counsel their patients about physical activity. However, the evidence is mixed as to whether such counseling actually motivates individuals to exercise more.[50] Studies of the effectiveness of counseling find that counseling practices of primary care physicians are highly variable, from a brief recommendation to be more active to a referral for intensive counseling by health educators. Somewhat more effective are community-wide campaigns that include improving access to places for physical activity and using group settings to help people set individual goals, teaching skills for incorporating activity into daily routines, and providing social support to people trying to adopt healthier behaviors.[50]

The suburban lifestyle, which requires people to drive to wherever they want to go, is a major barrier that is very hard to overcome. As part of health promotion programs, some communities build walking trails or persuade shopping malls to open early for "mall walkers." Schools are a greatly underused resource for community recreation. Surveys of bicycle riders suggest that many more people would commute to work by bicycle if safe bike paths or bike lanes were available, and some communities have responded to this evidence by building such routes. Community trials designed to increase physical activity—usually as part of a "healthy heart" program—have incorporated such environmental modifications while also employing communications strategies, from public service announcements about physical activity to signs that provide cues to action. In one study, signs that said, "Stay Healthy, Save Time, Use the Stairs," were placed next to an escalator. This measure increased the percentage of people who used the stairs from 8 percent to 17 percent.[30]

Pedometers are increasingly being used in campaigns to motivate people to increase their physical activity. Generally, it is recommended that healthy adults should walk about 10,000 steps a day, which is about 5 miles, a requirement that would fulfill the federal recommendation of about 60 minutes of leisure time physical activity. The recommendation for less active people is to measure their current number of steps and gradually increase the number by about 2000 a day. A 2007 review of the effectiveness of pedometers in increasing physical activity found that people who wore the instruments did, in fact, increase the number of steps they took by an average of about 27 percent. Moreover, these individuals significantly reduced their BMI and blood pressure.[51]

Many public health advocates believe that the best hope for increasing population-wide physical activity is to focus on developing the habit of exercise in children and adolescents. Most young children engage in physical activity because they enjoy it. One strategy for promoting exercise is to encourage children to play outdoors.[52] This can be a problem for families living in poor urban neighborhoods, where children's risk of obesity is high. A Census Bureau report published in 2007 found that 34 percent of black and 39 percent of Hispanic parents keep their children inside because they believe it is too dangerous to allow them to play outside.[53] A potential solution is described in a study conducted in two low-income neighborhoods in New Orleans. Researchers opened a schoolyard and provided attendants to ensure children's safety. They observed that the number of children who were outdoors and physically active in the schoolyard and the surrounding neighborhood was 84 percent higher than in a comparison neighborhood. Surveys found that the children in the intervention neighborhood spent less time watching television or movies or playing video games than children in the comparison school. The authors commented that providing safe play spaces holds promise as a simple, inexpensive measure that should be applied more widely.[54]

Walking or biking to school is another straightforward way to increase children's physical activity. Less than 16 percent of students aged 5 to 15 years walked or biked to school in 2001, in contrast to 48 percent of children in 1960.[55] Much of this difference is determined by the distance a child must travel to get to school, a factor that communities could consider when new schools are built. However, when distances are manageable, parents and schools can encourage children to walk by participating in public health programs such as the Walking School Bus or the Safe Routes to School program. In both of these programs, groups of children from the same neighborhood walk or bike together under the supervision of one or more adults, who ensure that the route is safe, that children are protected from traffic, crime, and aggressive dogs.

The CDC recommends that physical education classes teach school-age children about the health benefits of physical activity and help them to develop skills that can be applied in lifelong physical fitness activities, such as jogging, tennis, and aerobic dance. These programs can be more effective if they are culturally appropriate for the targeted population. For example, one experimental program in a California middle school with predominantly black and Hispanic students was called "Dance for Health." Regular physical education classes were replaced with moderate- to high-intensity aerobic dance, accompanied by popular music recommended by the students themselves. At the end of the 3-month program, participating students had lower BMIs and a more positive attitude toward physical activity than a control group. The program was especially popular and effective with girls.[56]

A youth development program focused on American Indian young people, who are particularly prone to obesity, type 2 diabetes, and suicide, is called Wings of America. Given that many American Indian communities include running in some of their celebrations, Wings of America uses running as a catalyst for empowering youth to take pride in themselves and their culture. The organization sponsors cross-country teams, runs youth development summer camps, and provides speakers and other assistance for wellness programs, conferences, clinics, and fairs.[57]

Despite such efforts, Americans' lack of exercise is one of the most intractable problems facing public health today. Very little is known about psychosocial, cultural, environmental, and public policy factors that may influence physical activity. The surgeon general's *Physical Activity and Health* report called for more research on various interventions and their long-term effects.[30] There is much to learn about how to motivate Americans to exercise adequately. In the words of one researcher, "The return of physical activity as the norm in everyone's everyday life—the 'restoration of biological normality'—will require cultural change on a scale similar to that which has occurred with smoking."[30(p.253)]

Confronting the Obesity Epidemic

The prevalence of overweight and obesity has increased so rapidly over recent decades (see Figures 16-1 and 16-2) that public health professionals have begun calling it an epidemic. The health risks caused by overweight and obesity threaten to reverse many of the improvements in public health that were achieved in the 20th century. In fact, an analysis published in 2005 projected that life expectancy of Americans will decline in the future due to obesity.[58] The authors predict that if current trends continue, the next generation will be the first to die younger and sicker than their parents. They suggest that concerns about bankruptcy of the Social Security system are overblown, because fewer people will be around to collect the checks. However, the costs of treating obesity-related diseases, especially diabetes, will put increased strain on Medicare.

Costs of treating the diseases caused by overweight and obesity are estimated to account for up to 20.6 percent of total U.S. medical expenditures and may have reached as high as $190 billion annually from 2000 to 2005.[59] About half of the costs are paid by Medicare and Medicaid, the government health insurance plans, and the other half by private health insurance and by individuals.

In 2000, then surgeon general David Satcher organized a public "listening session" on the problem, which led to the publication of the *Surgeon General's Call to Action to Prevent and Decrease Overweight and Obesity*.[60] The purpose was to develop a national plan and to forge coalitions of governments, organizations, and individuals to "promote healthy eating habits and adequate physical activity, beginning in childhood and continuing across the lifespan." As Dr. Satcher states in the report's foreword, "Many people believe that dealing with overweight and obesity is a personal responsibility. To some degree they are right, but it is also a community responsibility. When there are no safe, accessible places for children to play or adults to walk, jog, or ride a bike, that is a community responsibility. When school lunchrooms or office cafeterias do not provide healthy and appealing food choices, that is a community responsibility. When new or expectant mothers are not educated about the benefits of breastfeeding, that is a community responsibility. When we do not require daily physical education in our schools, that is also a community responsibility. There is much that we can and should do together."[60(p.xiii)]

The health consequences of obesity are serious, and the ineffectiveness of simply advising people to change their diet and exercise habits has led to the acceptance of more drastic measures. Bariatric surgery, which involves reducing the size of the stomach through implanting a gastric band or by surgically removing or bypassing part of the stomach, has been found effective in helping obese people to lose weight and to control diabetes. The National Institutes of Health recommends bariatric surgery for obese people with a BMI of at least 40 and for people with a BMI of 35 together with serious coexisting medical conditions such as diabetes.[61]

An effective diet pill might be a less drastic approach than bariatric surgery in helping people to lose weight. In recent decades, the FDA was reluctant to approve weight-loss drugs because of fear of side effects. A drug combination called fen-phen introduced in the 1990s had to be removed from the market because it caused heart valve problems and pulmonary hypertension. More recently, the FDA has concluded that obesity has become such an important public health concern that pharmaceutical and approaches to controlling it are badly needed and need not be risk-free. It has now approved two new drugs.[62]

Conclusion

Poor diet and physical inactivity have been ranked second among the behavioral factors identified as the leading actual causes of death in the United States. The combination of eating too much and exercising too little causes a very high prevalence of obesity among Americans. Obesity contributes to many health problems, including cardiovascular disease, diabetes, and most kinds of cancer. It is not only the extra pounds, but how the weight is distributed that adversely affects health. Extra weight in the hips and buttocks is less harmful to health than extra weight in the midsection.

Americans eat too much protein and fat and too few fruits and vegetables. This pattern of eating is itself unhealthy even if it did not lead to obesity. Increases in the consumption of sweetened beverages and decreases in the consumption of milk over the past several decades, especially among children, have contributed to the obesity epidemic.

Recommendations for a healthy diet call for people to eat more vegetables, fruits, whole grains, and low-fat milk products. However, people have great difficulty in changing their eating patterns, as seen from the large numbers who are trying to lose weight, most of them without success. Public health programs to promote healthy eating employ the ecological model, trying to create a favorable social environment by conducting media campaigns, encouraging the ready availability of nutritious foods, and providing nutritional information so that people will choose their foods wisely.

Exercise helps to protect against cardiovascular disease, diabetes, and some forms of cancer, in addition to helping to control weight. People who are physically active live longer than those who are inactive. Americans get far too little exercise, a factor that contributes to the high prevalence of obesity. Most public health interventions to promote physical activity apply the ecological model of behavior, using interpersonal and media messages to motivate people to exercise and removing environmental barriers that hinder them.

Because of the difficulty in changing diet and physical activity patterns of adults, the best hope of improving the population's behavior may be to focus on children. The prevalence of obesity in children is increasing in the United States. Breastfeeding can help protect children against being overweight. Some studies have shown that interventions that involve the whole family can be effective in reducing children's obesity. Encouraging children to play outside and to walk or bike to school can help increase their physical activity. In school, physical education classes that help children develop skills they can use later in life may encourage them to develop the habit of being physically active. One of the most important obstacles to the development of healthful diet and activity patterns in children is television watching, which not only promotes inactivity but also tempts children with advertisements for non-nutritious snacks.

References

1. U.S. Centers for Disease Control and Prevention, *Health, United States, 2011.* http://www.cdc.nchs/data/hus/hus11.pdf, accessed July 4, 2012.
2. U.S. Centers for Disease Control and Prevention, "QuickStats: Percentage of Adults Aged >20 Years Who Said They Tried to Lose Weight During the Preceding 12 Months, by Age Group and Sex—National Health and Nutrition Examination Survey, United States, 2005–2006," *Morbidity and Mortality Weekly Report* 57 (2008): 1155.
3. Institute of Medicine, *Weighing the Options: Criteria for Evaluating Weight-Management Programs* (Washington, DC: National Academies Press, 1995).
4. U.S. Centers for Disease Control and Prevention, "Defining Overweight and Obesity." http://www.cdc.gov/obesity/adult/defining.html, accessed July 4, 2012.
5. K. R. Fontaine et al., "Years of Life Lost Due to Obesity," *Journal of the American Medical Association* 289 (2003): 187–193.
6. World Health Organization Expert Consultation, "Appropriate Body-Mass Index for Asian Populations and Its Implications for Policy and Intervention Strategies," *Lancet* 363 (2004): 157–163.
7. U.S. Centers for Disease Control and Prevention, "Basics About Childhood Obesity." http://www.cdc.gov/obesity/childhood/basics.html, accessed July 4, 2012.
8. C. B. Ebbeling and D. S. Ludwig, "Tracking Pediatric Obesity," *Journal of the American Medical Association* 299 (2008): 2442–2443.

9. C. Ogden, M. D. Carroll, and K. M. Flegal, "High Body Mass Index for Age Among U.S. Children and Adolescents, 2003–2006," *Journal of the American Medical Association* 299 (2008): 2401–2405.

10. A. Sinaiko et al., "Relation of Weight and Rate of Increase in Weight During Childhood and Adolescence to Body Size, Blood Pressure, Fasting Insulin, and Lipids in Young Adults: The Minneapolis Children's Blood Pressure Study," *Circulation* 99 (1999): 1471–1476.

11. A. Fagot-Campagna et al., "Type 2 Diabetes Among North American Children and Adolescents: An Epidemiologic Review and a Public Health Perspective," *Journal of Pediatrics* 135 (2000): 664–672.

12. D. S. Ludwig, "Childhood Obesity—The Shape of Things to Come," *New England Journal of Medicine* 357 (2007): 2325–2527.

13. U.S. Department of Agriculture, "Dietary Guidelines, 2010." http://www.choosemyplate .gov/dietary-guidelines.html, accessed July 2, 2012.

14. M. Nestle, *Food Politics: How the Food Industry Influences Nutrition and Health* (Berkeley, CA: University of California Press, 2002).

15. S. Kumanyika, "Improving Our Diet—Still a Long Way To Go," *New England Journal of Medicine* 335 (1996): 738–739.

16. S. J. Nielsen and B. M. Popkin, "Changes in Beverage Intake Between 1977 and 2001," *American Journal of Preventive Medicine* 27 (2004): 205–210.

17. J. M. Chrisler, "Adherence to Weight Loss and Nutritional Regimens," in D. S. Gochman, ed., *Handbook of Health Behavior Research II: Provider Determinants* (New York: Plenum Press, 1997), 323–333.

18. D. S. Ludwig and H. A. Pollack, "Obesity and the Economy: From Crisis to Opportunity," *Journal of the American Medical Association* 301 (2009): 532–535.

19. D. S. Ludwig and M. Nestle, "Can the Food Industry Play a Constructive Role in the Obesity Epidemic?" *Journal of the American Medical Association* 300 (2008): 1808–1811.

20. S. Chan, "A Tax on Many Soft Drinks Sets off a Spirited Debate," *The New York Times*, December 16, 2008.

21. M. Warner, "Kellogg and Viacom to Face Suit Over Ads for Children," *The New York Times*, January 19, 2006.

22. K. Zernike, "Lawyers Shift Focus from Big Tobacco to Big Food," *The New York Times*, April 9, 2004.

23. L. M. Grummer-Strawn and Z. Mei, "Does Breastfeeding Protect Against Pediatric Overweight? Analysis of Longitudinal Data from the Centers for Disease Control and Prevention Pediatric Nutrition Surveillance System," *Pediatrics* 113 (2004): 81–86.

24. L. M. Maynard, D. A. Galuska, H. M. Blanck, and M. K. Serdula, "Maternal Perceptions of Weight Status of Children," *Pediatrics* 111 (2003): 1226–1231.

25. J. Kantor, "As Obesity Fight Hits Cafeteria, Many Fear a Note from School," *The New York Times*, January 8, 2007.

26. American Academy of Pediatrics, "Policy Statement: Prevention of Pediatric Overweight and Obesity," *Pediatrics* 112 (2003): 424–430.

27. S. E. Barlow et al., "Medical Evaluation of Overweight Children and Adolescents: Reports from Pediatricians, Pediatric Nurse Practitioners, and Registered Dietitians," *Pediatrics* 110 (2002): 222–228.

28. Institute of Medicine, *Preventing Childhood Obesity: Health in the Balance* (Washington, DC: National Academies Press, 2005).

29. J. N. Morris, "Exercise Versus Heart Attack: History of a Hypothesis," in M. Marmot and P. Elliott, eds., *Coronary Heart Disease Epidemiology: From Aetiology to Public Health* (Oxford, England: Oxford Medical Publications, 1992), 242–255.

30. U.S. Department of Health and Human Services, *Physical Activity and Health: A Report of the Surgeon General* (Atlanta, GA: Centers for Disease Control and Prevention, National Center for Chronic Disease Prevention and Health Promotion, 1996).

31. R. S. Paffenbarger, Jr. et al., "Physical Activity, All-Cause Mortality, and Longevity of College Alumni," *New England Journal of Medicine* 314 (1986): 605–613.

32. R. S. Paffenbarger, Jr. et al., "The Association of Changes in Physical Activity Level and Other Lifestyle Characteristics with Mortality Among Men," *New England Journal of Medicine* 328 (1993): 538–545.

33. W. B. Kannel and P. Sorlie, "Some Health Benefits of Physical Activity: The Framingham Study," *Archives of Internal Medicine* 139 (1979): 857–861.

34. J. Boone-Heinonen et al., "Walking for Prevention of Cardiovascular Disease in Men and Women: A Systematic Review of Observational Studies," *Obesity Reviews* 10 (2009): 204–217.

35. A. D. Tsopanakis et al., "Lipids and Lipoprotein Profiles in a 4-Hour Endurance Test on a Recumbent Cycloergometer," *American Journal of Clinical Nutrition* 49 (1989): 980–984.

36. D. M. Kramsch et al., "Reduction of Coronary Atherosclerosis by Moderate Conditioning Exercise in Monkeys on an Atherogenic Diet," *New England Journal of Medicine* 305 (1981): 1483–1489.

37. T. J. Orchard et al., "Diabetes," in R. B. Wallace, ed., *Maxcy-Rosenau-Last Public Health and Preventive Medicine* (Stamford, CT: Appleton and Lange, 1998), 973.

38. J. E. Manson et al., "Physical Activity and Incidence of Non-Insulin-Dependent Diabetes Mellitus in Women," *Lancet* 338 (1991): 774–778.

39. J. E. Manson et al., "A Prospective Study of Exercise and Incidence of Diabetes Among U.S. Male Physicians," *Journal of the American Medical Association* 268 (1992): 63–67.

40. National Cancer Institute Fact Sheet: "Physical Activity and Cancer: Questions and Answers." http://www.cancer.gov/cancertopics/factsheet/prevention/physicalactivity, accessed July 3, 2012.

41. J. E. Manson et al., "Walking Compared with Vigorous Exercise for the Prevention of Cardiovascular Events in Women," *New England Journal of Medicine* 347 (2002): 716–725.

42. M. Barinaga, "How Much Pain for Cardiac Gain?" *Science* 276 (1997): 1324–1327.

43. Institute of Medicine, *Dietary Reference Intakes for Energy, Carbohydrate, Fiber, Fat, Fatty Acids, Cholesterol, Protein, and Amino Acids* (Washington, DC: National Academies Press, 2002).

44. U.S. Centers for Disease Control and Prevention, *Health, United States, 2009.* http://www.cdc.gov/nchs/data/hus/hus09.pdf, accessed July 4, 2012.

45. U.S. Department of Health and Human Services, "Physical Activity Guidelines for Americans At-A-Glance: A Fact Sheet for Professionals" http://www.health.gov/paguidelines/factsheetprof.aspx, accessed June 1, 2012.

46. U.S. Centers for Disease Control and Prevention, "Physical Activity Facts." http://www.cdc.gov/HealthyYouth/physicalactivity/facts.htm, accessed July 3, 2012.

47. T. N. Robinson, "Reducing Children's Television Viewing to Prevent Obesity," *Journal of the American Medical Association* 282 (1999): 1561–1567.

48. W. H. Dietz and S. L. Gortmaker, "Do We Fatten Our Children at the Television Set? Obesity and Television Viewing in Children and Adolescents," *Pediatrics* 75 (1985): 807–812.

49. B. A. Dennison, T. A. Erb, and P. L. Jenkins, "Television Viewing and Television in Bedroom Associated with Overweight Risk Among Low-Income Preschool Children," *Pediatrics* 109 (2002): 1028–1035.

50. U.S. Preventive Services Task Force, "Behavioral Counseling in Primary Care to Promote Physical Activity: Recommendations and Rationale," *American Family Physician* 66 (2002): 1731.

51. D. M. Bravata et al., "Using Pedometers to Increase Physical Activity and Improve Health: A Systematic Review," *Journal of the American Medical Association* 298 (2007): 2296–2304.

52. R. C. Whitaker, "Obesity Prevention in Pediatric Primary Care: Four Behaviors to Target," *Archives of Pediatrics and Adolescent Medicine* 157 (2003): 725–727.

53. S. Roberts, "Census Reveals Fear Over Neighborhoods," *The New York Times*, November 1, 2007.

54. T. A. Farley et al., "Safe Play Spaces to Promote Physical Activity in Inner-City Children: Results from a Pilot Study of an Environmental Intervention," *American Journal of Public Health* 97 (2007): 1625–1631.

55. K. K. Davidson, J. L. Werder, and C. T. Lawson, "Children's Active Commuting to School: Current Knowledge and Future Directions," *Preventing Chronic Disease: Public Health Research, Practice, and Policy* 5 (July 2008): A100.

56. R. Flores, "Dance for Health: Improving Fitness in African American and Hispanic Adolescents," *Public Health Reports* 110 (1995): 189–193.

57. J. Spring, "Running from Despair: A Collection of American Indian Athletes Has Risen to Prominence," *The New York Times*, February 16, 2008.

58. S. J. Olshansky et al., "A Potential Decline in Life Expectancy in the United States in the 21st Century," *New England Journal of Medicine* 352 (2005): 1138–1145.

59. Institute of Medicine, "Accelerating Progress in Obesity Prevention: Solving the Weight of the Nation," (Washington, DC: National Academies Press, 2012).

60. U.S. Department of Health and Human Services, *Surgeon General's Call to Action to Prevent and Decrease Overweight and Obesity* (Rockville, MD: U.S. Government Printing Office, 2001).

61. U.S. National Institutes of Health, "Weight Loss for Life." http://win.niddk.nih.gov/publications/for_life.htm#wtlosslife, accessed September 15, 2012.

62. A. Pollack, "F.D.A. Approves Qsymia, a Weight-Loss Drug," *The New York Times*, July 17, 2012.

Injuries Are Not Accidents

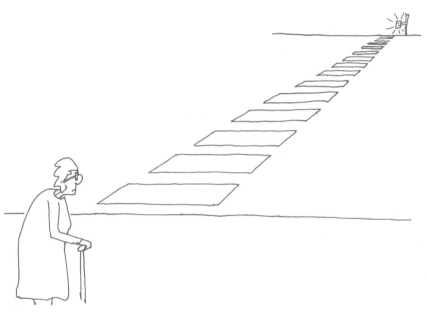

An "Accident" Waiting to Happen

Injuries are the fifth leading cause of death in the United States.[1(Table 27)] They are even more important than statistics suggest because injuries disproportionately affect young people and thus cause many years of potential life lost (YPLL). Injuries are the number one cause of death among people ages 1 to 44.[1(Table 27)] In addition to the people killed by injuries, there are almost as many survivors left with permanent disabilities, a major economic and emotional drain on families and on society in general.

Traditionally, injuries have been thought of as "accidents," unavoidable random occurrences, or the results of antisocial or incautious behavior. It is only recently that public health practitioners have recognized that injuries can and should be treated as a public health problem, analyzable by epidemiologic methods and amenable to preventive interventions. While most injuries are caused to some extent by individual behavior, they are also influenced by the physical and social environment. Public health programs to prevent injury must find ways to change people's behavior by the classic methods of education and regulation, but for many types of injuries, prevention by changing the environment may be more effective.

Epidemiology of Injuries

Prevention of injury, like the prevention of most diseases, is based on epidemiology. Data are needed to answer the questions of who, where, when, and how, looking for patterns and connections that suggest where the greatest needs for prevention are as well as ways to intervene to prevent the injury. Fatal injuries are generally categorized as unintentional (sometimes referred to as "accidental") or intentional (homicide or suicide).

Injuries are an especially important cause of death in young people. In 2008, unintentional injuries caused 31 percent of deaths in children aged 1 to 4, 33 percent of deaths in children aged 5 to 14, and 41 percent of deaths in young people aged 15 to 24.[1(Table 31)] An additional 30 percent of deaths in the 15 to 24 age group were caused by suicide or homicide.

Race and gender affect injury rates. Males are more likely to sustain injuries than females, with a fatal injury rate more than 2.1 times higher than that of females for all age groups combined. African Americans have lower rates of injury mortality than whites, except for the high rates of homicide among young black males, which is more than five times the rate for white youths.[1(Table 44)]

Injury rates, like other indicators of poor health, are higher in groups of lower socioeconomic status. The death rate from unintentional injury is twice as high in low-income areas as in high-income areas. House fires, pedestrian fatalities, and homicides are all more common among the poor.[2] The poor are more likely to have high-risk jobs, low-quality housing, older, defective cars, and such hazardous products as space heaters, all of which contribute to higher injury risks.

Figure 17-1 shows the leading categories of injury deaths in the United States. Poisoning leads the list, followed by motor vehicle injuries, with firearms fatalities third. As a result of the high priority the federal government has placed on prevention of motor vehicle–related injuries, as described in a following section, highway fatalities have declined over most of the past four decades. Firearm fatalities increased between 1968 and 1994, and the Centers for Disease Control and Prevention (CDC) predicted that if trends continued, the number of firearm-related deaths would surpass those related to motor vehicles by the year 2003.[3] The trend in firearm injuries reversed in the early 1990s, however, while traffic fatalities remained steady, and motor vehicle deaths continued to dominate the injury statistics, as shown in Figure 17-2.[4]

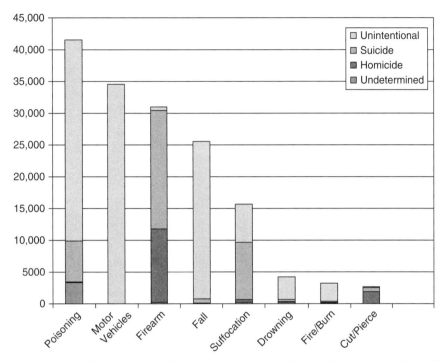

FIGURE 17-1   Leading Causes of Injury Death, 2009. *Source:* Reproduced from Centers for Disease Control and Prevention, "National Vital Statistics Report: Deaths: Final Data for 2009." http://www.cdc.gov/nchs/data.nvsr/nvsr60, accessed September 27, 2012.

Death rates from poisoning overtook traffic fatalities in 2009, however, becoming the leading cause of injury death in the United States. Deaths due to prescription drugs almost doubled between 1999 and 2008,[5] Other major causes of injury deaths that have drawn significant public health attention are falls and jumps, suffocation, drowning, and fires and hot objects.

Many injuries are not fatal, of course, but fatal injuries are the ones that are most reliably reported. While data on nonfatal injuries are less complete, these injuries can have serious and even devastating effects. In the year 2009, for every fatal injury reported, 11 individuals were hospitalized for nonfatal injuries, and 182 were treated in the emergency department.[5] These numbers are illustrated in the "injury pyramid" shown in **Figure 17-3**, from which it is possible to estimate the impact of nonfatal injuries when data on fatal injuries are known.

Injuries that result in long-term disability, especially head and spinal cord injuries, are particularly costly to society. An estimated 1.7 million Americans each year sustain a traumatic brain injury (TBI).[6] Of these, about 52,000 die, and 275,000 are hospitalized and survive, often with lifelong disabling conditions. Many of these victims are young. Caring for these patients costs billions of dollars, much of it paid for with public funds.

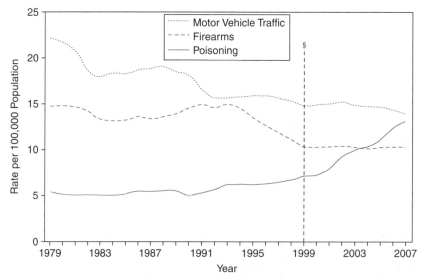

§ In 1999, *International Classification of Diseases, 10th Revision* (ICD-10) replaced the previous revision of the ICD (ICD-9). This resulted in approximately 5 percent fewer deaths being classified as motor vehicle traffic–related and 2 percent more deaths being classified as poisoning-related. Therefore, death rates for 1998 and earlier are not directly comparable with those computed after 1998. Little change was observed in the classification of firearm-related deaths from ICD-9 to ICD-10.

In 2007, the three leading causes of injury deaths in the United States were motor vehicle traffic, poisoning, and firearms. The age-adjusted death rate for poisoning more than doubled from 1979 to 2007, in contrast to the age-adjusted death rates for motor vehicle traffic and firearms, which decreased during this period. From 2006 to 2007, the age-adjusted poisoning death rate increased 6 percent, whereas the motor vehicle traffic death rate decreased 4 percent, and the firearm death rate did not change.

Sources: National Vital Statistics System, mortality data, available at http://www.cdc.gov/nchs/deaths.htm. CDC WONDER, compressed mortality file, underlying cause-of-death, available at http://wonder.cdc.gov/mortsql.html.

FIGURE 17-2   Death Rates* for the Three Leading Causes of Injury Death[†]—United States, 1979–2007. *Source:* Reproduced from U.S. Centers for Disease Control and Prevention, *Morbidity and Mortality Weekly Report* 59 (2010): 957. http://www.cdc .gov/mmwr/preview/mmwrhtml/mm5930a6.htm, accessed October 1, 2012.

* Per 100,000 population. Age-adjusted to the 2000 U.S. standard population.
[†] Injuries are from all manners, including unintentional, suicide, homicide, undetermined intent, legal intervention, and operations of war. Poisoning deaths include those resulting from drug overdose, those resulting from other misuse of drugs, and those associated with solid or liquid biologic substances, gasses or vapors, or other substances such as pesticides or unspecified chemicals.

Alcohol is a significant factor in a very high percentage of injuries. Thirty-one percent of traffic fatalities in 2010 involved alcohol.[7] High alcohol levels are found in the blood of more than one-third of adult pedestrians killed by motor vehicles.[8] Many of those fatally injured in falls, drownings, fires, and suicides are under the influence of alcohol, as are many of the

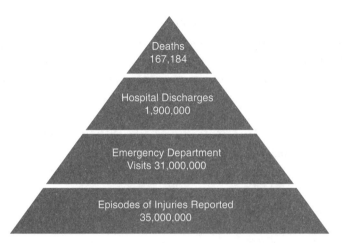

FIGURE 17-3   Burden of Injury: United States, 2004. *Source:* Data from U.S. Centers for Disease Control and Prevention, Injury in the United States: 2007 Chartbook. http://www.cdc.gov/nchs/data/misc/injury2007.pdf, accessed October 1, 2012.

perpetrators and victims of homicides. Other drugs may play a role in injury, but because blood alcohol tests are much more commonly done than tests for other drugs, the role of alcohol in injury is better documented.

The importance of alcohol's contribution to injury accounts for its high placement on the list of "actual causes of death." To stress the importance of driving while intoxicated as a cause of death, the authors counted alcohol-related motor vehicle deaths in both the alcohol and the motor vehicle categories, making alcohol the third leading cause and motor vehicles the sixth.[9]

Analyzing Injuries

While injuries are generally brought on by human behavior, injury researchers have increasingly sought to understand the role of the environment in causing an injury-producing event and in influencing the severity of the resulting injury. The public health approach to injury control analyzes injuries, like the approach to infectious diseases, in terms of a chain of causation: the interactions over time between a host, an agent, and the environment. To analyze an injury-causing event requires information about the person who initiates the event and/or suffers the injury, the agent (automobile, firearm, swimming pool), and the environment (road conditions, weather, involvement of other people) before, during, and after the event.

To prevent certain injury-causing events from occurring in the first place—primary prevention—analysts seek to understand the conditions prevailing before each such event. For example, characteristics of the host (e.g., alcohol intoxication), the agent (e.g., defective brakes), and the environment (e.g., a dark and rainy night) are all relevant to whether a motor vehicle crash occurs. Conditions prevailing during the event affect the outcome of the crash. Thus, wearing a seat belt (host), equipping a car with an airbag (agent), and driving on a divided highway (environment) may allow the driver to avoid serious injury during a crash—secondary prevention. Tertiary prevention depends on conditions after the crash that determine whether the victim survives the injury and the extent of any resulting disability. The availability and quality of emergency care are major factors in tertiary prevention.

Because motor vehicle injuries cause so many deaths, they were the first category of injuries to be analyzed and subjected to systematic prevention efforts. Much data are available on conditions surrounding motor vehicle crashes, and methods for preventing motor vehicle injuries are highly developed. National highway safety programs were launched 2 decades before Congress identified injury as a general public health problem and established the National Center for Injury Prevention and Control at the CDC.

Injury-control efforts developed for motor vehicle injuries have served as a model for more embryonic efforts to control other categories of injury. Early prevention strategies focused on changing people's behavior by the classic public health methods of education and regulation. As with many public health issues related to behavior, regulation is usually more effective than education in getting people to change their behavior. In the earliest days of traffic safety efforts, for example, society learned that laws regarding speed limits and traffic lights were necessary to control the chaos on the roadways.

Modern injury control began, however, with the recognition that engineering plays an important role in the causation of injuries and their severity. Sharp objects cause more damage to the human body than blunt ones; an impact distributed over a broad surface results in a less severe injury than that to a smaller surface; if deceleration can be controlled and made less sudden, the body can better withstand the force. In general, automatic protections are more effective than measures that require effort, and the more effort a measure requires, the less likely it is to be employed. Thus the "three Es" of injury prevention are education, enforcement, and engineering.

These insights, first applied in the auto industry, have also been applied to prevention of many other kinds of injury—especially childhood injuries—with considerable success. For example, when the New York City Health Department noted that a large number of children died from falls out of windows, it instituted the "Children Can't Fly" program, requiring landlords to install window guards, and the number of fatal falls was reduced by half.[10] The number of children that drown in swimming pools has been reduced by laws requiring pools to be fenced. Poisonings in children can be prevented by childproof caps on medicine containers and some household chemicals. The use of smoke detectors has reduced the number of deaths from fires. State and federal regulation of the flammability of fabrics has also saved lives, especially those of children—due to laws on children's sleepwear. As a result of these measures and others, fatal injury rates among small children have declined markedly in recent years.[1(Table 31),11]

Motor Vehicle Injuries

Attention was focused on the problem of motor vehicle injuries by Ralph Nader's indictment of the automobile industry in his book, *Unsafe at Any Speed: The Designed-In Dangers of the American Automobile*, published in 1966. Congress responded by passing the National Traffic and Motor Vehicle Safety Act of 1966, which established the National Highway Traffic Safety Administration (NHTSA) and empowered it to set safety standards for new cars, such as installation of seat belts, laminated windshields, collapsible steering assemblies, and dashboard padding. Hundreds of thousands of drivers had died from being impaled on unyielding steering columns. Heads and faces of front-seat passengers had been cut by sharp dashboard edges and by glass from broken windshields. The safer designs mandated by the 1966 legislation led to an enormous reduction in both injury and mortality.[10]

The NHTSA was also required to collect data on motor vehicle–related deaths and to conduct research aimed at prevention of motor vehicle collisions and amelioration of their effects. Among other activities, the NHTSA has an ongoing program of crash-testing various vehicle models, seeking to understand how further improvements in engineering could protect occupants during a crash. These studies have led to further improvements in automobile design— including headrests that protect their occupants during rear-end collisions, strengthened side bars to protect occupants during side crashes, and airbags—now required by federal law.[12]

While requirements that vehicles more effectively protect their occupants during a crash are an important part of injury control (secondary prevention), preventing crashes from occurring in the first place (primary prevention) is the highest priority. Characteristics of the vehicle such as turn signals and brake lights help prevent crashes. State laws that require annual inspections of these devices, as well as of brakes and tires, are aimed at ensuring that defects in vehicles do not lead to injuries. Beginning with 2011 models, the NHTSA rates cars with a 5-star safety ratings system that includes crash avoidance technology such as electronic stability control, lane departure warnings and forward collision warnings.[12] Environmental features, especially improvements in highway design, have been shown to prevent crashes. Divided highways, raised lane dividers embedded in road surfaces, rumble strips at road edges, and "wrong-way" signs at off ramps can help to prevent mistakes by drivers.

Injury control methods that target the driver depend on both education and enforcement, and they exemplify the typical difficulties in getting people to practice healthier behaviors. Because alcohol plays such a major role in fatal crashes, laws against drinking and driving are virtually universal. Their effectiveness depends on how well they are enforced, however. The activism of volunteer groups such as Mothers Against Drunk Driving (MADD) has helped to raise public consciousness about the extent of the problem, and tolerance for drinking and driving has declined in recent years. In addition to imposing severe penalties for being caught driving drunk, many states have expanded legislation to make establishments that serve alcohol liable for serving minors or persons already obviously intoxicated.

After alcohol, the second most important factor in fatal crashes is youth: 13 percent of drivers in fatal crashes are under the age of 20, even though those under 20 make up only 6.4 percent of all drivers.[13] According to the NHTSA, 16-year-old drivers have crash rates that are three times more than 17-year-olds, five times greater than 18-year-olds, and twice those of 85-year-olds.[14] This is believed to be due in part to inexperience: driving is a complex task, and new drivers are more likely to make mistakes. These crashes are also due to risk-taking behavior and poor judgment.

Some states are addressing the issue by implementing graduated driver-licensing systems by which young drivers must pass through one or two preliminary stages over a period of time before they are allowed a full license. The NHTSA has developed a model law that includes the following provisions: With a learner's permit, a licensed adult must be in the vehicle at all times; the young person must remain crash-free and conviction-free before being allowed to take a road test for a provisional license. Nighttime driving is restricted for those with a provisional license. Young drivers must remain crash-free and conviction-free for a year before moving to a full license. As of 2008, all states have adopted some form of the graduated system: 46 states have a three-stage system and the other four states use a two-stage system. Graduated licensing has been successful in preventing traffic fatalities among young people: states that have adopted the system have experienced significant reductions in crashes by drivers less than 20 years old.[14]

In addition to being inexperienced, young drivers may also be just starting to drink, and learning how to do both together can be fatal. In 2007, 31 percent of drivers 15 to 20 years old who were killed in crashes had alcohol in their blood.[13] The federal government and many states have made concerted efforts to reduce drinking and driving among young people. One attempt to deal with the problem was a federal law requiring states to increase the drinking age to 21 to receive highway funds (the law became effective in 1988).[10] In 1995, a similar federal law required states to pass zero tolerance laws for drivers under 21 years old. Since 1998, all states and the District of Columbia have laws setting a limit of 0.02 percent blood-alcohol concentration or below, suspending driver's licenses for those found in violation. The evidence indicates that this is an effective approach to saving lives.[15]

Speed limits are an important factor in highway injuries. In 1974, Congress imposed a national speed limit of 55 miles per hour to conserve fuel at the time of the Arab oil embargo. That law, which contributed to a 16 percent decline in traffic fatalities between 1973 and 1974, was revoked in 1995 as part of the deregulation trend.[10] Many states have raised their speed limits as a result, including 35 states that have limits of 70 miles per hour or above on rural interstates.[16]

The use of seat belts has been shown to reduce fatalities by 40 to 50 percent. Child-safety seats can reduce the risk of a child's being killed during a collision or sudden stop by 71 percent.[10]

These engineering measures require people to use them correctly, however, and even state laws requiring the use of seat belts and child safety seats are widely ignored. In states that have primary seat belt laws—laws allowing police officers to pull over drivers and ticket them merely for not wearing a seat belt—the rate of seat belt use is higher than it is in states that have secondary laws—laws that permit police to issue tickets for seat belt violations only after stopping a driver for another reason. As of July 1, 2012, 32 states and the District of Columbia have primary laws, and 17 have secondary laws. New Hampshire has no seat belt law for adults. All states and the District of Columbia have child restraint laws, though the types of restraints for various age children varies among the states.[17]

An issue that has recently come to the attention of traffic safety advocates is cell phone use while driving. The NHTSA collects data on distracted driving, which includes using a cell phone, eating, reading, and using a navigational system, all of which degrade the driver's performance. The NHTSA estimates that distraction from all sources, including cell phones, contributes to 18 percent of all police-reported traffic crashes.[18] As of August 1, 2012, 10 states and the District of Columbia had laws banning the use of handheld cell phones while driving, and an additional 24 states ban their use by novice drivers.[19] No state has banned use altogether, although the evidence indicates that even hands-free phones can cause significant distraction to the driver. Even more risky than talking on a cell phone is text messaging, which has become increasingly common, especially among younger drivers. A study that used video cameras installed in the cabs of long-haul trucks found that when drivers texted, their risk of a collision increased 23-fold.[20] Other studies suggest that the risk among drivers of passenger cars is similar. Thirty-nine states and the District of Columbia ban text messaging while driving, and an additional five states ban the practice for novice drivers.[19]

In 1968, when implementation of federal traffic safety legislation began, almost 55,000 Americans died each year from motor vehicle–related injuries. The national effort to reduce this toll has had significant success. By 1993, the number had declined to just over 40,000 fatalities per year despite the fact that many more cars were on the roads and that the number of miles driven has more than doubled.[3] Since then, the downward trend halted for over a decade and then dropped dramatically to 32,885 in 2010. The fatality rate per 100 million vehicle miles of travel was at an all-time low in 2009 and 2010.[21] Future progress in traffic safety could depend on factors such as the price of gasoline. High gas prices tend to lead people to drive less. They also encourage people to buy smaller cars. When gas prices are low, heavier vehicles such as minivans, pickup trucks, and sport utility vehicles are popular, contributing to increases in traffic fatalities because crashes between vehicles of widely disparate size and weight cause high risk to the occupants of the smaller vehicle. Sport utility vehicles, vans, and pickup trucks, with their higher center of gravity, are more likely to roll over in crashes than sedans, however, offsetting the advantage occupants get from their size.

Pedestrians, Motorcyclists, and Bicyclists

About 13 percent of people killed in motor vehicle crashes are pedestrians, and public health efforts are also directed at preventing these injuries.[22] Elderly people have the highest risk for being killed by a motor vehicle while walking. Nineteen percent of pedestrians killed by motor vehicles are over 65.[22] Most of these injuries occur in urban areas. A 1985 study investigated reasons for a high fatality rate among older pedestrians along Queens Boulevard in a part of New York City inhabited by large numbers of senior citizens. It was found that elderly persons took an average of 50 seconds to cross the 150-foot wide boulevard, while the "walk" sign allowed only 35 seconds. Moreover, because of the boulevard's width and because vision loss is common among the elderly, many pedestrians could not read the "walk/don't walk" signs, which were located on the far side of the boulevard. The traffic safety unit installed additional signs on the median strips so that they could be more easily seen, and they reset the signs to allow more time for crossing. After implementation of these and other measures, such as stricter enforcement of speed limits, the rate of death and severe injuries among pedestrians fell by 60 percent.[10]

Public health professionals viewed the Queens Boulevard story as a success, but residents of the neighborhood still call that stretch of roadway the "Boulevard of Death." The city's Department of Transportation has continued to make safety improvements, including more fences to curtail jaywalking, restricting vehicle U-turns and left turns, and posting safety signs to remind pedestrians about the danger.[23]

In 2010, 4502 motorcyclists and 618 bicyclists are killed in crashes.[24,25] Children younger than 16 years of age account for 11 percent of the bicycle-related fatalities, making this one of the leading causes of injury-related death in children.[25] Over the last decade, an increasing proportion of bicyclists killed are ages 25 to 64. The most important protective measure for bicycle and motorcycle riders is to wear a helmet. Ninety-one percent of bicyclists killed and 58 percent of fatally injured motorcyclists were not wearing helmets.[24,26] Head injuries also cause profound, permanent disability in many survivors.

Public health advocates have devoted considerable efforts to promote the use of bicycle and motorcycle helmets. Congress (as part of the 1966 National Highway Safety Act) mandated that states pass laws requiring motorcyclists to wear helmets, leading to a dramatic decline in motorcycle fatalities.[12] Because of vigorous objections on grounds of personal liberty, the federal law was changed in 1976. In response, 27 states repealed or weakened their laws, and by 1980 motorcycle fatalities increased dramatically.[27] As of September 2012, 19 states and the District of Columbia required helmet use for all motorcycle operators and their passengers. In another 28 states, only those under a certain age, usually 18, are required to wear helmets.[28] In states where only minors are required to wear helmets, laws are difficult to enforce. Data on crashes in these states show that, despite the law, fewer than 40 percent of fatally injured minors wore helmets.[29] Only 21 states and the District of Columbia have laws requiring bicycle helmets, and these laws apply only to children, although some local governments have laws that apply to riders of all ages.[28] The bulk of the public health effort regarding bicycle helmets focuses on community education programs.

Poisoning

Poisoning surpassed firearms as a cause of injury death in 2004, as shown in Figure 17-3. In fact, the death rate from poisoning almost doubled between 1999 and 2008. In 2009, drug poisoning became the leading cause of injury death in the United States.[5]

In trying to understand the dramatic increase in poisoning fatalities, scientists at the CDC analyzed death certificates recorded at the National Center for Health Statistics and found that the vast majority of them listed drugs, legal and illegal, as the cause of death.[30] Opioid pain medications were most commonly involved in the unintentional deaths, followed by cocaine and heroin. Suicide by poisoning most commonly involved psychoactive drugs, such as sedatives and antidepressants, followed by opiates and other prescription pain medications.

The CDC scientists noted that during the 1990s, pain specialists were arguing that opioid pain medications were being underprescribed because of fear of addiction, leading to suffering by patients who were being denied relief from chronic pain. In response, between 1990 and 2002 there was a dramatic increase in prescriptions written for these drugs, including hydrocodone, oxycodone, and methadone. The increase in sales of methadone was explained by prescriptions filled at pharmacies for pain management rather than distribution of the drug through narcotics treatment programs. The scientists' conclusion was that the increase in unintentional poisoning deaths was largely a result of nonmedical, recreational use of prescription pain relievers. Further evidence for this explanation is the age and sex distribution of the individuals who died, primarily middle-aged and male, rather than older females who typically suffer from chronic pain, and many of them had a history of drug abuse.[30]

The CDC analysis leads to the conclusion that the medical prescription of opioid painkillers is being diverted for illegitimate and dangerous uses. The authors note that corrective actions may be necessary to reduce deaths without diminishing the quality of care for patients who need the drugs for pain relief. This may include better communication and education of healthcare providers to warn them of the risks and inform them how to recognize patients who may be prone to abuse. There may be a need for stricter regulation of opiates by the Drug Enforcement Agency, which registers physicians and pharmacies that handle opiates and tracks the buying and selling of these drugs.

The New York State Attorney General, Eric Schneiderman, has proposed an online drug tracking system for the state that would reduce the risk of patients' obtaining multiple prescriptions for opiate drugs. The system would require physicians to check a patient's prescription history before writing a new prescription and require pharmacists to confirm prescriptions before filling them.[31]

The age group with the lowest poisoning mortality rates is children under 15 years old, in part thanks to public health measures designed to protect curious youngsters from ingesting toxic substances. Childproof caps on pharmaceuticals and cleaning products have helped to keep poisons out of the hands and mouths of toddlers, and poison control centers staff emergency phone lines 24 hours per day. Nevertheless, parents are advised to be alert to the risks of childhood poisonings.

Firearms Injuries

In 1994, firearms injuries had surpassed motor vehicle injuries as the leading cause of injury death in eight states and the District of Columbia. It appeared that firearms would soon become number one nationwide, as seen in Figure 17-2. However, the number of homicides dropped dramatically in 1994 and 1995, and suicides and unintentional gun deaths fell slightly. The number of deaths caused by firearms continued to decline, falling from almost 40,000 in 1993 to below 30,000 in 2004. A number of reasons have been proposed for the decline, including tougher gun control laws, community policing, and demographic changes.[32] Since 2004, the number of firearms deaths increased slightly, reaching 31,347 in 2009.[33]

Violence is traditionally thought of as a criminal justice issue rather than a public health issue. Certainly no one is arguing that the criminal justice system should abandon its mission. But public health has a different mission: it focuses on prevention as opposed to punishment. The relative success of the public health approach against motor vehicle injuries has inspired calls for it to be applied against violence, especially against firearm violence, the behavior that has the most severe consequences for health.

There are plenty of grim statistics showing that America's permissive attitude toward guns is harmful to people's health. In 2009, firearms killed 31,347 Americans.[33] Of these, almost 60 percent were suicides, 37 percent were homicides, and the rest were caused by unintentional shootings, legal intervention, or unknown causes. Teenagers and young adults are especially at risk. Twenty percent of people who die from firearms are between the ages of 15 and 24. Almost one in three of these deaths among youths were suicides, and almost two-thirds were homicides. The death rate from firearms is six times higher for males than that for females. Young African American males are especially at risk, especially for homicide.[33]

Homicide rates in the United States are two to four times higher than those in other developed countries.[34] Although suicide rates among Americans are comparable to those in other developed countries, a high percentage of them are committed with firearms. The easy availability of guns in the United States is believed responsible for many of these deaths. Homicide and suicide are more likely to succeed if guns are used rather than less lethal weapons. In 2009, 51 percent of suicides and 68 percent of homicides were committed with guns.[33] Suicide among young people is especially tragic. While rates of suicide among people 15 to 24 years old have declined since 1990, suicide is still the third leading cause of death in this age group.[1(Table 27)] Almost half of these suicides are committed with firearms.[33]

About one-third of U.S. households possess firearms, and half of the guns are handguns, the weapon most likely to be used in a fatal injury.[35] While many people own a handgun because they believe it will protect them, a number of case-control studies have shown that the opposite is true. One study found that the relative risk of death by an unintentional gunshot injury is 3.7 for people living in a home with at least one gun, compared to a home without guns.[36] Another study found that residents of a household with a gun present in the home are three times more likely to die in a homicide[37] and five times more likely to commit suicide[38] than when no gun is available. In another study, a gun kept at home was found to be 43 times more likely to kill its owner, a family member, or a friend than an intruder.[39] An analysis by the National Academy of Sciences, however, cast doubt on whether the relationship between gun ownership and homicide or suicide represents cause and effect. The report stated that the data were too unreliable to draw firm conclusions and noted that information such as that collected on guns traced to crimes by the Bureau of Alcohol, Tobacco and Firearms is inaccessible to researchers.[34]

The CDC has been collecting data on patterns of violence for almost 2 decades, and in the early 1990s the agency stepped up its efforts to identify and evaluate interventions to prevent and reduce the impact of violence. Politically, however, guns have been a much more difficult issue to deal with than motor vehicles. Many conservative politicians, with the support of the National Rifle Association (NRA), regard any attempt to control access to firearms as an attack on the Second Amendment to the Constitution. Limits on the depiction of violence in the media are also vigorously opposed in the name of protecting freedoms, although there is some evidence that viewing violent episodes on television or in the movies increases the cultural acceptance of violence and makes children and youths more likely to behave in aggressive ways.

Opponents of gun control have even gone so far as to try to prevent the CDC from conducting research on violence as a public health problem. In 1995 and 1996, conservative members of the House of Representatives, backed by the NRA, tried first to eliminate the CDC's National Center for Injury Prevention and Control and then to cut from the center's budget the exact amount—about $2.4 million—that it had proposed for research on firearms injury.[40] President Clinton supported the CDC's work, and attempts to cut the center's budget failed.

However, the political opposition had an impact. Legislation passed in 1996 explicitly forbade the CDC from using any of its funding "to advocate or promote gun control."[41(p.190)]

Efforts to reduce firearms injuries are continuing nonetheless. The Harvard Injury Control Research Center, with funding from private foundations, developed a National Violent Injury Statistics System in 1999, modeled after the NHTSA's reporting system for motor vehicle injuries. This became a pilot for what is now the National Violent Death Reporting System (NVDRS), established in 2002 by the CDC with support from a new Congress. The NVDRS is a state-based system that collects detailed data on homicides and suicides in order to better inform policy on violence and suicide.[42,43] As of 2011, the program operated in 18 states.

The successful passage of the Brady Handgun Violence Prevention Act and the federal assault weapons ban in 1994 showed that there could be political support for limiting access to firearms even in an antiregulatory climate. However, the assault weapons ban expired in 2004 and the fact that it has not been renewed by Congress shows that the NRA still has clout in Washington. Some states and communities have similar bans, as well as violence prevention and youth development programs, including education to promote nonviolent resolution of arguments. The economic cost of gun violence in medical care—calculated at about $2.3 billion per year[44]—has helped to persuade some states to pass stricter gun control regulations. About half the medical costs of firearms injuries are borne by taxpayers.

Public health advocates note that guns need not be banned in order to make them safer. The third "E" of injury prevention—engineering—has not been widely applied in the prevention of firearms injuries. Safety catches can be used to make guns childproof, for example, and there are even ways to personalize guns so that they can be used only by the owner. Safety features are required by law for many consumer products that are much less dangerous than guns. When the political climate is ready to support major efforts to prevent firearms-related injuries, the public health approach has much to offer.[45]

Occupational Injuries

Workplace injuries have been a significant public health problem since the Industrial Revolution, if not before. In 1907, over 15,000 American workers were reported to have died on the job. Many states implemented occupational safety laws in the late 19th and early 20th centuries. In 1970, the Congress passed a federal law creating the Occupational Safety and Health Administration (OSHA), empowered to set standards, inspect workplaces, and impose penalties for workplace hazards. The law also created the National Institute for Occupational Safety and Health (NIOSH) to conduct research, recommend standards, and conduct hazard evaluations.[12]

The workplace is safer now, with 4690 fatal injuries reported by the Bureau of Labor Statistics in 2010, despite a large increase in the number of workers.[46] In part, this improvement reflects mandated safety measures and educational programs; in part, it reflects an economy less dependent on heavy industry. However, in addition to the deaths, almost one million Americans suffer an injury each year that leads to lost work days.

As in the pattern of injuries overall, motor vehicles are the leading occupational cause of death, with highway crashes accounting for 22 percent of all worker deaths.[46] The second leading cause of injury mortality in 2010 was falls, at about 14 percent of deaths. Workplace homicides, which ranked fourth in 2010, have declined to about half of the over 1000 in 1994, following the general trend of decreasing firearms deaths. In fact, the number of workplace homicides was the lowest reported since the Bureau of Labor Statistics started keeping track. Other commonly reported causes of occupational fatality were "struck by falling object or equipment," which ranked third, "overturned farm or industrial vehicle," "caught or compressed by equipment or objects," and "contact with electric current."

Not surprisingly, workers in some types of jobs have higher risks of occupational fatality than others. Fishing and logging are the most dangerous occupations, with the highest rate of deaths per 100,000 workers. Loggers are likely to be struck by falling trees. Construction workers have a high risk of falls. Agricultural workers are at risk for amputations by machinery, electrocutions, and pesticide poisoning. Police officers have a high risk of homicide. Aircraft pilots and flight engineers had a high fatality rate in 2010.[46]

Injury from Domestic Violence

All too often, family conflict leads to violence against children or spouses. In 2010, an estimated 1560 children under age 18 died from child maltreatment; 80 percent of the deaths occurred in children younger than age 4. Moreover, 740,000 children and youth are treated each year in hospital emergency departments as a result of violence, and more than 3 million reports of child maltreatment are received by state and local agencies.[47] Most of the victims were maltreated by a parent.

Intimate partner violence, including rape, physical violence, or stalking, is another serious problem in the United States, affecting more than 12 million women and men each year. In 2007, intimate partner violence resulted in 2300 deaths. A number of surveys provide data on the extent of domestic violence in the United States. For example, in 1996 the CDC collaborated with the National Institute of Justice to sponsor the Violence Against Women Survey and, together with the Department of Defense, conducts an ongoing National Intimate Partner and Sexual Violence Survey. The CDC's Behavioral Risk Factor Surveillance System includes questions about intimate partner violence, and the Pregnancy Risk Assessment Monitoring System collects data about physical abuse during and after pregnancy.[48]

The risk factors for domestic violence victimization and perpetration are often the same. For example, childhood physical or sexual victimization is a risk factor for future victimization and perpetration. Other factors include low self-esteem, low income, young age, and heavy alcohol and drug use. The CDC puts a high priority on preventing domestic violence, but little is known on how to accomplish this goal. The agency conducts and supports research on how to reduce or eliminate risk factors and increase protective factors.

Nonfatal Traumatic Brain Injuries

In addition to the 52,000 deaths annually, an estimated 1.4 million Americans are treated in hospital emergency departments for nonfatal traumatic brain injuries (TBIs), and uncounted others sustain the injury but are treated elsewhere or do not seek care.[49] TBIs may be mild, such as a concussion, or severe. Severe TBIs may cause permanent disability, but even mild ones can lead to changes in thinking, sensation, or language, and may increase the risk later in life for Alzheimer's or Parkinson's Disease. A well-known example of the latter is the boxer Mohammed Ali, who was diagnosed with Parkinson's Syndrome at the age of 43 after years of enduring blows to the head.[50]

The CDC gathers information on TBI by funding selected states to report data on individuals who are treated in hospital emergency departments for these injuries. The data revealed that in all states, males were twice as likely as females to suffer a TBI, but the rates varied significantly among states. The age group at highest risk for hospitalization and death was individuals 75 years and older, while the greatest number of emergency department visits were by children aged 4 and under.[6] The two leading causes of these injuries were falls and motor vehicle incidents, the latter including drivers, passengers, pedestrians, motorcyclists, and bicyclists.[51]

The Consumer Product Safety Commission (CPSC) administers another surveillance system that collects data from a nationally representative sample of 66 hospital emergency rooms. This system focuses on injuries associated with consumer products and identifies TBIs associated with products such as bicycles, swing sets, or inline skating equipment. Accordingly, the injuries identified through this system have different causes and affect younger individuals than those included in the CDC system. The group found at highest risk by the CPSC are aged 10 through 14 years, and the leading causes of the injury involve bicycles, football, playground activities, basketball, and riding all-terrain vehicles. Like the CDC system, the CPSC found that boys are more than twice as likely as girls to suffer a TBI.[52] The CDC recommends primary and secondary prevention to minimize TBI. Primary prevent calls for participants in such activities to wear protective equipment such as helmets. Secondary prevention provides that anyone suspected of having a TBI should be removed from play and allowed to return only after being evaluated by a healthcare provider experienced in diagnosing and managing TBI.[52]

Recently, attention has been drawn to the TBI risks from playing football, both professionally and as students. In October 2008, a 16-year-old high school football player in New Jersey died after suffering a brain hemorrhage during a game, the fourth high school player to die of a head injury in the United States that year.[53] The New Jersey student had had a concussion during a practice 3 weeks earlier, but had been cleared by a doctor to return to play. Young brains are especially vulnerable to repeat mild TBIs within a short period of time, and the question of how long young athletes need to recover is controversial. Sports physicians note that athletes of all ages, eager to return to the game, tend to deny symptoms, and it is difficult for doctors to determine when it is safe for them to return.[54]

Similar issues have troubled the National Football League (NFL) in trying to develop a policy on when players may return to the game after a head injury. Several observations have suggested that professional football players may suffer a high rate of brain damage due to repeated head trauma. A study of retired players found a statistical link between multiple concussions and later-life depression. After evidence accumulated that retired football players had a higher than average risk of dementia, an NFL program to assist these retirees was launched, and dozens more candidates than expected signed up. Another red flag was that when autopsies were done on five retired NFL players who had died before age 51, degenerative brain damage was found similar to that found in boxers with dementia. At a meeting of NFL officials, Troy Vincent, veteran player who is president of the players' union, noted that most players don't worry about concussions. He himself had had six documented concussions, he said, but possibly dozens more. "Outside of me being knocked out, asleep, I went back in the game on all the other occasions. And 50 or 60 times, I'm in the huddle, I don't know where I'm at, don't know the call, and I've got a player holding me up. I'm not sure if athletes really know what a concussion is—get some smelling salts and back in the game."[55]

The CDC, together with the NFL and other football organizations, have developed a poster on concussions to be displayed in all NFL locker rooms, cautioning players about the importance of recognizing a concussion, taking time to recover, and not returning to play too soon. A similar poster has been developed for young athletes to be posted in team locker rooms, gymnasiums, and schools.[56]

Tertiary Prevention

For any kind of serious injury, the promptness and quality of emergency medical aid play a significant role in whether a victim survives as well as in the extent of permanent disability. Lack of prompt emergency care accounts for the fact that death rates from motor vehicle crashes are higher in rural areas than in more populated ones. The establishment of special trauma centers and the use of helicopters to transport injured patients over long distances have improved the prospects in some locations, but many parts of the country still lack integrated trauma-care programs. Well-trained emergency medical technicians and well-equipped ambulances can make the difference between life and death. There is still a need for research to better understand the biomedical aspects of injury and to devise better treatments.

Conclusion

Injuries are a major cause of death and disability in the United States. They are of particular concern to public health because they disproportionately affect young people, and many injuries are preventable. Fatal injuries are categorized as unintentional—commonly called "accidents"—and intentional, a category that includes homicide and suicide. Poisoning has recently surpassed motor vehicle crashes as the leading cause of injury deaths. Injuries caused by firearms are third. Alcohol is a significant factor in a very high percentage of injuries. The number of deaths caused by injuries is just the tip of the injury pyramid, which shows that for every death there are many injuries resulting in hospitalizations, many more injuries requiring treatment in emergency rooms and physicians' offices, and even more injuries treated at home.

Analysis of injuries provides guidelines for prevention. The analysis involves considerations of the host, agent, and environment and how they may be altered to prevent an injury from occurring (primary prevention), to minimize the damage (secondary prevention), or to prevent resulting disability by providing prompt treatment (tertiary prevention). This kind of analysis was pioneered in the analysis of motor vehicle injuries, which focused not only on the driver (host) but on making the vehicle (agent) safer and on developing safer highways (environment). Tertiary prevention included the provision of ambulances and trauma centers.

Prevention of motor vehicle injuries also includes campaigns to change people's behavior by persuading them, or requiring them by law, to wear seat belts when riding in motor vehicles and to wear helmets when riding on motorcycles. Bicycle helmets, which are underutilized, are also an important safety measure.

The number of poisoning fatalities has increased dramatically over the last decade. Much of the increase is due to misuse of prescription drugs, especially painkillers. Regulatory approaches to reducing poisoning risks must be balanced against evidence that patients suffering from chronic disease have sometimes been denied the relief of appropriate medications.

Due to large numbers of firearms injuries, the United States has higher rates of homicides and childhood suicides than other industrialized nations. The easy availability of guns in the United States contributes to the high death rate from firearms injuries. Some studies have suggested that the presence of a gun in the home increases the risk that a resident will be a victim of homicide or suicide. However, data to support such studies is unreliable because of opposition by the gun lobby to the collection of such data.

Public health has made progress in preventing childhood injuries from falls, drowning, poisoning, and fires and burns. Much of this progress comes from laws requiring safety features such as window guards in apartment buildings, fencing around swimming pools, childproof caps on medicine containers, and fireproofing of children's sleepwear.

Domestic violence, including child abuse and domestic partner violence, is a significant problem in the United States. Surveys sponsored by the CDC and other organizations provide evidence on the prevalence of these problems. The CDC has placed a high priority on prevention and sponsors and conducts research on how to reduce risk factors and enhance protective factors.

Because TBI, in addition to causing deaths, can have serious consequences, including lifelong disability, the federal government has surveillance systems in place to identify such injuries and their risk factors. Young people are especially vulnerable to TBI, because their brains are more easily damaged and take longer to heal than adult brains. Recently football injuries have drawn public health attention. There is evidence that professional football players may suffer degenerative changes to the brain because of repeated blows to the head, putting them at risk of depression and dementia. High school football players are even more vulnerable to serious consequences if they return to the playing field too soon after suffering a concussion.

References

1. National Center for Health Statistics, *Health, United States, 2008, with Special Features on the Health of Young Adults* (Hyattsville, MD: Public Health Service, 2009).
2. S. P. Baker, B. O'Neill, and R. S. Karpf, *The Injury Fact Book* (New York: Oxford University Press, 1992).
3. U.S. Centers for Disease Control and Prevention, "Deaths Resulting from Firearm- and Motor-Vehicle-Related Injuries—United States, 1968–1991," *Morbidity and Mortality Weekly Report* 43 (1994): 37–42.
4. U.S. Centers for Disease Control and Prevention, "QuickStats: Death Rates for the Leading Causes of Injury Death—United States, 1979–2007," *Morbidity and Mortality Weekly Report* 59 (2010): 957.
5. U.S. Centers for Disease Control and Prevention, NCHS Fact Sheet: "NCHS Data on Injuries." http://www.cdc.gov/nchs/data/factsheets/factsheet_injury.htm, accessed July 5, 2012.
6. U.S. Centers for Disease Control and Prevention, "Traumatic Brain Injury in the U.S." http://www.cdc.gov/Features/dsTBI_BrainInjury/, accessed July 5, 2012.
7. National Highway Traffic Safety Administration, "Traffic Safety Facts 2010 Data—Alcohol-Impaired Driving," April 2012. http://www-nrd.nhtsa.dot.gov/Pubs/811606.pdf, accessed July 5, 2012.

8. National Highway Traffic Safety Administration, "Traffic Safety Facts, 2010 Data—Overview," June 2012. http://www-nrd.nhtsa.dot.gov/Pubs/811630, accessed July 5, 2012.

9. A. H. Mokdad, J. S. Marks, D. F. Stroup, and J. L. Gerberding, "Actual Causes of Death in the United States, 2000," *Journal of the American Medical Association* 291 (2004): 1238–1245.

10. National Committee for Injury Prevention and Control, "Injury Prevention: Meeting the Challenge," *American Journal of Preventive Medicine* 5 (1989), (Supplement 3): 1–303.

11. U.S. Centers for Disease Control and Prevention, "Vital Signs: Unintentional Injury Deaths Among People Aged 0–19 Years—United States, 2000–2009," *Morbidity and Mortality Weekly Report* 61 (2012): 270–276.

12. National Highway Traffic Safety Administration, "Quick Reference Guide to Federal Motor Vehicle Safety Standards and Regulations." http://www.safercar.gov/, accessed July 6, 2012.

13. National Highway Traffic Safety Administration, "Traffic Safety Facts: 2007 Data—Young Drivers." http://www-nrd.nhtsa.dot.gov/Pubs/811001.PDF, 2007, accessed September 18, 2012.

14. National Highway Traffic Safety Administration, "Traffic Safety Facts: Laws. Graduated Driver Licensing System," January 2008. http://www.nhtsa.gov//Teen-Drivers/, accessed July 6, 2012.

15. National Highway Traffic Safety Administration, "Countermeasures That Work: A Highway Safety Countermeasure Guide For State Highway Safety Offices, 3rd ed." http://www.nhtsa.dot.gov/people/injury/airbags/Countermeasures/pages/0Introduction.htm, accessed July 6, 2012.

16. Insurance Institute for Highway Safety, "Maximum Posted Speed Limits." http://www.iihs.org/laws/speedlimits.aspx, accessed July 6, 2012.

17. Insurance Institute for Highway Safety, "Safety Belt and Child Restraint Laws." http://www.iihs.org/laws/SafetyBeltUse.aspx, accessed July 6, 2012.

18. National Highway Traffic Safety Administration, "What Is Distracted Driving?." http://www.distraction.gov/content/get-the-facts/facts-and-statistics.html, accessed September 18, 2012.

19. National Highway Traffic Safety Administration, "State Laws," http://www.distraction.gov/content/get-the-facts/state-laws.html, accessed September 18, 2012.

20. M. Richtel, "In Study, Texting Lifts Crash Risk by Large Margin," *The New York Times*, July 28, 2009.

21. National Highway Traffic Safety Administration, "Traffic Safety Facts: 2010 Motor Vehicle Crashes: Overview." http://www-nrd.nhtsa.dot.gov/Pubs/811552.pdf, accessed July 6, 2012.

22. National Highway Traffic Safety Administration, "Traffic Safety Facts: 2010 Data—Pedestrians." http://www-nrd.nhtsa.dot.gov/Pubs/811625, accessed September 18, 2012.

23. R. F. Worth and J. Steinhauer, "New Traffic Rules for a Dangerous Street," *The New York Times*, April 6, 2004.

24. National Highway Traffic Safety Administration, "Traffic Safety Facts: 2010 Data—Motorcycles." http://www-nrd.nhtsa.dot.gov/Pubs/810639.pdf, accessed September 18, 2012.

25. National Highway Traffic Safety Administration, "Traffic Safety Facts: 2010 Data—Bicyclists and Other Cyclists." http://www-nrd.nhtsa.dot.gov/Pubs/811624, accessed September 18, 2012.

26. Bicycle Helmet Safety Institute, "Helmet-Related Statistics from Many Sources," June 18, 2012. http://www.helmets.org/stats.htm accessed September 18, 2012.

27. G. S. Watson, P. L. Zador, and A. Wilks, "Helmet Use, Helmet Use Laws, and Motorcyclist Fatalities," *American Journal of Public Health* 71 (1981): 297–300.

28. Insurance Institute for Highway Safety, "Motorcycle and Bicycle Helmet Use Laws." http://www.iihs.org/laws/HelmetUseCurrent.aspx, accessed September 18, 2012.

29. National Highway Traffic Safety Institute, "Traffic Safety Facts: Motorcycle Helmet Use Laws," http://www.nhtsa.gov/DOT/NHTSA/Communication%20&%20Consumer%20Information/Articles/Associated%20Files/810887.pdf, accessed September 18, 2012.

30. L. J. Paulozzi, D. Budnitz, and Y. Xi, "Increasing Deaths from Opioid Analgesics in the United States," *Pharmacoepidemiology and Drug Safety* 15 (2006): 618–627.

31. N. R. Kleinfeld, "Oxycodone Prescriptions Rose Sharply in New York," *New York Times* January 11, 2012.

32. Associated Press, "Death Rate Up for Car Crashes, but Down for Shootings in 95," *The New York Times*, July 27, 1997.

33. U.S. Centers for Disease Control and Prevention, National Vital Statistics Reports, "Deaths: Final Data for 2009," Volume 60, Number 3, December 29, 2011, Table 18. http://www.cdc.gov/nchs/data/nvsr/nvsr60/nvsr60_03.pdf, accessed September 19, 2012.

34. National Research Council (U.S.), *Firearms and Violence: A Critical Review* (Washington, DC: National Academies Press, 2005).

35. R. M. Johnson, T. Coyne-Beasley, and C. W. Runyan, "Firearm Ownership and Storage Practices, U.S. Households, 1992–2002: A Systematic Review," *American Journal of Preventive Medicine* 27 (2004): 173–182.

36. D. J. Wiebe, "Firearms in US Homes as a Risk Factor for Unintentional Gunshot Fatality," *Accident Analysis and Prevention* 35 (2003): 711–716.

37. A. L. Kellermann et al., "Gun Ownership as a Risk Factor for Homicide in the Home," *New England Journal of Medicine* 329 (1993): 1084–1091.

38. A. L. Kellermann et al., "Suicide in the Home in Relation to Gun Ownership," New Eng*land Journal of Medicine* 237 (1992): 467–472.

39. A. L. Kellermann and D. T. Reay, "Protection or Peril? An Analysis of Firearm-Related Deaths in the Home," *New England Journal of Medicine* 314 (1986): 1557–1560.

40. N. A. Lewis, "N.R.A. Takes Aim at Study of Guns as Public Health Risk," *The New York Times*, August 26, 1995.

41. J. Rovner, "U.S. House Refuses Point-Blank to Restore CDC Gun-Research Funds," *Lancet* 348 (1996) 190.

42. Harvard Injury Control Research Center, "Research to Practice," 2012. http://www.hsph.harvard.edu/research/hicrc/research-to-practice/, accessed September 19, 2012.

43. U.S. Centers for Disease Control and Prevention, "National Violent Death Reporting System." http://www.cdc.gov/ViolencePrevention/NVDRS/, accessed September 19, 2012.

44. P. J. Cook, B. A. Lawrence, J. Ludwig, and T. R. Miller, "Medical Costs of Gunshot Injuries in the United States," *Journal of the American Medical Association* 281 (1999): 447–454.

45. S. B. Sorenson, "Regulating Firearms as a Consumer Product," *Science* 286 (1999): 1481–1482.

46. U.S. Department of Labor, Bureau of Labor Statistics, "National Census of Fatal Occupational Injuries in 2007," press release. http://www.bls.gov/news.release/pdf/cfoi.pdf, accessed June 27, 2012.

47. U.S. Centers for Disease Control and Prevention, "Child Maltreatment Prevention." http://www.cdc.gov/ViolencePrevention/childmaltreatment/index.html, accessed September 15, 2012.

48. U.S. Centers for Disease Control and Prevention, "Intimate Partner Violence." http://www.cdc.gov/ViolencePrevention/intimatepartnerviolence/index.html, accessed September 15, 2012.

49. U.S. Centers for Disease Control and Prevention, "Traumatic Brain Injury in the United States: Emergency Department Visits, Hospitalization and Deaths, 2001–2006." http://www.cdc.gov/traumaticbraininjury/tbi_ed/html, accessed November 10, 2012.

50. R. McG. Thomas, Jr., "Change in Drugs Help Ali Improve," *The New York Times*, September 9, 2004.

51. U.S. Centers for Disease Control and Prevention, "Rates of Hospitalization Related to Traumatic Brain Injury—Nine States, 2003," *Morbidity and Mortality Weekly Report* 56 (2007): 167–170.

52. U.S. Centers for Disease Control and Prevention, "Nonfatal Traumatic Brain Injuries from Sports and Recreation Activities," *Morbidity and Mortality Weekly Report* 56 (2007): 733–737.

53. M. S. Schmidt and D. Caldwell, "High School Football Player Dies," *The New York Times*, October 16, 2008.

54. A. Schwarz, "New Guidelines on Young Athletes' Concussions Stir Controversy," *The New York Times*, June 7, 2009.

55. A. Schwarz, "Player Silence on Concussions May Block NFL Guidelines," *The New York Times*, June 20, 2007.

56. A. Schwarz, "N.F.L. Asserts Greater Risks of Head Injury," *The New York Times*, July 26, 2010.

Maternal and Child Health as a Social Problem

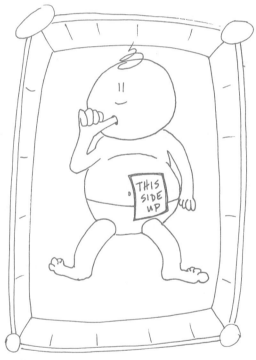

The "Back to Sleep" Campaign

The health of pregnant women and children is traditionally one of the highest priorities of public health. In a society concerned with the welfare of its population, everyone should be guaranteed adequate conditions for the best possible start in life. The fetal and infant stages of development provide the foundations of good health throughout life. There is increasing evidence that conditions in utero and during early life play a powerful role in increasing individuals' susceptibility to the chronic diseases that plague American adults, including high blood pressure, obesity, cardiovascular disease, and diabetes.[1] Moreover, because children are the most vulnerable segment of the population, like canaries in the coal mine, they are the first to suffer from any adverse conditions that affect human health in general.

Children's health first became a public concern in the United States at the end of the 19th century, prompted by alarm at the high infant and child death rates in the summer from diarrheal diseases.[2] Heat, poor sanitation, and lack of refrigeration contributed to heavy microbial contamination of milk, which was sickening poor children. In 1893, New York City established milk stations that provided safe milk. Similar programs soon followed in other cities. The success of the milk programs in improving children's health inspired the formation of voluntary infant welfare societies with the mission of teaching poor and immigrant mothers about nutrition and hygiene. The federal government got involved in 1912 with the establishment of the Children's Bureau, mandated to "investigate and report on all matters affecting children and child life."[2(p.8)] In 1921, Congress first provided grants to states to develop health services for mothers and children. During the same period, advocates for child health and welfare were fighting to protect children from oppressive and exploitive labor, which was not regulated by the federal government until the 1930s.

Child health programs have, since the beginning, been plagued by a basic philosophical and political conflict: society's responsibility for the well-being of infants and children was sometimes in conflict with the presumed right of parents to provide for, or neglect, their own children.[3] Until the 20th century, children were regarded as the property of their parents. Passage of the 1912 legislation establishing the Children's Bureau reflected a new view that children were a national resource and that their health and vigor were important for the progress of society. In recent decades, children have increasingly been viewed as having rights on their own, independent of their parents or their prospective role in society. Current controversies concerning the role of government in the protection of children—issues that range from the removal of children from abusive parents to medical treatment for the children of Christian Scientists—are a continuation of a century-long tradition of conflict.

Maternal and Infant Mortality

The infant mortality rate (IMR) is a gauge of a society's attention to children's health and is, in fact, an indicator of the health status of a population as a whole. This rate is a particular concern for American public health professionals because the infant mortality rate in this country is very high compared with that of other industrialized countries. As shown in Table 18-1, the United States ranks 27th after many industrialized Asian and European countries. Sweden and Japan, for example, both have infant mortality rates less than half of that in the United States.

Table 18-1 IMRs in OECD Countries (Deaths per 1000 Live Births), 2008

Iceland	2.5	Israel	3.8
Sweden	2.5	Netherlands	3.8
Finland	2.6	Denmark	4.0
Japan	2.6	Switzerland	4.0
Greece	2.7	Australia	4.1
Norway	2.7	United Kingdom	4.7
Czech Republic	2.8	New Zealand	5.0
Italy	3.3	Canada	5.1
Portugal	3.3	Hungary	5.6
Spain	3.3	Poland	5.6
Germany	3.5	Slovak Republic	5.9
S. Korea	3.5	United States	6.6
Austria	3.7	Chile	7.8
Belgium	3.7	Turkey	14.9
France	3.8	Mexico	15.2
Ireland	3.8		

Source: Data from National Center for Health Statistics, *Health, United States*, 2011, Table 20.

The IMR, defined as the number of infant deaths within the first year of life for every 1000 live births, has been declining in the United States over the course of the century, as seen in Figure 18-1. The rate fell from 100 in 1915 to 6.6 in 2008. Reasons for the decline include improved socioeconomic status (SES), housing, and nutrition; immunization; clean water and pasteurized milk; antibiotics; and better prenatal care and delivery. The availability of family planning services and legalized abortion in the United States contributed to the lowering of IMR during the 1970s because wanted babies are more likely to thrive than unwanted ones.[4] Progress in recent years is largely credited to technological advances in caring for premature infants and infants with low birth weight.

A very disturbing feature of the trends in infant mortality in the United States is the disparity according to race. The IMR for black Americans is more than double that for white Americans.[5(Table 17)] While the high infant mortality among blacks accounts in part for this country's dismal showing on an international scale, the rate for white Americans is worse than that of 24 other countries seen in Table 18-1.

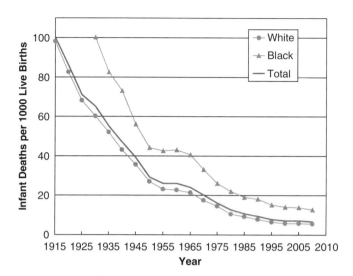

FIGURE 18-1   U.S. Infant Mortality Rates Between 1915 and 2008. *Source:* Data from U.S. Bureau of the Census and Centers for Disease Control and Prevention, *Health, United States*, 2011, Table 18.

Maternal mortality rates also declined dramatically in the United States during the 20th century, so that today the death of a woman in childbirth is a very rare event. Between 1998 and 2005, an average of 14.5 women have died each year from causes related to childbirth for every 100,000 live births, as compared with 850 in 1900. Like IMRs, maternal mortality rates are significantly higher for black women than for white women—three to four times higher.[6]

Infant Mortality—Health Problem or Social Problem?

"Infant mortality is not a health problem; it is a social problem with health consequences," in the words of a former director-general of the World Health Association.[7(p.473)] In seeking reasons to explain the high IMR in the United States, epidemiologists find that the number one risk factor for infant mortality is poverty. The generally lower SES of African Americans in the United States accounts in large part, but not entirely, for their higher IMR. There are a variety of reasons—environmental, nutritional, behavioral, medical, and social—that poverty leads to high infant mortality. These same factors that raise the risk of infant death also have a more general harmful impact on the health of the children that survive, leading to increased rates of chronic illness and disability, both physical and mental.

An extreme example of an environmental cause of infant mortality is the epidemic of birth defects in Minamata, Japan, caused by mercury contamination of the bay from an industrial source. Poor families are more likely to live in such industrial areas, exposing pregnant women and their fetuses to the harmful effects of polluted air and water. Lead, which is highly toxic to the developing nervous system, is a common contaminant in the American inner city, both from deteriorating paint and old plumbing. Other environmental chemicals known to harm the developing fetus are pesticides and organic solvents. More generally, to the extent that air or water pollution or substandard housing harm a mother's health, they harm her ability to give birth to a healthy infant. They may then cause further harm to a sickly infant who is brought home to an unhealthy environment.

Poverty may interfere with a prospective mother's ability to consume an adequate diet for nourishing her fetus. Poor women may lack the knowledge, time, or energy to prepare nutritious meals for themselves and their children. They may live in rural or inner-city areas where fresh fruits and vegetables are not readily available or are too expensive. Ignorance or lack of financial resources may carry over to how a baby is fed. Breastfeeding, which provides the best nutrition for an infant [unless the mother is infected with human immunodeficiency virus (HIV)], is less commonly practiced among poorly educated women than it is among those of higher SES.

Maternal behaviors that can harm the health of an infant include smoking, drinking alcohol, and the use of legal and illegal drugs. Women who smoke during pregnancy substantially increase their risk of giving birth to an infant of low birth weight. Moreover, infants are more likely to develop respiratory infections or die of SIDS when family members smoke in the home. Alcohol is a teratogen, and fetal alcohol syndrome is a risk for children of mothers who are problem drinkers. The use by inner-city pregnant women of illegal drugs, especially crack cocaine, became a major concern in the late 1980s and early 1990s. So-called "crack babies" were born addicted to the drug, suffered withdrawal symptoms after birth, and some sustained permanent neurological impairment. Unhealthy behaviors are not limited to poor women, of course: affluent women may smoke, drink alcohol, use drugs, and eat unhealthy diets while pregnant. However, these behaviors are more common among poor women.

Social factors that contribute to high-risk pregnancies are those common in poor neighborhoods: young maternal age and low maternal education, out-of-wedlock birth, and violence. Teenage mothers are more likely to deliver premature infants than older women of the same SES, apparently for biological reasons.[8] Poor women are more likely to be single mothers, thus lacking social support. Infants and children of poor families are at greater risk from violence, both the impersonal violence of the neighborhood and child abuse by family members. Poor children are also more likely to die from unintentional injuries, including fires and falls.

The lack of prenatal care has been linked with high risk of infant mortality. Poor women, who are more likely to lack access to medical care for financial and other reasons, are less likely to get prenatal care. However, it is not clear to what extent the lack of medical attention in itself contributes to the risk for poor women, since women who do not receive adequate prenatal care are likely to have other risk factors for infant mortality.[9]

Underlying and bound up with these factors that link poverty to infant mortality is the fact that poor women suffer higher levels of stress and lower levels of social support than most women of higher SES. According to one definition, stress is "a state that occurs when persons perceive that demands exceed their ability to cope."[10(p.19)] Poor women may find that even such modest demands as paying the rent and the food bill, getting to work, or finding daycare are too much. Poor housing increases stress when leaky plumbing, malfunctioning appliances, and infestations of vermin must be dealt with. A mother's ability to cope with the needs of a sick child is limited when she has no health insurance, no transportation to a doctor's office, and no one to help her care for other children in the family. A poor, young, single mother may not have the coping skills that might come from experience, education, and the support of the child's father. To make matters worse, this mother is likely to seek stress relief through maladaptive behavior such as smoking, drug use, or entering into abusive relationships.

Preventing Infant Mortality

The United States has been successful in substantially reducing IMRs over the past 3 decades, as seen in Figure 18-1. However, much of this success is due to improved medical treatments for highly vulnerable infants after they are born.[11] The disadvantages of the technological approach are obvious: it disrupts normal bonding between parents and infants; it leaves a significant number of the survivors with long-term developmental disabilities, even severe handicaps; and it is very expensive. The countries that have better IMRs than the United States are generally much less dependent on neonatal intensive care for achieving their successes.

The public health approach to the prevention of infant mortality focuses on two groups: pregnant women in general, most of whom are highly motivated to bear a healthy child and are receptive to information on how to avoid risks; and high-risk women—the poor, young, minority, unmarried women whose infants are most likely to suffer from their socioeconomic disadvantages. Prenatal care provides women with information on how to have a healthy pregnancy and bear a healthy child. Thus prenatal care is the most public health–oriented kind of care the medical profession provides. Prenatal visits also provide the opportunity to diagnose problems that need medical intervention. For example, bacterial infections of the genital tract increase a mother's risk of giving birth prematurely, and treatment with antibiotics can reduce that risk.

The Centers for Disease Control and Prevention (CDC) recommends that all pregnant women should be screened for common infections and treated if infected.[12] Beginning prenatal care as early as possible—preferably even before a woman conceives—greatly enhances a woman's prospects of bearing a healthy infant.

Prenatal care is especially important for the women with the lowest SES. Visits to a health-care provider may be the only source of the education, services, and social support these women need. Most states recognize the importance of prenatal care and have tried to remove financial barriers by providing insurance or other sources of payment and by establishing prenatal clinics at health departments, hospital outpatient departments, and community health centers. In 2008, not quite 71 percent of pregnant women received prenatal care in the first trimester of pregnancy.[5]

A number of barriers remain that discourage the women at highest risk from seeking prenatal care, including lack of information about available services, inconvenient hours of service, rudeness and long waits at the clinics, inadequate transportation, and lack of child care for older children. The percentage of black and Hispanic women who receive prenatal care in the first trimester is significantly lower than that for white women (59.1 percent for blacks and 64.7 percent for Hispanics in 2008, compared with 72.2 percent for whites).[5] Reaching women who do not seek early prenatal care requires active outreach programs including hotlines, community canvassing, and the provision of incentives to the expectant mother.[11] A new barrier arose in the wave of anti-immigrant sentiment and policies included in the 1996 federal welfare reform bill, which resulted in denial of prenatal care for immigrants in some states. From a public health perspective, this is a foolish and expensive policy, since the infants—U.S. citizens—born to these women will be more likely to be premature, unhealthy, and in need of neonatal intensive care.[13]

To be effective in reducing infant mortality, prenatal care for high-risk women should include a broad array of medical, educational, social, and nutritional services. However, political realities too often mean that, although major efforts are made to increase the number of women who receive prenatal care, the clinics that provide it are understaffed, rushed, and not financed adequately to provide the services that could really make a difference in the health of the mother and infant.

Congenital Malformations

The leading specific causes of infant mortality, according to the listings on death certificates, are the following: congenital malformations, disorders related to short gestation and low birth weight, and sudden infant death syndrome (SIDS).[14] Congenital anomalies, which account for more than 20 percent of infant deaths, are preventable in many cases. Some disorders, such as Tay-Sachs disease, hemophilia, and Down syndrome have a well-known genetic basis and can be prevented by genetic screening and/or prenatal diagnosis. Newborn screening programs are designed to identify infants born with defects in body chemistry such as phenylketonuria and hypothyroidism that can be remedied by early diagnosis and treatment. Other congenital anomalies may be caused by known environmental exposures, such as tobacco smoke, viruses, heavy metals, or the use of legal or illegal drugs. Public health intervention includes Food and Drug Administration (FDA) regulation of teratogenic drugs such as thalidomide or warnings to pregnant women such as those required on alcoholic beverage containers and on the packaging of legal teratogenic drugs such as the acne drug Accutane or the epilepsy drug Dilantin. Infection with the rubella virus—German measles—once a common cause of deafness and mental retardation, is prevented by immunization. However, the causes of more than 70 percent of birth defects are unknown. It is believed that many defects are caused by a combination of genetic and environmental factors.

In an attempt to identify causes, the CDC is coordinating the ongoing National Birth Defects Prevention Study, a case-control study involving 10 states. Mothers of infants with birth defects are interviewed about their own health, pregnancy history, diet, medication and substance use, work history, drinking water sources, and other questions thought to be relevant. They are also asked to provide DNA samples, which can help identify the role of genetics. Infants in the control group for the study are chosen at random from birth certificates of live-born infants with no major birth defects, and their mothers are similarly interviewed and asked for DNA samples.[15] Among the study's findings to date are that women with uncontrolled diabetes or who are obese are at increased risk for bearing a child with a broad range of birth defects. Smoking during pregnancy increases the risk of premature birth and certain birth defects such as cleft lip and cleft palate. Drinking alcohol during pregnancy may cause fetal alcohol syndrome.[16]

Nutritional factors are known to contribute to the risk of some defects. Two of the most severe—anencephaly (a lethal condition in which all or most of an infant's brain is missing) and spina bifida (protrusion of the spinal cord from the spinal column accompanied by paralysis of the lower body) are caused in part by a deficiency in folic acid, a B vitamin present in green leafy vegetables, dried beans, liver, orange juice, and grapefruit juice. The damage occurs early in the pregnancy, when the developing spinal column is being formed. Dietary supplementation with folic acid has been shown to reduce the incidence of these neural tube defects by 50 percent or more, but the supplementation must happen during the first month of pregnancy, even before the woman may recognize she is pregnant.[17] Public health campaigns to encourage all women of childbearing age to take folic acid supplements have had only modest success, and poor, high-risk women are probably the least likely to comply with the recommendation. In order to remedy the problem, the FDA decided to require that foods such as flour, corn meal, pasta, and rice be fortified with folic acid, effective January 1, 1998. As a result of the fortification, the number of affected pregnancies in the United States declined by 26 percent by 2000 and has continued to decline.[18] The amount of folic acid used for fortification is not sufficient to provide a maximum protective effect, however, and young women are still advised to take supplements.

Preterm Birth

An analysis by CDC scientists, published in 2006, proposed that preterm birth is responsible for many more infant deaths than are indicated on the death certificates. The scientists noted that 6 of the 11 leading causes listed on the death certificates, including three separate diagnoses involving respiratory distress, are entirely attributable to preterm birth. When this information is taken into account, prematurity—disorders of short gestation and low birth weight—becomes the leading cause of infant death, causing over one-third of these deaths. Thus reducing infant mortality rates in the United States will require "a comprehensive agenda to identify, to test, and to implement effective strategies for the prevention of premature births."[19(p.1573)] The percentage of infants born prematurely amounted to over 12 percent of all births in 2009.[20] This indicates a public health failure and an increasing reliance on high-technology medical care to maintain the continued decline in IMRs. Black infants are more than twice as likely to be born too small as are white infants. This disparity has decreased slightly in recent years, not because African-American mothers are having healthier pregnancies, but because many white women are postponing conception until they are older, when they are more likely to have difficult pregnancies or need assisted reproduction technology, increasing the risk of multiple births.

While the causes of premature labor and delivery are not well understood, many of the environmental, behavioral, nutritional, and social factors previously discussed can contribute. In trying to understand how to reduce the mortality and disability caused by preterm births, scientists classify preventive measures as primary, secondary, or tertiary.[21] In the United States, most of the efforts have been focused on tertiary prevention, aimed at improving the outcomes for infants born prematurely, and requiring expensive use of neonatal intensive care. Secondary prevention is aimed at identifying women at risk of giving birth too early and reducing their risk. For example, maternal smoking causes a 25 percent increased risk of preterm birth; the CDC monitors the prevalence of smoking among pregnant women, which has declined significantly since 1990 but is still over 10 percent.[5(Table 8)] Other risk factors include previous preterm births, carrying more than one fetus, obesity, diabetes, and bacterial infections of the genital tract. Recent evidence suggests that gum disease is associated with preterm births, and that periodontal treatment may reduce the risk.[22] Some of these factors can be helped by timely prenatal care. However, as many as half of preterm infants in the United States are born to women considered to be low risk.

Primary prevention of preterm birth is, from a public health perspective, the most desirable strategy. Many European countries accomplish this by providing social and financial support for low-risk pregnant women, but this might be politically difficult to implement in the United States.[21] Preterm birth, of the various causes of infant mortality, is clearly a social problem rather than a health problem, as discussed earlier in this chapter. The reason the United States has such a poor record in preventing infant mortality is that we have tried to approach it as a medical problem.

Sudden Infant Death Syndrome

Sudden Infant Death Syndrome (SIDS), the third leading cause of infant death overall, is also not well understood. Almost always the death is unexpected; usually the infant appeared to be healthy before he or she died, and an autopsy fails to establish the cause of death. While SIDS is more common in infants of low birth weight and in infants of smokers or drug users, it is not limited to infants with these risk factors.[23] Until recently, because of the lack of understanding about the causes of SIDS, there was not much parents could do to reduce the risk. Then, in the early 1990s, studies done in New Zealand, Australia, and the United Kingdom reported that SIDS occurred more frequently in infants that were sleeping on their stomachs. The American Academy of Pediatrics and the National Institute of Child Health and Human Development began a "Back to Sleep" campaign to educate maternity wards, doctors and nurses, and parents that infants should be put to sleep on their backs. Since the campaign was launched, the number of deaths from SIDS has declined dramatically: by 2005, the SIDS death rate had fallen by over 50 percent.[24] There is still room for improvement: surveys of infant sleeping positions have found that almost 20 percent of American infants continue to sleep on their stomachs, and only 31 percent of black infants are put to sleep on their backs.[23] The SIDS death rate for black and American Indian infants is two to three times the rate for white infants.[23] Public health agencies and medical care providers are working with communities of minority groups to educate them about the importance of putting infants to sleep on their backs. Other factors that increase the risk of SIDS are soft bedding, being overheated, and bed sharing.

SIDS is a diagnosis of exclusion, meaning that any unexplained death is thoroughly investigated and SIDS is listed as the cause of death only if no other explanation is found. Law enforcement officials participate in the investigation, which includes an autopsy as well as interviews with family members and other caregivers. The CDC publishes guidelines recommending how these investigations should be done, with the aim of better understanding causes and risk factors for SIDS.[25]

Family Planning and Prevention of Adolescent Pregnancy

Because pregnancy is not good for the health of either a teenager or her infant, preventing adolescent pregnancy is a high public health priority. In addition to the health risks, pregnancy during the teen years has many harmful consequences, including interference with the young mother's education and career prospects, economic hardship, and interference with the formation of a strong family unit. Thus adolescent pregnancy, and all the accompanying socioeconomic consequences, increases the health risks to the child for all the reasons previously described as causes of infant mortality. Teenage mothers are less likely to seek prenatal care than older women and are more likely to have no care at all. They are more likely to smoke and less likely to gain adequate weight during pregnancy. Infants of teenage mothers are at greatly increased risk of low birth weight, serious and long-term disability, and dying during the first year of life.[26]

Rates of adolescent pregnancy in the United States have declined since the 1950s, but in those days, social pressure forced marriage on many girls who became pregnant, producing a more stable economic and family environment for the young child. Today, most teenage mothers are unmarried, and a large increase in adolescent births in the late 1980s alarmed public health advocates and policy makers.[26] However, after peaking in 1991, rates declined steadily through 2005 and have remained level through 2008.[5(Table 6),27] Birth rates have consistently been higher among African American and Hispanic teenagers than among white teenagers, and rates have been lowest among Asian Americans and Pacific Islanders. U.S. adolescent pregnancy rates are the highest in the industrialized world.

Unintended pregnancy in older women is also a matter of concern to public health because it is more likely to lead to poorer health outcomes for mother and child. Some unintended pregnancies are merely mistimed, but many are unwanted, leading to some of the same risks as occur in teenage pregnancies. Surveys have shown that only about half of the pregnancies among American women are planned. A frequent consequence of unintended pregnancy is induced abortion. In the United States, there is approximately one abortion for every four live births.[28] This is a decrease from the ratio of more than one in three live births in the 1980s. From a public health perspective, every pregnancy should be an intended pregnancy.

Adequate access to contraception could go a long way toward reducing rates of unintended pregnancy and abortion. Americans' ambivalent feelings about sex probably contribute to the fact that many women lack access to comprehensive family planning services. Even private health insurance plans often do not provide coverage for contraception. Unmarried women, poor women, adolescents, and African-American women are especially likely to encounter difficulty in obtaining and paying for services. A number of federal programs provide financing for family planning services, as do many state programs. However, availability of services varies widely from one state to another and, in many areas, well under half of those in need of sub-sidized services receive them.[29] President Obama's Affordable Care Act requires new health insurance plans to cover birth control without a deductible or co-payment, a measure that should help prevent many unintended and unwanted pregnancies. Government financing for contraception is opposed by many Republicans, however, and there was real concern about whether the new law would survive the 2012 election.[30]

Female sterilization and vasectomy for men are the most effective methods of contraception and are commonly used in the United States, but they are permanent and thus inappropriate for young people. Other highly effective methods—for women—are intrauterine devices (IUD) and some hormonal implants. These methods have a failure rate of less than 1 pregnancy per 100 women per year. Equally effective when used correctly are combination oral contraceptives—"the pill"—and other hormonal contraceptives, such as Depo-Provera shots and the hormone-laden vaginal ring. Pills must be taken every day, however, and the other hormonal methods must be renewed at regular intervals.

All of these methods have drawbacks, although the health risks tend to be overestimated by the general public. Barrier methods, including the male and female condoms and the female dia-phragm and cervical cap, can be fairly effective if used correctly (failure rates of 2 to 6 pregnancies per 100 women per year) and condoms have the added advantage of reducing the risk of sexually transmitted diseases. However, barrier methods are often used inconsistently and incorrectly. Spermicides used alone (foams, creams, and jellies) have failure rates of 15 pregnancies per 100 women per year for perfect use and much worse for typical use.[31]

The "morning after pill,"—also known as "Plan B"—is a mixture of estrogen and progestin to be used within 72 hours of unprotected intercourse— the sooner, the better. It is an effec-tive backup method, reducing the risk of pregnancy by up to 94 percent, although the mecha-nism is not well understood.[32] This emergency method has not been widely used, apparently because many women and even some medical providers are not aware of its potential. In 2003, the drug's manufacturer requested the FDA to approve the sale of emergency contraceptives without a prescription, which would make the medication more easily and rapidly available to women who need it. An FDA advisory committee, after reviewing the evidence for safety, recommended that the request be approved. However, in an unusual move widely interpreted as being motivated by political pressure by the Bush administration, the FDA rejected the com-mittee's recommendation. Availability of emergency contraception would be expected to sig-nificantly reduce the number of unwanted pregnancies, including the 25,000 that result from rape, and the rate of abortions in the United States. After 3 years of pressure from Congress, including a threat to hold up confirmation of the next FDA commissioner, the FDA finally approved Plan B sale without a prescription to women 18 and older. In 2009, a judge ordered the FDA to allow sale of the pill to 17-year-olds, and the FDA complied.[33]

Public health programs specifically aimed at preventing teenage pregnancy include comprehensive sex education in the schools, which has been found to be effective in delaying young people's initiation of intercourse and increasing their use of contraception when they do have sex.[34] There is considerable controversy about the exact message that should be conveyed in pregnancy prevention programs. The federal welfare reform bill that was implemented in 1998 included funding for programs that teach sexual abstinence only. Many states were reluctant to apply for the money because they believe such programs are much less effective than those that include education on contraception as well. A 2004 congressional review found that commonly used abstinence-only curricula contained "multiple scientific and medical inaccuracies."[34(p.2014)] For example, they teach that condoms are ineffective. Some programs encourage teenagers to sign virginity pledges; studies have shown that those who do sign may delay sex, but when they do initiate intercourse they are less likely to use protection.[35]

Abstinence-only advocates took credit for the significant decline in adolescent pregnancy rates since 1991 described previously. However, despite hundreds of millions of dollars of federal funds spent on abstinence-only programs each year, studies have found no measurable impact on teen sexual behavior. An analysis of data from national surveys of young women ages 15 to 19 found that only 14 percent of the decline in pregnancy could be attributed to delayed initiation of sexual activity, while 86 percent of the decline was due to increased use of contraceptives.[36] The authors concluded that "abstinence promotion is a worthwhile goal, particularly among younger teenagers."[36(p.155)] However, it is insufficient to help adolescents prevent unintended pregnancies and sexually transmitted diseases. "Public policies and programs... should vigorously promote provision of accurate information on contraception and on sexual behavior and relationships, support increased availability and accessibility of contraceptive services and supplies for adolescents, and promote the value of responsible and protective behaviors, including condom and contraceptive use and pregnancy planning."[36(p.155)]

Nutrition of Women and Children

Since the establishment of milk stations in the 1890s, nutrition has been an important component of maternal and child health programs. At first, the emphasis was on breastfeeding and the safety of milk and baby foods. Public health is still concerned with promoting breastfeeding, which offers most infants the healthiest start in life, reducing risks of infectious diseases, ear infections, respiratory infections, obesity, and chronic diseases such as asthma and allergies. Medical and public health organizations recommend that infants be exclusively breastfed for the first 6 months of their lives and then breastfed with supplemental baby food at least until their first birthday. The CDC tracks rates of breastfeeding at discharge from the hospital, but data at 6 months is sparse. Rates of initiation of breastfeeding have increased, but they vary depending on age and education of the mothers, with rates of only 61 percent among women without a high school diploma, compared with 91.5 percent among those with a bachelor's degree. Seventy-three percent of women under 20 years old initiate breastfeeding, but that rate falls to 61 percent after 3 months.[5(Table 14)]

During the Great Depression of the 1930s, the federal government established several food assistance programs to ensure adequate nutrition for poor families. They formed the basis of current federal programs, run by the Department of Agriculture, which originated in the 1960s.[37] The Special Supplemental Nutrition Program for Women, Infants, and Children (WIC), provides vouchers for milk, fruit juice, eggs, cereals, and other nutritious foods for pregnant women, lactating mothers, infants, and children up to 5 years old. Nutrition education is also provided, and WIC centers often become a source of many support services for poor, young families. The Department of Agriculture has evaluated the WIC program and found it to be effective in saving medical costs for the women and infants who participated.

The nutritional needs of older children are addressed through the School Meals Program. School lunches, provided at most schools, must meet certain nutritional standards, including offering a meat or meat alternative, fruit and/or vegetables, bread, and milk. Children from households with incomes at or below 185 percent of the poverty level receive the lunches free or at reduced prices. Children from families with higher incomes pay more. A more limited number of children receive free or reduced price school breakfasts, and some schools offer after-school snacks. There is also a Summer Food Service Program, which provides meals during school vacation periods.

A third federal program designed to help low-income families afford adequate food is the Supplemental Nutrition Assistance Program (SNAP), formerly the Food Stamp Program. Based on the household's size and income, families are issued an electronic benefits transfer card that can be used like a credit card to buy nutritious foods at grocery stores. The Food Stamp Program, which cannot be used for alcohol, tobacco, or nonfood items, has come under fire, in part because of some well-publicized abuses. There are some limitations on immigrant families' eligibility to receive SNAP benefits.[38]

Despite food assistance programs, children are at risk of going hungry in the United States. Department of Agriculture surveys have found that 11 percent of households are food insecure, meaning that they have limited or uncertain access to nutritionally adequate foods. Families headed by single women with children and black and Hispanic households are the most likely to experience food insecurity. Poor nutrition increases children's risks of stunting, inadequate cognitive stimulation, iodine deficiency, and iron deficiency anemia. It also increases the risk of overweight and obesity, in that high-calorie processed foods are often less expensive than fresh, perishable foods such as fruits, vegetables, and low-fat dairy products.[39,40]

While undernutrition is a real concern for the poorest American families, overeating is a more widespread problem.

Children's Health and Safety

Deaths in childhood from infectious diseases have been vastly reduced because of widespread immunization programs. Virtually all children are vaccinated against diphtheria, tetanus, pertussis (whooping cough), polio, measles, rubella (German measles), mumps, and hepatitis B before they enter school, because most of these immunizations are required by law. However, many preschool children are at risk because they do not receive immunizations at the recommended ages. Well-baby care is almost as important as prenatal care for child health, but children of poor families often miss out on these visits to the doctor for the same reasons that their mothers missed prenatal visits, including lack of affordable health care.

In 1993, the federal government launched a childhood immunization initiative aimed at increasing vaccination coverage among children ages 19 months to 35 months. The federal government began to provide free vaccines for children who were uninsured or whose insurance did not cover vaccines. Public and private sector organizations and healthcare providers at the national, state, and local levels were enlisted to implement the goals of the initiative, in the hope of virtually eliminating many of the traditional childhood diseases. In addition to the eight diseases listed above, four more recent vaccines are covered by the Vaccines for Children Program: Haemophilus influenzae type b (spinal meningitis), varicella (chicken pox), pneumococcal disease, and hepatitis A.[41]

In 2008, the FDA approved a vaccine that has proven uniquely controversial. Human papilloma virus (HPV) is a group of sexually transmitted viruses that will, at some time in their lives, infect about half of all people who have ever had sex. Although some infections do not cause symptoms and are cleared by the immune system, others may lead to genital warts in men and women or cause cancers of the cervix or other genital organs. The new vaccine prevents infection with the types of the virus that cause most cervical cancers and genital warts. It is ineffective, however, in people who are already infected. Thus vaccination is recommended for 11- and 12-year-old girls, to reach them before they become sexually active, but they are approved for women up to age 26. The vaccine is expensive, with a cost of $125 for each dose, and it is designed to be given as 3 doses within 6 months. The Vaccines for Children Program will pay for poor and uninsured young people to be vaccinated. Many states have considered making the vaccine mandatory.[42]

The controversy about the HPV vaccine stems from several factors.[43] There is the question of whether the expense is justified to prevent a disease, cervical cancer, which is relatively rare in the United States. Because the vaccine prevents only 70 percent of cancer cases, women will continue to need regular Pap smears to screen for the disease. Moreover, it is unclear how long immunity persists, so there may be a need for booster shots. Some parents are reluctant for their daughters to be vaccinated because they fear it may encourage promiscuity. There is also concern about side effects of the vaccine. The greatest value of the vaccine would be in developing countries, where screening is rare and the death rate from cervical cancer is high, but the vaccine is too expensive to be used in third-world countries.

Immunization rates are tracked by the CDC. In 2009, 90 percent of children aged 19 months to 35 months had received the recommended doses of the most highly recommended six vaccines.[44] In recent years, there have been shortages of some vaccines. Manufacturers have left the market or produced insufficient supplies because they conclude that profits are not high enough, and they fear lawsuits over possible side effects. How to respond to these shortages is a challenge to the public health system.

Other preventive services of concern to public health because they may be missed by children of low SES who do not get regular well-baby care include screening for tuberculosis, problems with vision and hearing, and scoliosis, or curvature of the spine. Because recognizing these problems as early as possible is important for ensuring a child's future health and ability to learn, these services are usually provided in schools. Diagnosing a problem in a school screening program does not guarantee that the problem will be corrected, however. Children who are uninsured or underinsured may be unable to obtain treatment even after the problem is identified repeatedly.

Childhood asthma is a significant public health concern, affecting 9.5 percent of children. Prevalence is higher among blacks (16.0 percent) than whites (8.2 percent).[45] Asthma prevalence grew dramatically between 1980 and 1996 for reasons that are not well understood.[46] Since then, rates appear to have reached a plateau. Deaths from asthma are rare among children, but African-American children have a risk four times higher than white children of dying from the disease. Environmental factors in the inner city are believed to be responsible, at least in part, for the increase in asthma prevalence. Because asthma can generally be controlled by medication when patients and their parents are educated about self-management techniques, hospitalizations, and deaths are thought to be due to lack of access to regular, appropriate medical care.

Although fluoridation of community water supplies and other sources of fluoride have reduced tooth decay among children by more than 50 percent since the 1960s, some children still suffer from painful and debilitating tooth decay. Poor children are especially likely to suffer from dental decay when the water is not fluoridated, and communities vary in the extent to which they provide dental services through clinics or local health departments. The CDC has identified fluoridation of drinking water as one of the 10 great public health achievements of the 20th century. In 2010, about 74 percent of the population served by public water systems received fluoridated water.[47]

The fact that most mothers now work outside the home, a major change from the norm in previous decades, means that young children are increasingly being cared for in day care centers. Suddenly, the need for safe and affordable day care has become a public health issue. Infectious diseases spread rapidly among young children, and adequate hygiene when changing diapers is especially important. There are also risks of injury because of an unsafe physical plant or play equipment, inadequate staffing, or unqualified caregivers. These risks can be reduced by state licensing of day care centers, requiring them to meet basic health and safety standards.

Injuries constitute the main risk to the life and health of children once they pass their first year. Public health efforts to prevent childhood injury include education and regulations that encourage use of seat belts, child safety seats, and bicycle helmets. The U.S. Consumer Products Safety Commission monitors toys and children's furniture for safety hazards, issuing warnings and ordering recalls of products that are found to be dangerous to children.

While maternal and child health services, like public health in general, focus on prevention of death and disability, there is a long tradition of public concern about the care of children with handicaps. Beginning in 1935, the federal government funded state "crippled children's programs" that provide diagnosis, treatment, and rehabilitative services for children with special needs, many of whom are also eligible for support through Social Security.[2] While in the past many of these children might have been institutionalized, current programs try as much as possible to keep them at home, supporting families and preparing disabled young people to live independent lives.

In order to better understand factors that influence children's health and development, Congress in 2000 authorized the National Institutes of Health, the CDC, and the Environmental Protection Agency to conduct the largest long-term study on children ever done in the United States.[48] The National Children's Study is a longitudinal cohort study, comparable to the Framingham Heart Study and the Nurses' Health Study. The study will follow 100,000 children, from before birth to age 21, to better understand the link between children's genes, the physical, chemical, and psychosocial environments in which they are raised, and their physical and mental health and development. The study is designed to answer questions such as the following:

- Is preterm birth caused by inflammation and infection?
- Does repeated head trauma adversely affect neurodevelopment?
- Is early-life infection associated with asthma risk?
- Does impaired maternal glucose metabolism (diabetes) during pregnancy cause children to be overweight?
- Does breastfeeding reduce the risk of obesity?
- How does routine low-level pesticide exposure interact with genes to affect neurobehavior and cognitive development?

- Does household mold exposure in the first year of life lead to asthma?
- Does prenatal infection and inflammation increase the risk of cerebral palsy and autism spectrum disorders?[49]

The National Children's Health Study recruited its first patients in January 2009. Plans call for 40 study centers that will coordinate the research at 105 sites around the country, locations chosen to be representative of children in the United States.[50]

Conclusion

Maternal and child health is one of the highest priorities for public health. In the United States, city, state, and local governments have for over a century conducted programs and enforced legislation aimed at protecting children and promoting their health.

Infant mortality is a gauge of society's attention to children's health and is often used as an indicator of the health status of a population as a whole. The United States compares poorly with other countries on infant mortality, ranking 27th overall. IMRs, along with other public health improvements, have greatly improved since the beginning of the 20th century. Like other indicators of health, infant mortality is higher among African Americans than among whites and declines with increasing SES.

The three leading causes of infant mortality overall are congenital anomalies, low birth weight, and SIDS. Public health programs to prevent infant mortality because of congenital anomalies, or birth defects, include pre- and postnatal screening and diagnostic programs. They also include protection of pregnant women from exposure to environmental teratogens. Dietary supplementation with folic acid has been found to prevent some birth defects.

Low birth weight, caused by preterm birth, is closely linked to SES. Because pregnant adolescents are especially likely to give birth to infants of low birth weight, prevention of pregnancy in teenagers is a high priority for public health.

SIDS deaths declined dramatically during the 1990s after it was found that babies who were put to sleep on their stomachs were at increased risk of sudden death. An educational campaign about infant sleeping positions cut SIDS deaths by over 50 percent.

Adequate family planning services are important for public health. Pregnancy in adolescence is risky for both mothers and infants. Comprehensive sex education is effective in preventing teen pregnancy. Political conservatives promote abstinence-only programs, which are less effective than programs that include information on contraception. Unintended pregnancy also increases health risks in older women and their infants. While a variety of effective contraceptive methods are available, many women do not have access to affordable family planning services. Nutrition is an important component of maternal and child health programs. The federal government has, since the 1930s, supported a number of programs that provide supplemental foods for pregnant women, infants, and children.

Other public health initiatives that have a significant impact on children's health include immunization requirements, fluoridation of community water supplies, and injury-prevention measures. Regular access to medical care is important for the health of children, but many poor and minority children do not have this access.

The National Children's Study, a cohort study linking genes and the physical, chemical, and psychosocial environment of children to their physical and mental health and development, started recruiting subjects in 2009. It will track 100,000 American children from birth to age 21.

References

1. P. D. Gluckman et al., "Effect of In Utero and Early-Life Conditions on Adult Health and Disease," *New England Journal of Medicine* 359 (2008): 61–73.
2. W. M. Schmidt and H. M. Wallace, "Development of Health Services for Mothers and Children in the United States," in H. M. Wallace, G. M. Ryan, Jr., and A. C. Oglesby, eds., *Maternal and Child Health Practices* (Oakland, CA: Third Party Publishing, 1988), 3–21.
3. C. A. Miller, "Development of MCH Services and Policy in the United States," in H. M. Wallace, G. M. Ryan, Jr., and A. C. Oglesby, eds., *Maternal and Child Health Practices* (Oakland, CA: Third Party Publishing Company, 1988), 39–45.
4. W. S. Nersesian, "Infant Mortality in Socially Vulnerable Populations," *Annual Review of Public Health* 9 (1988): 361–377.
5. U.S. Centers for Disease Control and Prevention, *Health, United States, 2011*. http://www.cdc.gov/nchs/data/hus/hus11.pdf, accessed July 15, 2012.
6. C. J. Berg et al., "Pregnancy-Related Mortality in the United States, 1998–2005," *Obstetrics and Gynecology* 116 (2010):1302–1309.
7. M. G. Wagner, "Infant Mortality in Europe: Implications for the United States," *Journal of Public Health Policy* (Winter 1998): 473–484.
8. A. M. Fraser, J. E. Brockert, and R. H. Ward, "Association of Young Maternal Age with Adverse Reproductive Outcomes," *New England Journal of Medicine* 332 (1995): 1113–1117.
9. J. Huntington and F. A. Connell, "For Every Dollar Spent—The Cost-Savings Argument for Prenatal Care," *New England Journal of Medicine* 331 (1994): 1303–1307.
10. N. Adler et al., "Socioeconomic Status and Health: The Challenge of the Gradient," *American Psychologist* 49 (1994): 15–24.
11. S. S. Brown, "Preventing Low Birthweight," in H. M. Wallace, G. M. Ryan, Jr., and A. C. Oglesby, eds., *Maternal and Child Health Practices* (Oakland, CA: Third Party Publishing, 1988), 307–324.
12. U.S. Centers for Disease Control and Prevention, "STDs and Pregnancy—CDC Fact Sheet," http://www.cdc.gov/std/pregnancy/STDFact-Pregnancy.htm, accessed July 15, 2012.
13. S. Sengupta, "Legislators Seek Way to Restore Prenatal Care for Immigrants," *The New York Times*, May 24, 2001.

14. U.S. Centers for Disease Control and Prevention, "QuickStats: Infant Mortality Rates for 10 Leading Causes of Infant Death—United States 2005," *Morbidity and Mortality Weekly Report* 56 (2007): 1115.

15. P. W. Yoon et al., "The National Birth Defects Prevention Study," *Public Health Reports* 116 (2001), Supplement 1: 32–40.

16. U.S. Centers for Disease Control and Prevention, "National Birth Defects Prevention Study (NBDPS)." http://www.cdc.gov/ncbddd/birthdefects/NBDPS.html, accessed July 15, 2012.

17. U.S. Centers for Disease Control and Prevention, "Spina Bifida and Anencephaly Before and After Folic Acid Mandate—United States, 1995–1996 and 1999–2000," *Morbidity and Mortality Weekly Report* 53 (2004): 362–365.

18. U.S. Centers for Disease Control and Prevention, "Folic Acid: Data and Statistics." http://www.cdc.gov/ncbddd/folicacid/data.html, accessed July 15, 2012.

19. W. M. Callaghan et al., "The Contribution of Preterm Birth to Infant Mortality Rates in the United States," *Pediatrics* 118 (2006): 1566–1573.

20. U.S. Centers for Disease Control and Prevention, "National Vital Statistics Report: Births: Final Data for 2009." http://www.cdc.gov/nchs/data/nvsr/nvsr60/nvsr60_01.pdf, accessed July 15, 2012.

21. J. D. Iams et al., "Primary, Secondary, and Tertiary Interventions to Reduce the Morbidity and Mortality of Preterm Births," *Lancet* 371 (2008): 164–175.

22. N. P. Polyzos et al., "Effect of Periodontal Disease Treatment During Pregnancy on Preterm Birth Incidence: A Meta-Analysis of Randomized Trials," *American Journal of Obstetrics and Gynecology* 200 (2009): 225–232.

23. SIDS Mid Atlantic, "Sudden Infant Death Syndrome." http://www.sidsma.org/professionals/documents/SIDSforhealthcare.pdf, accessed July 16, 2012.

24. National SUID/SIDS Resource Center, "Statistics." http://www.sidscenter.org/sytatistics/table1.html, accessed July 16, 2012.

25. Centers for Disease Control and Prevention, "Sudden Unexpected Infant Death and Sudden Infant Death Syndrome: Infant Death Scene Investigation." http://www.cdc.gov/sids/SceneInvestigation.htm, accessed July 16, 2012.

26. S. J. Ventura, S. C. Curtin, and T. J. Mathews, "Teenage Births in the United States: National and State Trends, 1990–96," *National Vital Statistics System* (Hyattsville, MD: National Center for Health Statistics, 1998).

27. L. Gavin et al., "Sexual and Reproductive Health of Persons Aged 10–24 Years—United States, 2002–2007," *Morbidity and Mortality Weekly Report* 58 (2009): SS-6.

28. U.S. Centers for Disease Control and Prevention, "Abortion Surveillance—United States, 2005," *Morbidity and Mortality Weekly Report* 57(2008): SS-13.

29. J. J. Frost, L. Frohwirth, and A. Purcell, "Availability and Use of Publicly Funded Family Planning Clinics: U.S. Trends, 1994–2001," *Perspectives in Sex and Reproductive Health* 36 (2004): 206–215.

30. Editorial, "Birth Control and Teenage Pregnancy," *The New York Times,* April 18, 2012.

31. Planned Parenthood, "Birth Control." http://www.plannedparenthood.org/health-topics/birth-control-4211.htm, accessed July 11, 2009.

32. F. Davidoff and J. Trussell, "Plan B and the Politics of Doubt," *Journal of the American Medical Association* 296 (2006): 1775–1778.

33. G. Harris, "FDA Easing Access to 'Morning After' Pills," *The New York Times*, April 22, 2009.

34. T. Hampton, "Abstinence-Only Programs Under Fire," *Journal of the American Medical Association* 299 (2008): 2013–2015.

35. H. Bruckner and P. S. Bearman, "After the Promise: The STD Consequences of Adolescent Virginity Pledges," *Journal of Adolescent Health* 36 (2005): 271–278.

36. J. S. Santelli et al., "Explaining Recent Declines in Adolescent Pregnancy in the United States: The Contribution of Abstinence and Improved Contraceptive Use," *American Journal of Public Health* 97 (2007): 150–156.

37. J. T. Dwyer and J. Freedland, "Nutrition Services," in H. M. Wallace, G. M. Ryan, Jr., and A. C. Oglesby, eds., *Maternal and Child Health Practices* (Oakland, CA: Third Party Publishing, 1988), 261–282.

38. U.S. Department of Agriculture Food and Nutrition Services: Programs and Services. http://www.fns.usda.gov/fns/services.htm, accessed July 17, 2012.

39. T. Hampton, "Food Insecurity Harms Health, Well-being of Millions in the United States," *Journal of the American Medical Association* 298 (2007): 1851–1853.

40. U.S. Department of Agriculture. Economic Research Service. *Household Food Security in the United States in 2010*, September 2011. http://www.ers.usda.gov/media/121066/err125_reportsummary.pdf, accessed July 17, 2012.

41. U.S. Centers for Disease Control and Prevention, "Vaccines for Children Program (VFC)." http://www.cdc.gov/vaccines/programs/vfc/default.htm, accessed July 17, 2012.

42. U.S. Centers for Disease Control and Prevention, "Sexually Transmitted Diseases: Human Papilloma Virus (HPV)." http://www.cdc.gov/hpv, accessed February 19, 2010.

43. E. Rosenthal, "Drug Makers' Push Leads to Cancer Vaccines' Rise," *The New York Times*, August 19, 2008.

44. U.S. Centers for Disease Control and Prevention, "National, State, and Local Area Vaccination Coverage Among Children Aged 19–35 Months—United States, 2009, *Morbidity and Mortality Weekly Report* 59 (2010): 1171–1177.

45. U.S. Centers for Disease Control and Prevention, "Summary Health Statistics for U.S. Children: National Health Interview Survey, 2010." http://www.cdc.gov/nchs/data/series/sr_10/sr10_250.pdf, accessed July 17, 2012.

46. U.S. Centers for Disease Control and Prevention, "National Surveillance for Asthma—United States, 1980–2004," *Morbidity and Mortality Weekly Report* 56 (SS08): 1–14; 18–54.

47. U.S. Centers for Disease Control and Prevention, "Community Water Fluoridation: 2010 Water Fluoridation Statistics." http://www.cdc.gov/fluoridation/statistics/2010stats.htm, accessed July 17, 2012.

48. "Children's Health Act of 2000." http://www.nationalchildrensstudy.gov/about/funding/Pages/childrenshealthact.aspx, accessed July 18, 2012.

49. U.S. Department of Health and Human Services, "Growing Up Healthy: An Overview of the National Children's Study." http://www.nichd/nih.gov/publications/pubs/upload/growing_up_healthy.pdf, accessed July 18, 2012.

50. National Institutes of Health, "NIH News: National Children's Study Begins Recruiting Volunteers." http://www.nichd.nih.gov/news/releases/jan12-09-NCS-Recruiting.cfm, accessed July 18, 2012.

Mental Health: Public Health Includes Healthy Minds

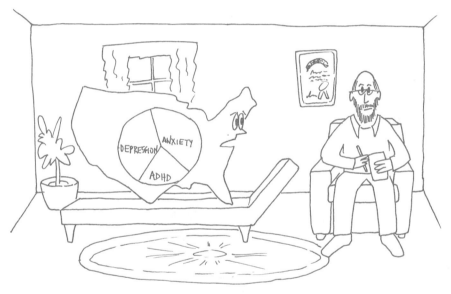

A Country in Distress

According to the World Health Organization, mental illnesses account for more disability in developed countries than any other group of illnesses, including cancer and heart disease. In 2004, an estimated 25 percent of adults in the United States reported having a mental illness in the previous year.[1] Nearly half of adult Americans will develop at least one mental illness during their lifetime.

The most common mental illnesses in adults are anxiety and mood disorders. These disorders are often associated with chronic diseases, including cardiovascular disease, diabetes, asthma, epilepsy, and cancer. People with mental illness have an increased risk of injuries, both intentional and unintentional. They are also more likely than people without mental illness to use tobacco products and to abuse alcohol and other drugs.

Categories of mental disorders, such as anxiety, psychosis, mood disturbance, and cognitive deficits, are broad, heterogeneous and somewhat overlapping. Any particular patient may manifest symptoms from more than one of these categories. Thus mental illnesses are sometimes hard to diagnose and, consequently, hard for epidemiologists to count.

Anxiety

Anxiety is a vitally important physiological response to dangerous situations that prepares one to evade or confront a threat in the environment. However, inappropriate expressions of anxiety exist if the anxiety experienced is disproportionate to the circumstance or interferes with normal functioning. Examples include phobias, panic attacks, and generalized anxiety. Other manifestations of anxiety include obsessive-compulsive disorder and post-traumatic stress disorder (PTSD).

Psychosis

Disorders of perception and thought process are considered to be symptoms of psychosis. They are most characteristically associated with schizophrenia, but psychotic symptoms can also occur in severe mood disorders. Among the most commonly observed psychotic symptoms are hallucinations—sensory impressions that have no basis in reality—and delusions—false beliefs held despite evidence to the contrary, such as paranoia.

Disturbances of Mood

Disturbances of mood characteristically manifest themselves as a sustained feeling of sadness—major depression—or sustained elevation or fluctuation of mood—bipolar disorder. Mood disturbances are also associated with symptoms like disturbances in appetite, sleep patterns, energy level, concentration, and memory. Perhaps most alarming, major depression is often associated with thoughts of suicide.

Disturbances of Cognition

The ability to organize, process, and recall information, as well as to execute complex sequences of tasks, may be disturbed in a variety of disorders. Notably, Alzheimer's disease is a progressive deterioration of cognitive function, or dementia.

Epidemiology

A number of surveys of the U.S. population have yielded estimates of the prevalence of mental illness. The most comprehensive, the National Comorbidity Survey (NCS), conducted from the fall of 1990 to spring of 1992, was sponsored by the National Institute of Mental Health, the National Institute of Drug Abuse, and the W. T. Grant Foundation. Researchers at Harvard Medical School interviewed 10,000 adults asking questions designed to diagnose specific mental and substance use disorders.[3] The same respondents were reinterviewed in 2001–2002 to study patterns and predictors of the course of mental disorders and their relation to substance use. The NCS is the source of the commonly cited findings about the high incidence and prevalence of mental illness in the United States.

Some of the surveys conducted by the Centers for Disease Control and Prevention (CDC) include questions on mental health. The Behavioral Risk Factor Surveillance System (BRFSS), a state-based telephone survey, conducts approximately 450,000 adult interviews each year. One question asked every year of all respondents is the number of mentally unhealthy days they experienced. Individual states may choose optional modules, including some that address other mental health issues in depth. For example, in 2006, 2008, and 2010, an optional module included one question on lifetime diagnosis or anxiety and one on lifetime diagnosis of depression.[1]

The National Health Interview Survey, which conducts in-person interviews with carefully selected representative households, has since 1997 asked a question designed to identify serious psychological distress in the past 30 days. In 2007, the survey included three questions on lifetime diagnoses: "Have you EVER been told by a doctor or other health professional that you had bipolar disorder? Schizophrenia? Mania or psychoses?"[1]

The National Health and Nutrition Examination Survey, participants chosen from a carefully selected representative households are asked questions on number of mentally unhealthy days, as well as questions designed to measure depression. A survey of women who have recently given birth, the Pregnancy Risk Assessment Monitoring System (PRAMS) asks questions about postpartum depression. Surveys on healthcare utilization gain information about mental health issues from data provided by hospitals, community health centers, office-based providers, and nursing homes.

The NCS provides data on the lifetime prevalence of mental disorders broken down by types of disorder—anxiety disorders, mood disorders, impulse-control disorders, and substance disorders—and for each, sex and age cohort of people suffering from each type. The total percentage of the populations that has had an anxiety disorder is 31.2 percent; 21.4 percent have had a mood disorder; 25.0 percent an impulse control disorder; and 35.3 percent a substance disorder. There is significant overlap among the specific disorders, with the total prevalence of any mental disorder amounting to 57.4 percent. Table 19-1 shows details of the lifetime prevalence of various mental disorders by sex and age group.

Table 19-1 Lifetime Prevalence of Mental Disorders by Sex and Cohort

Lifetime	Total %	SE	Female %	SE	Male %	SE	18–29 %	SE	30–44 %	SE	45–59 %	SE	60+ %	SE
			Sex				**Cohort**							
I. Anxiety Disorders														
Panic disorder	4.7	(0.2)	6.2	(0.3)	3.1	(0.3)	4.2	(0.5)	5.9	(0.6)	5.9	(0.4)	2.1	(0.4)
Agoraphobia without panic[6]	1.3	(0.1)	1.6	(0.2)	1.1	(0.2)	1.2	(0.3)	1.4	(0.2)	1.8	(0.3)	0.9	(0.2)
Specific phobia	12.5	(0.4)	15.8	(0.6)	8.9	(0.6)	13.0	(0.9)	13.9	(0.7)	14.4	(1.0)	7.7	(0.6)
Social phobia	12.1	(0.4)	13.0	(0.6)	11.1	(0.6)	13.3	(0.7)	14.5	(0.9)	12.6	(0.9)	6.8	(0.5)
Generalized anxiety disorder[6]	5.7	(0.3)	7.1	(0.3)	4.2	(0.4)	4.3	(0.4)	6.5	(0.5)	7.6	(0.7)	4.0	(0.4)
Post-traumatic stress disorder[2]	6.8	(0.4)	9.7	(0.7)	3.6	(0.3)	6.3	(0.6)	8.1	(0.9)	9.2	(0.8)	2.8	(0.5)
Obsessive-compulsive disorder[3]	2.3	(0.3)	3.1	(0.5)	1.6	(0.3)	3.1	(0.7)	3.0	(0.9)	2.4	(0.8)	0.6	(0.3)
Adult/Child separation anxiety disorder[2]	9.2	(0.4)	10.8	(0.6)	7.4	(0.5)	12.4	(0.9)	11.1	(0.7)	9.2	(0.8)	3.1	(0.5)
Any anxiety disorder[5]	31.2	(1.0)	36.4	(1.1)	25.4	(1.2)	32.9	(1.3)	37.0	(1.5)	34.2	(1.7)	17.8	(1.4)
II. Mood Disorders														
Major depressive disorder[6]	16.9	(0.5)	20.2	(0.5)	13.2	(0.8)	16.0	(0.8)	19.3	(0.9)	20.1	(1.2)	10.7	(0.7)
Dysthmia[6]	2.5	(0.2)	3.1	(0.3)	1.8	(0.2)	1.8	(0.3)	2.8	(0.4)	3.8	(0.6)	1.3	(0.2)
Bipolar I-II-sub disorders	4.4	(0.3)	4.5	(0.3)	4.3	(0.4)	7.0	(0.8)	5.3	(0.4)	3.7	(0.4)	1.3	(0.3)
Any mood disorder	21.4	(0.6)	24.9	(0.6)	17.5	(0.9)	22.6	(1.0)	24.5	(1.0)	24.2	(1.2)	12.2	(0.9)

(Continued)

Lifetime	Total		Sex				Cohort							
			Female		Male		18–29		30–44		45–59		60+	
	%	SE	%	SE	%	SE	%	SE	%	SE	%	SE	%	SE
III. Impulse-control Disorders														
Oppositional-defiant disorder[4,6]	8.5	(0.7)	7.7	(0.9)	9.3	(0.8)	9.9	(1.0)	7.3	(0.8)	–	–	–	–
Conduct disorder[4]	9.5	(0.8)	7.1	(0.9)	12.0	(1.0)	10.8	(1.1)	8.4	(0.7)	–	–	–	–
Attention-deficit/hyperactivity disorder[4]	8.1	(0.6)	6.4	(0.7)	9.8	(1.0)	7.8	(0.8)	8.3	(0.8)	–	–	–	–
Intermittent explosive disorder[6]	7.4	(0.4)	5.7	(0.4)	9.2	(0.6)	12.6	(1.1)	8.8	(0.7)	5.3	(0.5)	2.4	(0.5)
Any impulse-control disorder[4]	25.0	(1.1)	21.6	(1.4)	28.6	(1.5)	27.0	(1.6)	23.4	(1.6)	–	–	–	–
IV. Substance Disorders														
Alcohol abuse with/without dependence[2]	13.2	(0.6)	7.5	(0.5)	19.6	(0.9)	14.5	(1.0)	16.4	(1.1)	14.1	(1.0)	6.3	(0.7)
Drug abuse with/without dependence[2]	8.0	(0.4)	4.8	(0.4)	11.6	(0.7)	11.1	(0.9)	12.1	(1.0)	6.8	(0.7)	0.3	(0.1)
Nicotine dependence[2]	29.6	(0.8)	26.5	(1.3)	33.0	(1.0)	26.5	(1.8)	29.5	(1.5)	34.3	(1.6)	27.3	(1.7)
Any substance disorder[2]	35.3	(0.9)	29.6	(1.3)	41.8	(1.1)	33.2	(1.9)	37.1	(1.8)	39.8	(1.5)	29.6	(1.7)
V. Any Disorder														
Any[5]	57.4	(1.1)	56.5	(1.5)	58.4	(1.4)	58.7	(2.2)	63.7	(1.9)	60.0	(1.6)	44.0	(2.3)

[1] This table includes updated data as of July 19, 2007. Updates reflect the latest diagnostic, demographic and raw variable information.
[2] Assessed in the Part II sample (n = 5692).
[3] Assessed in a random one-third of the Part II sample (n = 2073).
[4] Assessed in the Part II sample among respondents in the age range 18–44 (n = 3197).
[5] Estimated in the Part II sample. No adjustment is made for the fact that one or more disorders in the category were not assessed for all Part II respondents.
[6] Disorder with hierarchy.

Source: Reproduced from Ronald C. Kessler, Harvard Medical School (2005). National Comorbidity Survey (NCS). http://www.hcp.med.harvard.edu/ncs/ftpdir/NCS-R_Lifetime_Prevalence_Estimates.pdf, accessed September 27, 2012.

When broken down by sex, females reported more anxiety disorders and mood disorders than males, while males have more impulse-control disorders and substance disorders. It is notable that for all the disorders, younger cohorts have a higher prevalence than those over 60 years. In fact, the prevalence of anxiety disorders and mood disorders is only half among those over 60 as it is among those 18 to 59. Only nicotine dependence is comparable among the older cohort to the younger groups; in fact it is higher among those over 60 than it is among those 18 to 29.[1]

Two CDC surveys (BRFSS and PRAMS) collect data at the state or substate level, and the prevalence of some disorders varies substantially across regions of the country. Southeastern states generally have the highest prevalence of depression, serious psychological distress, and mean number of mentally unhealthy days. This finding likely reflects the association between mental illness and certain chronic diseases, such as obesity, diabetes, and cardiovascular disease, which are also more prevalent in the Southeast.

Causes and Prevention

The precise causes of most mental disorders are not known, but much is known about the broad forces that shape them. The causes of mental disorders are viewed as a product of the interaction between biological, psychological, and sociocultural factors. Genetic factors are important in some mental disorders, including schizophrenia, bipolar disorder, autism, and attention deficit hyperactivity disorder (ADHD). However, in the case of schizophrenia, for example, studies of identical twins find that in only half the cases where one twin has the disorder, does the second twin also have it, even though both twins have the same genes. This implies that environmental factors exert a significant role, and therefore there is a possibility of intervening to prevent the development of the disorder. PTSD is clearly caused by exposure to an extremely stressful event, although not everyone develops PTSD after such exposure. Again appropriate treatment may prevent the disorder.[2]

Prevention of mental illness may depend on identification of risk factors that can be targeted, especially in children. Risk factors that are common to many disorders include individual factors, family factors, and community factors. An individual may be put at risk by neurophysiological deficits, difficult temperament, chronic physical illness, or below-average intelligence. Family factors that increase risk are severe marital discord, social disadvantage, overcrowding or large family size, paternal criminality, maternal mental disorder, and admission into foster care. Community factors such as living in an area with a high rate of disorganization and inadequate schools may also increase risk.[2]

Children

Both biological factors and adverse psychosocial experiences during childhood may influence the risk that a child will develop a mental disorder. A risk factor may have no, little, or a profound impact depending on individual differences among children and the age at which the child is exposed to it, as well as whether it occurs alone or in association with other risk factors.

Biological risk factors that may lead to mental illness in children include intrauterine exposure to alcohol or cigarettes, environmental exposure to lead, malnutrition of pregnancy, birth trauma, and specific chromosomal syndromes. The quality of the relationship between infants or children and their primary caregiver is believed to be of primary importance to mental health across the lifespan. Maternal depression increases the risk of depressive and anxiety disorders, conduct disorder, and alcohol dependence in the child. Child abuse and neglect is a widespread problem in the United States, and is associated with depression, conduct disorder, delinquency, and impaired social functioning with peers.[2]

Autism is a severe, chronic developmental disorder characterized by severely compromised ability to engage in, and by a lack of interest in, social interaction. Affected children may have a wide range of symptoms, skills, and levels of disability, and thus they are referred to as being on the autism spectrum. A 2009 CDC survey found that the rate of autism spectrum disorders was about 1 in 110 children. The prevalence in boys is about four to five times higher than in girls.[4]

The evidence for a genetic influence includes twin studies, which find that identical twins of autistic individuals will also have autism in 9 out of 10 cases. Researchers are starting to identify particular genes that may increase the risk of autism. Because autism results in significant lifelong disability, intensive special education programs in highly structured environments are recommended to help autistic children to acquire self-care, social, and job skills.

Mood disorders, including bipolar disorder, major depression and suicide are a matter of serious concern for anyone who cares about the mental health of children and adolescents. Mortality from suicide increases steadily through the teen years, and suicide is the third leading cause of death at that age. Suicide is rare for preteens and young adolescents, but much higher in 15- to 19- year olds and even higher in young adults ages 20 to 24. Among older teens, boys are nearly five times as likely to commit suicide as girls, while girls are twice as likely to attempt suicide.[2,5]

ADHD is the most commonly diagnosed behavior disorder of childhood, with a prevalence four times higher in boys than in girls. Twin studies have shown that when ADHD is present in one twin, it is significantly more likely also to be present in an identical twin than in a fraternal twin, supporting the view that genes are important in the disorder. ADHD is often treated with psychoactive stimulants. Pharmaceutical treatment is more effective when accompanied by behavioral therapy aimed at helping a child organize tasks, follow directions, and monitor his or her own behavior.[6]

Concerns have been raised that children, especially active boys, are being overdiagnosed with ADHD and thus receiving psychostimulants unnecessarily. This view is supported by findings of one study that, although many children who do meet the full criteria for ADHD are not being treated, the majority of children and adolescents who are receiving stimulants did not fully meet the criteria. This reflects a failure of proper, comprehensive evaluation and diagnosis. The long-term safety of psychostimulant treatment has not been established.[2]

Disruptive disorders, such as oppositional defiant disorder and conduct disorder, are frequently found in children who suffer from ADHD. Other mental illnesses generally diagnosed in childhood include anxiety disorders, including separation anxiety, social phobia, eating disorders, and obsessive-compulsive disorder, which has a strong familial component.[2]

Several interventions that focus on enhancing mental health and preventing behavior problems have been found to be effective in enhancing children's success in the classroom and minimizing their involvement in the juvenile justice system, indicators of mental health. Project Head Start is probably the country's best-known prevention program. Although originally designed to improve academic performance of economically disadvantaged preschool children, its advantages are mainly social and include better peer relations, less truancy, and less antisocial behavior. A number of other early childhood programs for high-risk children, many of which involve home visits by nurses, are effective in part because they include a parental education component.[2]

Mental Health in Adulthood

Mental health in adulthood is characterized by the successful performance of mental function, enabling individuals to cope with adversity and to flourish in their education, vocation, and personal relationships. Traits or personal characteristics that contribute to mental health include self-esteem, optimism, and resilience traits that are needed to deal with stressful life events. Confidence in one's own abilities to cope with adversity is a major contributor to mental health in adulthood.[2]

The most common psychological and social stressors in adult life include breakup of intimate romantic relationships, death of a family member or friend, economic hardships, racism and discrimination, poor physical health, and accidental and intentional assaults on physical safety. Such events are more likely to cause mental disorders in people who are vulnerable biologically, socially, and/or psychologically.

There are effective treatments for mental disorders, contrary to what many think. A variety of psychotherapy approaches have been found effective, from Freudian psychoanalysis to cognitive-behavioral therapy, which strives to alter faulty cognitions and replace them with thoughts that promote adaptive behavior. Drugs for the treatment of depression, anxiety, and schizophrenia have also been found effective in correcting biochemical alterations that accompany these mental disorders.

Anxiety disorders are the most prevalent mental disorders in adults. These include panic disorders, agoraphobia (anxiety about being in situations from which escape might be difficult), generalized anxiety disorder, specific phobia, social phobia, obsessive-compulsive disorder, acute stress disorder, and PTSD. One-year prevalence of anxiety disorders among adults is about 18 percent, and there is significant overlap with mood and substance abuse disorders. Females have a higher rate than males of most anxiety disorders. Some anxiety disorders, like panic disorder, appear to have a strong genetic basis. Others are more rooted in stressful life events. Anxiety disorders are treated with some form of counseling or psychotherapy or drug treatment.[2,7]

Many veterans of the Iraq and Afghanistan wars suffer from PTSD. They may experience flashbacks to the traumatic events, have nightmares, or feel stressed and angry during the day, making it hard for them to do daily tasks, such as sleeping, eating, or concentrating. In August 2012, President Obama signed an executive order to strengthen access to mental health care for veterans, including suicide prevention efforts. The president also ordered the Department of Defense, the Department of Veterans Affairs, and the Department of Health and Human Services to conduct research programs on how to better prevent, diagnose, and treat these disorders. Strategies for promoting evidence-based PTSD treatments are urgently needed.[8]

Two types of psychotherapies are currently being evaluated: prolonged exposure (PE) therapy and cognitive processing therapy (CPT). PE involves helping people confront their fear and feelings about the trauma they experienced in a safe way through mental imagery, writing, or other ways. In CPT, the patient is asked to recount his or her traumatic experience and a therapist helps the patient redirect inaccurate or destructive thoughts about the experience.[9]

Mood disorders, including major depression and bipolar disorder, are a major cause of disability. The prevalence of bipolar disorder does not differ by sex, but major depression is more prevalent in women than men. The most dreaded consequence of mood disorders is suicide. About 10 to 15 percent of patients formerly hospitalized with depression commit suicide. In the United States, men complete suicide four times as often as women; women attempt suicide four times as often as men. About half of those with a primary diagnosis of major depression also have an anxiety disorder. Substance use disorders are also common in individuals with mood disorders. The relative importance of biological and psychosocial factors varies across individuals and across different types of mood disorders. Genetic factors are strongly implicated in bipolar disorder.[2,5,10]

Several types of medications have been found effective in treatment of mood disorders, including four major classes of antidepressants and mood stabilizers such as lithium. Psychotherapy is often added to pharmaceutical treatment. Electroconvulsant shock therapy is sometimes used for severe mood disorders.[11]

Schizophrenia, which affects about 1 percent of the population, is characterized by profound disruption in cognition and emotion, affecting language, thought, perception, affect, and sense of self. Symptoms frequently include hearing internal voices (hallucinations) and holding fixed false personal beliefs (delusions). Onset generally occurs during young adulthood, although earlier and later onset do occur. Twin and other family studies support the role of genetics in schizophrenia. Immediate biological relatives of people with the condition have about

10 times greater risk than that of the general population. However, only about 40 to 65 percent of identical twins of someone diagnosed with schizophrenia have the disorder, indicating that environmental factors play a likely role.[2,12]

Treatment of schizophrenia generally includes some form of antipsychotic medication, of which a variety have been shown to be effective, combined with psychotherapy and family intervention programs.

Mental Health in Older Adults

A substantial proportion of the population 55 and older experience specific mental disorders that are not part of "normal" aging. These include depression, Alzheimer's disease, alcohol and drug misuse and abuse, anxiety, late-life schizophrenia, and other conditions. Of all age groups, older adults have the highest rates of suicide, frequently a consequence of depression.[2,5]

Risk factors for mental illness in the elderly include general medical conditions, admission to a nursing home, the high number of medications taken by many older individuals, and psychosocial stressors such as bereavement or isolation. Depression is particularly prevalent among older people, especially after loss of a spouse. Prevention through grief counseling or through participation in self-help groups is effective in improving social adjustment and reducing the use of alcohol and other drugs of abuse. Depression and suicide prevention strategies are also important for nursing home residents.

Anxiety symptoms not specific to any identified syndrome are prevalent in older adults, affecting up to about 20 percent of the elderly. Schizophrenia is commonly regarded as an illness of young adulthood, but it can both extend into and first appear in later life. Some younger patients who have received early intervention with antipsychotic medications demonstrate remarkable recovery after many years of chronic dysfunction. Symptoms of late-onset schizophrenia are similar to those in younger patients, and the risk factors are also similar.

Treatment of mental illness in older adults is similar to that for younger patients. However, physiological changes due to aging increases the risk of side effects of drug treatments. Interactions with medications used for other disorders of aging also complicate effective treatment for mental illness, both by increasing side effects and decreasing efficacy of one or both drugs.

Treatment

Most people with mental disorders do not seek treatment. In part this is because they do not know that there are effective treatments. In part it is fear of the stigma of acknowledging the problem. Above all, the major deterrent is the cost of care. In general, insurance coverage of mental health care is inferior to that of physical health.

In the past, hospitalization was the norm for serious mental illness. People were sent to asylums, where they frequently endured poor and occasionally abusive condition. Patients became excessively dependent and lost connection to the community. More recently, inpatient units are used for crisis care, focusing on reducing the risk of danger to self or others and rapid return of patients to the community. Housing is often a major problem for people with severe mental illness, who often tend to be poor. It is estimated that up to one in three individuals who experience homelessness has a mental illness.

Conclusion

Mental illnesses account for more disability in developed countries, including the United States, than any other group of illnesses. Nearly half of adult Americans will develop at least one mental illness during their lifetime. The most common mental illnesses in adults are anxiety and mood disorders. Schizophrenia, which occurs in about 1 percent of the population, is characterized by profound disruption in cognition and emotion and often includes hallucinations and delusions. Genetic factors are important in some mental disorders, including schizophrenia, autism, bipolar disorder, and ADHD. Most mental disorders are also influenced by environmental factors. PTSD is clearly caused by extremely stressful events. Most people with mental disorders do not seek treatment, although effective treatments do exist, including medications and psychotherapy.

References

1. U.S. Centers for Disease Control and Prevention, "Mental Illness Surveillance Among Adults in the United States," *Morbidity and Mortality Weekly Report* 60 (2011): 1–32.
2. U.S. Department of Health and Human Services, *Mental Health: A Report of the Surgeon General*, 1999. http://profiles.nlm.nih.gov/ps/access/NNBBHS.pdf, accessed September 8, 2012.
3. National Comorbidity Survey (NCS) and National Comorbidity Survey Replication (NCS-R). http://www.hcp.med.harvard.edu/ncs/index.php, accessed September 3, 2012.
4. National Institute of Mental Health, "A Parent's Guide to Autism Spectrum Disorder." http://www.nimh.nih.gov/health/publications/a-parents-guide-to-autism-spectrum-disorder/index.shtml, accessed September 14, 2012.
5. National Institute of Mental Health, "Suicide in the U.S.: Statistics and Prevention." http://www.nimh.nih.gov/heatlh/publications/suicide-in-the-us-statistics-and-prevention/index.shtml#intro, accessed September 14, 2012.
6. National Institute of Mental Health, "Attention Deficit Hyperactivity Disorder (ADHD)." http://www.nimh.nih.gov/health/publications/attention-deficit-hyperactivity-disorder/index.shtml, accessed September 14, 2012.
7. National Institute of Mental Health, "Anxiety Disorders," November 2, 2010. http://www.nimh.nih.gov/health/publications/anxiety-disorders/complete-index.shtml, accessed September 14, 2012.

8. The White House, "Executive Order—Improving Access to Mental Health Services for Veterans, Service Members, and Military Families." http://www.whitehouse.gov/Zthe-press-office/2012/08/31/executive-order-improving-access-mental-health-services-veterans-service, accessed November 11, 2012.

9. National Institute of Mental Health, "PTSD Treatment Efforts for Returning War Veterans to be Evaluated." http://www.nimh.nih.gov/science-news/2009/ptsd-treatment-efforts-for-returning-war-veterans-to-be-evaluated.shtml, accessed September 14, 2012.

10. National Institute of Mental Health, "Bipolar Disorder," May 16, 2012. http://www.nimh.nih.gov/health/publications/bipolar-disorder/index.shtml, accessed September 14, 2012.

11. National Institute of Mental Health, "Depression." http://www.nimh.nih.gov/health/publications/depression/index.shtml, accessed September 14, 2012.

12. National Institute of Mental Health, "Schizophrenia," 2009. http://www.nimh.nih.gov/health/publications/schizophrenia/complete-index.shtml, accessed September 14, 2012.

Environmental Issues in
Public Health

A Clean Environment: The Basis of Public Health

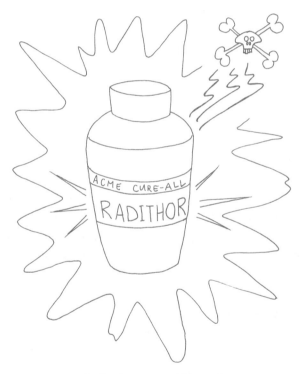

An Environmental Hazard

Humans are designed by eons of evolution to live on the earth: to breathe the earth's air, to drink the earth's water, to eat the plants and animals that grow on the earth's surface. People are adapted to the earth's environment. While there is considerable variation in that environment in different parts of the planet, and while humans have found ways to live in many different climates and habitats, people's health depends on the presence of these basic ingredients of life—air, water, and food. There are also natural phenomena in the environment that can harm human health: extremes of heat and cold, ultraviolet rays of the sun, toxic minerals and plants, and other living organisms, from pathogenic bacteria to predatory mammals.

Human beings are social creatures, dependent upon other people to help them navigate the earth's environment. All humans in all parts of the world live in groups, from small bands of hunters and gatherers to the residents of teeming cities. When groups of people settle down to live together in one place, they change their shared environment: the larger the group, the greater the effect on the environment. Some of these changes may be made deliberately, to improve life for everyone; some are the inadvertent results of crowding, with harmful effects on people's well-being.

Archaeological evidence shows that the earliest cities were designed with consideration for the health of their inhabitants. As early as 2000 B.C., cities in India, Egypt, Greece, and South America had devised ways of providing clean water and draining wastes. These ancient systems of water supply, drains, and sewers are the first evidence of public health measures: organized community efforts to provide healthy conditions for the population.

Ensuring a clean water supply and the safe disposal of wastes—functions that fall into the category of environmental health—are still among the most important responsibilities of government. Other environmental health functions necessary in industrial countries are measures to ensure clean air and safe food. All these concerns arise because of the human tendency to live in groups. Most people do not have the means or the desire to grow their own food, draw water from their own well, and dispose of wastes in their own yard. Because people live together in cities and suburbs, they rely on others to provide their food and water and to dispose of their wastes. Because there are so many people on earth today, and because of the prodigality of the modern lifestyle, the wastes people produce have unprecedented potential to pollute the air and litter the earth.

Role of Government in Environmental Health

Environmental health is clearly the responsibility of government. Many environmental exposures, such as air pollution, are beyond the control of the individual. Others can be avoided only at significant trouble and expense, for example, if people grow their own vegetables, or buy them from farmers whose agricultural methods they have inspected themselves. Governments ensure a healthy environment by various means, sometimes providing services directly, in other cases by setting standards and regulating how the services should be provided.

Traditionally in the United States, local governments have provided water for their citizens. They are required by law to meet standards set by state and federal governments. Local governments also traditionally provide sewage systems to dispose of wastes from individual households and to handle runoff from the land.

In the 1960s, Americans became increasingly aware that the environment was deteriorating. Lakes and streams were choked with sewage and chemical wastes that killed fish and other wildlife. Cities were overhung with smog. Citizens were outraged by news stories of neighborhoods poisoned by long-dormant toxic waste dumps. State and federal governments were pressured to assume more responsibility for the environment. In the late 1960s and early 1970s, many new laws set standards for air, water, and waste disposal. The first Earth Day, celebrated in the United States on April 22, 1970, marked the beginning of the modern environmental movement with coast-to-coast rallies and teach-ins.

Perhaps the most difficult environmental health issue people face today is the threat that human activities worldwide are changing the climate of the earth. The major concerns are depletion of the earth's ozone layer and the accumulation of "greenhouse gases" in the atmosphere. These problems, both of which may significantly affect human health, transcend national boundaries. While the United Nations has sponsored international meetings on these issues and governments have signed treaties designed to bring the problems under control, there is no way of enforcing these agreements.

Identification of Hazards

A major role of the federal government in environmental health is to identify hazards in the environment and to set safety standards that must be met by industry and by state and local governments to protect people from these hazards. Both the identification of a substance as hazardous and the setting of standards are often difficult and controversial. The risks posed by most synthetic chemicals that are discharged into the environment by industrial processes or that are disposed of by consumers are unknown. Testing for potential harmful effects is expensive and time-consuming, and the choice of chemicals to test may be politically controversial. Even in cases where the health risk is obvious—such as the discharge of raw sewage into waterways or the air pollution caused by America's dependence on the private automobile—local governments, industry, and even the average citizen may resist requirements to meet standards because of the expense and inconvenience of cleaning up the environment.

Radiation is an environmental health hazard that people tend to worry about only when it is artificially produced. However, all people are exposed to cosmic radiation in varying amounts depending on where they live, and natural radioactive materials are found in soils and rocks in many parts of the world. Radon gas, produced by the natural radioactive decay of uranium, is present in many homes, a fact that was recognized only in the mid-1980s. Prolonged exposure to radon is potentially a cause of lung cancer, although the risks from radon in the home are not well understood. Ultraviolet radiation from the sun is a significant cause of skin cancer and melanoma. There is no way these exposures can be regulated by government, except for some testing requirements concerning radon.

The discovery in the mid-1890s of x-rays, which could pass through flesh and reveal bones, aroused great public excitement and led to extensive human exposures before the danger was recognized. During the early decades of the 20th century, x-ray treatments were popular as cure-alls for a variety of ailments, and radioactive ingredients were added to patent medicines. The first alarm was raised in the mid-1920s, with the deaths from kidney and bone disease of a number of workers who painted watch dials with radium so they would glow in the dark. They had been touching the paintbrushes to their lips to sharpen the points, thereby ingesting toxic quantities of the chemical. Then in 1932, a rich, socially prominent businessman died agonizingly from the same mysterious ailment, which was diagnosed on autopsy as radium poisoning. He had been dosing himself over a 5-year period with hundreds of bottles of Radithor, a radium-containing patent medicine. The publicity surrounding the Radithor scandal led to strengthened Food and Drug Administration (FDA) powers to regulate patent medicines as well as specific limitations on radioactive pharmaceuticals.[1]

Evidence that chronic exposure to low levels of x-radiation caused cancer came from epidemiologic studies that began in the 1930s. One study compared death rates of radiologists with those of other medical specialists and found that the average age at death for radiologists was 5 years younger than that of other specialists.[2] Radiation's damaging health effects were confirmed by long-term follow-up studies of survivors of the atomic bombings of Hiroshima and Nagasaki, Japan, which ended the Second World War. The incidence of leukemia and other cancers was significantly increased among these people. Today, medical and dental x-rays constitute the largest source of nonbackground radiation exposure, although equipment has been continuously improved to reduce the hazard. Since about one-third of the medical and dental x-rays that Americans receive are estimated to be unnecessary, patients are advised to question whether each exposure is essential.

That some metals have harmful health effects has been common knowledge for decades or longer. This is the case with mercury, which was recognized in the 19th century to cause neurological damage in workers who made felt hats—the origin of the expression "mad as a hatter" and the inspiration for the character the Mad Hatter in Lewis Carroll's *Alice in Wonderland*. The devastating effects of the mercury discharged by a plastics factory into Japan's Minamata Bay in the 1950s caused some 700 deaths and varying degrees of paralysis and brain damage in 9000 other people. The mercury accumulated in fish, which were the staple of the community's diet. Another well-known episode of mercury poisoning occurred in Iraq in 1972, when the substance was used as a fungicide on seed grain. The contaminated wheat was turned into bread, which poisoned more than 6500 people, 459 of whom died.[3]

In the United States, mercury enters the environment mainly by emissions from coal-burning power plants. The heavy metal falls to earth and becomes a hazard to humans mainly by getting into fish. Because the developing brain is most sensitive to the toxic effects of mercury, pregnant women and women who may become pregnant, as well as nursing mothers and young children are advised to avoid eating fish species that have the highest average amounts of mercury in their flesh: tilefish, swordfish, king mackerel, and shark. Up to 12 ounces per week of other species of fish are considered safe. Mercury is regulated under both the Clean Air Act and the Safe Drinking Water Act.

People may be exposed to mercury when the liquid metal is spilled, releasing toxic vapors, for example after a glass thermometer breaks. Mercury may also be found in equipment used in school science labs, and exposure may occur if the equipment breaks or is mishandled. The Environmental Protection Agency (EPA) recommends that mercury-containing products be removed from homes and schools. The sale of mercury-containing fever thermometers is banned in many states; safer alternatives are available. Cleanup of mercury spills requires great caution in order to prevent droplets of the metal from accumulating in small spaces and releasing vapors into the air. The EPA cautions against trying to clean up mercury with a vacuum cleaner or broom, or pouring it down a drain, because these methods are likely to put more of the toxic vapors into the air.[4]

Lead is another metal known to harm the brain and nervous system, especially those of children. It also damages red blood cells and kidneys. Lead is believed to be the single most important environmental threat to the health of American children, who may be exposed to it from a variety of sources. Over the past 3 decades, evidence has accumulated that even low levels of lead can slow a child's development and can cause learning and behavior problems. The federal government recommends that all young children poor enough to be eligible for Medicaid be screened for lead in the blood, and some states have extended the mandate to children of all income levels. Permissible levels of lead have been steadily lowered from 60 micrograms per deciliter of blood in 1970 to 10 micrograms at present.[5]

Lead has been used—and has been causing lead poisoning—since the time of the Roman Empire, when it was a component of wine casks, cooking pots, and water pipes. In fact, the Latin word for lead is "plumbum," the origin of the English word "plumbing." Even today, a major source of lead exposure for millions of Americans is water contaminated with lead from lead pipes or from lead solder used with copper pipes. The use of lead in pipes was phased out in the 1980s, and newer homes use plastic plumbing.

Until the 1980s, lead was a significant air pollutant, emitted from the tailpipes of motor vehicles that burned leaded gasoline. As a result of the phasing out of leaded gas, lead levels in the air have dropped to negligible amounts. Lead was also a component of paint, both interior and exterior, until its use was banned in 1977. Children—especially those who live in old, substandard housing—are still significantly exposed when they chew on chips of old peeling paint or when they put dirty hands in their mouths if the dirt is contaminated with dust from deteriorating paint. Attempts to remove old lead-containing paint can sometimes be even more hazardous if it turns to airborne dust as it is sanded or sandblasted off a surface and is inhaled.

New alarms about lead surfaced in 2007, when the Consumer Product Safety Commission (CPSC) recalled millions of wooden toys that had been painted with lead paint, including the popular Thomas the Tank Engine. It turned out that the toys had been manufactured in China, which produces 70 percent to 80 percent of the toys sold in the United States. Consumer advocates note that toy safety is largely the responsibility of the companies that import them. The Commission suffered cuts during the Bush administration and did not have the staff to monitor the safety of so many imports, although the budget has increased significantly during the Obama administration.[6,7] Lead in toys is of special concern because young children often put them in their mouths. A list of recalled toys posted on the CPSC website shows that lead paint on toys continues to be a major risk in the United States.[8]

Arsenic, "the king of poisons," is well known as a common means of homicide through the centuries. It was not recognized as an important environmental toxin until the United Nations Children's Fund inadvertently turned it into one in the 1970s in India and Bangladesh.[9] Concerned about epidemics of cholera, dysentery, and other waterborne diseases, the organization led a campaign to drill millions of wells so that the population would no longer need to drink contaminated surface water. However, it soon became apparent that people began to develop symptoms such as abdominal pain, vomiting, diarrhea, pain and swelling in the hands and feet, and skin eruptions. In some cases, symptoms progressed to progressive nervous system deterioration and death. Children of poor nutritional status proved to be especially susceptible to these problems. The well water, while free of disease-causing bacteria, was found to contain very high concentrations of arsenic. With 80 percent of Bangladeshis affected, the World Health Organization has labeled this "the worst mass poisoning in history."[9(p.A386)] Developing effective strategies for mitigating the effects of arsenic has been called one of the most important environmental health challenges of our time.

Studies have shown that, at somewhat lower concentrations, long-term exposure to arsenic in drinking water increases risk of diabetes and cancer. In the United States, regulations call for public water systems to contain no more than 10 micrograms per liter of arsenic, well below levels known to cause harm. However, people in some parts of the country who have private wells may be drinking water that contains 50 to 90 micrograms per liter of arsenic. The risks from chronic exposure to these amounts are not known.[9]

Asbestos is a fibrous mineral valuable for a variety of uses because of its strength and fire resistance. The hazards of asbestos were first recognized in an occupational setting: Inhalation of high concentrations of asbestos dust caused stiffening and scarring of the lungs of miners and other asbestos workers, a condition known as asbestosis, which can be disabling and eventually fatal. Regulations limiting exposure were instituted, but as workers began to live longer, many of them developed cancer. They were especially likely to get lung cancer or mesothelioma, a rare cancer of the lining of the chest or abdominal cavity that seems to be caused exclusively by inhalation of asbestos. As a result of a succession of lawsuits brought by injured workers and their families in the 1960s and 1970s, the Manville Corporation—the largest asbestos company in the United States—filed for bankruptcy in 1982.[10] Once the dangers of asbestos were recognized, many uses of the material were banned, and standards for occupational exposure were tightened. However, asbestos can still be found in brake linings and a number of construction materials.[3]

The general public is most likely to be exposed to asbestos fibers released into the air in the dust from crumbling walls and ceilings of old, deteriorating buildings. This is a special concern in schools, since all schools built or renovated between 1940 and 1973 were required to install asbestos insulation as a fire safety measure. Children's exposure is of special concern because they would live for many years with the fibers lodged in their lungs, and the likelihood of developing cancer would increase with time. In 1986, the Asbestos Hazard Emergency Response Act was passed. It required all primary and secondary schools to be inspected and, if loose asbestos was found, to carry out plans for removing, enclosing or encapsulating material. Unfortunately, the removal was often done improperly, causing more asbestos to be released into the air than if the material had been left intact. Other schools, unable to afford the expense of asbestos removal, ignored the rulings.[3] There is no evidence thus far that exposure to asbestos has been a significant cancer risk to the general population.

However, the population of Libby, Montana, was clearly harmed by decades of exposure to asbestos. The vermiculite ore that had been mined in the Libby area since the 1920s was heavily contaminated with asbestos. A study by the National Institute of Occupational Safety and Health found that among 1,675 Libby workers, 15 died of mesothelioma, a very rare disease, and the death rate from asbestosis was 165 times higher than expected. Death rates from asbestosis among residents of the area were approximately 40 times higher than the rest of Montana and 60 times higher than the rest of the United States.[11] Follow-up studies found abnormalities in the chest x-rays of household contacts of asbestos workers who presumably were exposed to asbestos dust brought home on the clothes of the workers. Abnormalities were also found in the x-rays of children who had played in piles of vermiculite at the processing facilities.[12]

The fallout from the Libby crisis continues. A disease registry has been established to track individuals who were exposed, in order to learn more about asbestos-related illnesses, and to share information on new therapies and diagnostic tools. A community health center has been established with federal funds to provide medical services. Libby has been declared a Superfund site and is being cleaned up. In fact, in June 2009 the EPA declared a public health emergency under the Superfund law, the first time such an emergency has been declared.[13] W. R. Grace, the company that operated the mine, has been overwhelmed with lawsuits by injured residents, and the company filed for bankruptcy protection in 2001.[14] It has been ordered to pay $250 million to the EPA for environmental cleanup. The EPA has warned that asbestos-containing vermiculite from Libby was used as insulation in millions of homes and businesses across the country and that asbestos fibers could pose a health threat if the insulation is disturbed.

Asbestos exposure is also a concern as a result of the 9/11 attacks on the World Trade Center. Beginning a few days after the collapse of the towers, the EPA and the New York City and New York State Health Departments monitored pollutants in the air, including asbestos. Concentrations near Ground Zero were quite high in the first few days and weeks after 9/11, but they decreased to background levels by January or February 2002.[15] These exposures were most likely to affect the thousands of rescue and recovery workers, who are now being monitored for long-term health effects by the New York City Fire Department and the Centers for Disease Control and Prevention. One study of over 3700 firefighters who worked at the site found that almost 40 percent of them continued to have respiratory symptoms 3 years later.[16]

Pesticides and Industrial Chemicals

Rachel Carson's best-selling book *Silent Spring*, published in 1962, was a wake-up call to the American public, a warning that chemicals in the environment cause harm. The publication of her book, more than any other single event, launched the environmental movement that led to sweeping legislation in the 1970s. *Silent Spring* called attention to the harmful effects of the virtually ubiquitous pesticide DDT. The chemical could be found in lakes and streams, plants and insects. When eaten or drunk by fish and birds, it accumulated in their flesh, to be eaten in turn by predators, which concentrated these chemicals further in their own bodies. A world-wide survey measuring chemicals in the body fat of people on six continents found DDT in all of them.[17] The use of DDT was banned in the United States in 1972. A number of other insecticides chemically related to DDT were also banned in the 1970s. These chemicals—including chlordane, aldrin, mirex, and Kepone—shared common features of solubility in fatty tissue and persistence in the environment; they break down very slowly, so they continue to cause harm long after their use is halted.

Studies looking for environmental pesticides discovered that a related group of chemicals, polychlorinated biphenyls (PCBs), also turned up often. Unlike pesticides, these chemicals were used mainly in sealed systems—capacitors, transformers, and heat exchangers—but they were still entering the environment in large quantities and getting into the food chain. PCBs frequently entered the environment through discharge of industrial wastes, a route similar to the mercury at Minamata. The contamination of New York's Hudson River with PCBs, discovered by environmentalists in 1975, was traced to two General Electric Company capacitor plants that had been discharging large volumes of PCBs into the river for more than 25 years.[18] Although the discharge was halted, the chemicals, unless cleaned up, would persist in the soil of the riverbed indefinitely. Fish caught in the Hudson River still contain PCBs at concentrations considered unsafe for women of childbearing age and children under 15 to eat at all, and for others to eat more than once a week.[19] The EPA developed a plan to clean the river by dredging the contaminated soil, a plan that generated controversy both because it will stir up the chemicals and cause more contamination of the river water in the short term, and because of vigorous objections by the communities proposed as disposal sites for the contaminated soil. After years of dispute, the dredging began in May 2009; the contaminated soil is to be transported by train to a hazardous waste landfill in Texas.[20] The dredging is expected to continue for 5 to 7 years over a 40-mile stretch of the river north of Albany.[21]

Environmental scientists believe that PCBs are the most widespread chemical contaminant worldwide. Although production was halted in the United States in 1977, they and their chemical relatives, called persistent organic pollutants (POPs), are carried to remote regions of the globe, including the Arctic, by air, water, and migratory species. The effects on human health of exposure to these chemicals at the levels commonly found in the environment are still uncertain. However, people exposed to large doses of PCBs by a number of industrial accidents were made ill by the chemicals. In western Japan in 1968, a leak at a cooking oil factory contaminated a batch of the rice oil with heat exchanger fluids containing PCBs and related chemicals. Eighteen hundred people were sickened in what became known as the "Yusho" incident ("Yusho" means oil disease in Japanese).[22] Eleven years later, a similar accident occurred in Taiwan, affecting 2000 people with "Yu-cheng," which means oil disease in Chinese.[23] Two well-known incidents in the United States during the 1970s—a warehouse fire in Puerto Rico that caused PCB contamination of tuna meal used for animal and fish feeds, and a labeling mixup in Michigan that contaminated cattle feed with polybrominated biphenyls, a chemical similar to PCBs—resulted in human exposure to this type of chemicals through the food supply.[24]

Victims of the Yusho, Yu-cheng, and other accidents have been the subjects of epidemiologic studies tracking the victims' health over the years since their exposure. The most conspicuous and consistent symptom is chloracne, severe skin rashes and discoloration that show up soon after exposure and may persist for years. Other effects include endocrine and immune system defects, fatigue, headaches, and aching joints. Many of these symptoms still persist more than 30 years after the original exposure.[25] An increased risk of some forms of cancer is now becoming apparent; the EPA has declared PCBs to be a probable human carcinogen.[26] Infants born to Yusho and Yu-cheng mothers were small at birth and had dark discoloration of the skin—leading to the nickname "Coca Cola babies"—which faded after a few months.[27] These infants suffered developmental delays and persistent cognitive deficits that were still apparent decades later.[28]

Some of the POPs, including dioxins and furans, are not manufactured intentionally but are byproducts of some industrial processes. They were contaminants of PCBs and may have been responsible for some of the toxic effects observed in the Yusho and Yu-cheng incidents. Common pollutants of air and water, they are also produced by the burning of forests or household trash. They are highly toxic, and even relatively small exposures are thought to cause adverse effects on people's immune, endocrine, and neurological systems. POPs are very stable, remaining in the fatty tissues of fish, animals, and humans indefinitely. Although levels of these chemicals are high in the blood and fatty tissues of people who eat fish from contaminated waters, in most Americans the levels appear to be declining.[29] In 2001, the United States joined 90 other nations in signing the Stockholm Convention on Persistent Organic Pollutants, agreeing to reduce and/or eliminate the production, use, and release of 12 of the POPs of greatest concern. However, the convention has not yet been ratified in the United States Senate.[30,31]

Other chemicals that have stimulated concern in the last few years are bisphenol A (BPA) and phthalates. Both are components of plastics commonly used in food and drink containers, capable of leaching into the containers' contents and being consumed. Traces of these chemicals are found in the blood of almost everyone in the United States.[32] BPA is found in hard plastics used to make everything from compact discs to baby bottles and linings of soft drink and food cans.[33] Phthalates are used to produce soft and flexible materials such as vinyl flooring, shower curtains and some water bottles; they are also used in personal-care products such as soaps, shampoos, hair sprays, and nail polishes.[34] Although government agencies have affirmed the safety of both chemicals at the low levels commonly found in humans, there is evidence that they may be especially harmful to infants and developing fetuses.

BPA and phthalates, as well as some POPs, have been shown to be endocrine disruptors in humans and wildlife, meaning that they interfere with normal hormone action in the body. BPA can mimic estrogen, causing early puberty in females and abnormalities in male and female sex organs. Phthalates interfere with testosterone synthesis in males, causing low sperm counts and abnormalities in the development of male sex organs. Some endocrine disruptors may interfere with the activities of the pancreas and thyroid glands, increasing the risk of obesity and diabetes.[32] A study using 1999–2002 data from the National Health and Nutrition Examination Survey found that concentrations of phthalates in the urine of adult American men were associated with increased waist circumference and insulin resistance. Although this does not prove cause and effect, the finding adds to evidence that exposure to phthalates may contribute to the growing prevalence of obesity and diabetes.[35]

The Endocrine Society, the world's oldest and largest organization devoted to research on hormones and the clinical practice of endocrinology, has issued a Scientific Statement on Endocrine-Disrupting Chemicals that details known evidence about the health effects of these substances and strongly recommends that more research should be done to understand their role in the chronic diseases that are so common in the world today.[32] In contrast, the FDA's website states that it has "performed extensive research on BPA, has reviewed hundreds of other studies, and is continuing to address questions and potential concerns raised by certain studies." The FDA's assessment is that the "scientific evidence at this time does not suggest that the very low levels of human exposure to BPA through the diet are unsafe."[36] However, a July 17, 2012, *New York Times* article reported that the agency had banned BPA in baby bottles and drinking cups. FDA officials were quoted as saying that manufacturers had stopped using the chemical some time ago because of consumer concerns.[37]

Occupational Exposures—Workers as Guinea Pigs

Workers are regularly exposed to larger amounts of toxic substances on the job than most of the population is ever likely to encounter. Consequently, workers tend to be the first and foremost to suffer from any harmful health effects caused by their exposures. Many chemicals that all people encounter in everyday life may have unrecognized effects at low doses, causing unexplained cancer, neurological disorders, and reproductive disorders in susceptible individuals. Workers, exposed to larger quantities, may inadvertently serve as the guinea pigs that call attention to the dangers.

That certain occupations carry an increased risk of certain kinds of cancer has long been known, and the information has been helpful in understanding some of the causes of cancer. The first environmentally caused cancer to be recognized was from an occupational exposure: scrotal cancer was common in 19th century English chimney sweeps. The soot to which they were exposed contained the same carcinogens found in tobacco smoke—chemicals that are now known to cause lung cancer. Few other cancers can be clearly linked to specific causative agents. Because most exposures are relatively low, and because the time lag between exposure and the development of cancer is long, cause and effect are difficult to establish. Workers are effective though unintentional guinea pigs because exposure on the job is likely to be much higher than that in the general environment. An obvious increase in the rate of a specific cancer in a group of workers who have all been exposed to the same substance clearly throws suspicion on that substance as the cause.

Chemicals identified as carcinogens through occupational exposures include benzidine, which caused bladder cancer in dye factory workers; arsenic, which caused lung and lymphatic cancer in copper smelters; and vinyl chloride, used to make some plastics, which causes angiosarcoma, a rare cancer of the liver.[3] Evidence that radiation exposure causes cancer came from the higher incidence of cancer among radiologists, as discussed earlier. Mesothelioma occurs almost exclusively in asbestos workers, who were also found to have high rates of lung cancer.

Neurotoxins, like carcinogens, may be hard to recognize because they act over a long period of time. In fact, nerve poisons may be even more insidious than carcinogens, because the damage they do—deterioration of vision, muscle weakness, failure of memory—may mimic common aspects of aging. Neurological disorders that typically strike workers with specific exposures call attention to those chemicals as neurotoxins. Starting with Mad Hatter's disease from mercury, nerve damage was found in shoemakers exposed to hexane-containing solvents, dry cleaners exposed to trichloroethylene, pesticide applicators, and many other workers exposed to neurotoxins.[38]

New Source of Pollution—Factory Farms

Over the past few decades, there has been a revolution in farming that threatens to overwhelm the system for regulating environmental pollution. Thousands of hogs, cattle, and poultry are crowded into confined spaces where they can be fed and tended to by automated systems. The environmental problems caused by this approach to farming are the huge volumes of waste produced by these animals, which must be disposed of on a relatively limited amount of land. According to the Sierra Club, factory farms produce an estimated 500 million tons of manure every year, three times the total waste produced by the U.S. human population.[39] The farms deal with waste by creating "lagoons" in which the liquids are allowed to evaporate or from which they are sprayed on fields. Lagoons at many of these operations have broken, failed, or overflowed. They emit gases—including ammonia, hydrogen sulfide, and methane—that can be toxic to humans. People living near the farms suffer from symptoms caused by the lagoon gases: headaches, runny noses, sore throats, coughing, respiratory problems, nausea, diarrhea, dizziness, burning eyes, depression, and fatigue. Seepage from the lagoons pollutes groundwater that feeds wells used for drinking water. After heavy rains, lagoons may overflow or burst, spilling thousands of gallons of manure into rivers, lakes, streams, and estuaries; such spills have caused massive fish kills in at least 10 states.[39]

Most of these farms are owned by a very few major corporations, which have great economic and political power. Some state legislatures have passed laws protecting the industry from regulation. State universities receive funding from the industry and may discourage research that makes the companies look bad.[40] Under the Bush administration, the EPA and the Department of Agriculture halted enforcement investigations of the farms and suppressed research results unfavorable to the industry.[41] The farms should be regulated under the Clean Air Act, but the law has never been enforced. The Clean Water Act requires large livestock operations to obtain permits, but this law has also been widely ignored.

Congress has repeatedly attempted to protect the corporations against enforcement of existing laws on clean air, clean water, and toxic chemicals. For example, the 2009 bill in the House of Representatives that appropriated funds for the EPA included provisions to block the Agency from requiring factory farms to report greenhouse gas emissions.[42] Meanwhile, a number of environmental advocacy organizations, including the Sierra Club, the Environmental Integrity Project, and the Natural Resources Defense Council, sued the EPA in an attempt to force concentrated animal feeding operations to obey environmental laws. In 2010, the EPA agreed to strengthen the rules.[43,44]

Setting Standards—How Safe Is Safe?

Tens of thousands of synthetic chemicals have been manufactured since World War II and, in the United States alone, three to four billion pounds of them are released into the environment each year. Most have not been tested for the capacity to cause cancer, birth defects, neurological damage, or other harmful effects on health. Because of the sheer number of chemicals, it is unrealistic to require testing them all.

The environmental legislation of the 1960s and 1970s tried to establish guidelines for identifying environmental hazards and required standards to be set that protected human health and the environment. Standard setting was required for air quality, water quality, radiation safety, food and drug safety, and the disposal of hazardous wastes. The Occupational Safety and Health Act of 1970 empowered the federal government to set standards for workers' exposure to toxic substances, and the Toxic Substances Control Act of 1976 allowed the government to require testing of potentially hazardous substances before they go on the market and to ban them in certain instances. The Federal Insecticide, Fungicide, and Rodenticide Act, originally passed in 1947 and amended several times since, requires government approval of these substances before they can be used. Congress required a variety of federal agencies to set standards for exposure to toxic substances via various routes: the EPA, the FDA, the Department of Agriculture, the Department of Transportation, the Nuclear Regulatory Commission, the Consumer Product Safety Commission, and the Occupational Safety and Health Administration (OSHA) are among those responsible for various aspects of environmental health.[3]

Standard setting progressed very slowly, however, after these laws were passed. For example, the Clean Air Act of 1970 required the EPA to develop a list of industrial pollutants that can cause serious health damage and set emission standards for them; as of 1993, only eight had been regulated.[3] The Clean Air Act amendments of 1990 introduced measures designed to speed up the process.

There are a number of reasons why regulation tends to progress slowly. One factor is the sheer volume of potentially toxic chemicals being manufactured in the United States. Today there are more than 80,000 chemicals registered for use, with about 2000 new ones introduced each year.[45] Another problem is that toxicity testing on any single chemical can be expensive and time-consuming. The EPA has information suggesting that 10 to 15 percent of the newly introduced chemicals each year need more extensive toxicological evaluation. The National Toxicology Program (NTP), an interagency program within the Department of Health and Human Services, can test only a few dozen agents each year, based on the extent of human exposure and/or suspicion of toxicity. One of the NTP's major goals for the 21st century is to develop and validate improved testing methods that will reduce the need for animal testing.

Another reason for the delays in standard setting is that each chemical must be regulated separately, each with the potential for controversy, legal challenge, and extensive litigation over each proposed regulation. Each standard is likely to have significant economic impact on some industry, whose members will naturally fight against the potential threat to their businesses and jobs. Emotions on the part of the public often run high, since citizens believe that their health and the health of their children is endangered, and their demands for safety may be perceived as unreasonable.

Risk–Benefit Analysis

The question "How safe is safe?" has been debated in connection with one potential health threat after another. Increasingly, policy analysts have come to agree that absolute safety is an impossible goal and that attempting to avoid risk of one sort may increase risks of other kinds. Furthermore, as one analyst asks and answers in the affirmative, "Does overregulation cause underregulation?"[46] He argues that too much effort is expended setting very strict standards for too few substances. By battling to achieve zero exposure to one carcinogen, for example, public health agencies may be neglecting to investigate other chemicals that are potentially more hazardous. Public health may be better served by aiming for looser, more easily achieved standards. This approach would generate less controversy and opposition, allowing for a stepped-up pace of standard setting.

The argument is also made that prevention of risk must be balanced against other societal goals, including economic well-being. Until recently, the public health approach has been to ignore economic factors in seeking risk reduction. However, an increasing understanding of the fact that economic factors are significant to people's health and well-being has led to greater willingness on the part of public health advocates to consider costs as well as benefits in evaluating risks.

The Republican Congress elected in 1994 tried to roll back all kinds of regulations under the argument that they were irrational and expensive, examples of government interference that had negative economic impacts on business. The fact that most of these initiatives failed demonstrated that most Americans want the government to protect their health and environment. But the initiatives made people ask how regulations could become more rational, less cumbersome, and more balanced. During the Clinton administration, the political debate focused on how to achieve effective environmental protection while minimizing red tape and government intrusiveness. The Bush administration was even more inclined to favor economic and business interests in policy making on environmental and public health issues. There is hope that President Obama will again place a priority on the health of the population and the environment.

Conclusion

Providing a clean environment, a necessity for human health, is one of the most important functions of government. When people began to live together in cities and towns, they were dependent on the government—traditionally the local government—to provide clean drinking water and safe disposal of wastes. As the American population grew, municipalities and industry discharged their wastes into the air, water, and land, and it became apparent that the environment was deteriorating. Pollution tends to spread beyond local areas, requiring state and federal intervention to be effective. In the late 1960s and early 1970s, a number of significant federal laws were passed that set standards for air, water, and waste disposal aimed at protecting human health and cleaning up the environment.

Identification of hazards is an important first step in creating a safe environment. While environmental health has traditionally focused on microbial pathogens, many other phenomena can also threaten human health. Radiation, both natural and manmade, can be highly dangerous to living organisms, something that was not recognized when x-rays were first discovered. Many metals and minerals, including lead, mercury, and asbestos, are toxic to humans. Pesticides and some industrial chemicals have been widely disseminated in the environment and have been absorbed into the fatty tissues of animals and humans, where they persist indefinitely, sometimes with harmful effects. Recently, concern has been raised about endocrine disruptors, including BPA and phthalates, common contaminants of plastics, which are suspected to cause problems with development in fetuses and infants and to increase the risk of common chronic diseases.

Sometimes hazards of environmental exposures are recognized first in workers who develop occupational illnesses after being exposed on the job. The effects of a number of cancer-causing and neurotoxic substances have been recognized because workers have served as "guinea pigs," the first humans to test the safety of new chemicals.

Federal legislation in the 1960s and 1970s established a number of agencies charged with identifying environmental hazards and setting standards to protect human health. These include OSHA and the EPA. Standard setting was required for air quality, water quality, radiation safety, food and drug safety, the control of toxic substances, and the disposal of hazardous wastes.

Many of these mandates have been politically controversial, in that they have economic impact on various industries. Recent trends have brought greater willingness by public health advocates to weigh costs against benefits in evaluating risks.

Recently, environmentalists have recognized a new hazard—animal wastes from factory farms. These wastes are collected in "lagoons" and may be sprayed on fields, causing air and water pollution. Nearby residents and communities are often powerless to object to the unpleasant odors and, sometimes, toxic fumes. Because of the economic power of agricultural companies, federal and state governments have done little to regulate them.

References

1. R. M. Macklis, "The Great Radium Scandal," *Scientific American* (August 1993): 94–99.
2. R. Seltser and P. E. Sartwell, "The Influence of Occupational Exposure to Radiation on the Mortality of American Radiologists and Other Medical Specialists," *American Journal of Epidemiology* 81 (1965): 2–22.
3. A. Nadakavukaren, *Our Global Environment: A Health Perspective*, 6th ed. (Prospect Heights, IL: Waveland Press, 2005).
4. U.S. Environmental Protection Agency, "Mercury: Spills, Disposal and Site Cleanup." http://www.epa.gov/mercury/spills/index.htm, accessed July 20, 1012.
5. U.S. Centers for Disease Control and Prevention, "Preventing Lead Poisoning in Young Children." http://www.cdc.gov/nceh/lead/publications/prevleadpoisoning.pdf, accessed July 20, 2012.
6. E. S. Lipton and D. Barboza, "As More Toys Are Recalled, Trail Ends in China," *The New York Times*, June 19, 2007.
7. L. Layton, "Obama 2011 Budget Request: Consumer Product Safety Commission," *Washington Post*, February 1, 2010.
8. U.S. Consumer Safety Commission. "Toy Hazard Recalls." http://www.cpsc.gov/cpscpub/prerel/category/toy.html, accessed July 20, 2012.
9. M. N. Mead, "Arsenic: In Search of an Antidote to a Global Poison," *Environmental Health Perspectives* 113 (2005): A379–A386.
10. P. Brodeur, *Outrageous Misconduct: The Asbestos Industry on Trial* (New York: Pantheon Books, 1985).
11. U.S. Agency for Toxic Substances and Disease Registry, "Asbestos: Libby, Montana." http://www.atsdr.cdc.gov/asbestos/sites/libby_montana/, accessed July 20, 2012.
12. L. A. Peipins et al., "Radiographic Abnormalities and Exposure to Asbestos-Contaminated Vermiculite in the Community of Libby, Montana, USA," *Environmental Health Perspectives* 111 (2003): 1753–1759.
13. C. Dean, "U.S. Cites Emergency in Asbestos-Poisoned Town," *The New York Times*, June 17, 2009.
14. J. M. Broder, "$250 Million Settlement Over Asbestos Is Announced," *The New York Times*, March 12, 2008.

15. M. Lorber et al., "Assessment of Inhalation Exposures and Potential Health Risks to the General Population That Resulted from the Collapse of the World Trade Center Towers," *Risk Analysis* 27 (2007): 1203–1221.

16. M. P. Webber et al., "Trends in Respiratory Symptoms of Firefighters Exposed to the World Trade Center Disaster: 2001–2005," *Environmental Health Perspectives* 117 (2009): 975–980.

17. M. Wasserman et al., "World PCBs Map: Storage and Effects in Man and His Biologic Environment in the 1970s," *Annals of the New York Academy of Science* 320 (1979): 69–124.

18. E. G. Horn et al., "The Problem of PCBs in the Hudson River System," *Annals of the New York Academy of Science* 320 (1979): 591–609.

19. New York State Department of Health, "Health Advice on Eating Sportfish and Game." http://www.health.state.ny.us/environmental/outdoors/fish/health_advisories/pdf, accessed July 20, 2012.

20. A. C. Revkin, "Dredging of Pollutants Begins in Hudson," *The New York Times*, May 15, 2009.

21. M. Navarro, "Under Stricter Rules, Dredges Return to Hudson," *The New York Times,* June 6, 2011.

22. Y. Masuda, "The Yusho Rice Oil Poisoning Incident," in A. Schecter, *Dioxins and Health* (New York: Plenum Press, 1994), 633–659.

23. C. C. Hsu et al., "The Yu-cheng Rice Oil Poisoning Incident," in A. Schecter, *Dioxins and Health* (New York: Plenum Press, 1994), 661–684.

24. M. J. Schneider, *Persistent Poisons: Chemical Pollutants in the Environment* (New York: New York Academy of Sciences, 1979).

25. Y. Kanagawa et al., "Association of Clinical Findings in Yusho Patients with Serum Concentrations of Polychlorinated Biphenyls, Polychlorinated Quarterphenyls, and 2,3,4,7,8-Pentachlorodibenzofuran More Than Thirty Years After the Poisoning Event," *Environmental Health* 7 (2008): 47.

26. Environmental Protection Agency, "Health Effects of PCBs." http://www.epa.gov/osw/hazard/tsd/pcbs/pubs/effects.htm, accessed July 23, 2009.

27. F. Yamashita and M. Hayashi, "Fetal PCB Syndrome: Clinical Features, Intrauterine Growth Retardation and Possible Alteration in Calcium Metabolism," Environmental Health Perspectives 59 (1985): 41–45.

28. Y.-L. Guo et al., "Growth Abnormalities in the Population Exposed In Utero and Early Postnatally to Polychlorinated Biphenyls and Dibenzofurans," *Environmental Health Perspectives* 103 (Supplement 6) (1995): 117–122.

29. U.S. Environmental Protection Agency, "The Foundation for Global Action on Persistent Organic Pollutants: A United States Perspective." http://www.epa.gov/nceawww1/pdfs/pops/POPsa.pdf, March 2002, accessed July 20, 2009.

30. E. Schor, "Obama Administration Steps Up Pressure to Ratify Treaties on Toxics," *The New York Times*, September 24, 2010.

31. Stockholm Convention on Persistent Organic Pollutants, "Status of Ratifications." http://chm.pops.int/Countries/StatusofRatification/tabid/252/language/en-US/Default.aspx, accessed July 20, 2012.

32. E. Diamanti-Kandarakis et al., "Endocrine-Disrupting Chemicals: An Endocrine Society Scientific Statement," *Endocrine Reviews* 30 (2009): 293–342.

33. Centers for Disease Control and Prevention, "Factsheet: Bisphenol A (BPA)." http://www .cdc.gov/biomonitoring/BisphenolA_FactSheet.html, accessed July 20, 2012.

34. Centers for Disease Control and Prevention, "Factsheet: Phthalates," April 2, 2012. http:// www.cdc.gov/biomonitoring/Phthalates_FactSheet.html, accessed July 20, 2012.

35. R. W. Stahlhut et al., "Concentrations of Urinary Phthalate Metabolites Are Associated with Increased Waist Circumference and Insulin Resistance in Adult U.S. Males," *Environmental Health Perspectives* 115 (2007): 876–882.

36. U.S. Food and Drug Administration, "FDA Continues to Study BPA." http://www.fda .gov/ForConsumers/ConsumerUpdates/ucm297954.htm, accessed July 21, 2012.

37. S. Tavernise, "FDA Makes It Official: BPA Can't Be Used in Baby Bottles and Cups," *The New York Times*, July 17, 2012.

38. P. Spencer and H. H. Schaumburg, eds., *Experimental and Clinical Neurotoxicology* (Baltimore, MD: Williams & Wilkins, 1980).

39. Sierra Club, "Water Sentinels: Factory Farms." http://www.sierraclub.org/watersentinels/ factoryfarms.aspx, accessed July 21, 2012.

40. S. Wing, "Social Responsibility and Research Ethics in Community-Driven Studies of Industrialized Hog Production," *Environmental Health Perspectives* 110 (2002): 437–444.

41. R. F. Kennedy, Jr. and E. Schaeffer, "An Ill Wind from Factory Farms," *The New York Times*, September 20, 2003.

42. R. Bravender et al., "Farm Interests Use EPA Spending Bill to Fight Climate Regs," *The New York Times*, June 19, 2009.

43. S. N. Bhanoo, "Tougher E.P.A. Action on Factory Farms," *The New York Times*, May 28, 2010.

44. Environmental Integrity Project, ""EPA Report: Iowa Factory Farm Program Shown to Violate Federal Clean Water Act." http://www.environmentalintegrity.org/news_ reports/07_13_2012.php, accessed July 21, 2012.

45. Department of Health and Human Services, National Toxicology Program, "About the NTP." http://ntp.niehs.nih.gov/?objectid=7201637B-BDB7-CEBA-F57E39896A08F1BB, accessed July 22, 2012.

46. J. Mendeloff, "Does Overregulation Cause Underregulation? The Case of Toxic Substances," *Regulation* (September–October 1981).

Clean Air: Is It Safe to Breathe?

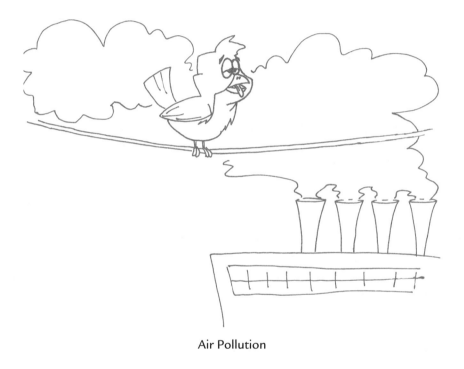

Air Pollution

Air pollution caused by coal burning was a problem in London as early as the 17th century. With the advent of the Industrial Revolution in the 18th and 19th centuries, the air of many cities was blackened with smoke from industrial and household furnaces and railroad locomotives. In 1952, an unusual weather pattern caused a particularly severe air pollution crisis in London. A layer of cold, moist air hung motionless over the city for 5 days, and smoke, fumes, and motor vehicle exhaust accumulated. More than 4000 deaths from both respiratory and heart disease were attributed to the foul air. Britain's first clean air act was passed soon afterward.[1]

Earlier, in 1948, the United States had been shocked by a similar deadly air pollution crisis caused by a similar weather pattern. A 5-day atmospheric inversion trapped the smoke and fumes of a heavily industrialized Pennsylvania valley. In the small town of Donora, population 14,000, residents suffered eye, nose, and throat irritation and breathing difficulties resulting in 20 deaths.[1] The event gained national attention and helped raise awareness about the health consequences of air pollution. In 2008, on the 60th anniversary of the event, the town opened the Donora Smog Museum with the slogan "Clean Air Starts Here."[2]

For most cities, the effects of air pollution were not so dramatic, but air quality was noticeably deteriorating in the United States during the 1950s and 1960s. Increasingly, this was due to automobiles. Los Angeles became known for its photochemical smog, the yellowish-brown haze caused by intense sunlight acting on the complex mix of chemicals emitted in motor vehicle exhaust. The irritating effects of air pollution were obvious to everyone and were especially harmful to the health of children and people with heart and lung diseases.

Efforts by cities and states to regulate pollutant emissions proved unsuccessful, and the federal government began attacking the problem in the mid-1960s. The first emission standards for automobiles were passed in 1965, to take effect with 1968 model-year cars. The Clean Air Act of 1970 established strict air quality standards, set limits on several major pollutants, and mandated reduction of automobile and factory emissions. Since then, improving air quality has been an almost constant political battle. Environmental and public health groups have pressed for compliance and even stricter standards, while industries, supported by political conservatives, argue that the cost of pollution control is too high, hurting the nation's economy. Amendments to the Clean Air Act, strengthening some air quality regulations, were passed in 1977 and 1990. In general, the United States has cleaner air now than it did in 1970, but the battle is far from over.[1]

Criteria Air Pollutants

The Clean Air Act and its amendments require monitoring and regulation of six common air pollutants, called criteria air pollutants, known to be harmful to health and the environment: particulates, sulfur dioxide, carbon monoxide, nitrogen oxides, ozone, and lead.[1] All of these substances enter the air as a result of combustion—for energy in power plants or motor vehicles, or for solid waste disposal or industrial processes.

Particulate matter is the most visible form of air pollution—the smoke, soot, and ash that were so typical of the Industrial Revolution. Aesthetically, particulate matter is objectionable because it reduces visibility, forms layers of grime on buildings and streets, and corrodes metals. Epidemiologic studies have shown that particulates in the air also have harmful health effects. A groundbreaking cohort study conducted by Harvard epidemiologists compared the health of adults and children over the period 1975 to 1988 in six cities with markedly different amounts of particulate pollution in their air.[3] Residents of Steubenville, Ohio, the most polluted city in the study, were more likely to suffer from respiratory symptoms and had poorer lung function than residents of Portage, Wisconsin, the least polluted city. Death rates in Steubenville were 26 percent higher than those in Portage. In a larger study of 151 cities, death rates were increased by 15 percent in the cities with the dirtiest air.

Early air pollution regulation focused on limiting total particulate matter. However, a number of studies, including the study of six cities, suggest that the smallest particles are the most dangerous because they can evade the body's natural defenses and penetrate deeply into the lungs, becoming a chronic source of irritation. In 1987, the Environmental Protection Agency (EPA) revised the standard so that the smaller particles—those with a diameter less than 10 micrometers (PM_{10})—were limited. In 1997, and again in 2006, the EPA focused on even smaller particles, issuing increasingly stringent limits for particles smaller than 2.5 micrometers ($PM_{2.5}$). In 2012, the agency proposed a further strengthening of $PM_{2.5}$. States will have until 2020 to meet the new standards.[4]

Opponents of stricter regulations tried hard to discredit the six-city study and other data, but the evidence has continued to strengthen, showing increased hospitalizations and deaths associated with higher levels of the smallest particles. Opponents of the 1997 $PM_{2.5}$ standard sued the EPA, demanding a cost–benefit analysis for implementing the new rules.[5] In 2001, the Supreme Court ruled unanimously that a cost–benefit analysis was not necessary and that the EPA must consider only public health and safety in setting the standards.[6] The importance of $PM_{2.5}$ was affirmed in several other studies, including the Women's Health Initiative, which in 2007 found that every increase of 10 micrograms per cubic meter in $PM_{2.5}$ almost doubled the risk of death from cardiovascular disease.[7]

Sulfur dioxide is produced by combustion of sulfur-containing fuels, especially coal. It irritates the respiratory tract, but its most significant impact is as a precursor to acid rain, a major threat to the environment. Sulfur dioxide reacts with water vapor to form sulfuric acid; it also tends to stick to fine particulates in the air, both mechanisms that increase this pollutant's potential for causing respiratory damage.[1] Sulfur dioxide levels, which are highest in the vicinity of large industrial facilities, declined by 83 percent between 1980 and 2010.[8]

Carbon monoxide is a highly toxic gas, most of which is produced in motor vehicle exhaust. It interferes with the oxygen-carrying capacity of the blood and is therefore especially harmful to patients with cardiovascular disease, who are more likely to suffer heart attacks when exposed to higher concentrations of the pollutant. Carbon monoxide also affects the brain, causing headaches and impairing mental processes. Average carbon monoxide levels, which generally are highest in areas of high traffic congestion, decreased by 82 percent between 1980 and 2010.[9]

Nitrogen oxides are the chemicals responsible for the yellowish-brown appearance of smog. Like sulfur dioxide, nitrogen oxides are respiratory irritants that contribute to acid rain. They also contribute to the formation of ozone. The main sources of nitrogen oxides are on-road motor vehicle exhaust, off-road equipment, and power plant emissions.[9] Nitrogen oxides levels declined by 52 percent between 1980 and 2010.[10]

Ozone, a highly reactive variant of oxygen, is produced by photochemical reactions in which sunlight acts on other air pollutants including nitrogen oxides. It is very irritating to the eyes and to the respiratory system, and chronic exposure can cause permanent damage to the lungs. A study of 95 large urban communities in the United States, published in 2004, found that even short-term increases in ozone levels lead to increases in mortality from cardiovascular and respiratory diseases.[11]

Ozone levels in the air are an indicator of various other chemicals produced by motor vehicles, and they are often used as a general measure of air pollution. As discussed later, ozone is an important protective component of the upper atmosphere, but at low altitudes its effects are harmful. Although ozone levels tend to be high in many urban areas, many rural and wilderness areas may also be affected, because the wind carries the pollutants hundreds of miles from their original source.[12] In 2008, the National Parks Conservation Association and the Environmental Defense Fund filed suit to force the EPA to clean up emissions responsible for the haze that obscures the views in many national parks.[13] Maximum ozone levels in the United States decreased 28 percent between 1980 and 2010.[12]

Lead is a highly toxic metal that can damage the nervous system, blood, and kidneys, posing a special risk to the development of children's intellectual abilities. The main source of lead as an air pollutant was the use of leaded gasoline, which was phased out in the United States during the 1980s.[1] While environmental lead from other sources is still a threat to children, the amount of lead in the air has decreased dramatically, having dropped by 89 percent between 1980 and 2010.[14]

When an area does not meet the air quality standard for one of the criteria pollutants, the EPA may designate it a nonattainment area and may impose measures designed to force the area to attain the standard. According to the EPA, 125 areas in 37 states, Puerto Rico, and the District of Columbia were classified as nonattainment areas for one or more criteria pollutant in 2010.[15] Poor air quality that is due to ozone levels is especially widespread, affecting broad areas in California, Texas, the East Coast from Boston to Atlanta, and parts of the Midwest. In 2010, approximately 124 million people lived in counties with poor air quality.[16]

In addition to the criteria air pollutants, which are widespread, a large number of other toxic and carcinogenic chemicals are released into the air by local factories, waste disposal sites, and other sources. The Clean Air Act of 1970 directed the EPA to identify and set emission standards for such hazards, but as of 1993, only eight had been acted upon: asbestos, mercury, beryllium, benzene, vinyl chloride, arsenic, radionuclides, and coke-oven emissions.[1] Legal battles over each standard have made progress painfully slow.

Clean Air Act amendments passed in 1990 contained a number of provisions designed to speed up the process. Congress identified 187 specific chemicals for the EPA to regulate. Rather than addressing each chemical individually, however, the agency was to identify major sources that emit these pollutants and to develop technical standards that will reduce the emissions. Since then, the EPA has issued rules covering over 80 categories of major industrial sources, including chemical plants, oil refineries, aerospace manufacturers, and steel mills, as well as categories of smaller sources such as dry cleaners.[17] It has also identified 33 toxic air pollutants that pose the greatest threats to public health in the largest number of urban areas and developed health risk assessments on them, producing maps of county-level risk for cancer, respiratory effects, and neurological effects.[17]

Strategies for Meeting Standards

Motor vehicles are the primary source of air pollution in urban areas, and the number of motor vehicles is increasing far more rapidly than the population. The standard approach for limiting air pollution from motor vehicles has been limitation of tailpipe emissions by mandating changes both in automobile engineering and in fuel. Significant improvement was achieved by the use of catalytic converters, devices that have been repeatedly improved to meet increasingly strict standards. The newest cars have reduced emissions of carbon monoxide and ozone-producing chemicals by about 90 percent and nitrogen oxides by 70 percent below those of cars without emission controls.[1] The ban on leaded gasoline has almost eliminated lead as an air pollutant.

Because of the continuing increase in the number of cars, however, and because older cars and poorly maintained vehicles continued to emit high levels of pollutants, a number of other requirements were included in the 1990 Clean Air amendments. Special attention was paid to geographic areas that fail to meet standards for one or more criteria pollutants. These requirements include use of less polluting alternative fuels such as ethanol and reformulated gasoline, installation of vapor recovery systems on gasoline pumps, and inspection and maintenance programs that require annual measurement of tailpipe emissions on each car, with mandatory remediation on cars that fail the test. Another mandate was that automakers should develop and market "zero-emission" vehicles—electric cars—a goal that is beginning to be achieved, beginning with the increasingly popular hybrid vehicles. Complicating efforts to reduce tailpipe emissions has been the increase in the number of pickup trucks and SUVs, for which the standards for passenger cars did not apply. The rules were changed in the 1990s to require all new vehicles to meet the same standards by 2009, but vehicles manufactured under the old rules will still be on the road for years.[1]

Ideally, the number of cars on the road in highly populated areas should be reduced. Public transportation undoubtedly benefits air quality in New York City and Washington, D.C., but too many American cities—including Los Angeles—are not designed for efficient public systems. While Americans support most measures to ensure cleaner air, they consistently resist efforts to move them out of their private automobiles. Many urban areas have developed, with modest success, policies to encourage carpooling by providing high-occupancy vehicle lanes and by taxing parking spaces. Substantially higher taxes on gasoline, such as those in most European and Asian countries, would undoubtedly discourage unnecessary driving; but raising gas taxes seems to be considered political suicide by most politicians. Efficient public transport systems require some assistance from public funds—the dreaded increase in taxes. Spikes in gasoline prices in recent years due to market forces have had some beneficial effects in encouraging people to buy smaller, more fuel-efficient and less polluting vehicles.

A variety of strategies have been effective in reducing industrial sources of pollution. Foremost among them have been installation of scrubbers on smokestacks and a move to less polluting fuels, especially away from high-sulfur coal. A new approach included in the 1990 Clean Air Act amendments is the creation of pollution allowances that can be bought and sold. Instead of requiring each factory or power plant to meet defined standards, an overall national or regional emissions goal is set, and that goal is set lower each year. Each potential polluter is assigned a fraction of that amount as an allowance, which can be used or sold. Plants that choose to clean up their technology can recoup some of their investment by selling their allowances to plants that find cleanup too expensive. This market approach was expected to achieve Clean Air Act goals with a maximum of flexibility and a minimum of political pain.[1]

A provision of the 1977 Clean Air Act Amendments that has generated a great deal of controversy is called "New Source Review." When the original Act was passed in 1970, it set standards for newly built power plants but did not require changes to existing plants. Because this provision led the companies to improve existing facilities without cleaning up their emissions, the 1977 rules required that companies that substantially upgraded their old plants had to bring them into compliance with the standards. Many companies, however, ignored the rules. In the mid-1990s, after years of negotiations with the industry, the Clinton administration sued seven electric utility companies in the Midwest and the South to force them to comply with the law and launched investigations of dozens of others.

When the younger President Bush took office in 2001, his administration responded to the complaints of the utilities by setting out to weaken the environmental laws. In 2002, the president proposed the "Clear Skies Initiative," which replaced the New Source Review requirement with a market-based trading system that clearly set weaker emissions standards than those required by the Clean Air Act. Congress did not act on the proposal, so the Bush administration began to administratively change the rules. It also dropped the investigations of noncompliant companies. In late 2003, attorneys general of 15 states, in cooperation with national environmental organizations, filed their own lawsuits against a number of the polluting power plants. Most of the states that sued were in the Northeast, where air is polluted by emissions blown in from the Midwest. The legal battles continued throughout Bush's term in office; by the end of his term, the New Source Review rule was still in place, but power plant emissions were still major sources of pollution.[18,19]

The Bush administration also issued rules on mercury pollution by coal-burning power plants that were later found by the courts to be inadequate and ineffective. The Bush rules used the cap-and-trade system that has been effective for air pollutants that disperse in the atmosphere; but mercury is heavy and tends to settle near the source of emission, causing local deposits that pollute soil and surface waters. Power plants, which produce more than 40 percent of mercury emissions, had lobbied heavily against strict rules requiring state-of-the-art technology at each site. The Obama administration promised to tighten the rules for mercury in accordance with the court order.[20] Accordingly, the EPA in 2011 proposed stricter rules for emissions of mercury and other pollutants from coal-burning power plants.[21]

There was one exception to Bush's attempts to weaken air quality rules; however, in May 2004, the administration announced rules that require vehicles using diesel fuel to meet stricter standards on emissions. Engine makers are required to install emission control systems, and refineries are required to produce cleaner-burning diesel fuel. The new regulations, which were scheduled to take effect by 2012, apply to nonroad vehicles such as tractors, bulldozers, locomotives, and barges, as well as to buses and trucks. The change was expected to significantly cut emissions of particulate matter and also, because diesel fuel contains high concentrations of sulfur, to reduce levels of sulfur dioxide in the air, helping to reduce acid rain.[1] The program has been something of a disappointment, however, because there are many more older, polluting, diesel engines in use than new clean ones. In 2005, Congress authorized funding to retrofit old engines with a filter that reduces soot emissions. Due to budget-cutting fervor, however, the funding has not been sufficient to significantly reduce the health risks from diesel exhaust.[22]

A modest law that took effect in 1988, the Emergency Planning and Community Right-to-Know Act (EPCRA), has had unexpectedly beneficial effects in prodding companies to voluntarily restrict their discharge of air pollutants. The law was passed in response to the infamous Bhopal disaster of 1984, in which a leak of isocyanate gas occurred at a Union Carbide pesticide factory in India, killing over 10,000 people who lived nearby. EPCRA requires businesses to report the locations and quantities of chemicals stored at their sites. This allows communities to prepare for emergencies such as leaks and chemical spills. The law also requires that manufacturers disclose information on the kinds and amounts of toxic pollutants they discharge into the local environment each year.[23] Frequently, local communities, alarmed by the information, pressure the industry to cut back on their emissions. The program, known as the Toxics Release Inventory, is credited with reducing industrial releases of toxic chemicals in the United States by 54.5 percent between 1988 and 2001 and another 30 percent between 2001 and 2010.[24,25]

Even before September 11, 2001, some industries were pressuring the EPA to relax requirements of EPCRA, claiming, among other reasons, that publication of such information would increase communities' vulnerability to terrorism. After September 11, the EPA has gone much further in trying to restrict public access to environmental information. Some critics claim that the terrorism argument is being used as a smokescreen to protect industry from lawsuits or bad publicity. As one of these critics is quoted as saying, "What's tricky is finding the right balance between protection from terrorists on one hand and providing information for the neighbors so they can be safe."[26(p.107)]

Urban areas that are having the most difficulty meeting air quality standards by requiring controls on motor vehicles and factories must consider regulating sources of pollution that have thus far been left alone. For example, Los Angeles banned the use of charcoal lighter fluid for barbecues and regulates the exhaust of gas-powered lawnmowers. Dry cleaners, auto body shops, and furniture refinishers are also significant sources of toxic air pollutants that are regulated in the Los Angeles area.[27] In 2004, the region announced a program through which residents could turn in old gasoline lawnmowers in exchange for new, nonpolluting electric mowers.[28] California still struggles with pollution associated with its ports, caused by cargo ships and the trucks that crowd the dock areas to move imported goods inland. The area's air pollution control agency is taking measures to replace some of the older diesel trucks with newer, cleaner models.[29] On a national scale, the Obama administration's 2009 program, nicknamed "Cash for Clunkers," which provided rebates to people who turn in old vehicles for new, more fuel-efficient ones, proved popular and helped to reduce pollution in areas with high emissions from motor vehicles.[30]

Overall, the United States has made substantial progress in fighting air pollution. As shown in Figure 21-1, emissions of most common pollutants have decreased significantly since 1970 despite significant increases in the nation's population and economic growth. In Los Angeles, concentrations of ozone, historically the most difficult pollutant to control, are now only one half of what they were in the mid-1970s; still, ozone levels in Los Angeles air violated federal standards on 109 days in 2010.[31]

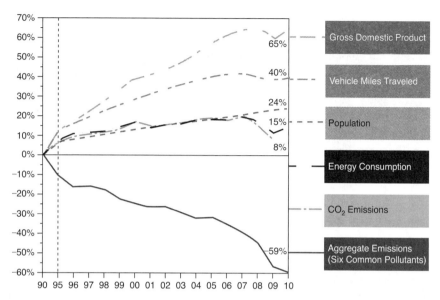

FIGURE 21-1   Comparison of Growth Measures and Emissions, 1990–2010.
Source: Reproduced from U.S. Environmental Protection Agency. http://www.epa.gov/
air/airtrends/2011/report/airpollution.pdf, accessed September 27, 2012.

Indoor Air Quality

While most public concern and political action have focused on outdoor air pollution, the 1980s saw increased attention paid to indoor air quality. In fact, most people spend more time indoors than out, and concentrations of many pollutants trapped inside a building may exceed those outdoors in all but the most polluted cities. The problem is exacerbated by energy conservation measures that minimize the quantity of outdoor air allowed inside. In the extreme, the lack of sufficient ventilation may lead to "sick building syndrome," in which building occupants develop an array of symptoms that disappear when they go outdoors.

The most common indoor air pollutants are tobacco smoke, other products of combustion, radon gas, consumer products that release chemicals into the air, and biological pollutants, including bacteria, mold, dust mites, and animal dander. "Secondhand smoke" has become a political issue in recent years, and many states now ban smoking in various public places. In the homes of smokers—beyond the arm of laws and regulations—tobacco smoke may be the most significant air pollutant and the main source of particulate pollution for children. Smoking also increases levels of carbon monoxide in indoor air and is a source of benzene, which is toxic and carcinogenic. Wood-burning stoves and fireplaces emit significant amounts of particulate matter and gases into the air. Gas ranges and furnaces burn more cleanly than wood stoves, but they produce carbon monoxide and nitrogen oxides.[1]

Radon is a radioactive gas emitted by the decay of radium and uranium. Radon has long been known to be a major health threat to uranium miners, who had a high risk of developing lung cancer. Then in 1984, a nuclear power plant worker set off radiation detection alarms on his way into the plant, near Philadelphia.[1] Investigation of his home found that radon gas levels there were 1000 times higher than normal. Since that discovery, elevated radon levels have been found in homes in most states; an estimated 1 of 15 homes in the United States has concentrations above the standard set by EPA.

The health threat from indoor radon pollution is not clear. The EPA and most other public health agencies believe that, extrapolating from the evidence obtained by studying uranium miners, radon in the home must be regarded as a serious cancer threat, causing an estimated 7000 to 30,000 lung cancer deaths annually.[1] Skeptics believe that these estimates are too high, noting that miners' effective exposure is much greater than what is measured, because the radon adheres to dust particles that lodge in the lungs. In miners, smoking acts synergistically with radon to cause lung cancer, meaning that the risk to miners who smoke is many times greater than that of the average smoking nonminer or nonsmoking miner. By analogy, the danger of radon in homes would be greatly enhanced if the residents are smokers.

Radon enters homes by seeping up from the soil and rock through dirt floors, crawl spaces, cracks in cement floors and walls, and through sump holes and floor drains. It may dissolve in well water and be released into the air during showers or baths. Measurement of radon is easily done with inexpensive kits and, in most homes where elevated levels are found, measures to seal cracks and openings are effective in reducing levels.

Other common indoor air pollutants include formaldehyde, a possibly carcinogenic gas that irritates the respiratory system and is contained in insulation, particleboard, plywood, some floor coverings and textiles, and tobacco smoke. In the past, elevated levels of formaldehyde were common in prefabricated and mobile homes. Although the Department of Housing and Urban Development requires that plywood and particleboard must conform to specified emissions limits, formaldehyde turned out to be a significant problem in mobile homes supplied by the Federal Emergency Management Agency to victims of the 2005 hurricanes Katrina and Rita. Since then, the Sierra Club and other organizations have noted that high levels of formaldehyde are more widespread in manufactured housing than previously thought, and the organization has petitioned the EPA to tighten regulations.[32] Drywall imported from China turned out to be a significant source of foul odors and health complaints in newly built houses, especially in those built in 2006 and 2007 during the housing boom that resulted from the hurricanes. The problem with the drywall appears to be emissions of sulfur compounds that also cause corrosion of metal objects in the homes. Thousands of lawsuits were filed as a result. The Consumer Product Safety Commission conducted an investigation and confirmed the problems.[33,34] Other chemicals that may pollute indoor air and may have adverse health effects include pesticides, dry-cleaning solvents, paints and paint thinners, carpet glues, hair spray, and air fresheners. While most biological air pollutants, such as mold, house mites, and animal dander, are a problem only for people who are allergic to them, airborne microbes can pose serious health hazards: witness Legionnaire's disease, caused by bacteria vaporized from air-conditioning systems, and hantavirus released into the air from rodent urine or feces.

Global Effects of Air Pollution

Because air pollutants are the most mobile of all forms of pollution, their ill effects may spread far beyond the immediate area where they are released. In fact, evidence is mounting that human activities are actually changing the composition of the atmosphere. The ultimate effects on public health from these changes are still a matter of speculation and controversy, but it has become clear that the effects may be quite harmful.

Acid rain is produced when two common air pollutants—sulfur dioxide and nitrogen dioxide—react with water to form sulfuric acid and nitric acid. In the United States, the industrial areas of the Midwest are a major source of the pollutants that acidify rainfall in the East, since prevailing winds blow from west to east. Acid rain in eastern Canada resulting from U.S. air pollution has been a cause of diplomatic tension between the two countries. The environment in Europe, the former Soviet Union, and southern China—everywhere that coal and oil are intensively used—is also seriously affected by acid rain.

Acid rain damages forests, reduces crop yields, and corrodes surfaces of buildings and statuary. It turns the water in lakes and rivers acidic, killing freshwater shrimp, wiping out bacteria on lake bottoms, and interfering with fish reproduction. Some lakes are so acidic that they can no longer support life: all fish species disappear, as do most frogs, salamanders, and aquatic insects. Because many metals, such as aluminum, lead, copper, and mercury are soluble in acid, the increasing acidity of water may lead to toxic levels of metals in drinking water supplies. There is evidence that regulations on industrial pollutants in the United States have helped to bring down levels of sulfur dioxide in the air and have begun to reduce the acidity of rainfall in the Northeast. EPA data shows that 55 to 60 percent of monitoring sites in the Adirondack Mountains, the Catskills, and the North Appalachian Plateau have improving rates of acidification.[35]

Depletion of the ozone layer is another manifestation of the global effects of certain air pollutants. Ozone, which is so harmful to respiratory systems at ground level, is a natural component of the upper atmosphere that provides a layer of protection against ultraviolet radiation. The detection of chlorofluorocarbons (CFCs) in the ozone "hole" which opened over Antarctica in the early 1980s convinced scientists that these chemicals, which were used as refrigerants and spray can propellants, were responsible for the breakdown of ozone. Being very stable, CFCs drift upwards to the ozone layer, where they may cause damage for many decades. The increased ultraviolet radiation that reaches ground level is causing greatly increased rates of cataracts, already a major cause of blindness in the world, and skin cancer. It also has harmful effects on other organisms, including food crops, and could be a major threat to life on the planet.

This global problem clearly required international action. After several years of controversy and denial, diplomats from 29 nations met in Montreal, Canada, in 1987 to sign an agreement aimed at reducing the production and use of CFCs.[1] As evidence of ozone depletion continued to mount, the Montreal Protocol has been strengthened several times, now calling for the elimination of chemicals that deplete ozone.[1] The protocol has been signed by 191 nations.[36] The United States has ended production of CFCs and many other ozone-depleting substances. However, millions of pounds of CFCs already in use will continue to be released into the atmosphere for years. The ozone layer appears to have stabilized, and it is expected to recover by the middle of the 21st century.[37]

Carbon dioxide is not strictly an air pollutant—along with nitrogen, oxygen, and argon, it is one of the four major components of the atmosphere—but its increasing proportion in the air has ominous implications for the future of the earth's environment. Carbon dioxide levels have been rising since the beginning of the Industrial Revolution due to the burning of fossil fuels. They are now about 30 percent higher than they were at the beginning of the Industrial Revolution, and they are increasing rapidly.[1]

Atmospheric carbon dioxide acts like the glass of a greenhouse, allowing sunlight to enter but trapping the heat inside. The resulting "greenhouse effect" leads to warmer temperatures at the earth's surface. Evidence is growing that global warming is already under way. It has been hard to definitively prove that the average temperature of the earth's surface is increasing because of the normal fluctuations from year to year and even from one decade to another, but the evidence is now quite strong that the average temperature of the earth increased by about 1.3°F between 1906 and 2005.[37] The temperature is expected to continue increasing, and the extent of warming is dependent upon how successful we are in curbing further emissions of greenhouse gases.

Conclusion

Air pollution, while a conspicuous problem in cities for more than 2 centuries, was recognized as a severe threat to health in the 1940s and 1950s. Weather-related events together with smoke from the burning of fossil fuels in England and the United States caused local air pollution crises that led to deaths from respiratory and heart disease.

Because air pollution does not respect political boundaries, interventions, to be effective, must be implemented on a national and sometimes global scale. The United States began establishing regulations to control air pollution beginning in the 1960s. Regulations on both automobile and factory emissions have been repeatedly strengthened since the Clean Air Act of 1970. Each new standard has been highly controversial, opposed by industry, congressional conservatives, and the Bush administration. The Obama administration has signaled an intention to support stricter rules against air pollution.

Six criteria air pollutants were identified by the Clean Air Act: particulate matter, sulfur dioxide, carbon monoxide, nitrogen oxides, ozone, and lead. These pollutants must be monitored by the EPA, and levels in the air have fallen since 1970. A larger number of other chemicals have also been identified as toxic pollutants. The Clean Air Act amendments of 1990 required the EPA to identify major sources of these emissions and to set emission standards for the source categories rather than for individual pollutants.

Strategies for meeting air pollution standards include technological improvements in motor vehicles and factory smokestacks. Congress has encouraged a flexible approach by creating pollution allowances that can be bought and sold, permitting industries to cooperate in meeting the standards. Requirements that industries disclose information on their emissions often result in pressure on companies from local communities to reduce the pollution.

Indoor air may have even more significant effects on health than outdoor air, since most people spend more time indoors than out, and many indoor pollutants are trapped inside buildings at high concentrations. Common indoor air pollutants include tobacco smoke, radon gas, consumer products that release chemicals into the air, and biological pollutants such as bacteria and mold.

Air pollution can create acid rain, which profoundly affects the environment. Depletion of the ozone layer by CFCs increases risk of skin cancer and cataracts and has harmful effects on other organisms. Increases in carbon dioxide concentrations in the air lead to the greenhouse effect, resulting in global warming.

References

1. A. Nadakavukaren, *Our Global Environment: A Health Perspective*, 6th ed. (Prospect Heights, IL: Waveland Press, 2006).
2. S. D. Hamill, "Unveiling a Museum, a Pennsylvania Town Remembers the Smog That Killed 20," *The New York Times*, November 2, 2008.
3. D. W. Dockery et al., "An Association Between Air Pollution and Mortality in Six U.S. Cities," *New England Journal of Medicine* 329 (1993): 1753–1759.
4. U.S. Environmental Protection Agency, "Overview of EPA's Proposal to Revise the Air Quality Standards for Particle Pollution (Particulate Matter). http://www.epa.gov/pm/pdfs/PMNAAQSProposalOVERVIEW61512UPDATED.pdf, accessed July 24, 2012.

5. J. H. Ware, "Editorial: Particulate Air Pollution and Mortality—Clearing the Air," *New England Journal of Medicine* 343 (2000): 1798–1799.

6. L. Greenhouse, "E.P.A.'s Right to Set Air Rules Wins Supreme Court Backing," *The New York Times*, February 28, 2001.

7. W. Dockery and P. H. Stone, "Cardiovascular Risks from Fine Particulate Air Pollution," *New England Journal of Medicine* 365 (2007): 511–513.

8. U.S. Environmental Protection Agency, "Air Trends: Sulfur Dioxide." http://www.epa.gov/airtrends/sulfur.html, accessed July 24, 2012.

9. U.S. Environmental Protection Agency, "Air Trends: Carbon Monoxide." http://www.epa.gov/airtrends/carbon.html, accessed July 24, 2012.

10. U.S. Environmental Protection Agency, "Air Trends: Nitrogen Dioxide." http://www.epa.gov/airtrends/nitrogren.html, accessed July 24, 2012.

11. M. L. Bell et al., "Ozone and Short-Term Mortality in 95 U.S. Urban Communities, 1987–2000," *Journal of the American Medical Association* 292 (2004): 2372–2378.

12. U.S. Environmental Protection Agency, "Air Trends: Ozone." http://www.epa.gov/airtrends/ozone.html, accessed July 24, 2012.

13. Environment News Service, "EPA Sued for Allowing Haze to Obscure National Parks," October 22, 2008. http://www.ens-newswire.com/ens/oct2008/2008-10-22-091.html, accessed July 24, 2012.

14. U.S. Environmental Protection Agency, "Air Trends: Lead." http://www/epa.gov/airtrends/lead.html, accessed July 25, 2012.

15. U.S. Environmental Protection Agency, "Currently Designated Nonattainment Areas for All Criteria Pollutants." http://www.epa.gov/air/oaqps/greenbk/ancl3.html, accessed July 24, 2012.

16. U.S. Environmental Protection Agency, "Our Nation's Air—Status and Trends Through 2010." http://www.epa.gov/airtrends/2011/index.html, accessed July 25, 2012.

17. U.S. Environmental Protection Agency, "About Air Toxics." http://www.epa.gov/ttn/atw/allabout.html, accessed July 25, 2012.

18. B. Barcott, "Changing All the Rules," *New York Times Magazine*, April 4, 2009.

19. J. M. Broder et al., "Environmental Views, Past and Present," *The New York Times*, February 7, 2009.

20. Editorial, "Mercury and Power Plants," *The New York Times*, July 24, 2009.

21. J. M. Broder and J. C. Rudolf, "E.P.A. Proposes New Emission Standards for Power Plants," *The New York Times,* March 16, 2011.

22. J. P. Jacobs, "EPA Toxics Report Sparks Fight Over Diesel Emissions," *The New York Times* March 17, 2011.

23. G. E. R. Hook and G. W. Lucier, "The Right to Know Is for Everyone," *Environmental Health Perspectives* 108 (2000): A160–A162.

24. U.S. Environmental Protection Agency, "2001 Toxics Release Inventory (TRI): Public Data Release." http://www.epa.gov/tri/NationalAnalysis/archive/2001_National_Analysis_Executive_Summary.pdf, accessed November 17, 2012.

25. U.S. Environmental Protection Agency, "2010 Toxics Release Inventory National Analysis Overview." http://www.epa.gov/tri/tridata/tri10/nationalanalysis/index.htm, accessed July 25, 2012.

26. R. Dahl, "Does Secrecy Equal Security? Limiting Access to Environmental Information," *Environmental Health Perspectives* 112 (2004): A104–A107.

27. W. Boly, "Smog City Wants to Make This Perfectly Clear," *Health* (San Francisco, CA) 6, No. 2 (1992): 54.

28. B. Bergman, "To Cut Smog, Los Angeles Places a Bounty on Mowers," *The New York Times*, May 5, 2004.

29. South Coast Air Quality Management District, "Board Meeting Date: July 10, 2009, Agenda No. 4." http://www.aqmd.gov/hb/2009/July/09074a.htm, accessed July 26, 2012.

30. M. L. Wald, "In Congress, a Jump Start for Clunkers," *The New York Times*, July 31, 2009.

31. South Coast Air Quality Management District, "Historic Ozone Air Quality Trends." http://www.aqmd.gov/smog/o3trend.html, accessed July 26, 2012.

32. B. M. Kuehn, "Stronger Formaldehyde Regulation Sought," *Journal of the American Medical Association* 299 (2008): 2015.

33. L. Wayne, "The Enemy at Home: Thousands in U.S. Attribute Ailments to Chinese Drywall," *The New York Times*, October 8, 2009.

34. U.S. Consumer Product Safety Commission, "Summary of Revision 1 to the Interim Guidance—Identification of Homes with Corrosion from Problem Drywall." http://www.cpsc.gov/info/drywall/guidance0827.pdf, accessed July 26, 2012.

35. U.S. Environmental Protection Agency, "Clean Air Interstate Rule, Acid Rain Program, and Former NO_x Budget Trading Program 2010 Progress Report." http://www.epa.gov/airmarkt/progress/ARPCAIR10.html, accessed July 26, 2012.

36. National Oceanic & Atmospheric Administration, Earth System Research Laboratory, "Twenty Questions and Answers About the Ozone Layer: 2010 Update." http://www.esrl.noaa.gov/csd/assessments/ozone/2010/twentyquestions/, accessed July 26, 2012.

37. Intergovernmental Panel on Climate Change, "Climate Change 2007: Synthesis Report." http://www.ipcc.ch/pdf/assessment-report/ar4/syr/ar4_syr_spm.pdf, accessed July 26, 2012.

Clean Water: A Limited Resource

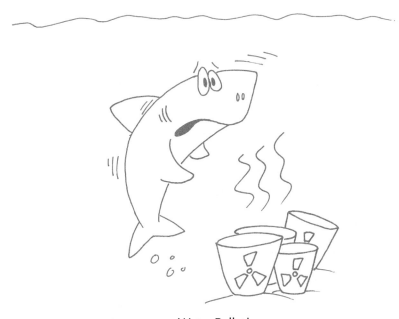

Water Pollution

The importance of safe drinking water to public health has been clear since John Snow identified polluted water as the source of London's cholera epidemic in 1855. Major epidemics of cholera and other waterborne diseases broke out periodically in the United States until the end of the 19th century. Ninety thousand people died of cholera in 1885 in Chicago, persuading city officials to stop discharging the city's sewage into Lake Michigan, which was also the source of municipal drinking water.[1] While contaminated water is still a major cause of disease and death in developing countries, Americans expect that their tap water will be safe to drink and, for the most part, it is. Nevertheless, 647 outbreaks of waterborne diseases were documented by the Centers for Disease Control and Prevention (CDC) between 1971 and 1994, including the

1993 cryptosporidiosis outbreak in Milwaukee.[2] Each year between 1991 and 2002, the CDC and the Environmental Protection Agency (EPA) recorded an average of 17 outbreaks associated with contaminated drinking water.[3] Such outbreaks continue, as will be seen later in this chapter.

Common water pollutants include, in addition to microbial pathogens, a wide range of chemicals that may not only be toxic in drinking water, but have harmful effects on fish and wildlife. Many chemicals have been discharged into waterways as industrial wastes, such as the mercury in Minamata Bay or the polychlorinated biphenyls (PCBs) in the Hudson River. People may then be poisoned by eating the fish that have accumulated these toxins in their flesh. Other sources of pollution include deposition from the air, as in acid rain, or runoff from the land.

Until the early 1970s, individual states were responsible for the quality of their waterways and the purity of their drinking water. This arrangement did not control water pollution for the same reason that it could not control air pollution: the sources of pollution and the communities affected by the pollution may be under different political jurisdiction. For example, New Orleans draws its drinking water from the Mississippi River, yet it was helpless to stop cities upstream, located in other states, from discharging sewage and industrial wastes into the river.

A number of infamous pollution cases occurred in the United States in the 1960s and 1970s that inspired the passage of federal legislation. The discovery of PCBs in the Hudson River led to a ban on commercial fishing there because the chemicals were so concentrated in the flesh of the fish. Residents of Duluth, Minnesota, were alarmed to learn that the Reserve Mining Company had been dumping asbestos-containing wastewater into Lake Superior, the source of municipal water, for more than 20 years.[4] While no one knew whether asbestos was as carcinogenic when drunk as it was when breathed, bottled water was distributed to the population for over a year until a new water-filtration plant was completed. The James River was so badly polluted with the insecticide Kepone, discharged from a manufacturing plant in Hopewell, Virginia, between 1966 and 1975, that no practical way has ever been proposed to clean it up. The plant was closed, not because of the environmental damage it caused, but because so many of its employees suffered neurological, liver, and other damage from Kepone poisoning.[5] Perhaps the most dramatic call to action occurred in 1969, when the Cuyahoga River in Ohio caught fire because it had so much oil floating on its surface.[4]

The two goals of cleaning up lakes and rivers and ensuring safe drinking water are distinct but related, and Congress has addressed them in separate legislation: the Clean Water Act of 1972, amended in 1977 and several times since, and the Safe Drinking Water Act of 1974, which was rewritten in 1996.[1] Since half of the drinking water in the United States comes from lakes and rivers, success in meeting the goals of the Clean Water Act is obviously a help in achieving the goals of the Safe Drinking Water Act.

Clean Water Act

The Clean Water Act set national goals that lakes and rivers should be "fishable" and "swimmable" and that all pollutant discharges should be eliminated. First attempts at cleaning up the nation's waterways focused on "point-source" pollution—well-defined locations that discharge pollutants into lakes and rivers. Most point-source pollution comes from municipal sewage and industrial discharges. The 1972 and 1977 legislation imposed strict controls on these sources; it also provided billions of dollars of funding to assist municipalities in building wastewater treatment facilities. With the success of these efforts, it became apparent that a great deal of pollution washed into waterways from the air and the land. The 1987 reauthorization of the Clean Water Act focused on cleaning up nonpoint-source pollution, which has proven to be a much more difficult task.[1]

Laws governing point-source pollution set requirements for treating wastewater so that it can be discharged into waterways without causing human health problems or disrupting the aquatic environment. In the case of sewage treatment plants, this requires several steps. The primary step is to remove suspended solids by screening them and then allowing them to settle out by gravity in settling tanks. The secondary stage is to break down the remaining organic material using biological processes: the wastewater is mixed with bacteria and plenty of oxygen, resulting in conversion of the organic wastes into carbon dioxide, water, and minerals. The wastewater is then usually disinfected with chlorine before being discharged into the environment.[1]

While the treatment process produces a liquid discharge that meets standards of environmental safety, it also generates "sludge," the solid waste left behind on screens and at the bottom of settling tanks. Enormous amounts of sludge are generated by municipal sewage plants, creating a major disposal problem. In the past, sludge was often dumped in the ocean or incinerated, but these methods create other pollution problems. Congress prohibited the ocean dumping of sludge in 1992. Some communities bury it in landfills, but landfill space is running low. Since sludge is rich in nutrients, the EPA encourages the use of treated sludge as a fertilizer and soil conditioner to improve marginal lands and increase forest productivity. The EPA has developed strict regulations on sanitizing and removing hazardous contaminants from the sludge—known after treatment as biosolids—before it can be used on land. Currently, 54 percent of the six million tons of sewage sludge generated every year is used as fertilizer.[1]

About 70 percent of the U.S. population is served by sewage treatment plants. Most of the other 30 percent use onsite septic systems, which function as miniature sewage treatment plants including the use of bacteria to break down organic wastes. Like the larger plants, septic systems produce sludge, which must be pumped out periodically. Improperly constructed and poorly maintained septic systems contribute to pollution of waterways and often result in public health problems.[1]

Despite the laws and some occasional funding from the federal government, many cities have inadequate sewer systems that back up into basements or overflow and dump untreated sewage into waterways. In part the problems are due to population growth, which has placed additional burden on aging systems, and in part they occur because most systems combine rainwater runoff with sewage, overwhelming the system when it rains. According to an analysis of EPA data by *The New York Times*, sewage systems are the nation's most frequent violators of the Clean Water Act. The EPA and the Government Accountability Office have estimated that $400 million in extra spending is needed over the next decade to fix the nation's sewage infrastructure.[6]

Discharges from industrial sources are the second major category of point-source pollution, which is strictly regulated by the Clean Water Act. The EPA is required to develop standards for the release of various categories of pollutants into the environment. Industries that discharge directly into the nation's waterways are required to obtain a permit specifying allowable amounts and constituents of pollutants they may discharge. They must routinely monitor their discharges, and they must report regularly to the EPA.[1]

Industrial wastes may cause special problems if they are discharged into sewer systems and pass through a municipal sewage treatment plant, occasionally with disastrous consequences. In 1977, pesticide wastes illegally dumped into the sewers of Louisville, Kentucky, killed all the microbes responsible for the secondary treatment process, rendering the plant ineffective. For nearly 2 years while the plant was being cleaned up at a cost of millions of dollars, 100 million gallons of untreated sewage were discharged into the Ohio River every day. In 1981 in Cincinnati, a paint factory discharged hydrochloric acid into the city sewers, corroding the sewer pipe and causing it to collapse, leaving a hole in the street 24 feet in diameter.[7]

To prevent such problems, the Clean Water Act requires pretreatment of industrial wastes that are discharged into sewers. But standards have not been set for many smaller commercial establishments, including car washes and photo processing plants. Hazardous chemicals also enter sewer systems from residences, when people dispose of bleaches, toilet bowl cleaners, paint thinners, and other household substances by flushing them down the drain.

As strict limits have been set on pollution from sewage systems and industry, nonpoint-source pollution has become an increasingly important threat to water quality. These contaminants come from stormwater runoff from farmland, construction sites, and urban streets. Agriculture is the leading source of water pollution in the United States, contributing soil, manure fertilizers, and pesticides that wash into streams and lakes. Agricultural runoff is believed to have been the source of the Milwaukee cryptosporidiosis outbreak. Construction activities also contribute soil to runoff water, together with oil, tar, paint, and cleaning solvents. Contaminants contributed by urban street runoff include sand, dirt, road salt, oil, grease, heavy metal particles, pesticides and fertilizers from lawns, and animal and bird droppings.

A variety of approaches must be used to minimize pollution caused by stormwater runoff. These include preventing soil erosion by planting vegetation on exposed soil, incorporating more green space into urban areas, minimizing the use of chemical fertilizers and pesticides, and controlling litter.

Air pollution is also a source of water pollution. In addition to acid rain, a number of other chemicals are deposited into lakes, rivers, and oceans from the air. These include lead, asbestos, PCBs, and various pesticides. It has been shown that the major portion of PCBs in the Great Lakes comes from the air. Industrial accidents and spills also contribute to pollution of waterways.

To conform to the requirements of the Clean Water Act, the EPA regularly collects data from the states on water quality of rivers, lakes, and estuaries. The most recent report available, using data from 2004, showed that the nation still has a long way to go meet the fishable and swimmable requirements. Forty-four percent of river miles, 64 percent of lake acres, and 33 percent of bay and estuaries square miles were found to be unfit for fishing and swimming.[8]

Safe Drinking Water

Almost half of the drinking water in the United States comes from rivers and lakes. Thus it is likely to be contaminated by the point-source and nonpoint-source pollutants discussed above. The other half comes from underground aquifers; these are generally of better quality but are increasingly susceptible to contamination by leaching from landfills, leaky oil and gas storage tanks, and other sources of toxic chemicals. Improvements in surface-water quality brought about by the Clean Water Act make the job easier for community water systems, which must, however, meet much higher standards to produce potable water—water that is safe for human consumption.

All community systems need to treat their water so that, theoretically, all contaminants are removed. The steps needed to produce potable water vary depending on the source of the water and the type of contaminants. The basic steps common to most systems include sedimentation, coagulation, filtration, and disinfection. Incoming water is first allowed to sit quietly while suspended material settles out. Then alum is added, causing small particles to coagulate and settle out. Filtration through beds of sand or similar materials removes the smaller particles that do not settle, and chlorine is added to kill remaining pathogens. In areas of the country where water is "hard"—containing high concentrations of dissolved calcium or magnesium—or where it has objectionable tastes or odors due to dissolved iron or gases, additional treatments may be used. As a last step, fluoride is often added to protect community residents from tooth decay. A typical drinking-water purification plant is diagrammed in **Figure 22-1**.

Typical Municipal Water Treatment Plant

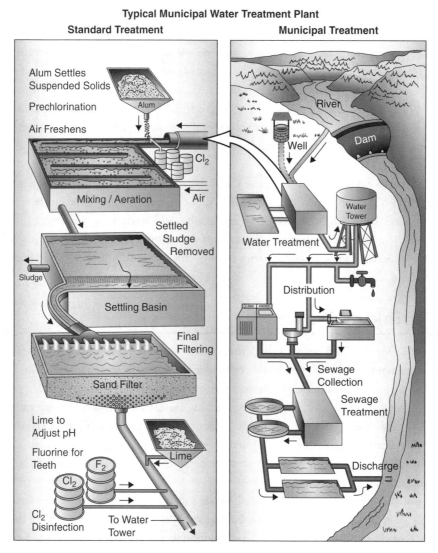

FIGURE 22-1   Drinking and Wastewater Treatment. *Source:* Reproduced from U.S. Environmental Protection Agency, "The Water Sourcebooks," p. 236. http://water.epa.gov/learn/kids/drinkingwater/upload/The-Water-Sourcebooks-Grade-Level-9-12.pdf, accessed September 27, 2012.

To ensure that the treatment process is working effectively, regular laboratory tests are generally done on the final product. The traditional measures of water purity are turbidity and coliform levels. Turbidity indicates the presence of suspended particles, a failure of the sedimentation and filtration steps. Suspended particles may interfere with the germicidal action of the chlorine. After the cryptosporidiosis outbreak, which accompanied an increase in the turbidity of Milwaukee's water, national turbidity standards were tightened. If coliform bacteria are detected, there has probably been a failure of disinfection. These bacteria are common inhabitants of the intestines of humans and other animals and, while they are usually not pathogenic themselves, their presence indicates that other, more harmful microorganisms may have survived the treatment process.[1]

The general approach to water treatment described above is directed primarily against bacterial diseases, the most common and historically devastating type of waterborne disease. It is not very effective, however, against viruses and the parasites *Cryptosporidia* and *Giardia*, which are resistant to chlorine. Furthermore, it does nothing to address the problem of contamination with common chemical pollutants such as pesticides, herbicides, fertilizers, PCBs, lead, and other metals that may be harmful to health. Most community water systems are totally unprepared even to test for these pollutants.

The Safe Drinking Water Act of 1974 required the EPA to set standards for local water systems and mandated that states enforce the standards. Uniform guidelines were set for drinking-water treatment, and regular monitoring and testing were required, with the results to be reported to state governments. However, no deadlines were established for the standard setting, and state agencies were lax in enforcing the requirements that were in place. The 1986 reauthorization of the Safe Drinking Water Act specified 83 contaminants to be regulated by the EPA and set deadlines for action. In addition, it required water systems to take measures to prevent contamination with *Giardia* and *Cryptosporidia*.[1] The EPA stepped up the pace of regulation. Now, maximum contaminant levels have been set for 87 identified contaminants, including microorganisms, disinfectants, disinfection byproducts, inorganic chemicals, organic chemicals, and radionuclides. A selected list of these contaminants is shown in Table 22-1. In addition, secondary standards have been set for 15 contaminants that do not cause health risks but that may affect taste, odor, or color, or that cause discoloration of skin or teeth.

In 1996, Congress again strengthened the Safe Drinking Water Act. New measures required that community water systems provide annual Consumer Confidence Reports to their customers on the source of the water, water contaminants, and the health effects of these contaminants.[9] The law also included requirements for source water protection, tightened standards for training and certification of operators, and provided funding to help localities improve their systems. The "right-to-know" measure was expected to evoke public pressure that would result in better compliance with standards.

Ongoing surveillance for waterborne disease by the CDC provides data useful for evaluating the adequacy of existing water treatment technologies and the effectiveness of drinking water regulations. The CDC publishes its findings every 2 years, analyzing the outbreaks by causative

Table 22-1   EPA National Primary Drinking Water Standards

Contaminant	MCLG[1] (mg/L)[2]	MCL or TT[1] (mg/L)[2]	Potential Health Effects from Long-Term Exposure Above the MCL (unless specified as short-term)	Sources of Contaminant in Drinking Water
Microorganisms				
Cryptosporidium	zero	TT[3]	Gastrointestinal illness (e.g., diarrhea, vomiting, cramps)	Human and animal fecal waste
Giardia lamblia	zero	TT[3]	Gastrointestinal illness (e.g., diarrhea, vomiting, cramps)	Human and animal fecal waste
Heterotrophic plate count	n/a	TT[3]	HPC has no health effects; it is an analytic method used to measure the variety of bacteria that are common in water. The lower the concentration of bacteria in drinking water, the better maintained the water system is.	HPC measures a range of bacteria that are naturally present in the environment
Legionella	zero	TT[3]	Legionnaire's disease, a type of pneumonia	Found naturally in water; multiplies in heating systems
Total Coliforms (including fecal coliform and *E. Coli*)	zero	5.0%[4]	Not a health threat in itself; it is used to indicate whether other potentially harmful bacteria may be present[5]	Coliforms are naturally present in the environment; as well as feces; fecal coliforms and *E. Coli* only come from human and animal fecal waste.
Turbidity	n/a	TT[3]	Turbidity is a measure of the cloudiness of water. It is used to indicate water quality and filtration effectiveness (e.g., whether disease-causing organisms are present). Higher turbidity levels are often associated with higher levels of disease-causing microorganisms such as viruses, parasites and some bacteria. These organisms can cause symptoms such as nausea, cramps, diarrhea, and associated headaches.	Soil runoff
Viruses (enteric)	zero	TT[3]	Gastrointestinal illness (e.g., diarrhea, vomiting, cramps)	Human and animal fecal waste

	MCLG	MCL	Potential health effects	Sources
Disinfection Byproducts				
Bromate	zero	0.010	Increased risk of cancer	Byproduct of drinking water disinfection
Chlorite	0.8	1.0	Anemia; infants & young children: nervous system effects	Byproduct of drinking water disinfection
Haloacetic acids (HAA5)	n/a[6]	0.060[7]	Increased risk of cancer	Byproduct of drinking water disinfection
Total Trihalo-methanes (TTHMs)	--> n/a[6]	--> 0.080[7]	Liver, kidney or central nervous system problems; increased risk of cancer	Byproduct of drinking water disinfection
Disinfectants				
Chloramines (as Cl₂)	MRDLG =4[1]	MRDL=4.0[1]	Eye/nose irritation; stomach discomfort, anemia	Water additive used to control microbes
Chlorine (as Cl₂)	MRDLG =4[1]	MRDL=4.0[1]	Eye/nose irritation; stomach discomfort	Water additive used to control microbes
Chlorine dioxide (as ClO₂)	MRDLG =0.8[1]	MRDL=0.8[1]	Anemia; infants & young children: nervous system effects	Water additive used to control microbes
Inorganic Chemicals				
Antimony	0.006	0.006	Increase in blood cholesterol; decrease in blood sugar	Discharge from petroleum refineries; fire retardants; ceramics; electronics; solder
Arsenic	0[7]	0.010 as of 01/23/06	Skin damage or problems with circulatory systems, and may have increased risk of getting cancer	Erosion of natural deposits; runoff from orchards, runoff from glass & electronics production wastes

(Continued)

Table 22-1 EPA National Primary Drinking Water Standards (*Continued*)

Inorganic Chemicals

Contaminant	MCLG[1] (mg/L)[2]	MCL or TT[1] (mg/L)[2]	Potential Health Effects from Long-Term Exposure Above the MCL (unless specified as short-term)	Sources of Contaminant in Drinking Water
Asbestos (fiber >10 micrometers)	7 million fibers per liter	7 MFL	Increased risk of developing benign intestinal polyps	Decay of asbestos cement in water mains; erosion of natural deposits
Barium	2	2	Increase in blood pressure	Discharge of drilling wastes; discharge from metal refineries; erosion of natural deposits
Beryllium	0.004	0.004	Intestinal lesions	Discharge from metal refineries and coal-burning factories; discharge from electrical, aerospace, and defense industries
Cadmium	0.005	0.005	Kidney damage	Corrosion of galvanized pipes; erosion of natural deposits; discharge from metal refineries; runoff from waste batteries and paints
Chromium (total)	0.1	0.1	Allergic dermatitis	Discharge from steel and pulp mills; erosion of natural deposits
Copper	1.3	TT[7]; Action Level=1.3	Short term exposure: Gastrointestinal distress Long term exposure: Liver or kidney damage People with Wilson's Disease should consult their personal doctor if the amount of copper in their water exceeds the action level	Corrosion of household plumbing systems; erosion of natural deposits

Contaminant	MCLG	MCL	Potential Health Effects from Ingestion of Water	Sources of Contaminant in Drinking Water
Cyanide (as free cyanide)	0.2	0.2	Nerve damage or thyroid problems	Discharge from steel/metal factories; discharge from plastic and fertilizer factories
Fluoride	4.0	4.0	Bone disease (pain and tenderness of the bones); Children may get mottled teeth	Water additive which promotes strong teeth; erosion of natural deposits; discharge from fertilizer and aluminum factories
Lead	zero	TT⁷; Action Level=0.015	Infants and children: Delays in physical or mental development; children could show slight deficits in attention span and learning abilities. Adults: Kidney problems; high blood pressure	Corrosion of household plumbing systems; erosion of natural deposits
Mercury (inorganic)	0.002	0.002	Kidney damage	Erosion of natural deposits; discharge from refineries and factories; runoff from landfills and croplands
Nitrate (measured as Nitrogen)	10	10	Infants below the age of six months who drink water containing nitrate in excess of the MCL could become seriously ill and, if untreated, may die. Symptoms include shortness of breath and blue-baby syndrome.	Runoff from fertilizer use; leaking from septic tanks, sewage; erosion of natural deposits
Nitrite (measured as Nitrogen)	1	1	Infants below the age of six months who drink water containing nitrite in excess of the MCL could become seriously ill and, if untreated, may die. Symptoms include shortness of breath and blue-baby syndrome.	Runoff from fertilizer use; leaking from septic tanks, sewage; erosion of natural deposits
Selenium	0.05	0.05	Hair or fingernail loss; numbness in fingers or toes; circulatory problems	Discharge from petroleum refineries; erosion of natural deposits; discharge from mines
Thallium	0.0005	0.002	Hair loss; changes in blood; kidney, intestine, or liver problems	Leaching from ore-processing sites; discharge from electronics, glass, and drug factories

(Continued)

Table 22-1 EPA National Primary Drinking Water Standards (*Continued*)

Organic Chemicals

Contaminant	MCLG[1] (mg/L)[2]	MCL or TT[1] (mg/L)[2]	Potential Health Effects from Long-Term Exposure Above the MCL (unless specified as short-term)	Sources of Contaminant in Drinking Water
Acrylamide	zero	TT[8]	Nervous system or blood problems; increased risk of cancer	Added to water during sewage/wastewater treatment
Alachlor	zero	0.002	Eye, liver, kidney or spleen problems; anemia; increased risk of cancer	Runoff from herbicide used on row crops
Atrazine	0.003	0.003	Cardiovascular system or reproductive problems	Runoff from herbicide used on row crops
Benzene	zero	0.005	Anemia; decrease in blood platelets; increased risk of cancer	Discharge from factories; leaching from gas storage tanks and landfills
Benzo(a) pyrene (PAHs)	zero	0.0002	Reproductive difficulties; increased risk of cancer	Leaching from linings of water storage tanks and distribution lines
Carbofuran	0.04	0.04	Problems with blood, nervous system, or reproductive system	Leaching of soil fumigant used on rice and alfalfa
Carbon tetrachloride	zero	0.005	Liver problems; increased risk of cancer	Discharge from chemical plants and other industrial activities
Chlordane	zero	0.002	Liver or nervous system problems; increased risk of cancer	Residue of banned termiticide
Chlorobenzene	0.1	0.1	Liver or kidney problems	Discharge from chemical and agricultural chemical factories
2,4-D	0.07	0.07	Kidney, liver, or adrenal gland problems	Runoff from herbicide used on row crops
Dalapon	0.2	0.2	Minor kidney changes	Runoff from herbicide used on rights of way

Contaminant	MCLG	MCL	Potential Health Effects	Sources of Contaminant
1,2-Dibromo-3-chloropropane (DBCP)	zero	0.0002	Reproductive difficulties; increased risk of cancer	Runoff/leaching from soil fumigant used on soybeans, cotton, pineapples, and orchards
o-Dichlorobenzene	0.6	0.6	Liver, kidney, or circulatory system problems	Discharge from industrial chemical factories
p-Dichlorobenzene	0.075	0.075	Anemia; liver, kidney or spleen damage; changes in blood	Discharge from industrial chemical factories
1,2-Dichloroethane	zero	0.005	Increased risk of cancer	Discharge from industrial chemical factories
1,1-Dichloroethylene	0.007	0.007	Liver problems	Discharge from industrial chemical factories
cis-1,2-Dichloroethylene	0.07	0.07	Liver problems	Discharge from industrial chemical factories
trans-1,2-Dichloroethylene	0.1	0.1	Liver problems	Discharge from industrial chemical factories
Dichloromethane	zero	0.005	Liver problems; increased risk of cancer	Discharge from drug and chemical factories
1,2-Dichloropropane	zero	0.005	Increased risk of cancer	Discharge from industrial chemical factories
Di(2-ethylhexyl) adipate	0.4	0.4	Weight loss, liver problems, or possible reproductive difficulties.	Discharge from chemical factories
Di(2-ethylhexyl) phthalate	zero	0.006	Reproductive difficulties; liver problems; increased risk of cancer	Discharge from rubber and chemical factories
Dinoseb	0.007	0.007	Reproductive difficulties	Runoff from herbicide used on soybeans and vegetables
Dioxin (2,3,7,8-TCDD)	zero	0.00000003	Reproductive difficulties; increased risk of cancer	Emissions from waste incineration and other combustion; discharge from chemical factories
Diquat	0.02	0.02	Cataracts	Runoff from herbicide use

(Continued)

Table 22-1 EPA National Primary Drinking Water Standards (*Continued*)

Organic Chemicals

Contaminant	MCLG[1] (mg/L)[2]	MCL or TT[1] (mg/L)[2]	Potential Health Effects from Long-Term Exposure Above the MCL (unless specified as short-term)	Sources of Contaminant in Drinking Water
Endothall	0.1	0.1	Stomach and intestinal problems	Runoff from herbicide use
Endrin	0.002	0.002	Liver problems	Residue of banned insecticide
Epichlorhydrin	zero	TT[8]	Increased cancer risk, and over a long period of time, stomach problems	Discharge from industrial chemical factories; an impurity of some water treatment chemicals
Ethylbenzene	0.7	0.7	Liver or kidneys problems	Discharge from petroleum refineries
Ethylene dibromide	zero	0.00005	Problems with liver, stomach, reproductive system, or kidneys; increased risk of cancer	Discharge from petroleum refineries
Glyphosate	0.7	0.7	Kidney problems; reproductive difficulties	Runoff from herbicide use
Heptachlor	zero	0.0004	Liver damage; increased risk of cancer	Residue of banned termiticide
Heptachlor epoxide	zero	0.0002	Liver damage; increased risk of cancer	Breakdown of heptachlor
Hexachlorobenzene	zero	0.001	Liver or kidney problems; reproductive difficulties; increased risk of cancer	Discharge from metal refineries and agricultural chemical factories
Hexachlorocyclopentadiene	0.05	0.05	Kidney or stomach problems	Discharge from chemical factories
Lindane	0.0002	0.0002	Liver or kidney problems	Runoff/leaching from insecticide used on cattle, lumber, gardens
Methoxychlor	0.04	0.04	Reproductive difficulties	Runoff/leaching from insecticide used on fruits, vegetables, alfalfa, livestock

Contaminant	MCLG	MCL	Potential Health Effects	Sources
Oxamyl (Vydate)	0.2	0.2	Slight nervous system effects	Runoff/leaching from insecticide used on apples, potatoes, and tomatoes
Polychlorinated biphenyls (PCBs)	zero	0.0005	Skin changes; thymus gland problems; immune deficiencies; reproductive or nervous system difficulties; increased risk of cancer	Runoff from landfills; discharge of waste chemicals
Pentachlorophenol	zero	0.001	Liver or kidney problems; increased cancer risk	Discharge from wood preserving factories
Picloram	0.5	0.5	Liver problems	Herbicide runoff
Simazine	0.004	0.004	Problems with blood	Herbicide runoff
Styrene	0.1	0.1	Liver, kidney, or circulatory system problems	Discharge from rubber and plastic factories; leaching from landfills
Tetrachloroethylene	zero	0.005	Liver problems; increased risk of cancer	Discharge from factories and dry cleaners
Toluene	1	1	Nervous system, kidney, or liver problems	Discharge from petroleum factories
Toxaphene	zero	0.003	Kidney, liver, or thyroid problems; increased risk of cancer	Runoff/leaching from insecticide used on cotton and cattle
2,4,5-TP (Silvex)	0.05	0.05	Liver problems	Residue of banned herbicide
1,2,4-Trichlorobenzene	0.07	0.07	Changes in adrenal glands	Discharge from textile finishing factories
1,1,1-Trichloroethane	0.20	0.2	Liver, nervous system, or circulatory problems	Discharge from metal degreasing sites and other factories
1,1,2-Trichloroethane	0.003	0.005	Liver, kidney, or immune system problems	Discharge from industrial chemical factories

(*Continued*)

Table 22-1 EPA National Primary Drinking Water Standards (*Continued*)

Organic Chemicals

Contaminant	MCLG[1] (mg/L)[2]	MCL or TT[1] (mg/L)[2]	Potential Health Effects from Long-Term Exposure Above the MCL (unless specified as short-term)	Sources of Contaminant in Drinking Water
Trichloro-ethylene	zero	0.005	Liver problems; increased risk of cancer	Discharge from metal degreasing sites and other factories
Vinyl chloride	zero	0.002	Increased risk of cancer	Leaching from PVC pipes; discharge from plastic factories
Xylenes (total)	10	10	Nervous system damage	Discharge from petroleum factories; discharge from chemical factories

Radionuclides

Contaminant	MCLG[1] (mg/L)[2]	MCL or TT[1] (mg/L)[2]	Potential Health Effects from Long-Term Exposure Above the MCL (unless specified as short-term)	Sources of Contaminant in Drinking Water
Alpha particles	none[7] ------- zero	15 picocu-ries per Liter (pCi/L)	Increased risk of cancer	Erosion of natural deposits of certain minerals that are radioactive and may emit a form of radiation known as alpha radiation
Beta particles and photon emitters	none[7] ------- zero	4 millirems per year	Increased risk of cancer	Decay of natural and man-made deposits of certain minerals that are radioactive and may emit forms of radiation known as photons and beta radiation
Radium 226 and Radium 228 (combined)	none[7] ------- zero	5 pCi/L	Increased risk of cancer	Erosion of natural deposits
Uranium	zero	30 ug/L as of 12/08/03	Increased risk of cancer, kidney toxicity	Erosion of natural deposits

Sources: Reproduced from U.S. Environmental Protection Agency, "National Primary Drinking Water Regulations." June 5, 2012. http://water.epa.gov/drink/contaminants/index.cfm#list, accessed September 27, 2012.

agent, type of water system, type of deficiency in the system, and source of water. The data probably understate the incidence of waterborne diseases, because most cases go unrecognized or unreported.

The most recent available report found 36 outbreaks in the 2-year period 2007–2008, affecting 4128 people and causing three deaths.[10] Thirty-one of the outbreaks were caused by known infectious agents: five by viruses, three by parasites, 21 by bacteria, one by both viruses and bacteria, and one by bacteria and parasites. One outbreak was caused by a chemical. About one-third of the outbreaks in 2007–2008 were caused by *Legionella* bacteria, which caused respiratory disease. More than half of the outbreaks were associated with untreated or inadequately treated ground water, and most of these caused acute gastrointestinal illness.

In 1978, CDC's surveillance for waterborne disease outbreaks expanded to include outbreaks associated with recreational water, such as swimming pools, water parks, and beaches. These sources now account for more outbreaks than drinking water sources. In 2007–2008, there were 134 outbreaks, affecting 13,966 people and causing 17 deaths.[11] Most of the illnesses were gastrointestinal, caused by infectious agents or chemicals, but a significant number of cases were poisonings or respiratory irritation caused by pool chemicals.

Enforcement by state and local governments of safe drinking water laws has been spotty. An investigation by *The New York Times*, which analyzed data from the EPA and the states, found that 40 percent of the nation's community water systems violated the Safe Drinking Water Act at least once in just the one year of the study, 2008. More than 23 million people received substandard drinking water.[12] Many of the violations are due to chemicals that may, even at low concentrations, cause cancer or other chronic diseases that take years or decades to develop. Often politicians resist enforcing these laws, concerned about the economic impact or bad publicity. Under the Bush administration, the EPA did not push state and local governments to meet standards or punish industries that dumped pollutants into lakes and rivers.[12] Moreover, recent studies have found new, unregulated chemicals in water supplies and have revealed that some regulated chemicals are harmful at low concentrations that meet current federal standards. For example, according to *The New York Times* analysis, a community could drink perfectly legal water containing arsenic at a level such that roughly 1 in every 600 residents would likely develop bladder cancer over their lifetimes.[13]

In 2010, Lisa Jackson, the EPA administrator appointed by President Obama, announced that the agency had developed a new Drinking Water Strategy aimed at finding ways to strengthen public health protection from contaminants. Among the goals addressed in the new strategy are to address contaminants as groups rather than one at a time, foster development of new technology, and to develop closer relationships with states to share data on compliance and enforcement. The agency identified several groups of chemicals to focus on for regulation, starting with carcinogenic volatile organic compouds.[14]

Private wells are not regulated under the Safe Drinking Water Act, although the EPA issues recommendations for ensuring that wells are safe. About 43 million Americans get their drinking water from private wells and, according to a study by the U.S. Geological Survey, more than one in five of these wells contain at least one contaminant at a concentration high enough to be a health concern. Different contaminants are more common in different regions of the country. The study authors note that these findings underscore a continuing need for public education and for the testing of domestic wells.[15]

Many Americans choose to drink bottled water, believing that it is purer and tastes better than tap water. In most cases, this is not the case. According to a study published in 1999 by the Natural Resources Defense Council, many of the 103 brands tested contained chemical or biological contaminants, though not in concentrations high enough to cause health problems.[1] In 2000, however, CDC surveillance recorded a multistate outbreak affecting 84 people, caused by *Salmonella* in bottled water due to contamination at the water source.[16] Outbreaks associated with bottled water were also reported in 2001, 2003, 2004, and 2007.[17] Bottled water is regulated by the Food and Drug Administration (FDA), which requires it to meet EPA's drinking water standards. Enforcement is not strict, however. Many, but not all, states impose additional regulations. An estimated 25 to 30 percent of bottled water sold in the United States is obtained directly from municipal water supplies.[1]

Dilemmas in Compliance

A dilemma currently faced by New York City illustrates why it is so difficult to ensure safe drinking water for many Americans. New York gets most of its tap water from six reservoirs in the Catskill Mountains built in the 1950s and 1960s. For many years, the city was justly proud of the purity and taste of its water. However, the population in the watershed region has grown, and the quality of the water began to suffer in the 1970s and 1980s. More than 100 community sewage treatment plants discharged into the watershed area, many in violation of discharge permit standards. Substandard septic tanks also contributed to the problem. Dairy farms contributed tons of manure to the watershed. The amount of coliform bacteria measured in New York's water frequently violated EPA standards, and the amount of chlorine added to control bacteria increased to the level that it affected the water's taste. *Cryptosporidia* have also been found in the city's water. The EPA ordered New York to clean up the pollution or to build a filtration plant for the water from upstate reservoirs, setting a deadline of December 1996.[18]

New York City does not now filter the water from its upstate reservoirs, and the cost of constructing a filtration plant was estimated at up to $8 billion, a painful price for a city struggling with chronic financial difficulties. As an alternative, the city proposed a plan to protect the watershed by helping communities to upgrade their sewage plants, buying sensitive land near the reservoirs, and making changes in the way farmers dispose of manure. The upstate communities, already angry at the city for taking so much of their land for the reservoirs, were concerned that New York's plan would further harm the region's economy by discouraging development. While most experts believe that all water systems should include filtration, they agree that watershed protection is also important. Milwaukee's cryptosporidiosis outbreak occurred despite the fact that its system filters the water. In early 1997, New York City reached an agreement with the upstate region to implement the watershed protection plan.[19,20] After years of further negotiation, the City reached an agreement in 2007 with the EPA and the upstate counties for a 10-year Filtration Avoidance Determination.[21] The City has been buying land in the watershed region, which can be used for recreational purposes like hunting, fishing, and hiking, but cannot be developed. The agreement also calls for the City to work with communities to upgrade wastewater treatment plants and septic systems. It is also working with agricultural groups to develop pollution prevention programs for farmers. As an added protection, the city has built an untraviolet disinfection facility in Westchester County designed to kill *cryptosporidia* and *giardia* microorganisms.[21]

Meanwhile, New York City is under a court order to build a filtration plant for the older, more polluted reservoirs in the Croton system, located in suburban areas close to the city, which supply up to 10 percent of its water.[21] That plant, highly controversial, is now being built underground in the Bronx and is scheduled to be completed in 2012 at a cost of nearly $3 billion.[22]

The cost of ensuring safe drinking water is a major obstacle for many communities, large and small. While the federal government has provided some funds to assist states and localities in regulatory and remediation activities required by the Safe Drinking Water Act, the amount provided is never sufficient. In a report called *The Clean Water and Drinking Water Infrastructure Gap Analysis*, the EPA has shown that spending on water and sewage systems is inadequate to cope with such problems as leaks in aging water pipelines and failures in aging urban sewage systems.[23] In the absence of adequate funding, attempts to upgrade water supplies always involve disputes over who should pay for improvements.

Another dilemma concerning drinking water is that the very chemicals used to kill microbes in water may themselves be harmful to health. Chlorine, the most common disinfectant, reacts with organic matter to form byproducts that, some evidence shows, may be carcinogenic. Other, more expensive disinfection methods include bubbling ozone through the water, but these treatments tend to form other byproducts that may be equally harmful to health. There is no simple solution to this problem—even bottled water is required to meet only the same standards of purity as tap water, as discussed earlier in this chapter. General steps to prevent water pollution through eliminating point- and nonpoint-sources are helpful, however, since cleaner water sources require less treatment to meet drinking water standards.

A recent concern with implications that are still not known is the discovery in drinking water of trace amounts of a wide variety of hormones, pharmaceuticals, and household chemicals, most of which no one had thought to look for previously. Many of them probably get into wastewater when they are excreted by humans or animals and are not removed by sewage treatment systems. Some of the most frequently detected contaminants were steroids, insect repellants, antibiotics, and nonprescription drugs including caffeine and metabolites of nicotine. The health effects on humans of long-term exposure to low concentrations of these chemicals are not known, but there is evidence that they have ecological effects on fish and other aquatic species. For example, female hormones in very small concentrations have been found to cause feminization of male fish, and there is concern that human fetuses might similarly be affected.[24] It is not clear that this kind of contamination can be prevented, but it may be reduced by employing more care in disposal of medications and other chemicals, which should never be flushed down the drain.

Is the Water Supply Running Out?

Although water covers 71 percent of the earth's surface, most of it is in the form of salt water or ice in glaciers or polar ice caps. Less than 1 percent of the total amount consists of fresh water, potentially suitable for drinking, cooking, bathing, farming, and other human needs.[1] In many parts of the world, the supply of fresh water is inadequate for the demands of the local population. Already, political disputes are occurring in the United States over water shortages. Some heavily populated areas, including parts of Texas and New Mexico, are depleting finite underground water sources. In California, large quantities of water are transported to the central part of the state from the mountains for irrigation use while cities in the south complain of shortages. Water conservation measures of various kinds have been instituted throughout the United States, including legally mandated low-volume toilets and showerheads and limits on car washing and lawn watering in some areas during dry seasons.

As it becomes increasingly clear that pure water is a limited resource, it is also apparent that pure water is essential to public health.

Conclusion

Although Americans take it for granted that their tap water is safe to drink, outbreaks of waterborne illness are not uncommon in the United States; the 1993 cryptosporidiosis outbreak in Milwaukee is the most dramatic. Two federal laws are aimed at keeping the water supply clean and safe.

The Clean Water Act specifies that lakes and rivers should be fishable and swimmable. It imposes controls on point-source pollution, mainly discharges from municipal sewage systems and from industry, and nonpoint-source pollution, which is washed into waterways from the air and the land. Laws governing point-source pollution set requirements for treating wastewater before it can be discharged. Nonpoint-source pollution is more difficult to control.

The Safe Drinking Water Act requires the EPA to set standards for local drinking water systems and requires states to enforce the standards. However, the EPA was lax in setting the regulations, and states have been lax in enforcing them. Legislation passed in 1996 requires that community water systems provide annual reports to their customers on water contaminants, in hopes that public pressure will force better compliance with the standards.

Complying with federal drinking water standards is expensive, and many communities do not comply, including New York City, which spent years trying to find a way to clean up its reservoirs without building a multibillion-dollar filtration plant. In the most recent agreement with the EPA, reached in 2007, the City has agreed to work with upstate counties where its main reservoirs lie to protect the watershed. The City is also building a filtration plant in the Bronx to filter water from the more polluted reservoirs in areas closer to the City. Another dilemma concerning drinking water is that chlorine, the most common disinfectant used to kill microbes in the water, may itself cause harmful health effects. A recently discovered problem is that drinking water often contains pharmaceuticals and other household chemicals in low concentrations, the health effects of which are not known.

The supply of fresh water on earth is finite, and many areas of the world, including parts of the United States, suffer from shortages.

References

1. A. Nadakavukaren, *Our Global Environment: A Health Perspective*, 6th ed. (Prospect Heights, IL: Waveland Press, Inc., 2005).
2. U.S. Centers for Disease Control and Prevention, "Surveillance for Waterborne-Disease Outbreaks—United States, 1993–1994," *Morbidity and Mortality Weekly Report* 45 (1996): SS-1.
3. G. F. Craun et al., "Waterborne Outbreaks Reported in the United States," *Journal of Water and Health* 4 (2006), (Supplement 2): 19–30.
4. D. Zwick and M. Benstock, *Water Wasteland: Ralph Nader's Study Group Report on Water Pollution* (New York: Grossman Publishers, 1971).
5. W. J. Hayes, Jr., *Pesticides Studied in Man* (Baltimore, MD: Williams & Wilkins, 1982).
6. C. Duhigg, "Sewers at Capacity, Waste Poisons Waterways," *The New York Times*, November 23, 2009.
7. A. Nadakavukaren, *Our Global Environment: A Health Perspective*, 5th ed. (Prospect Heights, IL: Waveland Press, Inc., 2000).
8. U.S. Environmental Protection Agency, "National Water Quality Inventory: Report to Congress for the 2004 Reporting Cycle—A Profile." http://www.epa.gov/lawsregs/guidance/cwa/305b/upload/2009_01_22_305b_2004report_factsheet2004305b.pdf, accessed July 29, 2012.

9. U.S. Environmental Protection Agency, "Water on Tap: What You Need to Know." http://www.epa.gov/drink/guide/upload/book_waterontap_full.pdf, accessed July 29, 2012.

10. U.S. Centers for Disease Control and Prevention, "Surveillance for Waterborne Disease Outbreaks Associated with Drinking Water—United States, 2007–2008," *Morbidity and Mortality Weekly Report* 60 (SS12) (2011): 38–682.

11. U.S. Centers for Disease Control and Prevention, "Surveillance for Waterborne Disease Outbreaks and Other Health Events Associated with Recreational Water—United States, 2007–2008," *Morbidity and Mortality Weekly Report* 60 (SS12) (2011): 1–32.

12. C. Duhigg, "Clean Water Laws Neglected, at a Cost," *The New York Times*, September 13, 2009.

13. C. Duhigg, "That Tap Water Is Legal but May Be Unhealthy," *The New York Times*, December 17, 2009.

14. U.S. Environmental Protection Agency, "Basic Questions and Answers for the Drinking Water Strategy Contaminant Groups Effort," January 2011. http://www.epa.gov/lawsregs/rulesregs/sdwa/dwstrategy/upload/FactSheet_DrinkingWaterStrategy_VOCs.pdf, accessed November 17, 2012.

15. L. A. DeSimone, P. A. Hamilton, and R. J. Gilliom, "Quality of Ground Water from Private Domestic Wells," *Water Well Journal* 63 (2009), No. 4: 33–37.

16. U.S. Centers for Disease Control and Prevention, "Surveillance for Waterborne Disease Outbreaks in the United States, 1999–2000," *Morbidity and Mortality Weekly Report* 51(SS08) (2002): 1–28.

17. U.S. Centers for Disease Control and Prevention, "Drinking Water: Commercially Bottled Water." http://www.cdc.gov/healthywater/drinking/bottled/, accessed July 31, 2012.

18. A. Finder, "Delay Sought on Approving Watershed Plans," *The New York Times*, April 7, 1995.

19. A. Revkin, "New York Begins Spending to Save City's Reservoirs," *The New York Times*, January 22, 1997.

20. A. Revkin, "Billion-Dollar Plan to Clean New York City Water at Its Source," *The New York Times*, August 31, 1997.

21. New York City Department of Environmental Protection, "New York City 2011 Drinking Water Supply and Quality Report." http://nyc.gov/html/dep/pdf/wsstate11.pdf, accessed July 31, 2012.

22. A. DePalma, "For Bronx Water Plant Being Built 10 Stories Down, A Towering Price Tag," *The New York Times*, April 24, 2008.

23. U.S. Environmental Protection Agency, *The Clean Water and Drinking Water Infrastructure Gap Analysis*. http://www.epa.gov/owm/gapreport.pdf, accessed August 12, 2009.

24. B. M. Kuehn, "Traces of Drugs Found in Drinking Water," *Journal of the American Medical Association* 299 (2008): 2011–2013.

Solid and Hazardous Wastes: What to Do with the Garbage?

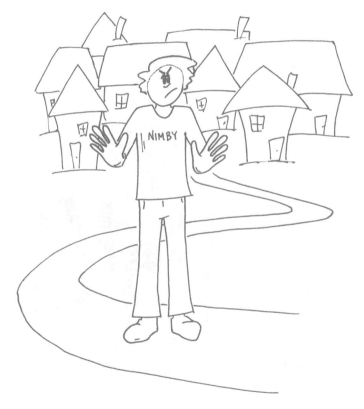

Not in My Backyard

In the spring and summer of 1987, the problem of solid waste disposal was brought to national attention by the plight of the "garbage barge" that could not find a place to unload its cargo. Carrying more than 3000 tons of commercial trash banned from the local landfill in Islip, New York, the barge's vain search for a disposal site somewhere along the Atlantic or Gulf coasts, Belize or the Bahamas, made national news over a 5-month period. Finally, the barge returned to New York, and the trash was incinerated.[1]

Americans dispose of about 250 million tons of municipal solid waste each year.[2] In 2010, this amounted to 4.43 pounds per person per day. Municipal solid waste includes durable goods, nondurable goods, containers and packaging, food scraps, yard trimmings, and miscellaneous inorganic wastes from residential, commercial, institutional, and industrial sources. It does not include construction and demolition debris, automobile bodies, municipal sludges, and industrial process wastes, all of which must also be disposed of in some way. Figure 23-1 gives a breakdown of the composition of municipal solid wastes. The greatest portion of it is paper; much of it is packaging.

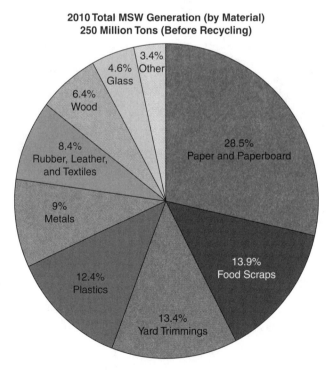

FIGURE 23-1   Composition of Municipal Solid Waste, 2010. *Source:* Reproduced from U.S. Environmental Protection Agency, "Municipal Solid Waste Generation," July 24, 2012. http://www.epa.gov/wastes/nonhaz/municipal/, accessed October 1, 2012.

Garbage collection has been an important responsibility of local governments since the late 19th century. At that time, it was recognized that rats, flies, and other vermin attracted by garbage carry diseases such as plague and typhus. Even earlier, enlightened cities—including ancient Athens—required that wastes be disposed of outside the city walls.

Until the 1970s, little attention was paid to what was done with the garbage after it was taken away from residential neighborhoods. Most often, it was disposed of in open dumps. Sometimes it was burned, either in incinerators or out in the open, at the dump. Another approach was to pour it into nearby rivers, lakes, or oceans. The drawbacks of these methods became obvious as the volume of garbage increased. Garbage washed up on beaches and contaminated drinking water. Incinerators emitted foul odors, noxious fumes, and black smoke. Dumps, in addition to supporting large populations of vermin, produced toxic leachates that seeped through the soil and contaminated groundwater.

Environmental protection laws banned these methods of waste disposal, which merely transferred garbage from one part of the environment to another. The Clean Air Act made most incinerators illegal; the Clean Water Act outlawed dumping into rivers and lakes; and the Marine Protection, Research, and Sanctuaries Act of 1972, with later amendments, prohibited most ocean dumping. Open dumps were outlawed by many states and then by the federal government in 1976 with the Resource Conservation and Recovery Act, RCRA ("rickra"), as it is known, also set standards for sanitary landfills, which have replaced dumps as the most common method of municipal waste disposal.[1]

Sanitary Landfills

Current standards for sanitary landfills require wastes to be confined in a sealed area. A properly designed landfill starts with an appropriate site, which should be dry and consist of impervious clay soil. A large hole is dug and lined with plastic. Refuse is spread in thin layers, compacted by bulldozers, and covered each day with a thin layer of soil. Since decomposing organic matter produces liquids, which may dissolve metals and other toxins, and potentially explosive gases, vents and drains must be constructed to control these hazards. In recent decades, some landfills have collected the gases and used them directly as an alternative fuel or burned them to produce renewable energy in the form of electricity.[2] When the landfill has reached its capacity, it is covered with a 2-foot layer of soil. The surface can then be used for a park, golf course, or other recreational facility.

The biggest drawback of sanitary landfills as a method of waste disposal is that they take up a lot of space. In many parts of the country there is no shortage of this commodity, but some urban areas are running out of land. It is expensive to transport garbage from crowded areas to disposal sites with plenty of free space. A measure of the availability of landfill space is the "tipping fee," the cost for disposing of a ton of municipal solid waste. In 2010, the average tipping fee in the United States for burial in a landfill was $43.99 per ton.[3] The northeast has the highest tipping fees; the fee in Massachusetts was $105.40.[4] Complicating the problem for cities is the phenomenon known as "NIMBY," meaning not in my backyard. People do not want a landfill in their neighborhood. Even people in areas of the country that have plenty of open space resist the idea of having to accept garbage sent from faraway cities.

The problem is epitomized by the garbage crisis in New York City, brought to a head by residents' complaints about the Fresh Kills landfill on Staten Island, a relatively rural borough located within city limits. Fresh Kills began taking garbage in 1948, and by 1996 it was accepting about 13,000 tons per day. It never met even minimal environmental standards, and in 1996 the Environmental Protection Agency (EPA) ordered it to cut down on emissions of noxious gases.[5] Meanwhile, the city's Department of Sanitation proposed to conduct regular tours of the site—"the world's largest dump"—a proposal which horrified city authorities and was promptly squelched.[6] Mayor Rudolph Giuliani then proposed to close it down. Fresh Kills was closed, with much fanfare, in March 2001. Except for its use to dispose of World Trade Center debris after September 11 of that year, the site has remained closed. Since then, the city has struggled with the difficulties of sending the wastes to landfills in other states, mostly Pennsylvania and Virginia. City sanitation trucks take the 12,000 tons of residential wastes per day to transfer stations in the five boroughs and New Jersey, where it is loaded onto tractor trailers for the trip. Roughly the same amount of commercial waste is managed by private carting companies, but it ends up in the same place. The total cost to the city of disposing of a ton of trash in 2004 had risen to $75—40 percent more than it cost in 1997, and there was concern about the willingness of Pennsylvania and Virginia to continue accepting New York's garbage.[7] In 2006, the city published a comprehensive solid-waste management plan, designed to address environmental issues, to increase reliability, and to reduce cost. The plan, which is now being implemented despite many controversies, includes an increase in recycling, a shift from reliance on trucks to trains and barges for carrying trash out of the City (to reduce pollution and fuel costs), and an attempt to find landfill space within New York State.[8]

Meanwhile, Fresh Kills is being turned into a park. The mountains of garbage need to settle and then will be capped with more than 2 feet of soil. Work is underway to turn the former landfill into acres of marshes and streams full of wildlife, as well as paths for hikers, bikers, horses, and cross-country skiers. The first phase is expected to be ready for use by 2014, but it may take another 30 years to complete the project.[9]

Alternatives to Landfills

Currently, about 54 percent of municipal solid waste, as well as wastes from other sources, is disposed of in landfills.[2] It is obvious that the garbage crisis could be eased if the volume that goes to landfills could be reduced. The only way to make landfills last longer is to apply the "three R's": reduce, reuse, and recycle. Prevention of a disposal problem by reducing waste materials at the source is obviously the most efficient approach. Consumer behavior holds the key to successfully reducing waste by this approach. It requires people to buy only the amount of a product that will be used, to choose items without excessive packaging, and to use reusable napkins, towels, diapers, dishes, and cups rather than the disposable variety. The popularity of yard sales is a favorable trend toward achieving reduction of waste through reuse. Although governmental action to encourage the reduction of wastes is still not widespread, there are steps that some communities have taken as incentives. Some residential garbage-pickup services charge by the bag, encouraging residents to cut down on volume. Some states impose taxes on hard-to-dispose-of items such as tires, batteries, and motor oil.

Recycling, technically called resource recovery, is rapidly growing as a method of reducing the amount of waste that must be put in landfills. In 2010, about 34 percent of municipal solid waste was recycled nationwide.[2] Providing curbside collection of separated recyclables is a way that communities encourage recycling. Having refundable deposits on bottles and cans is a very effective way to encourage recycling. As of 2010, 10 states require deposits; recycling rates are 70 to 90 percent in these states, about 2.5 times the rate in states without bottle bills. Michigan, which raised its deposit to 10 cents per bottle, the highest in the nation, has a recycling rate of 95 percent.[10]

The greatest obstacle to the growth of recycling is a lack of a market for used glass, metal, plastic, and paper. Paper is a special problem; it constitutes such a large proportion of trash, and yet it cannot be recycled indefinitely because the fibers break down. Some states require that newspapers contain a specified minimum percentage of recycled fiber. Since governments use large quantities of paper, they can make a significant impact on the recycled paper market. The U.S. government mandates that its agencies use paper containing at least 20 percent recycled content, and many states have similar requirements.[1] Because a healthy market for recyclables depends on their use for new products, the economic downturn in 2008 and 2009 had a negative impact on the market for all recycled materials. Recycling will remain cost-effective, however, as long as the price of placing trash in landfills remains high.[11]

Composting is a form of recycling that allows the natural decay processes to convert yard and food wastes to mulch, useful in gardening. Composting may be done on an individual or municipal level. Some communities mix their compost with sewage sludge to produce a rich fertilizer for agricultural uses.

Another approach to useful disposal of solid waste is waste-to-energy incineration, which both reduces solid waste and produces heat and energy. Special incinerators for this purpose have been designed to minimize the emission of air pollutants. However, the possibility still exists that they may emit toxic gases, including dioxins and furans from the burning of plastics, lead, cadmium, and mercury vapors from batteries mixed in with municipal wastes. Incinerator ash must be disposed of as a hazardous waste, because it frequently contains dangerous levels of heavy metals. NIMBY opposition tends to make finding a site for a waste-to-energy incinerator politically difficult, and building and operating one is expensive because of all the safety features required.[1] About 12 percent of municipal solid waste is disposed of by incineration.[2]

Hazardous Wastes

A small but significant percentage of solid waste is hazardous waste. These are materials that are toxic to humans, plants, or animals; are likely to explode; or are corrosive and thus likely to burn through containers or human skin. Two special categories of hazardous wastes that are regulated under separate laws are radioactive wastes and infectious medical wastes.

The problem of hazardous waste disposal first came to public attention in 1978 when Love Canal made the news. Residents of a 20-year-old housing development in the town of Niagara Falls, New York, had been noticing some alarming phenomena. After a season of heavy rains and snowfalls, noxious chemicals had begun to bubble up in backyards and seep into basements. Chemical odors were prevalent. Children developed rashes and watering eyes after playing outdoors. Heavy rains washed away soil to reveal buried metal drums, which were corroded and leaking. Reports began to circulate of cancer, birth defects, miscarriages, and other health problems among residents of the area. The alarmed citizens demanded that something be done.[1]

The New York State Health Department and the EPA began to investigate. Analyses of soil samples from backyards, air samples in the basements of homes, and water samples in sump pumps and storm sewers revealed contamination by more than 200 different chemicals, including benzene, dioxin, pesticides, and a number of other known carcinogens and teratogens. In August 1978, President Carter declared Love Canal a Federal Disaster Area. Over the next several years, hundreds of Love Canal families were evacuated from their homes.[1]

The source of the problem was an abandoned industrial dump, a trench originally intended to be a canal but never finished, which was used by a chemical company for disposal of its wastes over a 10-year period. In 1952, the trench was declared full and covered with soil. The city took over the property to build a school. By the time home building began in the neighborhood several years later, most people had forgotten about the former activities at the site, and it did not occur to anyone that the area might be hazardous.

Over much of the same period that the Love Canal problems were taking place, another hazardous waste drama was playing out in Missouri. The first act consisted of several episodes in 1971, when waste oil was sprayed on the floors of several horse arenas around the state, a practice used to keep the dust down. After the spraying, a wave of mysterious illnesses began affecting animals and people who came in contact with the dirt. Several children were sickened, some with chloracne, and some had to be hospitalized with severe flu-like symptoms. Horses were badly affected, and many died. Hundreds of dead birds were found in the area. The waste oil was suspected, but the hauler claimed there was nothing unusual about the oil. Investigators from the Missouri Department of Health and the Centers for Disease Control and Prevention (CDC) could find nothing unusual in the soil samples or in the blood of the victims. Meanwhile, the same hauler had been hired to spray oil on 23 miles of dirt roads in Times Beach, a community of about 2000 people near St. Louis, during the summer of 1972 and during each of the next four summers.[12]

CDC scientists continued to run tests on the soil from the horse arenas, and in 1974 they identified dioxin at concentrations as high as 31,000 parts per billion (ppb). This was more than high enough to cause human illnesses and the deaths of animals. Further investigation revealed that the oil hauler had been hired by a chemical company to dispose of wastes from the manufacture of Agent Orange, the herbicide used in the Vietnam War. The hauler was mixing this waste oil with used crankcase oil and using it for his spraying operations. The CDC was able to trace the hauler's activities and discovered Times Beach, among other places, where no problems had been suspected. That was in 1982, at just about the time when the community was inundated by a flood which, it was feared, spread the dioxin throughout the town. Tests found dioxin levels on the order of 100 ppb on roads and in yards. Residents panicked.[12]

In the end, Times Beach, like Love Canal, was evacuated. In retrospect, the decision has been widely criticized as an overreaction. The levels of dioxin in Times Beach were much lower than those in the horse arenas, and more modest remediation would probably have sufficed. However, little was known at that time about the toxicity and carcinogenicity of dioxin in humans. The effects on animals were certainly a cause of concern.

Love Canal residents have been carefully tracked for health outcomes that might be associated with the exposures. The New York State Department of Health interviewed over 6000 former residents between 1978 and 1982, and in 1996 it began searching records of births and deaths and state registries of cancer diagnoses and congenital malformations for evidence of health problems. In a report of the study published in 2008, there was clear evidence of adverse reproductive outcomes, including low birth weight and preterm birth, among women who had lived at Love Canal. Especially notable was the finding that women who had been exposed to waste at Love Canal as children were twice as likely to give birth to infants with congenital malformations than were comparable women who had grown up elsewhere. There were also indications of an increased risk of some forms of cancer, especially lung cancer.[13] The follow-up of these residents will be continued.

RCRA, the federal legislation first enacted in 1976 to deal with solid waste disposal, included special regulations on handling of wastes that potentially posed a hazard to health and the environment. These regulations, which were strengthened by amendments to RCRA in 1984 and 1992, can prevent future Love Canals and Times Beaches. They require that all hazardous wastes be accounted for "from cradle to grave," and there are criminal penalties for those who violate the laws. However, legal disposal of hazardous wastes is expensive, and no one knows how much illegal "midnight dumping" may actually go on today.[1]

RCRA lists many specific wastes that are regulated under the law, including wastes from petroleum refining, pesticide manufacturing, and some pharmaceutical products. Wastes are also considered hazardous if they are ignitable, corrosive, reactive, or toxic. The regulations are stricter for large-quantity generators, facilities that generate more than 2200 pounds per month, than for small-quantity generators, facilities that generate between 220 and 2200 pounds per month. Facilities that generate the smallest amounts of waste are subject to only minimal requirements. The RCRA regulations have two key elements: tracking and permitting. The tracking requirement, illustrated in **Figure 23-2**, mandates that paperwork document the progress of hazardous waste from its site of generation through treatment, storage, and disposal. Permitting means that any facility that treats, stores, or disposes of hazardous waste must be issued a permit from the EPA or the state; the permit prescribes standards for management of the waste. Transportation of hazardous waste, which must be clearly labeled, is regulated by the U.S. Department of Transportation.[14]

According to the EPA, over 40 million tons of hazardous wastes are managed annually under the RCRA regulations.[15] As with municipal solid waste, hazardous waste is managed by practicing the three R's: reduce, reuse, and recycle. One way of reducing the waste is by treating it to make it less hazardous; this can be done, for example, by biological or chemical treatment, by burning the waste at high temperatures, and by separating solids from wastewater to reduce the volume of waste that must be disposed of. A common method of disposing of liquid hazardous waste is by injecting it under pressure into underground wells encased with steel and concrete. Specially designed landfills are also used for disposing of hazardous waste. Efforts to reduce the generation of hazardous wastes have paid off, however, and the volume that needs to be disposed of is much reduced from previous decades.[16]

While RCRA was meant to control hazardous wastes as they are generated, it was inadequate to deal with old waste sites that kept turning up in the news after the public consciousness had been raised. In response, in 1980 Congress passed the Comprehensive Environmental Response, Compensation, and Liability Act, known as "Superfund." That law required the EPA to compile a priority list of waste sites that threatened the public health or environmental quality, and it authorized $1.6 billion over a 5-year period for emergency cleanup of these sites. The cleanup was paid for by a tax on industry, which created the trust fund that gave the program its name. Superfund was reauthorized in 1986 and 1990, allocating additional billions of dollars for cleanup.[1]

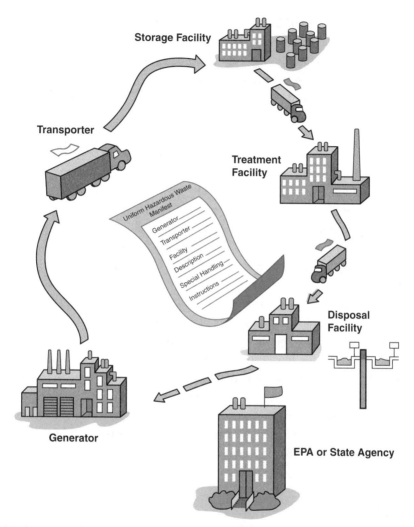

FIGURE 23-2   Tracking of Hazardous Wastes. *Source:* Reproduced from U.S. Environmental Protection Agency, "RCRA: Reducing Risk From Waste," p. 20, September 1997. http://www.epa.gov/epawaste/inforesources/pubs/risk/risk-1.pdf, accessed October 1, 2012.

The Superfund program has been mired in controversy from the beginning. The pace of the cleanup has been slow, and the cost has been very high. New sites are being added to the priority list more rapidly than old sites are being cleaned up and removed. As of 2005, there were 1242 sites on the list. Cleanup had been completed on 926 sites.[1] Because the legislation calls for polluters to pay, a great deal of effort has been spent on trying to establish who is liable. Congress did not reauthorize the corporate taxes that paid into the trust fund when the tax expired in 1995, and the fund has been exhausted. Although cleanup of many sites is going forward, paid for by the polluters—for example, General Electric Company is paying for the dredging of the Hudson River—cleanup of "orphan" sites, for which the responsible company could not be identified or could not pay, is now being paid for with taxpayer dollars. The amount of funds for this purpose in the federal budget has not grown in recent years, and many sites are far short of the funds that are needed.

Another problem faced by the Superfund program is the shortage of cleanup options: what to do with the toxic materials removed from a site. To prevent the mere removal of toxic materials from one place to another, Congress specified that cleanup actions should permanently and significantly reduce the volume, toxicity, or mobility of hazardous substances. Creative solutions are urgently needed. There are also disagreements over how clean is clean enough. The EPA's "Brownfields" initiative sets lower standards for sites designated for industrial use, an approach that makes cleanup easier but is less acceptable to some communities.[1]

Americans have been very concerned about hazardous waste disposal and cleanup, especially when it affects their neighborhoods. Some critics believe that the degree of concern is out of proportion to the actual risk to public health. While the release of toxic gases into the air and the leaching of toxic liquids into water supplies are important public health risks because many humans are likely to be exposed to the hazards, risks from toxic substances buried in the ground are much less certain. At times, close to one-quarter of the EPA's entire budget has been allocated to the Superfund program, and additional funds are contributed by industry. At present, it is not clear whether this is a rational allocation of the spending on the environment. Methods of analyzing risk and understanding the balance between benefits and costs can help make such decisions.

Coal Ash

A previously obscure category of waste hit the news just before Christmas 2008, when a dam on the banks of a Tennessee River tributary broke, spilling a billion gallons of toxic sludge across 300 acres of East Tennessee. The earthen dam was holding back millions of cubic yards of wet coal ash, waste from a Tennessee Valley Authority power plant that burned 14,000 tons of coal per day and supplied enough electricity for 670,000 households. In addition to destroying and damaging homes in the area, the spill polluted the river water with thousands of pounds of arsenic, lead, and other toxic and carcinogenic metals.[17]

It turns out that coal ash was not regulated by the EPA, which had been studying the issue for over 28 years amid controversy about whether to consider it hazardous or nonhazardous waste. Meanwhile, the volume of ash produced grew from less than 90 million tons in 1990 to 121 million tons in 2007. Most of the waste is stored in more than 1300 open dumps around the country, where heavy metal contaminants have been leached into water in at least 26 states. The results have been decimated fish, bird, and frog populations and contaminated drinking water for an unknown number of people. Coal ash has also been used for construction landfill, mine reclamation, and "improvement" of soil for agricultural and golf courses.[18] The Obama administration promised to propose new regulations on coal ash by the end of 2009, but in 2010 EPA Administrator Lisa Jackson labeled coal ash nonhazardous, meaning that it will be regulated by the states.[19,20]

Conclusion

As concern about environmental pollution has grown, the problem of disposing of solid wastes has become more difficult to resolve. Traditional solutions, such as dumping garbage into waterways or incinerating it, can no longer be used because they increase water and air pollution. Old-fashioned open dumps cause noxious odors and attract vermin.

Solid-waste disposal is now confined to sanitary landfills, which must meet federal standards. But in many parts of the country, there is a shortage of space available for landfills. Communities resist having sanitary landfills sited near them—the NIMBY phenomenon.

The problem of finding space for garbage could be eased if the volume of garbage could be reduced, for example, by eliminating excessive packaging and charging consumers for disposal by volume. Recycling and use of reusable, as opposed to disposable, products also help to reduce the volume of garbage.

Hazardous wastes present an especially difficult disposal problem. Several environmental scandals in the 1970s and early 1980s, including Love Canal in New York State and Times Beach in Missouri, brought national attention to the need for regulation of hazardous waste disposal. Federal legislation known as RCRA requires that all hazardous wastes be accounted for "from cradle to grave." Superfund legislation provides for identification and cleanup of hazardous-waste sites dating from before RCRA. Although both programs have shortcomings, they have contributed—along with federal laws on air and water pollution—to a significant improvement in the environment. Congress has not reauthorized the corporate taxes to support cleanup under Superfund, but the program continues, paid for by polluters and taxpayers.

An environmental problem that has emerged recently is coal ash, waste from coal-burning power plants, which has not been regulated by law. Recent spills from coal ash dumps into rivers and other bodies of water have called attention to the toxic contaminants contained in the ash, poisoning wildlife and threatening human health.

References

1. A. Nadakavukaren, *Our Global Environment: A Health Perspective*, 5th ed. (Prospect Heights, IL: Waveland Press, 2000).
2. U.S. Environmental Protection Agency, "Municipal Solid Waste Generation, Recycling, and Disposal in the United States: Facts and Figures for 2010." http://www.epa.gov/epawaste/nonhaz/municipal/pubs/msw_2010_rev_factsheet.pdf, accessed August 1, 2012.
3. National Solid Waste Management Association, "Municipal Solid Waste Landfill Facts." http://www.environmentalistseveryday.org/docs/research-bulletin/Municipal-Solid-Waste-Landfill-Facts.pdf, accessed August 1, 2012.
4. S. Wright, "Tipping Fees Vary Across the U.S.," *Waste and Recycling News*, July 20, 2012. http://www.wasterecyclingnews.com/article/20120720/NEWS01/120729997/tipping-fees-vary-across-the-u-s, accessed August 1, 2012.
5. I. Fisher, "EPA Tells Landfills to Curb Gas Emissions," *The New York Times*, March 3, 1996.
6. B. Weber, "Broadway, Statue of Liberty and Fresh Kills? World's Biggest Garbage Dump Hopes to Draw Tourists as Well as Gulls," *The New York Times*, March 27, 1996.
7. W. C. Thompson, Jr., City of New York, Office of the Comptroller, "No Room to Move: New York City's Impending Solid Waste Crisis." http://old.gothamgazette.com/comptrollertrash.pdf, accessed August 1, 2012.
8. New York City Department of Sanitation, "Comprehensive Solid Waste Management Plan." http://www.nyc.gov/html/dsny/html/swmp/swmp-4oct.shtml, accessed August 1, 2012.
9. J. S. Russell, "Garbage Mountains Slowly Morph Into $160 Million New York Park," *The New York Times*, September 23, 2010.
10. Container Recycling Institute, "Bottle Bill Resource Guide." http://www.bottlebill.org, accessed August 2, 2012.
11. M. Richtel and K. Galbraith, "Back at Junk Value, Recyclables Are Piling Up," *The New York Times*, December 8, 2008.
12. M. J. Schneider, *Persistent Poisons: Chemical Pollutants in the Environment* (New York: The New York Academy of Sciences, 1979).
13. New York State Department of Health, "Love Canal Follow-up Health Study," October 2008. http://www.health.state.ny.us/environmental/investigations/love_canal/docs/report_public_comment_final.pdf, accessed September 27, 2012.
14. U.S. Environmental Protection Agency, *RCRA: Reducing Risk from Waste*. http://www.epa.gov/epawaste/inforesources/pubs/risk/risk-1.pdf, accessed August 2, 2012.
15. U.S. Environmental Protection Agency, "Hazardous Wastes." http://www.epa.gov/wastes/basic-hazard.htm, July 24, 2012, accessed September 27, 2012.
16. U.S. Environmental Protection Agency, "25 Years of RCRA: Building on Our Past to Protect Our Future." http://www.epa.gov/wastes/inforesources/pubs/k02027.pdf, accessed August 2, 2012.
17. S. Dewan, "At Plant in Coal Ash Spill, Toxic Deposits by the Ton," *The New York Times*, December 30, 2008.

18. S. Dewan, "Hundreds of Coal Ash Dumps Lack Significant Regulation," *The New York Times*, January 7, 2009.

19. S. Dewan, "Administration Plans New Regulations On Coal-Ash Ponds by End of the Year," *The New York Times*, March 8, 2009.

20. P. Reis, "EPA Backs Off 'Hazardous' Label for Coal Ash After White House Review," *The New York Times*, May 7, 2010.

Safe Food and Drugs: An Ongoing Regulatory Battle

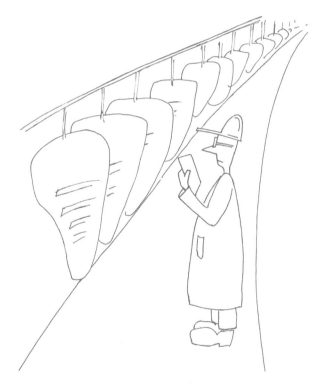

Meat Inspection

Americans are very concerned about the safety of their food. Although Americans used to think of their food supply as the safest in the world, this confidence has been shaken in the last few years by widely publicized outbreaks of illnesses caused by foods ranging from bagged spinach to peanut butter.

Since only the most serious cases of foodborne disease are reported, the extent of the problem is unclear. The Centers for Disease Control and Prevention (CDC) has estimated that 48 million people contract foodborne diseases each year, with 3000 deaths, an estimate that has declined since the early 2000s.[1] With some 300 million people eating three meals per day, not counting snacks, however, the likelihood of getting sick from eating a single meal is extremely small. Many government agencies—local, state, and federal—are involved with regulating food safety. The challenge is enormous: an analysis published in 1992 estimated that some 6100 meat and poultry plants, more than 50,000 food processing establishments, about 537,000 commercial restaurants, 172,000 institutional food programs, 190,000 retail food stores, and 1 million food vending locations are subject to government inspection, and the numbers have certainly grown.[2]

The need for government oversight of the food supply, like many other public health measures, arose with the urbanization of the population. City dwellers neither grew their own food nor knew its source and history. Demands for action arose as the public became aware of unhygienic conditions such as those in meatpacking plants—conditions revealed in Upton Sinclair's 1906 novel, *The Jungle*. Other widespread practices that outraged the public included adulteration of supposedly pure food with cheaper materials and the use of sometimes toxic additives to improve color and conceal spoilage. The Federal Food and Drug Act and the Meat Inspection Act, both passed in 1906, established a program to supervise and control the circumstances of manufacture, labeling, and sale of food.[3]

Because similar abuses occurred in the sale of medicines, the 1906 Act included provisions to control manufacturing, labeling, and sale of drugs. The Food and Drug Administration (FDA), created to oversee regulation of food and drugs, was later given authority over cosmetics, medical devices, and feed and drugs for pets and farm animals.

Causes of Foodborne Illness

Foodborne diseases are most often caused by contamination of foods with bacteria, viruses, or parasites due to breakdowns in sanitation and/or proper food handling practices. *Salmonella* bacteria, for example, are common contaminants of poultry, meat, and eggs. Infected hens may transfer the pathogens to the eggs as they are being formed in the ovary. Although the bacteria are killed when the food is thoroughly cooked, people who prefer their meat rare or their egg yolks runny are at risk of salmonellosis, especially if the food has been kept at room temperature long enough for the bacteria to flourish. Caesar salad dressing made with raw eggs and homemade eggnog are particularly risky. The symptoms of salmonellosis, like symptoms of most types of food poisoning, include vomiting, diarrhea, and abdominal pain.

Like *Salmonella* in poultry and eggs, *Escherichia coli* 0157:H7 is widespread in beef, probably due to the way livestock are raised and processed. To prevent illness and deaths such as those that occurred in 1993 in Seattle, hamburgers must be cooked more thoroughly than the previous standard required. In addition to its occurrence in ground beef, *E. coli* 0157:H7 has also turned up in other foods, including salami, raw milk, lettuce, alfalfa sprouts, and unpasteurized apple juice. The bacteria are common in the intestinal tracts of cows and are excreted with their feces. The contaminated juice may have been made from apples that fell onto ground where cows had wandered, and the contaminated lettuce was prepared under unsanitary conditions near a cow pen.[4,5] The alfalfa sprouts could have been contaminated by being grown in fields near cattle feed lots and irrigated with water contaminated by manure.[6]

In fact, fresh produce is responsible for an increasing proportion of foodborne illness. In 2006, fruits and vegetables caused almost as many cases of illness as were caused by beef, poultry, and seafood combined.[7] A hepatitis A outbreak among people who had eaten at a Chi-Chi's restaurant in Pennsylvania in fall 2003 was traced to green onions imported from Mexico. More than 600 people were infected, and 3 people died.[8,9] In 2008, the largest foodborne disease outbreak in the previous decade was attributed to *Salmonella*-contaminated jalapeño and serrano peppers imported from Mexico. Investigators traced infection to two farms, where a pool of water used for irrigation was found to contain the bacteria. The investigation was made especially difficult because few of the interviewed victims recalled eating peppers, which were probably a minor ingredient in dishes that were remembered to contain tomatoes. The outbreak sickened 1442 people and contributed to 2 deaths in 43 states, the District of Columbia, and Canada.[10]

Fish and shellfish are likely to harbor pathogenic microbes if they are harvested from waters polluted by human sewage. Raw clams and oysters are especially dangerous: because they grow in shallow coastal waters, which are likely to be polluted, these shellfish may carry cholera and related bacteria, hepatitis A virus, and the common Norwalk virus, all capable of causing disease in humans. Fish used uncooked for Japanese dishes such as sushi and sashimi and South American ceviche may also carry parasites harmful to humans.[3]

Some bacteria cause illness by way of toxins they produce rather than by simple infection. Thus these contaminants are hazardous even after the food is cooked. The best known—and deadliest—of these are the bacteria that cause botulism. They flourish in the absence of oxygen and are most commonly associated with home-canned vegetables that were inadequately cooked before canning, although a number of botulism outbreaks have been traced to commercially canned foods. Once the toxin is formed, it can be destroyed only by boiling for 15 to 20 minutes, not a common practice with canned foods. Certain fish and shellfish may also contain toxins—for example, ciguatoxin or scombroid poison—produced by bacteria or algae that the fish feed on or that grow on them, thereby poisoning the flesh for human consumption.[3]

Food may also be contaminated by the actions of food handlers, either if they themselves are infected or if they transfer pathogens from one food to another. For example, a salad might be contaminated with *Salmonella* if the raw vegetables are chopped on a cutting board that had previously been used to cut up uncooked chicken. A number of other bacterial or viral infections tend to be transferred by infected food handlers to raw or cooked foods, such as salads, hot dogs, and delicatessen takeout items. The famous case of Typhoid Mary illustrates how an infected food handler can spread pathogenic bacteria even when she herself has no symptoms. Hepatitis A virus is also frequently transmitted by food handlers who are careless about hygiene. The disease is most contagious 10 to 14 days before the onset of symptoms.

Government Action to Prevent Foodborne Disease

A variety of federal, state, and local agencies are responsible for protecting the safety of the food supply. Because of patchwork legislation, division of responsibility, and lack of coordination, there are major inconsistencies among different types of food in the way food safety is regulated. Increasingly, it has become clear that the system depends too heavily on detecting and correcting problems after they occur rather than preventing them. As nutritionist Marion Nestle stated in her 2010 book, *Safe Food: The Politics of Food Safety*, "Today, an inventory of federal food safety activities reveals a system breathtaking in its irrationality."[11(p.55)] Some of the shortcomings were remedied by the FDA Food Safety Modernization Act, signed by President Obama in January 2011, though many problems remain.

The FDA and the Department of Agriculture (USDA) share the primary responsibility for ensuring that foods are safe, wholesome, and properly labeled. The laws governing the actions of the two agencies are highly inconsistent. The USDA is responsible for the safety of meat and poultry, including prepared products that contain more than 2 percent of cooked meat or poultry, as well as for processed eggs. The law requires inspection of all meat- and poultry-processing plants daily and that an inspector must be on site whenever a slaughtering plant is in operation. The plants that the USDA inspects account for about 20 percent of federally regulated foods and 27 percent of foodborne illness outbreaks. Its budget for food safety in 2009 was $972 million.[12]

The FDA is responsible for all other foods, including seafood and produce, which amount to about 80 percent of federally regulated foods, accounting for 67 percent of reported foodborne illness outbreaks. After increases in appropriations in 2008 and 2009, its annual budget for food safety had grown to $649 million, still far less than USDA's. Because of budgetary constraints, the FDA can inspect food-processing facilities under its jurisdiction only once every 10 years, on average. This leads to the paradox that a plant making frozen cheese pizza may be inspected (by the FDA) only once every 10 years, while a plant making frozen pepperoni pizza will be inspected (by the USDA) almost every day. The Food Safety Modernization Law put additional responsibilities on the FDA, including expanded inspections and setting standards for the safe growing, harvesting, sorting, packing, and storage of fresh fruits and vegetables.

However, in the climate of congressional budget cutting, it is not clear how adequate the FDA's budget will be for carrying out these tasks.

An increasing proportion of Americans' food is imported from other countries, especially developing countries, which is a challenge to the food safety system. About 40 to 45 percent of fresh fruits and vegetables and over 75 percent of seafood sold in the United States are imported.[13] The USDA has the power to bar importing of meat and poultry from countries with inferior food safety systems, a power the FDA lacked for fruits, vegetables, grains, and fish until the passage of the Modernization Act in 2011. It still must rely on port-of-entry inspections, an expensive and ineffective approach, but it now has the authority to deny entry of food from a facility that refuses to permit FDA inspection and it can detain for testing shipments of food that it has reason to believe may be harmful.[14]

Because they are eaten raw, fruits and vegetables imported from countries with inadequate safety systems are especially risky, causing, for example, the hepatitis A outbreak from Mexican green onions, the *Salmonella* outbreak from Mexican peppers, and an outbreak caused by the parasite *Cyclospora* on Guatamalan raspberries in the 1990s. As one CDC official is quoted as saying, "We used to believe you had to travel overseas to get travelers' diarrhea. It's a classic example of emerging infections common in Latin America becoming a problem here."[15]

Fish and shellfish cause more outbreaks than any other food category.[16] Regulation of the fish industry, which falls mainly under jurisdiction of the FDA, is especially difficult because most fish are caught in the wild by independent fishermen in relatively small boats. Fish may have been exposed to viruses or bacterial toxins in polluted waters, or they may have been contaminated with scombroid toxin due to inadequate cooling on the boat. Currently no techniques are available that would allow inspectors on the docks to test for these problems. Shellfish should, in theory, be easier to regulate because their source can be determined. However, much of the enforcement is left to the states, and some of them are lax about enforcing standards.

Fish also have the potential to be contaminated with nonmicrobial toxins. Research published in 2004 revealed that farmed salmon contained potentially dangerous levels of PCBs, as well as dioxin and several organochlorine pesticides. It turned out that farmed fish were fed a concentrated feed that was tainted with the chemicals. Since the news broke, fish farmers are experimenting with new feeds that will eliminate the PCB problem.[3] Another hazard from fish was revealed in 2008, when *The New York Times* published a report that it had found high levels of mercury in sushi made from tuna in 20 Manhattan stores and restaurants.[17] It has long been known that pregnant women and children should limit their consumption of some varieties of canned tuna because they contain mercury, but the levels found in the sushi were significantly higher. Mercury gets into the ocean from industrial sources, especially coal-burning power plants, is absorbed by bacteria and makes its way up the food chain to larger fish such as tuna. There is controversy about the extent of the risk from farmed salmon or tuna, because the risks must be balanced against the many health benefits of eating fish. A review of the evidence published in 2006 concluded that the cardiovascular benefits of modest fish consumption—one or two servings per week—far outweigh the possible increased cancer risk for adults. The authors recommended that pregnant women, women of childbearing age, and young children should avoid swordfish, shark, golden bass, and king mackerel and should eat no more than 6 ounces per week of albacore tuna.[18]

Because of concerns about seafood, as well as repeated outbreaks caused by meat, including the *E. coli* outbreak from Jack-in-the-Box hamburgers in 1993, the Clinton administration implemented a new preventive approach to meat and seafood safety, which took effect in December 1997.[11] Called HACCP ("hassip"), the new system was developed in the 1960s by food processors in cooperation with the National Aeronautics and Space Administration to ensure that foods prepared for the astronauts were safe. Rather than relying on inspections, which can never be done frequently or thoroughly enough to ensure complete safety, the HACCP system focuses on procedures, putting the responsibility on food businesses to analyze their procedures and requiring government inspectors to verify compliance. The system involves identifying potential sources of contamination and devising ways to avoid them. HACCP—which stands for "Hazard Analysis Critical Control Point"—requires an analysis of every step in the process of food production, processing, and preparation, as seen in **Box 24-1**. The purpose is to identify each possible hazard and, for each, one or more "control points," which are practices and procedures that will eliminate, prevent, or minimize the hazard.[11]

Box 24-1 HACCP Procedures

1. Conduct a hazard analysis
2. Determine the critical control points
3. Establish critical limits
4. Establish monitoring procedures
5. Establish corrective actions
6. Establish verification procedures
7. Establish record-keeping and documentation procedures

Source: Data from U.S. Food and Drug Administration, "Food: Hazard Analysis & Critical Control Point Principles and Application Guidelines," August 14, 1997. http://www.fda.gov/Food/FoodSafety/HazardAnalysisCriticalControlPointsHACCP/ HACCPPrinciplesApplicationGuidelines/default.htm, accessed October 10, 2012.

Many companies were already using HACCP, and the FDA and USDA in the late 1990s moved to encourage more reliance on the system. When fully implemented, HACCP is intended to reduce the need for inspections, relying instead on frequent reviews of procedures to make sure the system is being carried out. Although the meat and poultry industries resisted at first, the USDA reported that by 1999, 96 percent of federally regulated plants were using HACCP, including a requirement that the foods be tested for common pathogens. The FDA implemented HACCP for seafood, making it mandatory in 1998. Raw sprouts, eggs, and fresh juice were added later, but for them, use of the system is voluntary.[19] By 2004, a review by the General Accounting Office (GAO), the investigative arm of Congress (whose name was changed later in 2004 to the Government Accountability Office), reviewed the FDA's program for the safety of imported seafood, which accounts for 80 percent of the seafood Americans consumed. The review found that the FDA's procedures were still significantly deficient. The GAO made a number of recommendations for improvement, including developing agreements with trading partners that they maintain comparable food safety systems, requiring importers to ensure that foreign firms comply with HACCP regulations, and giving enforcement priority to violations posing the most serious risks.[14]

The FDA, in addition to its oversight of food production on a national scale, issues recommendations that state and local governments can use to regulate establishments that deal with food, including retail stores, restaurants, and institutions such as schools and nursing homes. These rules emphasize the importance of hand washing by food service workers and restricting sick workers from direct contact with food. They also include strict guidelines concerning the temperatures at which food may be stored, cooked, and kept in heating trays. To prevent bacterial growth, foods should be refrigerated at 40 degrees Fahrenheit or below, or heated thoroughly so that internal temperatures are above 140 degrees. Special rules apply to large pieces such as roast meats and stuffed poultry because their internal temperatures may lag behind the external changes in temperature, allowing pathogens to grow during roasting or after refrigeration.[3] Local health departments usually enforce these rules by conducting periodic inspections of stores, restaurants, and institutions, and they are usually authorized by local and state laws to close facilities that are significantly in violation.

One potential solution to the problem of foodborne disease is the use of radiation to kill microbial contaminants in food. The idea of irradiating food frightens many people, and the proposal has aroused great opposition among some consumer groups; yet it leaves no radioactive residue, and more than 40 years of research have shown it to be safe. It is already used for some foods in the United States and is widely used in some other countries. Radiation treatment kills pests in dried herbs, spices, and tea, controls insects in wheat and flour, and kills the parasites that cause trichinosis when undercooked pork is eaten. It has been shown to greatly reduce the contamination of chicken breasts with *Salmonella*, ground beef with *E. coli*

0157:H7, and shrimp with cholera bacteria. Because microbial contamination of food is such a common hazard, with potentially deadly consequences, many experts believe that widespread use of irradiation could greatly increase the safety of the food supply. The FDA has approved irradiation of red meat, poultry, pork, fruits and vegetables, seeds, herbs and spices, eggs, and wheat. In 2004, the USDA began to offer irradiated ground beef as part of the National School Lunch Program.[3,20] In 2008, the FDA approved irradiation for iceberg lettuce and fresh spinach to help protect consumers from *Salmonella* and *E. coli.*[21] All foods that have been irradiated are required to be labeled as such. Some experts believe that irradiation should be used routinely for many foods. The CDC has estimated that irradiation of high-risk foods could prevent up to a million cases of bacterial foodborne disease each year in North America.[22]

A very important component of any food safety program is epidemiologic surveillance and prompt follow-up of any foodborne outbreak to prevent further spread of disease. With a nationwide food distribution network, local public health authorities may not recognize that a number of seemingly isolated cases of an illness might be caused by contamination at a single source. The CDC has a program called PulseNet, consisting of public health laboratories in all 50 states and Canada that can do DNA "fingerprinting" on foodborne bacteria. The network permits timely comparisons of pathogens that may cause outbreaks in various parts of the country, identifying common sources and enabling public health officials to take action to halt distribution of a contaminated food.[23]

The system worked in November 2008, when PulseNet staff noted that an unusual strain of *Salmonella* had been reported from 12 states. As CDC epidemiologists, working with state and local health departments, began to investigate the cluster of cases, more case reports flooded in. Interviews with patients suggested an association with peanut butter. After noting that several of the patients had eaten in institutional settings, including nursing homes and an elementary school, the source of the problem was identified in early January 2009 as peanut butter produced by a Georgia company, which supplied the product to institutions and to producers of other foods, including cookies, crackers, cereal, candy, ice cream, and pet treats. The company voluntarily recalled all products, leading to a cascade of recalls of peanut butter–containing products made by other companies. As of the end of January 2009, 529 people from 43 states had been reported with laboratory-confirmed cases of the same unusual strain; 116 of them had been hospitalized and 8 had died. The outbreak was probably considerably larger than the official numbers, since only about 3 percent of *Salmonella* infections are laboratory confirmed. The Georgia plant was found to be severely deficient, with rodents, a leaky roof, demoralized workers, and previous evidence of *Salmonella* contamination that had not been addressed. The plant is now closed, and the business is under criminal investigation.[24,25]

Another program developed by the CDC is an active surveillance network, called FoodNet, designed to help public health officials better understand the epidemiology of foodborne diseases in the United States.[26] In contrast with the usual epidemiologic surveillance, called passive surveillance, in which the public health agency waits for information to be reported to it by doctors, hospitals, and laboratories, FoodNet investigators conduct active surveillance. They contact laboratories to ask about every case of diarrheal illness they conducted tests on; send surveys to physicians to determine how often and under what conditions they send stool specimens to laboratories; and even call members of the general population to ask if they have had recent diarrheal illnesses, what they think might have caused it, and whether they sought treatment. The data collected by these methods provide information on less severe foodborne illnesses that are often not reported to public health authorities and help officials at the USDA and FDA identify where their regulatory systems should be improved. The FoodNet network includes, in addition to the CDC, investigators at the USDA, the FDA, and 10 state health departments. After FoodNet was implemented in 1996, the incidence of infections caused by several pathogens declined. Salmonella, however, increased slightly, and the incidence of Vibrio, caused by eating contaminated seafood, more than doubled.[27]

Despite some signs of improvement, the patchwork system of federal food safety regulation remains, and there have been repeated calls to establish a single, independent agency that would administer a unified, science-based food safety system. The Institute of Medicine, the President's Council on Food Safety, and the GAO have each conducted studies on the current system and concluded that laws should be revised to give one federal official responsibility and authority to keep the nation's food supply safe. Part of the problem is resistance by the powerful food industry, which has great influence in Congress.[11] However, the need has become even more urgent since the threat of bioterrorism has become more prominent. In December 2004, when then Secretary of Health and Human Services announced his resignation, he warned of the problem. "For the life of me, I cannot understand why the terrorists have not attacked our food supply because it's so easy to do," Secretary Tommy Thompson said in his final press conference.[28]

Additives and Contaminants

Food safety standards include limits on unwanted substances that accidentally get into food—contaminants—as well as on additives, which are purposely incorporated into food to improve its taste, color, and resistance to deterioration. Contaminants that can be detected by inspection include dirt, hairs, rodent feces, and insect parts. Pesticide residues may be left on food as a result of crop spraying or when livestock eat pesticide-contaminated fodder. A pesticide law passed by Congress in 1996 requires the Environmental Protection Agency to establish tolerance levels—the maximum allowable residues—for all pesticides used on food crops. While earlier health concerns focused on cancer, the new law requires testing of pesticides for damage to the endocrine system and for effects on developing fetuses, infants, and young children. The FDA and the USDA are then required to monitor foods to ensure that pesticide residues are within the allowed tolerance levels.[29]

However, the monitoring system has been criticized because only a fraction of the food supply is tested, because tests are available for only some of the pesticides, and because when contaminants are detected, it is often too late to prevent the food from being marketed. This is especially a problem with imported foods, which may contain residues of pesticides that are banned in the United States.

Other possible contaminants include hormones and antibiotics. The use of antibiotics in livestock feed is believed to have led to increased antibiotic resistance in many bacteria. The sex hormone diethylstilbestrol, a form of estrogen, used to be fed to chickens to promote their growth. Because of concerns that hormone residues in the meat might increase human breast cancer risk, the practice was banned in 1977. In 1994, the FDA approved the use of bovine growth hormone in dairy cows to increase their milk production. Although hormone residues are generally not found in the milk, many consumers are concerned about the safety of the practice.[3]

Many people choose foods labeled "organic," believing that these foods are safer than foods grown by common commercial methods. Until 2000, however, there was no federal standard that regulated what foods could be labeled organic. A 1990 law required the USDA to set standards, but there was so much controversy and objections from the conventional food industry that it took over a decade for the standards setting process to be completed and the standards to finally become fully effective in 2002. The standards require that organic meat, poultry, eggs, and dairy products must be grown without antibiotics or growth hormones, and organic produce must be grown without pesticides, synthetic fertilizers, or sewage sludge. Genetically engineered products and radiation are also not allowed for organic foods. Then in early 2004, the Bush administration "clarified" the standards, weakening some of the prohibitions on antibiotics and pesticides.[30,31] There was such a clamor of protest that the agriculture secretary reversed the new ruling the next day. Studies have shown that organic produce contains only one-third as many pesticide residues as conventionally grown foods and that children fed organic produce and juice had only one-sixth the level of pesticide byproducts in their urine compared with those that ate conventionally farmed foods.[32,33]

Additives are put into food for a variety of reasons. One purpose is to prevent deficiency diseases that used to cause serious public health problems in the United States. For example, the addition of iodine to table salt has virtually eliminated goiter; vitamin D added to milk has done away with rickets; and niacin, a B vitamin, is added to bread to prevent pellagra. The FDA mandates that folic acid be added to flour and rice products to prevent some birth defects. Another purpose of food additives is as a preservative, to retard spoilage or prevent fats from turning rancid. Other additives are used to improve color or to enhance flavor or texture.[3]

Because of public concern about the safety of many food additives, Congress passed legislation in 1958 that required FDA approval for any proposed food additive. Additives already in use were exempted and placed on the GRAS list—"generally regarded as safe." Since then, several additives on the list have been removed because they turned out not to be safe, among them several food colors that were shown to be carcinogenic.

Drugs and Cosmetics

As its name makes clear, the FDA is also responsible for the safety of drugs. This responsibility includes both prescription drugs and over-the-counter drugs—those available without a prescription. Both types of drugs must be proven safe and effective before they can be approved by the FDA.

The FDA does not test drugs itself. Companies seeking to market new drugs are required by law to conduct the tests and submit the evidence to the agency. FDA staff then review the data and determine whether the evidence supports the new drugs' safety and efficacy.

There is an orderly procedure for collecting the evidence on new prescription drugs. Several stages of exchange of information between the pharmaceutical company and the FDA are required. The company files a new drug application (NDA) for an investigational new drug, providing evidence that the drug has the desired effect in animals and satisfies some basic safety criteria. If the FDA approves the NDA, the company is allowed to test the drug in humans in clinical trials. The trials go through three phases: In phase I, the new drug is given to a small number of people who are extensively tested to measure absorption, distribution, metabolism, and excretion, and to look for side effects and toxicities. Phase II tests a larger number of patients for signs that the new drug is effective. Phase III is a full-scale controlled trial in which patients are assigned randomly to two groups. People in the experimental group receive the new drug. Members of the control group receive either a placebo or standard treatment.[34]

The FDA also has a system of postmarketing surveillance, in which doctors and patients can report adverse reactions to an approved drug. On occasion, evidence arises after a drug is on the market that it has risks that were not recognized in preapproval studies. The FDA has revoked its approval of a number of drugs based on such evidence. For years, the Agency's drug approval process has involved great political controversy, as described later in this chapter.

Cosmetics are more loosely regulated by the FDA. They do not need preapproval. In fact, there is no requirement for safety testing of cosmetics, but a warning label must be attached to any product that has not been tested. A number of ingredients that were used in the past have been shown to be harmful to health, and their use is prohibited by law. These include several chlorinated compounds as well as some color additives and most compounds containing mercury.

Food and Drug Labeling and Advertising

The scandals that inspired passage of the original Pure Food and Drugs Act of 1906 were cases of economic fraud as much as they were threats to public health. Expensive imports such as tea, coffee, and spices were frequently adulterated with dried leaves of native trees or ground native nuts and berries.[35] Thus, accurate labeling was one of the important provisions of the 1906 act. Labeling requirements have become increasingly elaborate over the years. Recently, as it has become clear that overall dietary behavior has far more impact on health than food contamination does, the FDA has placed more emphasis on empowering consumers to eat a healthy diet. Regulations established in 1994 require labels on prepared foods to contain information on fats, fiber, vitamins, and other nutrients, along with recommended daily intakes for these nutrients. Because the kinds of fats in the diet have an important effect on health, especially heart disease, labels are required to list the amount of artery-clogging saturated fat, the kind found in butter, whole milk, beef, and pork. Then, since January 2006, foods have been required to add to their labels the amount of trans fats in a serving of the product. Trans fats, which have been used since the 1980s as substitutes for saturated fats in margarine, fried foods, and baked goods, have been found to be at least as harmful to arteries as saturated fats.[36]

Accurate labels on drugs are also required by the FDA. Here the emphasis is on ensuring that claims of safety and efficacy are accurate and communicate information about hazards directly to the consumer. This is especially important for over-the-counter drugs, for which the label may be the sole basis on which consumers choose to buy and consume the product. Oddly, advertising—a form of labeling—of over-the-counter drugs is regulated by the Federal Trade Commission rather than the FDA. However, the labeling of prescription drugs falls under the authority of the FDA. Prescription drugs are increasingly being advertised directly to consumers, and critics have become concerned that these ads are often misleading, overemphasizing the benefits and deemphasizing the risks. If the FDA determines that an ad is misleading, it may send a notice of violation to the drug company; however, the agency's authority is limited, and it has been criticized for not enforcing the law vigorously.[37]

Unfounded claims for health benefits from certain foods, drugs, and vitamins have had popular appeal in the United States since the nation's birth, despite governmental efforts to enforce accuracy in labeling and advertising. In the late 19th and early 20th centuries, patent medicines contained alcohol and sometimes opium, which helped patients feel better but did little to cure the underlying problems. Still today, desperate patients suffering from incurable diseases turn to quack therapies, at best just wasting their money, but in some cases turning their backs on therapies that might do some good. The FDA can act when labels on a food or drug contain false or misleading claims; accompanying leaflets are considered labels. However, nothing can be done to suppress articles and books containing unsubstantiated health claims about foods and "nutritional supplements" if the writings cannot be classified as labels.

Among the most persistent nutritional misconceptions has been the belief that if it is "natural," it must be safe. Accordingly, Congress in 1994 succumbed to intense lobbying by the health food industry and passed the Dietary Supplement Health and Education Act, which was signed by President Clinton. The Act forbids the FDA from requiring safety testing of herbs and food supplements. Consequently, a number of products known to have quite potent physiological effects are sold freely in health food stores, although they may turn out to be harmful once they are better understood. For example, melatonin, promoted as a sleep aid and treatment for jet lag, is sold as a nutritional supplement despite the fact that it is a hormone with unknown and potentially powerful effects on the brain and the reproductive and immune systems.

In 1996, people were shocked by news stories that a college student on spring break had died after taking an herbal product called "Ultimate Xphoria" (also called "Herbal Ecstasy"), which contained ephedra, a potent natural stimulant similar to amphetamines. Ephedra-containing compounds were marketed as energy boosters, aids to weight loss, as sexual stimulants, and as a way to get high.[38] Soon afterward, the CDC reported that 8 deaths and 500 adverse health affects including heart attacks, seizures, and psychoses, had occurred nationwide among people who had consumed ephedra-containing products.[39] While some state and local governments banned these products, the FDA could not stop their sale and use. Finally, after the highly publicized death in early 2003 of a 23-year-old Baltimore Orioles pitcher who used ephedra to lose weight at the beginning of spring training, the FDA banned the substance. It was the first time that the FDA had removed a dietary supplement from the market since 1994, and the action succeeded only after the agency had reviewed some 16,000 reports of adverse reactions, commissioned a study by a nonprofit research agency, and received tens of thousands of comments from the public.[40]

Ephedra is not the only natural substance that has proven to be unsafe. According to the American Association of Poison Control Centers, between the passage of the 1994 Act and 2007, poison control centers received more than 1.6 million reports of adverse reactions to vitamins, minerals, essential oils, herbs, and other supplements. In 2005 alone, there were 2001 reports of reactions to melatonin, including 535 hospitalizations and 4 deaths. A federal law passed in 2007 requires supplement manufacturers to report serious adverse effects to the FDA; whether the law will result in significant reporting remains to be seen.[41]

Politics of the FDA

The FDA regulates products amounting to over 25 percent of consumer dollars spent in the United States.[42] Not surprisingly, it has made itself unpopular with some of the industries financially impacted by its decisions. These industries can place intense political pressures on

Congress and the White House to rein in the agency's actions, as illustrated by the success of the dietary supplement industry in getting itself exempted from FDA oversight.

One of the most frequent criticisms of the FDA has been that it is too slow in approving new drugs. This complaint comes from the pharmaceutical industry, which argues that companies must wait too long to recoup their investments in research and development, as well as from patients with intractable diseases, who feel they are being denied promising new treatments. AIDS activists were especially critical of the FDA's caution, arguing that they would inevitably die if the process of new drug approval was not accelerated. Citing the thalidomide disaster that was averted in the United States by a cautious FDA official was no longer enough to deter calls for "reform." In 1992, Congress acted to speed up the approval process by requiring drug companies to pay a fee for the processing of NDAs, which allowed the agency to hire more reviewers, but this situation has given rise to other problems, as discussed below.

Consumer advocates claim that the FDA is now too ready to approve new drugs, a claim supported by the necessity in recent years to recall several drugs because of adverse effects that became evident only after they were on the market. For example, the diet drug known as "fen-phen," approved in 1996, had to be recalled a year later because it caused serious heart valve problems.[43,44] Other drugs that were withdrawn included the allergy drug Seldane in 1997 because of cardiac arrhythmias, the diabetes drug Rezulin in 2000 because of liver problems, and the cholesterol-lowering drug Baycol in 2001, because of injury to muscle tissue.

Further doubts about the drug-approval and -monitoring process surfaced in 2004 when the Merck pharmaceutical company withdrew from the market Vioxx, a pain killer that was one of the most widely advertised drugs in the world and had earned $2.5 billion for the company since it was approved by the FDA in 1999. Merck had found in a new study that people taking the drug doubled their risk of heart attacks and strokes. Questions were raised about why the FDA had not recognized the problems with Vioxx and recalled it earlier. In a hearing by the Senate Finance Committee, FDA employees disagreed with one another on whether the agency was too likely to surrender to the demands of the industry. As described in a *New York Times* news report on the hearing, "the clash was a rare public airing of tensions that have simmered in the agency for decades."[45] The conflict is clearly one that also reflects the opposing views Congress has held on the agency. After years of congressional pressure on the FDA to protect the interests of the pharmaceutical industry, the FDA is now accused of neglecting the safety of consumers.[45] As the newly appointed commissioner and principal deputy commissioner wrote in a 2009 article, "It has been said that the FDA has just two speeds of approval—too fast and too slow."[46]

Critics complain that since the 1992 law permitting pharmaceutical companies to pay "user fees" to speed up drug approval, the agency has become too cozy with the companies. They noted that the number of recalls of new drugs had increased dramatically, amounting to over 5 percent in the period 1997 to 2001, implying that the drugs were being approved too easily.[47]

Moreover, the law has forced the FDA to spend almost 80 percent of its budget, supplemented by the user fees, for drug approvals, with too little allocated for safety monitoring after the drugs have been approved. Postmarketing surveillance relies on the drug companies to report adverse effects, a system that is inadequate at best and rife with conflicts of interest on the part of the companies. In many cases, clinical trials do not include enough patients to detect rare responses that may become evident when large numbers of people take the drug after it has been approved.

Drugs sold in the United States, like food, are increasingly being manufactured in and imported from other countries, especially China and India. The FDA has a mandate to inspect producers of drugs and chemicals used to manufacture drugs for the American market, but it has been overwhelmed with the increasing number of foreign producers, estimated as between 3200 and 6800. That challenge was illustrated by the recall in 2008 of large quantities of heparin, a blood thinner commonly used to prevent clotting during surgery or other medical procedures, because of allergic reactions to an impurity introduced during manufacturing at a plant in China. At least 62 people in the United States died as a result. The Chinese plant had not been inspected by the FDA.[48]

The FDA's difficulties inspired a review by the Institute of Medicine, which recommended a number of reforms.[49] The report emphasized the need for improved monitoring of the safety of drugs after they have been approved and introduced into the marketplace. It recommended more funding for that purpose and greater authority for the FDA to require companies to conduct follow-up clinical studies on newly detected adverse effects. It also proposed that newly approved drugs should carry labeling that indicates safety information is incomplete, and that direct-to-consumer advertising should be banned for the first 2 years after approval. Another proposal was for the mandatory registration of clinical trials.[50]

Congress passed legislation in 2007 that addressed some but not all of the criticisms. It reauthorized the use of user fees for the drug approval process, and it also significantly increased funding for postmarketing studies of drugs already on the market. It granted the agency authority to require companies to do studies on approved drugs for adverse side effects. The law requires registration of all clinical trials and public posting of their results. It includes incentives for testing drugs in children, as well as provisions designed to limit conflicts of interest of advisors. However, it did very little to address concerns about the safety of imported foods.[51]

Conclusion

Confidence in the safety of the U.S. food supply has been shaken in recent years by widely publicized outbreaks of illnesses caused by foods, ranging from bagged spinach to peanut butter. Common sources of illness include *Salmonella* bacteria in poultry, meat, and eggs, as well as a variety of viruses and parasites in fish and shellfish. Over the past 2 decades, *E. coli* 0157:H7 has emerged as a serious threat in ground beef and other foods as well as in unpasteurized fruit juice.

Governmental responsibility for food safety is distributed among a variety of federal, state, and local agencies. The laws are inconsistent and, in many cases, paradoxical. The USDA has significant authority over meat and poultry safety. The FDA is responsible for most other foods, including fish and seafood, but its financial resources for inspection and monitoring are limited, and it has little power to act. The increasing proportion of imported foods in the American market has posed serious challenges to food safety regulation.

As the problem of food contamination became more apparent in the 1990s, the focus of the FDA and the USDA has fallen on a system for preventing problems before they occur rather than depending on inspections to detect food that is already contaminated. The system, called HACCP, analyzes every step in the process of food production, processing, and preparation, with the objective of identifying possible hazards and instituting practices that will eliminate or minimize them. The FDA has approved irradiation of many foods to kill microbial contaminants. Although many consumers are distrustful of irradiated food, the practice has been shown to be safe, and many experts believe routine irradiation would greatly improve the safety of our food supply. Strengthened surveillance for rapid detection of foodborne disease outbreaks is another feature of the food safety system; in the event of an outbreak, surveillance allows sources to be identified so that they can be halted rapidly.

In addition to its role in the prevention of microbial contamination of food, the FDA regulates food additives and chemical contaminants, as well as food labeling and advertising. It sets standards for foods to be labeled "organic."

The FDA also has oversight of the safety of drugs and medical devices. This responsibility has led to considerable controversy as the pharmaceutical industry and patient groups complain about the slow pace of new drug approval. Conservatives in Congress have made repeated efforts to weaken the agency's authority and to force it to act more quickly on drug approvals. One result was legislation passed in 1992 that allowed the FDA to assess fees on the pharmaceutical industry to be used for processing new drug approvals. Critics believe that this practice has led to too cozy a relationship between the agency and the drug companies. Another law that has been controversial is the Dietary Supplement Health and Education Act of 1994, which prohibits the FDA from regulating herbs and food supplements. Consumer groups are concerned that these laws, together with the climate of pressure to speed up drug approvals, endanger public health by allowing unsafe products on the market.

Several scandals occurred in the late 1990s and the 2000s that confirmed fears that drugs are approved too easily and that the system for detecting safety problems after approval is inadequate. Increasing importation of drugs from foreign countries has made regulation more difficult. Evidence that pharmaceutical companies selectively publicize clinical trials that show benefits of their drugs while suppressing negative results led to mandatory registration of clinical trials at the outset, so that all the evidence will be available publicly. This requirement was part of legislation passed in 2007 that also included a number of other measures designed to increase the FDA's funding and authority. Whether these measures will be effective in improving the safety of pharmaceuticals remains to be seen.

References

1. U.S. Centers for Disease Control and Prevention, "Food Safety at CDC." http://www.cdc.gov/foodsafety/facts.html#howmanycases, accessed August 4, 2012.
2. W. M. Laydon, "Food Safety: A Patchwork System," *GAO Journal* (Spring–Summer 1992): 48–59.
3. A. Nadakavukaren, *Our Global Environment: A Health Perspective*, 6th ed. (Prospect Heights, IL: Waveland Press, 2005).
4. C. Drew and P. Belluck, "Deadly Bacteria—a New Threat to Fruit and Produce in U.S.," *The New York Times*, January 4, 1998.
5. P. Belluck and C. Drew, "Tracing Bout of Illness to Small Lettuce Farm," *The New York Times*, January 5, 1998.
6. T. Breuer et al., "A Multistate Outbreak of *Escherichia coli* 0157:H7 Infections Linked to Alfalfa Sprouts Grown from Contaminated Seeds," *Emerging Infectious Diseases Journal* 7 (2001): 977–982.
7. Center for Science in the Public Interest, "CSPI Outbreak Alert Data: Info on Produce Outbreaks." http://www.cspinet.org/new/pdf/cspi_outbreak_alert.pdf, accessed August 3, 2012.
8. L. Polgreen, "Hepatitis Inquiry Moves Deliberately from Farm to Plate," *The New York Times*, November 18, 2003.
9. D. W. K. Acheson and A. E. Fiore, "Preventing Foodborne Disease—What Clinicians Can Do," *New England Journal of Medicine* 350 (2004): 437–440.
10. U.S. Centers for Disease Control and Prevention, "Outbreak of *Salmonella* Serotype Saintpaul Infections Associated with Multiple Raw Produce Items—United States, 2008," *Morbidity and Mortality Weekly Report* 57 (2008): 929–934.
11. M. Nestle, *Safe Food: The Politics of Food Safety* (Berkeley, CA: University of California Press, 2010).
12. C. S. DeWaal and D. W. Plunkett, Center for Science in the Public Interest, "Building a Modern Food Safety System for FDA Regulated Foods." http://www.cspinet.org/new/pdf/fswhitepaper.pdf, accessed August 4, 2012.
13. U.S. Food and Drug Administration, "Food and Drugs: Can Safety Be Ensured in a Time of Increased Globalization?" http://www.fda.gov/NewsEvents/Speeches/ucm242326, accessed August 3, 2012.
14. U.S. Food and Drug Administration, "For Consumers: The 'Teeth' of FDA's Food Safety Law." http://www.fda.gov/ForConsumers/ConsumerUpdates/ucm267460.htm, accessed August 4, 2012.

15. M. Burros, "President to Push for Food Safety," *The New York Times*, July 4, 1998.

16. Center for Science in the Public Interest, "Fish and Shellfish top CSPI Outbreak List." http://www.cspinet.org/new/200811251.html, accessed August 23, 2009.

17. M. Burros, "High Mercury Levels Are Found in Tuna Sushi Sold in Manhattan," *The New York Times*, January 23, 2008.

18. D. Mozaffarian et al., "Fish Intake, Contaminants, and Human Health: Evaluation the Risks and the Benefits," *Journal of the American Medical Association* 296 (2006): 1885–1899.

19. R. A. Robinson, "Food Safety and Security: Fundamental Changes Needed to Ensure Safe Food," General Accounting Office, Testimony Before the Subcommittee on Oversight of Government Management, Restructuring and the District of Columbia, Committee on Governmental Affairs, U.S. Senate. October 10, 2001. http://www.gao.gov/assets/110/109016.pdf, accessed August 5, 2012.

20. M. T. Osterholm and A. P. Norgan, "Role of Irradiation in Food Safety," *New England Journal of Medicine* 350 (2004): 1898–1901.

21. U.S. Food and Drug Administration, "Irradiation: A Safe Measure for Safer Iceberg Lettuce and Spinach." http://www.fda.gov/ForConsumers/ConsumerUpdates/ucm093651.htm, accessed August 5, 2012.

22. D. G. Maki, "Coming to Grips with Foodborne Infection—Peanut Butter, Peppers, and Nationwide Salmonella Outbreaks," *New England Journal of Medicine* 360 (2009): 949–953.

23. U.S. Centers for Disease Control and Prevention, "PulseNet?" http://www.cdc.gov/PULSENET, accessed August 5, 2012.

24. U.S. Centers for Disease Control and Prevention, "Multistate Outbreak of *Salmonella* Infections Associated with Peanut Butter and Peanut Butter-Containing Products—United States, 2008–2009," *Morbidity and Mortality Weekly Report* 58 (2009): 85–90.

25. M. Moss, "Peanut Case Shows Holes in Food Safety Net," *The New York Times*, February 9, 2009.

26. U.S. Centers for Disease Control and Prevention, "FoodNet—Foodborne Diseases Active Surveillance Network." http://www.cdc.gov/foodnet/, accessed August 5, 2012.

27. U.S. Centers for Disease Control and Prevention, "Trends in Foodborne Illness in the United States, 1996–2010." http://www.cdc.gov/foodborneburden/trends-in-foodborne-illness.html, accessed August 5, 2012.

28. R. Pear, "Departing Health Secretary Warns of Flu Risk and Attacks on Food," *The New York Times*, December 3, 2004.

29. U.S. Environmental Protection Agency, "Accomplishments under the Food Quality Protection Act (FQPA)." http://www.epa.gov/pesticides/regulating/laws/fqpa/fqpa_accomplishments.htm, accessed August 5, 2012.

30. M. Burros, "Last Word on Organic Standards, Again," *The New York Times*, May 26, 2004.

31. M. Burros, "Agriculture Dept. Rescinds Changes to Organic Food Standards," *The New York Times*, May 27, 2004.

32. M. Burros, "Study Finds Far Less Pesticide Residue on Organic Produce," *The New York Times*, May 8, 2002.

33. C. K. Yoon, "Exposure to Pesticides Is Lowered When Young Children Go Organic," *The New York Times*, March 25, 2003.

34. U.S. Food and Drug Administration, "The FDA's Drug Review Process: Ensuring Drugs Are Safe and Effective." http://www.fda.gov/Drugs/ResourcesForYou/Consumers/ucm143534.htm, accessed August 5 2012.

35. R. M. Deutsch, *The New Nuts Among the Berries: How Nutritional Nonsense Captured America* (Palo Alto, CA: Bull Publishing, 1977).

36. U.S. Food and Drug Administration, "Talking About Trans Fat: What You Need to Know." http://www.fda.gov/Food/ResourcesForYou/Consumers/ucm079609.htm, accessed August 5, 2012.

37. S. M. Wolfe, "Direct-to-Consumer Advertising—Education or Emotion Promotion?" *New England Journal of Medicine* 346 (2002): 524–526.

38. M. Burros and S. Jay, "Concern Grows Over Herb That Promises a Legal High," *The New York Times*, April 10, 1996.

39. U.S. Centers for Disease Control and Prevention, "Adverse Events Associated with Ephedrine-Containing Products—Texas, December 1993–September 1995," *Morbidity and Mortality Weekly Report* 45 (1996): 689–692.

40. S. G. Stolberg, "U.S. to Prohibit Supplement Tied to Health Risks," *The New York Times*, December 31, 2003.

41. D. Hurley, "Diet Supplements and Safety: Some Disquieting Data," *The New York Times*, January 16, 2007.

42. A. J. J. Wood, "Playing 'Kick the FDA'—Risk-free to Players but Hazardous to Public Health," *New England Journal of Medicine* 358 (2008): 1774–1775.

43. J. Couzin, "Gaps in the Safety Net," *Science* 307 (2005): 196–198.

44. W. A. Ray and C. M. Stein, "Reform of Drug Regulation—Beyond an Independent Drug-Safety Board," *New England Journal of Medicine* 354 (2008): 194–201.

45. G. Harris, "FDA Failing in Drug Safety, Official Asserts," *The New York Times*, November 19, 2004.

46. M. A. Hamburg and J. M. Sharfstein, "The FDA as a Public Health Agency," *New England Journal of Medicine* 360 (2009): 2492–2495.

47. P. B. Fontanarosa, D. Rennie, and C. D. DeAngelis, "Postmarketing Surveillance—Lack of Vigilance, Lack of Trust," *Journal of the Medical Association of America* 292 (2004): 2647–2650.

48. S. O. Schweitzer, "Trying Times at the FDA—The Challenge of Ensuring the Safety of Imported Pharmaceuticals," *New England Journal of Medicine* 358 (2008): 1773–1777.

49. Institute of Medicine, *The Future of Drug Safety: Preserving and Protecting the Health of the Public* (Washington, DC: National Academies Press, 2006).

50. G. D. Curfman, S. Morrissey, and J. M. Drazen, "Blueprint for a Stronger Food and Drug Administration," *New England Journal of Medicine* 355 (2006): 1821.

51. G. Harris, "House Passes Bill Giving More Power to the FDA," *The New York Times*, September 20, 2007.

Population: The Ultimate Environmental Health Issue

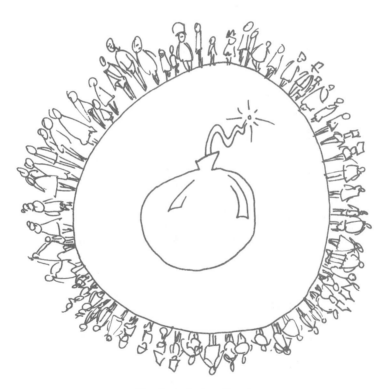

The Population Bomb

Population biology is a science in itself. Studies of animal, plant, and microorganism populations have yielded some concepts and insights that can be applied to human populations. However, application of these studies' findings to human populations is an inexact science, and predictions are always highly controversial. Interest in the dynamics of the human population arises from concern about its continuing growth and its increasing impact on the environment.

All organisms tend to produce more offspring than would be needed to maintain a stable population. Pressures from the environment, such as availability of food and prevalence of predators, tend to limit the survival of those offspring. The difference between the birth rate and the death rate is the population's rate of growth.

Studies of organisms newly introduced into a closed environment have shown two general patterns of population growth: the S curve and the J curve, illustrated in Figure 25-1. Both patterns start out with a rapidly expanding population, but they differ in their response to environmental limitations. In the more common S pattern, environmental pressures increase gradually as the population approaches the number known as the carrying capacity—the number of

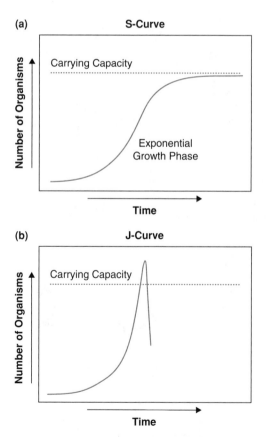

FIGURE 25-1   Patterns of Population Growth. *Source:* Reprinted by permission of Waveland Press, Inc. from A. Nadakavukaren, *Our Global Environment*, 6th ed. (Long Grove, IL: Waveland Press, Inc., 2006). All rights reserved.

organisms that can be supported in a given environment without degrading that environment. In the J pattern, the population expands rapidly past the carrying capacity and then crashes, because once the carrying capacity is exceeded, the environment is degraded, and the carrying capacity is reduced. For example, the J pattern is seen in lemmings and locusts, species famous for huge population explosions followed by massive numbers of deaths when the food supply is exhausted.[1]

It is not yet clear whether the human population is growing in an S or a J pattern. The world population has grown steadily, with minor irregularities, for the past million years, with a major surge beginning about 200 years ago. About that time, when the population of the Earth was about one billion, the British clergyman and economist Thomas Malthus raised an alarm that population growth was outpacing the food supply; he predicted that the resulting crowding would lead to famine, war, and disease. However, Malthus's dismal predictions did not come about, and his warnings were discredited. Progress in agricultural technology and migrations from highly populated areas in Europe to the open spaces of the Americas and southern Africa relieved pressures on populations, allowing the expansion to continue.[1]

In 1968, when the world's population was 3.5 billion, Paul Ehrlich, an American ecologist, published *The Population Bomb*, a best seller that repeated and expanded upon Malthus's warning.[2] Perhaps in part due to the attention paid to Ehrlich's book, the rate of the world's population growth has slowed since then, from an all-time high of 2.1 percent per year between 1965 and 1970 to 1.1 percent in 2012.[3] There is a tremendous momentum to population growth, however, and the numbers continue to increase dramatically. In 1990, when the population had reached 5.3 billion, Ehrlich and his wife, Anne, published another book, *The Population Explosion*, arguing that many of his dire predictions have already begun to be realized.[4] In 2004, with the world's population at 6.4 billion, they published *One with Nineveh*, which further examines the consequences of overpopulation and the linked problems of overconsumption and political and economic inequity—consequences that include the prospect of increasing terrorism.[5] Most recently, in 2010 when the population was approaching 7 billion, Paul Ehrlich, with Robert E. Ornstein, published *Humanity on a Tightrope* in which the authors argue that, in order to balance on the tightrope of sustainability suspended over the collapse of civilization, people need to recognize that we are all part of one family.[6]

Most environmentalists and public health experts agree with Ehrlich. However, like Malthus, he has his detractors. There are progrowth advocates—mostly economists—who argue that human ingenuity will always find ways of overcoming any problems created by crowding. In response, the Ehrlichs quote Kenneth Boulding: "Anyone who believes exponential growth can go on forever in a finite world is either a madman or an economist."[4(p.159)] Some of the world's major religions oppose population control measures, making it easier for politicians to listen to growth advocates and to simply ignore the problems created by overpopulation.

It is very difficult to predict what the world population will be in the future. There are indications, as the Ehrlichs point out, that environmental pressures opposing population growth are increasing, especially in developing regions of the world. There are also indications that international family planning efforts are paying off in slowing growth rates in many parts of the world. The United Nations predicted in 2010 that, if current trends continue, the population will reach 9.3 billion by 2050. The vast majority of the growth is in the poorest countries of Africa and southern Asia. Projections after that are uncertain, depending in part on the future of the AIDS epidemic.[7] It is not clear whether the Earth's carrying capacity is large enough to support so many people. If not, irreversible forces may be building for a sudden J-type population crash. By the time the Ehrlichs would be proved right, it would be too late to do anything to prevent the disaster.

Public Health and Population Growth

Public health has had a major role in bringing about the dramatic growth in the world's population over the past several decades. Public health improvements—clean water, immunization, pest control measures, inexpensive oral rehydration treatment of diarrheal diseases—in developing countries have led to major declines in death rates, especially among children. According to the United Nations Children's Fund (UNICEF) the number of children who die before reaching their fifth birthday declined by almost one-quarter between 1990 and 2010, and this number has continued to decline.[8] Because birth rates remained constant, populations grew rapidly in the developing countries.

In developed countries, which instituted public health measures over a period of many decades in the 19th and 20th centuries, birth rates tended to fall in response to falling death rates, a process known as the "demographic transition." The fall in birth rates is a rational response to parents' knowledge that their children are likely to survive to adulthood. In an industrialized, urban society, children are an economic liability—expensive to feed, clothe, and educate.

In the developing world, however, many public health measures were introduced by international agencies over a short period of time after World War II. International aid for population control efforts has not been as generous. This is, in part, because of cultural resistance to contraception within some societies and, in part, because of the religious and political controversy surrounding family planning, especially in the United States, which has limited the amount of aid this nation provides.

Because of continued high birth rates, the public health in many developing countries is now, ironically, threatened by the crowding that has resulted from public health improvements. In all parts of the world, there has been a trend toward urbanization, because rural areas whose main industries are agricultural do not need the increasing numbers of workers. This trend has been most marked in developing countries, where migrants from rural areas flock to the cities. From 1950 to 2008, the percentage of people living in cities increased from 29 percent to 50.5 percent.[1,9] According to the United Nations, the percentage of Africa's population living in cities is 40 percent and is increasing at 2.4 percent per year; Asia's rate of urbanization is 42 percent and is increasing at 2.3 percent per year.[10] Governments struggling to provide adequate drinking water and sewage services to their citizens cannot keep up with the influx. Many of the migrants settle on the outskirts of the cities in shantytowns totally lacking in water and sanitation. Others are completely homeless, simply living on the streets.

These conditions threaten to reverse all the progress in public health made through earlier efforts. Cholera and other diarrheal diseases are rampant in these third-world slums. Malaria, measles, whooping cough, and diphtheria are also common. Polio is still a threat in Africa. Cases of tuberculosis are surging, and AIDS rates are still increasing, although the epidemic appears to have stabilized. In sub-Saharan Africa, 6.1 percent of the adult population is infected with the human immune deficiency virus (HIV), and in some of these countries, prevalence is shockingly high: 26 percent in Swaziland and 24 percent in Botswana.[11] The number of children orphaned by AIDS reached 12 million in 2007.[11] In fact, AIDS has dwarfed all other public health problems in Africa. Life expectancy in several countries in southern Africa has fallen by 20 years or more, and the rate of population growth has dropped to almost zero, not because of low birth rates as in developed countries, but because death rates are almost equal to birth rates.

The desperate conditions in third-world urban slums lead to the disruption of traditional lifestyles and to the breakdown of normal social constraints, including sexual and parental restraints. Prostitution is common; children are abandoned to fend for themselves. These were the conditions that are believed to have led to the origin of AIDS as an epidemic threat, and they contribute to the continuing disaster of the epidemic. Such conditions may be the breeding ground for other emerging infections in the future. These conditions also encourage crime and violence. Even if, as predicted, population growth rates continue to decline, 95 percent of the 2 or 3 billion people added to the world in the next 25 to 50 years will be in the poorest countries, and most of that growth will occur in cities.[1]

Even the United States and other developed countries are affected by some of the pressures described above, although the rate of population growth in this country is under 1 percent, and in Japan and most European countries, it is close to zero. Russia and some other Eastern European countries have negative population growth. The American population is becoming increasingly urban, with over 75 percent living in communities with more than 2500 residents.[1] In 2010, 22 percent of American children lived in families with incomes below the poverty line; a high percentage of these children live with both housing and food insecurity.[12]

The United States is also affected by the social consequences of population growth in developing countries. Highly publicized problems with illegal immigration from Mexico and Central America are linked with poverty and with social problems caused by population growth in those countries. As conditions in those areas become more crowded and desperate in the future, the pressures on people to seek less crowded, more prosperous surroundings will increase, making it more difficult for the United States to remain isolated. Infectious diseases have no respect for political boundaries. With international travel and commerce so rapid and widespread, Americans are at risk from diseases imported from anywhere in the world. Furthermore, as discussed in the following section, human population growth threatens to change the environment of the entire globe, posing health threats that no one could escape, even if the nation's borders were sealed.

Global Impact of Population Growth—Depletion of Resources

The carrying capacity of the Earth—the population size that the Earth can support without being degraded—is determined by a number of factors, some of which can be altered by technological intervention and human behavior. These factors, which are related, include the availability of fresh water, the availability of fuel, the amount and productivity of arable land, and the amount and disposition of wastes, both biological and technological. There are signs that the carrying capacity is already exceeded in some parts of the world: as the environment is degraded, the size of the population that can be supported shrinks, leading to further environmental degradation and a vicious circle of hunger, disease, and death.

The supply of fresh water, which is basic to human life, is one of the factors that limits the Earth's carrying capacity. Water is essential for drinking, cooking, and washing. It is also used for agriculture, irrigating dry fields to grow the increasing amounts of food required by expanding populations. Water is a renewable resource, due to cycles of evaporation and precipitation, but the rate at which water supplies are renewed is fixed. Only a small percentage of the water on Earth is suitable for human use: while there are methods of removing the salt from sea water, the technology is expensive and uses large amounts of energy. Pollution resulting from the use of fresh water supplies for disposal of wastes also renders potential sources of water unsuitable for human use.

Availability of fresh water is highly variable according to geographic area and precipitation patterns. In drier parts of the world, especially the Middle East, water rights become volatile international issues because some countries depend on water sources that originate beyond their borders. For example, the Nile flows into Egypt from Ethiopia and Sudan, and the flow of the Tigris–Euphrates into Syria and Iraq may be altered by dam construction in Turkey.

In the United States, water supplies have been sufficiently plentiful so that Americans are accustomed to lavish consumption, watering lawns, washing cars, and filling private swimming pools, even in relatively dry areas of the Southwest. For example, much of the water used in that part of the country comes from the Ogallala Aquifer, the world's largest underground water reserve, which underlies portions of six southwestern states. This water accumulated during the last ice age and cannot be replenished. Yet it is being used, among other things, for industry and irrigation, attracting people to the area who will be left literally high and dry when the water runs out.[1]

The amount of fresh water on Earth is theoretically sufficient to support a population of 20 billion people if evenly distributed.[1] Many countries have taken steps to conserve fresh water supplies and to clean up the pollution. In poorer, drier countries, however, the available water is insufficient to support the growth in population that is occurring. The lack of water for cooking and washing, and the pollution of drinking water with human and industrial wastes, is already harming the public health. According to the United Nations, one-third of the world's people, mostly in Africa and south Asia, live in regions with water shortages, and that number will grow by one-half by 2025.[1]

Predictions about the Earth's carrying capacity have most often centered on food, attempting to estimate the limits of agricultural productivity. Malthus's warnings were built on concerns about limited growth in food supplies, which nevertheless continued to grow rapidly for almost 2 centuries. Now, unhappily, it is beginning to look as if Malthus may finally be proven right. According to a 2005 United Nations report, about 14 percent of the world's population are chronically or acutely malnourished. In sub-Saharan Africa, the prevalence of hunger is over 30 percent and increasing.[13]

With increasing populations needing greater amounts of food, the amount of land used for agriculture grew quickly during the period between 1850 and 1950. Then, despite continued population growth, the expansion of arable land slowed down and ceased altogether in the late 1980s.[14] Food production continued to keep pace with population growth during the 1960s and 1970s, however, because of the "green revolution," the development of genetic strains of wheat and rice that yielded harvests two to three times greater than conventional strains. Crop yields also grew because of increasing use of fertilizers, irrigation, and chemical pesticides.

Such increases in yields are unlikely to continue, however, because of water shortages, depletion of soil, and the development of resistance by pests to chemical pesticides. The amount of land under cultivation has declined in some parts of the world, especially Africa. According to one estimate, 10 percent of the Earth's vegetated surface is at least moderately degraded, and about 22 million acres are severely degraded. In part this is because of spreading urban centers, in part it is because the soil is depleted of nutrients or has become salty from irrigation. Erosion of topsoil due to overgrazing and poor agricultural practices contribute to the loss of arable land. The demand for agricultural land for farming has led to widespread clearing of forests, although forested land may be only marginally suitable for cultivation. Deforestation also occurs as a result of people gathering wood for fuel. The need by growing populations for firewood for cooking and, in colder climates and mountainous regions, heating as well, has resulted in vast treeless areas around towns and villages throughout Africa, Asia, and Latin America. The loss of forests increases soil erosion and contributes to catastrophic flooding in areas subject to monsoons.[1]

Population growth has also caught up with the seemingly limitless supply of food from the sea. Fish catches increased dramatically between 1950 and 1989 but have declined since then. The United Nations Food and Agriculture Organization has concluded that 75 percent of the major marine fish stocks are fully exploited, overexploited, or significantly depleted.[1] Pollution of coastal waters has also contributed to the decline of harvests, especially those of shellfish. On the bright side, the practice of aquaculture is growing rapidly, and by the early 21st century one out of every three fish eaten worldwide was raised on a fish farm.[1] There are drawbacks to fish farming, however. Farmed salmon, for example, are fed fish meal and fish oil made from large amounts of smaller fish such as sardines, anchovies and herring, thus depleting fisheries that might otherwise feed people. The waste from penned fish pollutes coastal waters. Saltwater fish farms incubate microbes and parasites that threaten to infect wild stocks.

Global Impact of Population Growth—Climate Change

Perhaps the most threatening effect of population growth is that it is beginning to change the composition of the Earth's atmosphere, with potentially drastic consequences. The depletion of the ozone layer, which protects the Earth's surface from ultraviolet radiation, is known to increase risks in humans of skin cancer, melanoma, and cataracts. It may also have a harmful impact on plant and animal life.

Although international agreements have led to policies effective in slowing and possibly even reversing damage to the ozone layer, there is less hope of preventing climate change caused by other human activities. Alteration in the relative concentrations of the four major constituents of air—nitrogen, oxygen, argon, and carbon dioxide—is causing global warming due to the "greenhouse effect," in which the energy of sunlight is absorbed by carbon dioxide in the air and turned into heat rather than radiating back into outer space.

The balance of atmospheric gases has been maintained over the millennia by the photosynthetic activities of green plants, which take up carbon dioxide and release oxygen. The reverse process occurs during combustion of wood, coal, oil, and gas: oxygen is consumed and carbon dioxide is released. Since the beginning of the Industrial Revolution, with the ever-increasing use of fossil fuels, the levels of carbon dioxide in the atmosphere have been rising. The trend is made worse by the loss of photosynthetic action that accompanies widespread destruction of forests through logging and, worse, by the burning of vegetation, including tropical rain forests, to clear land for agriculture and human settlement. Green plants are being lost from the ocean also, through poisoning of phytoplankton by pollution of the seas. The concentration of atmospheric carbon dioxide has grown by over 35 percent since the beginning of the Industrial Revolution and is continuing to grow at an increasing rate.[15] Other gases also contribute to the greenhouse effect, especially methane, which is released by microbial activity in the intestines of cattle and in paddy fields where rice is grown.

Although the evidence was strongly disputed for many years, it is becoming increasingly clear that global climate change has begun: the Earth's average temperature has risen by well over one full degree Fahrenheit over the past century, as seen in **Figure 25-2**. Predictions for the year 2100 range from 3 to 7 degrees Fahrenheit higher than today.[15] The temperature increase is widespread over the globe and is greatest in the northern arctic region. According to the Intergovernmental Panel on Climate Change (IPCC), which won the Nobel Peace Price in 2007, the effects of global warming are already being felt. Sea levels rose during the second half of the 20th century and have continued to rise as glaciers and Arctic ice sheets melt. The IPCC predicts a rise of 1 to 2 feet by the end of the 21st century. Shifting precipitation patterns have increased dryness in the southwestern United States, northern Mexico, the Mediterranean region, and sub-Saharan Africa, while increasing wetness in northern North America and northern Europe.[15]

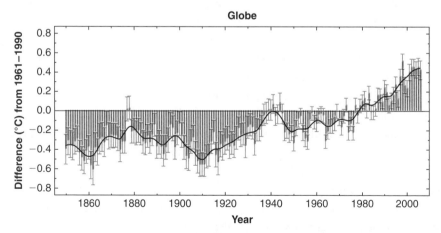

FIGURE 25-2   Global Temperature Change, 1850–2006. *Source:* Reproduced from the National Oceanic and Atmospheric Administration, "Global Warming: Frequently Asked Questions." www.ncdc.noaa.gov/img/climate/globalwarming/ar4-fig-3-6.gif, August 21, 2012, accessed September 28, 2012.

As oceans continue to rise, they will inundate coastal towns and cities, threatening tens of millions of people living in coastal regions of Africa, Asia, and small island nations.[16] The intensity of storms and hurricanes will increase. In the United States, 53 percent of the population lives in counties that include coastal areas, many of which, especially in the Southeast, Texas, and California, already suffer from the effects of hurricanes and tropical storms. The impact of higher sea levels will threaten many airports, rail lines, roads, ports, and pipelines.[17]

The implications for human health are complex and far-reaching. Food supplies will be affected, as optimal temperature and rainfall conditions for agriculture shift northward, and marginally dry lands turn to desert. Insect pests will become more active, adversely affecting crops even further. As temperate zones become hotter, vector-borne diseases that now plague tropical regions will enlarge their territory, spreading even to industrialized countries. Mosquitoes that carry the dengue and yellow fever viruses and malaria parasites threaten to move northward into the United States from Central America. A warmer climate may be responsible for the emergence of hantavirus infections in the United States, and the 1991 outbreak in South America of epidemic cholera, the first seen in the Western hemisphere in more than a century.[1] Extreme heat waves, such as the ones that occurred in Chicago in 1995, in Europe in 2003, and more than half of the United States in 2012 greatly increase the risk of death, especially among elderly city dwellers.

Prospects for slowing the process of global warming appear dim, in part because population pressures in developing countries contribute to continuing deforestation but, more importantly, because the United States and other industrialized countries contribute disproportionately to the production of greenhouse gases, as seen in **Figure 25-3**. The United States, with less than 5 percent of the world's population, contributes about 18 percent of the world's greenhouse emissions. By contrast, India has 17 percent of the people in the world while contributing only 5.5 percent of the world's greenhouse emissions.[18] The high per capita production of carbon dioxide is part of the affluent life style, one that poorer countries strive to emulate and may begin to achieve if they can control the growth of their populations. China, at almost 20 percent of the world's population, is rapidly improving the standard of living of its people and now contributes 24 percent of emissions, an amount that is growing. It is probable that environmental damage caused by the continued rise in the Earth's temperature will cause increases in human suffering, especially in the poorest countries.

Recognizing the dangers of global climate change, delegates to the United Nations' Earth Summit in 1992 negotiated an agreement that called for voluntary reductions in greenhouse gas emissions. It soon became obvious, however, that the nations were failing miserably at achieving any reduction in emissions, and negotiations were resumed in 1997 in Kyoto, Japan. At that conference, representatives from 171 nations agreed on mandatory reductions, with individualized goals for each country. The United States was assigned the goal of reducing its

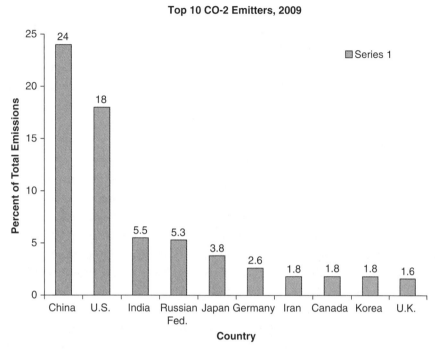

FIGURE 25-3   Top 10 CO-2 Emitters, 2009. *Source:* Data from International Energy Agency, "CO2 Emissions from Fuel Combustion: Highlights." www.iea.org/co2highlights/co2highlights.pdf, accessed October 10, 2012.

emissions to 7 percent below 1990 levels by 2012. The Kyoto Protocol was to become legally binding after being ratified by 55 countries representing 55 percent of the 1990 emissions.[1]

Prospects for ratification by the U.S. Congress looked bleak even when Bill Clinton was president, but upon the election of George W. Bush, it was clear that the United States would not participate. President Bush withdrew the nation from the Kyoto Protocol soon after he was inaugurated. He rejected evidence that global warming is occurring, to the extent that political pressures forced all reference to climate change to be removed from a major Environmental Protection Agency report on environmental quality.[19] In 2004, Russia became the 121st nation to ratify the Kyoto Protocol, allowing it to take effect in early 2005. However, without the participation of the world's leading emitters of greenhouse gases, the United States and China—which was not assigned limits under the Kyoto Protocol—the treaty was unlikely to make much difference. Even if all the signatories met their targets, the achievement would be only a small step toward reducing the impact of climate change.[1]

Another United Nations conference on climate change took place in Copenhagen in December 2009. Diplomats had worked hard over the preceding 2 years at negotiating a new treaty, which President Obama made a top priority. There were major differences between rich nations and poor nations, and no hard agreement was reached. Negotiators agreed to keep trying, but prospects for reaching an international agreement to control greenhouse gas emissions in the foreseeable future do not look promising.[20]

Dire Predictions and Fragile Hope

According to a moderate estimate, the United Nations expects the world's population to reach 9.3 billion in 2050 and be increasing by about 35 million persons annually at that time. Some countries are growing much more rapidly than others: The population of the 48 least developed countries is growing at 2.5 percent per year and is expected to double by 2050. The 10 countries with the highest fertility rates in 2005–2010 are all in Africa, except for Afghanistan and East Timor. Populations in the more developed regions are expected to increase only slightly by 2050, with most of the increase due to immigration. Most of the 10 countries with the lowest fertility rates are in East Asia and Eastern Europe.[7]

Many third-world countries are already suffering from shortages of natural and economic resources, including limited agricultural land and a lack of nonagricultural employment. Such regions may have already passed a threshold of irreversibility. The speed and magnitude with which populations are outstripping the available resources are unprecedented in history. The result is expected to be an increase in migrations and violent conflicts. Hundreds of millions of people may be compelled to relocate. Already, wars and civil violence are being fought over scarce resources such as water, farmland, forests, and fish. For example, the current violence in Darfur and Somalia is fundamentally related to food and water insecurity.[21] A comprehensive analysis of the economic effects of climate change, published in Great Britain in 2006, predicted that global warming could inflict worldwide disruption as great as that caused by the two World Wars and the Great Depression.[22] Some analysts predict a total breakdown in the social fabric of the planet.[23,24]

If there is any hope for saving the Earth from the direst of these predicted fates, it must come from control of population growth. Unfortunately, international agreement on this issue is exceedingly difficult. Three United Nations conferences on population were held at 10-year intervals, beginning in 1974; all were fraught with ethical, religious, and political controversy. Rich countries blamed poor countries for the destruction of natural resources, while poor countries blamed the rich for profligate consumption. Poor countries demanded help from the rich, which attached unwelcome conditions to the aid they provided. Opposition to contraception by Roman Catholic and Muslim authorities, as well as the incendiary politics of abortion in the United States, obstructed rational attempts at limiting population growth.

Although the 1994 conference held in Cairo was as contentious as the two previous meetings, a consensus emerged on a new approach to population policy, one that focused on individual rights, especially women's rights, including their right to make reproductive decisions. The conference produced a 20-year "Programme of Action" that included, among other goals, education for women.[25] Educated women prefer fewer children, and they have more bargaining power in the family and in society, studies have shown. Other goals agreed upon at Cairo were universal access to safe and reliable family-planning methods, universal access to and completion of primary education, reduction of infant mortality rates, reduction of maternal mortality rates, and increased life expectancy. The philosophy underlying the "Cairo Consensus" was that if needs for family planning and reproductive health care are met, along with other basic health and education services, then population stabilization will occur naturally, not as a matter of coercion or control.[26] Throughout 2009, a number of meetings were held to assess progress on implementing the goals, to reflect on emerging issues, to reaffirm commitments and to redouble efforts.

The United States is sheltered from some of the realities of the population problem because of the nation's relative isolation from the most crowded regions of the planet. However, Americans cannot afford to be complacent about the dangers posed by world crowding. Global warming, air and ocean pollution, and loss of biodiversity are environmental effects of overpopulation that are certain to affect public health in the United States, even if the nation could close its borders to all international travelers. Without global population control, other public health efforts would ultimately be a losing battle.

Population control cannot be imposed by force, however. As Paul and Anne Ehrlich point out in their book, *One with Nineveh*, stabilization of the world's population is closely tied to modernization and economic viability of the poorest countries.[5] This agrees with the conclusions of the 1994 Cairo conference, and it is the goal that the United States and other developed nations have agreed to strive toward. The Ehrlichs quote Lester Pearson, former prime minister of Canada and president of the United Nations General Assembly, "A planet cannot, any more than a country, survive half slave, half free, half engulfed in misery, half careening along toward the supposed joys of almost unlimited consumption. Neither our ecology nor our morality could survive such contrasts."[5(p.234)]

Conclusion

The Earth's human population has been growing rapidly and continuously for centuries. While the rate of growth appears to be slowing, the science of population biology suggests that a disastrous population crash is possible, a result of environmental pressures.

Paradoxically, public health measures such as clean water, immunization, and pest control have contributed to population growth by saving lives. While improved life expectancy has led to a fall in birth rates in industrialized countries, in the developing world population control efforts have not kept up with other public health efforts. The resulting crowding threatens to reverse the advances that have been made in public health. Migrants from rural areas, in search of jobs, settle in urban shantytowns that lack adequate drinking water and sewage services. These conditions lead to frequent epidemics of infectious diseases, and the accompanying social breakdown contributed to the rise of the AIDS epidemic. The AIDS epidemic in turn is so severe in parts of Africa that it has put a stop to population growth in those countries.

Many analysts believe that the carrying capacity of the Earth—the population size that the Earth can support without being degraded—is being reached. Factors that limit carrying capacity include the availability of fresh water, the availability of fuel, the amount and productivity of arable land, and the amount and disposition of wastes. Fresh water is already in short supply in some parts of the world, and many sources of fresh water are being degraded by pollution with human and industrial wastes. Arable land is being depleted through overcultivation and erosion. Deforestation is occurring on all continents, and even the sea is being depleted of fish.

In addition to the impact of resource shortages on human populations, overpopulation is bringing about global climate change. Increased atmospheric concentrations of greenhouse gases brought about by human activities are causing warming of the Earth's surface. This in turn causes melting of the polar ice caps and a rise in ocean levels. Weather patterns may already be changing. Warming of temperate zones may account for the recent emergence in the United States of a number of infectious diseases formerly confined to more tropical regions. At an international conference in Kyoto, Japan in 1997, an agreement was reached for countries to reduce their greenhouse gas emissions. However, President Bush tried to cast doubt on the evidence for global warming and withdrew U.S. support for the Kyoto Protocol. Now, with another climate conference that took place in December 2009, President Obama has expressed his support for climate control measures.

The United Nations has held three conferences on population, all fraught with ethical, religious, and political controversy. At the third conference, held in Cairo in 1994, a new approach to population control was agreed upon with a 20-year plan of action. This consensus builds on evidence that education and empowerment of women lead them to choose smaller families and brings a fragile hope that stabilization of the population may be achieved by helping the poorest nations to modernize and become economically stronger.

References

1. A. Nadakavukaren, *Our Global Environment: A Health Perspective*, 6th ed. (Prospect Heights, IL: Waveland Press, 2005).
2. P. R. Ehrlich, *The Population Bomb* (New York: Ballantine Books, 1975).

3. U.S. Central Intelligence Agency, *The World Factbook.* http://www.cia.gov/library/publications/the-world-factbook/fields/2002.html, accessed September 2, 2009.

4. P. R. Ehrlich and A. H. Ehrlich, *The Population Explosion* (New York: Simon and Schuster, 1990).

5. P. R. Ehrlich and A. H. Ehrlich, *One with Nineveh: Politics, Consumption, and the Human Future* (Washington, DC: Island Press, 2004).

6. P. R. Ehrlich and R. E. Ornstein, *Humanity on a Tightrope: Thoughts on Empathy, Family, and Big Changes for a Viable Future* (Lanham, MD: Rowman & Littlefield, Publishers, Inc., 2010).

7. United Nations Department of Economics and Social Affairs/Population Division, "World Population Prospects: The 2010 Revision." http://esa.un.org/wpp/Analytical-Figures/htm/fig_1.htm, accessed August 6, 2012.

8. United Nations Children's Fund, "State of the World's Children 2008." http://www.unicef.org/health/files/The_State_of_the_Worlds_Children_2008.pdf, accessed August 6, 2012.

9. United Nations Department of Economics and Social Affairs/Population Division, *Population Distribution, Urbanization, Internal Migration and Development: An International Perspective*, 2011. http://www.un.org/esa/population/publications//PopDistribUrbanization/PopulationDistributionUrbanization.pdf, accessed August 6, 2012.

10. United Nations Department of Economics and Social Affairs/Population Division, *Urban Population, Development and the Environment, 2011.* http://www.un.org/esa/population/publications/2011UrbanPopDevEnv_Chart/urbanpoopdevenv2011wallchart.html, accessed August 6, 2012.

11. United Nations Economic Commission for Africa, "Securing our Future: Report of the Commission on HIV/AIDS and Governance in Africa," 2008. http://www.unaids.org/en/regionscountries/regions/easternandsourthernafrica/, accessed August 6, 2012.

12. Federal Interagency Forum on Child and Family Statistics, "America's Children: Key National Indicators of Well-being, 2012." http://www.childstats.gov/americaschildren/eco.asp, accessed August 6, 2012.

13. P. A. Sanchez and M. S. Swaminathan, "Cutting World Hunger in Half," *Science* 307 (2005): 357–359.

14. J. Bongaarts, "Can the Growing Human Population Feed Itself," *Scientific American* (March 1994): 36–42.

15. Intergovernmental Panel on Climate Change, "Climate Change 2007: Synthesis Report—Summary for Policymakers." http://www.ipcc.ch/publications_and_data/ar4/syr/en/spm.html, accessed August 6, 2012.

16. R. A. Kerr, "Global Warming Is Changing the World," *Science* 316 (2007): 188–190.

17. National Research Council Transportation Research Board, *Potential Impacts of Climate Change on U.S. Transportation* (Washington, DC: National Academies Press, 2008).

18. International Energy Agency, "CO_2 Emissions from Fuel Combustion: Highlights," 2011. http://www.iea.org/co2highlights/co2highlights.pdf, accessed August 7, 2012.

19. E. Stokstad, "EPA Report Takes Heat for Climate Change Edits," *Science* 300 (2003): 201.

20. J. M. Broder, "Many Goals Remain Unmet in 5 Nations' Climate Deal," *The New York Times*, December 18, 2009.

21. J. D. Sachs, "Climate Change Refugees," *Scientific American* 296 (6) (June 2007): 43.

22. H. M. Treasury, "Stern Review on the Economics of Climate Change." http://www.hm-treasury.gov.uk/sternreview_index.htm, 2008, accessed September 8, 2009.
23. R. D. Kaplan, "The Coming Anarchy," *Atlantic Monthly* (February 1994): 44–76.
24. L. R. Brown, "Could Food Shortages Bring Down Civilization?" *Scientific American* 300 (5) (2009): 50–57.
25. J. DeJong, "Role and Limitations of the Cairo International Conference on Population and Development," *Social Science and Medicine* 51 (2000): 941–953.
26. United Nations, International Conference on Population and Development, "Programme of Action." http://www.unfpa.org/public/site/global/publications/pid/1973, accessed August 7, 2012.

Medical Care and
Public Health

Is the Medical Care System a Public Health Issue?

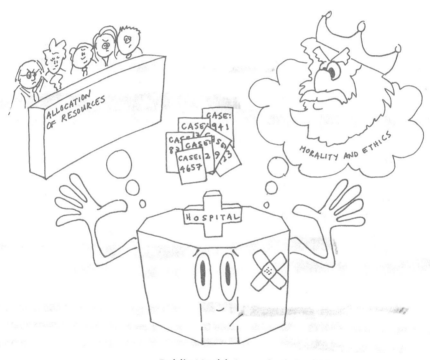

Public Health Issues?

Even in an ideal world, where public health functioned perfectly, there would be a need for medicine. The medical system provides preventive care: immunizations against infectious diseases, monitoring of pregnancies and provision of "well-baby care" to ensure that children develop normally, testing of adults for risk factors (such as high cholesterol and blood pressure) that lead to cardiovascular disease, and secondary prevention measures—screening for early detection of diabetes and cancer, for example, and early interventions to correct problems. Even people with the healthiest lifestyles get sick or injured. Medical care saves lives and prevents suffering and disability and, therefore, must be considered necessary for public health.

Medical care is even more necessary when public health is not functioning perfectly. There are many gaps in the public health system because of a lack of resources, lack of political will, and the emergence of new health threats. Also, competing values in society lead people to behave in unhealthy ways. The medical system is called upon to deal with the consequences of failures in public health. Doctors are asked to repair the damage when an unvaccinated child contracts an infectious disease, when a community is sickened by water or food contaminated because of deficiencies in sanitary practices, when someone is injured in a motor vehicle accident caused by a drunk driver, or when a smoker develops cancer after years of exposure to tobacco smoke.

The fact that medical care can and does make a difference in people's health raises a number of fundamental social questions. Who is responsible for providing medical care when it is needed? Medical care is expensive, and the costs have been rising dramatically over the past several decades. Who should pay for that care? Vastly greater sums of public money are spent each year on medical care than on public health measures aimed at preventing disease and disability. Is that a rational allocation of resources? Should U.S. citizens have the same right to medical care as they have to education in childhood? And, if there are limits on the community's responsibility for providing medical care, how should those limits be determined?

The medical profession has fought governmental involvement in addressing these questions, regarding itself as the ultimate authority over all matters of health.[1] However, public health concerns have repeatedly forced government action on a piecemeal basis to challenge medicine's sovereignty. Public health has always seen a role for itself as the provider of last resort, offering needed medical care to people who cannot afford to pay for it. This is part of the assurance function that the Institute of Medicine identified as one of public health's core functions. Government regulation has also been necessary to set standards for the practice of various healthcare services, to discipline medical professionals when they are thought to be acting unethically or incompetently, and to set policy when ethical dilemmas have arisen that transcend the individual sickroom.

When Medical Care Is a Public Health Responsibility

Some forms of medical care are more important to the health of the community than others. Medical treatment of communicable diseases is particularly important because of the possibility that one sick individual could infect many others. Consequently, public health has taken a major interest in all aspects of infectious disease control, from the early days when quarantines were the only effective way of controlling epidemics, to immunization programs, to the provision of free medical treatment for those who do not have health insurance and cannot afford to pay for care. City and county health departments have traditionally operated clinics for diagnosis and treatment of infectious diseases. Today, the threat of re-emerging tuberculosis is taken seriously enough that, for example, the New York City Department of Health provides a program of directly observed therapy in which public health nurses are sent to track down patients and make sure they take their medicine. The fact that AIDS is a communicable disease accounts, at least in part, for the major investment that the federal and some state governments have made not only in research, but also in providing treatment for patients.

A second area in which communities have an undisputed interest in the universal availability of medical care is the provision of emergency services. Emergencies are by definition unpredictable and can strike individuals at any time and in any place. In an increasingly mobile society, heart attacks and motor vehicle crashes may occur when people are far from home, with no family or friends present to provide first aid or call the doctor. It is in the interest of everyone to save lives first and ask questions later. Beginning with the Highway Safety Act of 1966, the federal government began to pressure states and localities to develop procedures for providing quick access to emergency care. Since then, in accordance with federal standards, communities have developed 911 phone-response networks, trained emergency medical technicians, dispatched ambulances using a centralized system, regulated the availability of hospital emergency rooms, identified trauma centers, and provided evacuation helicopters in rural areas. Still, the quality and the effectiveness of emergency response systems vary considerably in different parts of the country.[2]

A number of federal and state laws require that emergency rooms provide treatment to any patient that arrives with a life-threatening condition until he or she is stabilized, regardless of ability to pay. When the emergency situation has passed, however, many hospitals transfer poor and uninsured patients to public or charity hospitals. Some states have laws that prohibit hospitals from denying admission based solely on inability to pay, but in many parts of the country hospitals can and do turn away patients for financial reasons. Once medical treatment is under way, however, a patient's rights are greatly enhanced. There are laws against "abandonment," and hospitals cannot simply discharge patients because they are poor and uninsured.

Although most U.S. citizens do not have a general right to medical care, there are several exceptions, including veterans and prisoners. The hospitals and clinics of the Department of Veterans Affairs (VA) were designed to treat war-related injuries, but they also serve as a safety net for low-income veterans who do not have other sources of medical care. Funding for the VA system is chronically inadequate, however, and the agency has tightened its criteria for eligibility; except for those with combat injuries, only the poorest veterans can be served. Many veterans suffer from psychiatric disabilities or have substance abuse problems—conditions that the VA has special expertise to treat.[3] Prisoners are entitled to medical care because, as wards of the state, they are unable to seek care on their own. The courts have ruled that to deny them care would be the cruel and unusual punishment forbidden by the Constitution.[4] The medical care provided in prisons, however, is often substandard.

The Conflict Between Public Health and the Medical Profession

Most Americans get health insurance as part of an employee benefit package. The insurance covers the worker and his or her family. This approach to paying medical bills became dominant after World War II, when unions bargained actively to obtain health benefits for workers. The arrangement satisfied most groups over the next 3 or 4 decades. Workers and their families could receive necessary medical care without worrying about cost; doctors and hospitals were happy because they could provide care as they saw fit and not worry about getting paid; unions took credit for forcing employers to provide the benefits; employers did not object because the cost at first was modest and the benefits inspired loyalty in their workers.

Traditional health insurance, the kind of insurance provided by most employers until quite recently, is like car insurance. Regular premiums are paid to the insurance company to cover the worker and his or her family. When covered individuals get sick, they go to the doctor or other medical provider of their choice, and that provider then sends them bills for services rendered. The patients pay the bills and are reimbursed by the insurance company. Sometimes the policy, like many car insurance policies, calls for a deductible that the patient must pay first before the insurance kicks in. Sometimes the patients must also pay a flat fee or a fixed percentage of the remainder of the bill, called a copayment. This way of paying for medical care is called "fee-for-service." The fee-for-service approach permits doctors to make decisions about a patient's care with no consideration of cost. This freedom has led to escalating medical costs and increasing numbers of uninsured citizens whose access to care is limited.

The medical profession has strongly resisted efforts to be included in the domain of public services. Since the end of the 19th century, with the discovery of bacterial causes of diseases, public health has claimed the prevention and treatment of infectious disease as its responsibility, and doctors have resisted that claim. While tolerant of public health's efforts at cleaning up the environment, private practitioners regarded diagnosing and curing sick people as their domain. Early in the 20th century, they fought reporting requirements for cases of tuberculosis and venereal disease, and they opposed the creation of public health clinics and centers, which they perceived as an attack on their economic interests. This struggle continued throughout the century, and although public health had some victories, the medical establishment was able to prevent the United States from providing for its citizens the public assurance of needed medical care.[1]

Still, there is a long history of providing charity care for the nation's poor. Often, treatment was provided by part-time volunteer physicians who combined their services with research and the teaching of medical students. This practice began in the late 18th century, with the establishment of free dispensaries in eastern cities, many of them connected with medical schools. These services were controversial. Private practitioners were suspicious that free care was being provided to those who could afford to pay for it, and there was great concern about "dispensary abuse." The poor, on the other hand, were distrustful of the dispensaries, where they were forced to wait hours for hasty and superficial attention.[1]

In the early 20th century, city health departments began setting up clinics for the control of infectious diseases and the prevention of infant mortality. Baby clinics emphasized the teaching of hygienic practices and promotion of improvements in childcare, diet, and living patterns. Clinics for tuberculosis and venereal disease provided diagnosis and advice about hygiene and diet but left treatment to private physicians, who objected strongly when they felt that the clinics were trespassing on their territory. The New York City Department of Health ran into trouble when its diagnostic bacteriologic laboratory began producing diphtheria antitoxin, selling it to drugstores, and making it available to poor patients for free, prompting complaints of socialism and unfair competition that forced it to cease all sale of the antitoxin. Despite the early opposition of the medical profession, however, an uneasy truce has evolved that allows city and county health departments to provide treatment for the poor, often under the uncomfortable conditions that prevailed in the old dispensaries.[1]

Community health centers provide another source of basic medical care for the poor. These centers are supported by federal grants as well as by payments by public and private health insurance for services provided. There are about 1200 community health centers in the United States. They are located in inner cities and isolated rural areas where there are shortages of medical and social services. Community health centers provide primary and preventive care to people who might otherwise not be able to afford it. Services may be paid for by government programs (see the next section), or patients may pay a fee based on a sliding scale according to income. Community health centers serve as an important safety net for low-income families; the numbers served have been increasing, and they now serve about 20 percent of low-income uninsured persons.[5]

The health of schoolchildren has been a public health concern since the late 19th century. To control the spread of communicable diseases, cities began to employ medical inspectors to examine children who showed signs of illness and exclude them from school if they had a communicable disease. School doctors and nurses also began testing children for eye problems and other physical impairments that might interfere with learning. Because of the opposition of the medical establishment, they were not allowed to provide medical treatments. With the development of effective vaccines, the law began requiring that children be immunized—by their private physicians or in public clinics—before they started school, and the threat of epidemics in the schools has receded. In some cities, school health programs treat minor problems; sometimes they merely send notes recommending treatment home to parents. It is a source of frustration to public health practitioners that there is no integration of school health programs with medical services, leaving many children with health problems that are repeatedly diagnosed but untreated.[1]

Throughout the 20th century, there have been repeated attempts in the United States to provide some kind of national health insurance plan to ensure that everyone would have access to needed medical care. During this period, most industrialized countries were setting up such programs, some of them run by the national government, others more loosely organized. Germany established the first national system of compulsory sickness insurance in 1883. Over the next 30 years, Austria, Hungary, Norway, Serbia, Britain, Russia, and the Netherlands followed Germany's example. Canada implemented a national health insurance plan in the 1970s.[1]

In the United States, efforts to establish a national health program were made before World War I but were derailed by the war. Another attempt was made during the 1930s as part of President Franklin D. Roosevelt's New Deal, but health insurance was not included in the Social Security Act. After World War II, President Harry S. Truman proposed a single health insurance system that would apply to everyone; again the attempt failed. Each time, the medical profession opposed governmental involvement in medical care as "socialized medicine," and various other political interests joined to defeat the proposals.[1]

In 1965, a significant victory over the medical establishment's opposition was achieved under President Lyndon Johnson: legislation for Medicare, which provides insurance for the elderly, and Medicaid, a welfare-type program for the poor, were passed. These programs were designed to remedy what people considered the main problems with employer-based insurance: it stopped when a worker retired, and it left the poor and unemployed out of the system.[1]

Medicare, created in 1965 as a mandatory insurance program for people over the age of 65, is part of the Social Security system. (Younger people who are entitled to Social Security because of disability are also eligible for Medicare.) Workers pay into the system through deductions from their paychecks; employers pay a tax on their payroll; and workers are entitled to benefits when they reach retirement age. The Medicare program has two parts: Part A, which covers hospital insurance, and Part B, which pays doctor bills and other outpatient costs. Virtually all people are automatically enrolled in Medicare Part A when they reach age 65. Part B is voluntary and requires participants to pay a monthly premium. Medicare is much like traditional health insurance, in that most doctors and other providers are paid on a fee-for-service basis. Like private insurance, the patient is required to pay deductibles and copayments. In 2003, legislation was passed that created a new Medicare prescription drug plan. The new benefit, which became effective in 2006, is optional and requires an additional monthly premium.

Medicaid was created, also in 1965, as a welfare program for the poor, with costs shared by the federal government and the states. Eligibility is determined by income and varies from one state to another. Medical bills are paid directly by the state or local government to the provider, usually at a low, fixed rate for each service. Alternatively, states may fund managed care companies to cover Medicaid patients.

In the early 1970s, President Richard Nixon tried to expand these programs, proposing a national plan to cover everyone, but his efforts were derailed by the Watergate scandal. No further efforts were made until President Bill Clinton was elected in 1992, promising to provide health insurance for all; his proposal was also defeated. However, because of increasing concern about the problem of children without access to medical care, President Clinton and Congress negotiated a program called the Children's Health Insurance Program (CHIP). This is a joint federal–state program, similar to Medicaid, which expands coverage to children in families that earn too much to qualify for Medicaid, usually up to 200 percent of the federal poverty level.[6] Now, President Obama has succeeded in persuading Congress to pass the Affordable Care Act, an attempt to ensure that all Americans are covered by medical insurance. The new plan will be described later in this text.

Before the Affordable Care Act, the United States was the only industrialized nation, except South Africa, that did not have a national plan ensuring medical care for all its citizens. In 2008, over 20 percent of the American population ages 18 to 64 had no health insurance.[7] For many of these people, there was no guaranteed access to health care except for emergency care. While most public health advocates believe that the government should ensure access to basic medical care for anyone who needs it, the American political system had not supported that view. Clinical medicine, always more prestigious and more well financed than public health, was able to fend off public health's attempts to integrate medical treatment into a rational system that would maximize the health of all Americans. However, in response to increasing evidence that the U.S. healthcare system is dysfunctional, even the American Medical Association endorsed President Obama's efforts to change the system.[8]

Licensing and Regulation

While the medical profession, until recently, has resisted government efforts to ensure and fund medical care for all Americans, it has been willing to submit to some forms of government regulation. Licensure of qualified medical practitioners, including physicians, nurses, and other health professionals, protects the prerogatives of the professionals from encroachment by unlicensed practitioners and also ensures quality of care for patients. Physicians, nurses, and dentists must be licensed to practice in every state. Licensing requirements for other healthcare professionals vary from state to state. States may establish requirements, such as continuing medical education, for physicians and nurses to maintain or update their skills to retain their licenses. States also have the power to discipline medical professionals for incompetence or misconduct with the ultimate threat of revoking their licenses.

States also license and regulate medical facilities such as hospitals and nursing homes. To confirm that they provide high-quality care, healthcare institutions also may seek accreditation by a private organization, generally The Joint Commission (TJC). Since Medicare, Medicaid, and many private health insurers usually require institutions to be accredited in order to pay them for patient services, maintaining accreditation is important to them. Schools of medicine, nursing, and public health as well as training programs for advanced medical specialties also seek accreditation as a measure of their quality. As medical care is increasingly being provided by managed care organizations and as methods are developed to evaluate the quality of care provided by these organizations, accreditation of managed care organizations is becoming more widespread.

Governments have attempted to use regulatory approaches to restrain the growth of medical costs by requiring certificates of need before new facilities can be built or expensive new equipment purchased. These efforts have generally been ineffective and most have been abandoned.

Ethical and Legal Issues in Medical Care

Although the United States throughout the 20th century chose not to establish a broad right to medical care, it has been forced repeatedly to deal with individual cases that attract public attention and demand community response. Consequently, there are many legal requirements and restrictions on medical care that have arisen from specific cases. Usually, such cases have come to the attention of the courts when medical professionals disagreed with each other or with patients' families. Decisions in these cases have set legal precedents for how medicine can be practiced in certain situations. Many of these situations involve the beginning and end of life, and many of the precedents have profound implications for public health.

Abortion is one of the most controversial medico-legal issues, pitting the "right to life" of the fetus against the right of the pregnant woman to control her own body. Abortion was illegal in most states until 1973, when the Supreme Court decided in *Roe v. Wade* that women have a constitutional right to an abortion, at least in the first trimester of pregnancy. The controversy continues, however, with right-to-life activists trying, with some success in some state legislatures, to place limits on the circumstances under which women can exercise their rights. Similar controversy raged in the late 1990s over whether mentally competent, terminally ill patients have the right to physician-assisted suicide. Dr. Jack Kevorkian was making a career of helping to end the lives of people who were suffering or were afraid that they would suffer painful or degrading deaths. While laws were passed outlawing Dr. Kevorkian's activities, juries sympathized with the patients and refused to convict him. However, in 1999, he was convicted of second-degree murder because he went beyond assisting suicide and himself administered a lethal drug to a patient who wished to die. The death of a 52-year-old man with Lou Gehrig's disease was aired on the CBS program *60 Minutes*. Dr. Kevorkian served 8 years in prison and was released in 2007 after assuring authorities that he would never conduct another assisted suicide. He died of natural causes in 2011 at the age of 83.[9] Meanwhile, two states—Oregon in 1994 and Washington in 2008—have passed ballot measures that allow physicians to assist patients to commit suicide by prescribing lethal doses of drugs. The patients must be mentally competent adults, terminally ill with less than 6 months to live, and they must be capable of taking the medications by themselves.[10]

Ironically, while there is no legal requirement to provide medical care to people who want and could benefit from it, many of the most contentious legal cases have concerned the system's insistence on providing expensive, intrusive, and unwanted treatment to patients whose conditions are judged medically hopeless. In the 1976 case of Karen Ann Quinlan, a young woman left permanently unconscious from an overdose of drugs and alcohol, the New Jersey Supreme Court eventually ruled that she could be removed from a ventilator at the request of her parents over the objections of hospital personnel. However, in the 14 months of the court battle, the young woman had been weaned from the ventilator and was able to breathe on her own, although she remained unconscious. She was transferred to a nursing home where she survived for 10 years in a persistent vegetative state.[11]

In the similar case of Nancy Cruzan, a young Missouri woman in a persistent vegetative state resulting from an automobile crash, the Supreme Court decided in 1990 that states could set the standards for when life support could be removed. Cruzan's father had to move her to another state in order to remove the feeding tube and let her die.[12] Now, after a number of other cases have been tried in the courts, the precedent is well established that competent patients can refuse medical treatment and that life-support measures are not required for an incompetent patient who has specified in advance the conditions under which he or she would not want them. The most reliable way for an individual to ensure that his or her wishes would be followed is to sign a durable power of attorney over to a trusted friend or family member who can make medical decisions if he or she becomes incompetent.

The lack of such an advance directive led to the politically charged battle in early 2005 over removing a feeding tube from Terri Schiavo, a young Florida woman who had been in a persistent vegetative state for 15 years. Florida law provided that Ms. Schiavo's husband was entitled to decide that the feeding tube should be removed; he contended that she would not have wanted to be kept alive in this condition. However, Ms. Schiavo's parents objected, maintaining that she recognized them and that she might improve with treatment. Inspired by "right-to-life" political pressures, the Florida governor and legislature, the U.S. Congress, and President Bush attempted to block removal of the feeding tube, but the Florida courts, the federal appeals court, and the Supreme Court upheld the husband's right to decide. Ms. Schiavo died 13 days after the tube was removed. Such family disputes over withdrawing life support, while common, would be easily resolved if the individual had prepared a "living will" that specified her wishes.[13]

But what happens if a patient indicates that he or she wants all possible measures taken to preserve his or her life, even if there is no hope of regaining consciousness? This is what happened in 1991 in the case of Helga Wanglie, an 87-year-old woman in a persistent vegetative state who was being kept on a ventilator and feeding tube in a Minneapolis hospital. Her husband and children refused to allow life support to be removed, stating that they were praying for a miracle. The hospital went to court, claiming that the treatment was futile and merely prolonged death. The court refused to intervene, and the patient remained on life support until she died 3 days later.[14,15] In some states, including California and Texas, the law allows healthcare institutions to withdraw life support when further treatment is judged futile, even against the wishes of the patient as expressed in an advance directive.[13] Not often mentioned in the legal arguments is the cost of the care. Most often, the costs of caring for brain-damaged patients are borne by the taxpayer, since few families have the resources to pay for the necessary care.

Similar quandaries occur at the beginning of life, when decisions must be made about treating infants whose prospects are limited. Several notable cases occurred in the 1970s and 1980s involving babies born with Down syndrome, characterized by mental retardation and often accompanied by physical defects that are lethal but correctable by surgery. The difficult question with which parents are confronted, while still reeling from the news that their infant is not normal, is whether to authorize the surgery, allowing the infant a chance to live although his or her quality of life will be uncertain. In 1982, the Infant Doe case drew public attention to the problem. Infant Doe was a Down syndrome baby born in Bloomington, Indiana, with tracheoesophogeal fistula, a hole between the respiratory and digestive tracts. The parents chose not to operate, but hospital administrators and pediatricians went to court to force the surgery. The judge ruled that the parents had the right to make the decision; each level of appeal supported the parents, and the baby died before the case reached the Supreme Court.[11]

However, the publicity over Infant Doe attracted the attention of the Reagan administration, which firmly supported the right-to-life viewpoint. On the grounds that nontreatment of newborns constituted discrimination against people with disabilities, the Justice Department implemented the so-called Baby Doe rules, which mandated treatment of all newborns with birth defects. Large posters were to be displayed outside all neonatal intensive care units stating that "Discriminatory failure to feed and care for handicapped infants in this facility is prohibited by federal law." A toll-free 800 number, the "Baby Doe hotline," was posted to report abuses, and "Baby Doe squads," composed of lawyers, government administrators, and physicians, investigated complaints. Later court action struck down the Baby Doe rules; but in 1984, Congress passed a law declaring that nontreatment in Baby Doe cases is child abuse except when the child is chronically and irreversibly comatose, is inevitably dying, or when treatment would be "futile and inhumane."[11] The ethics of these rules are still being debated.[16]

It is not only Down syndrome infants that must be given aggressive medical treatment. Many of the 543,000 infants born preterm every year also must be provided with advanced, high-technology care. Although most of these infants survive to lead normal lives, many others—especially those with very low birth weight (less than 3.4 pounds) die or are left with permanent impairments. Infants with very low birth weight that survive are at increased risk of such long-term disabilities as cerebral palsy, autism, mental retardation, vision and hearing impairments, and other developmental problems.[17]

The costs of medical treatment for these infants, like the costs of providing life support for nearly dead adults, are not generally considered when decisions are made about whether aggressive treatment should be given. If these babies survive with major handicaps, medical and caretaking costs will continue throughout their lives. According to the Institute of Medicine, preterm births cost the nation an estimated $26 billion annually, mostly for medical care, but also for early intervention, special education, and lost productivity.[17] Much of the costs, like those for brain-damaged adults, is borne by taxpayers.

From a public health perspective, the American healthcare system is unfair and unethical. Vast resources are spent on a relatively few desperately ill patients, many of whom have no prospect of a reasonable quality of life, while millions of Americans have no access to the most basic medical services that could relieve pain and prevent long-term disability. Richard Lamm, a former governor of Colorado who has been an outspoken critic of the inequities of the system, laments that medical ethicists debate agonizingly over the treatment of a few individuals while little attention is paid to social ethics, a neglected and much needed examination of the allocation of resources for the entire system. Lamm argues that "it is axiomatic that public funds should buy the most health for the most people,"[18(p.14)] a view consistent with that of public health.

Ethical Issues in Medical Resource Allocation

While public health advocates believe that the inequities in access to care are the most important ethical dilemmas concerning the medical system, numerous other situations call for public participation in medical decisions. Sometimes the issue is access to scarce resources other than money. For example, when hemodialysis (blood-cleansing) was first developed in 1970 to help failing kidneys, there was a shortage of dialysis machines. To choose which patients should be dialyzed, "God Committees" were formed. The committees consisted of laypeople who would select the most worthy candidates for the life-saving treatment. The committees tended to favor those who had jobs, family responsibilities, youth, good general health, and strong motivation. The judgment process made many people uncomfortable.[11] After dramatic publicity about the plight of patients with kidney failure who were denied the dialysis treatment, Congress passed the 1972 End-Stage Renal Disease (ESRD) Act, which funded dialysis treatment for all Americans without selection criteria. Subsequently, the program's funding was extended to include kidney transplants, which can end patients' need for dialysis.

The ESRD Act created a new group of citizens with a right to medical care based on their diagnoses. Advocates for patients with other conditions, such as hemophilia and heart and lung disease, tried to persuade Congress to fund their diseases as well; however, the cost of kidney dialysis and transplants skyrocketed due in part to the open-ended funding, and Congress declined to extend the benefit to people other than kidney patients.[11]

As organ transplantation has became increasingly successful due to improved antirejection drugs, the problem of how to distribute scarce resources has resurfaced, since the number of donor organs is never adequate to fill the need. Livers are in especially short supply, and there is no substitute treatment, like kidney dialysis, for failing livers. More than 6000 patients receive liver transplants each year, but 2012, there were almost 16,000 people on regional waiting lists.[19]

The policy on distributing organs has been controversial. The task of matching available organs with waiting patients is handled by a nonprofit organization under contract with the Department of Health and Human Services. The organization, the United Network of Organ Sharing (UNOS), maintains a computerized network of 58 organ recovery centers in 11 geographic regions of the nation. When an organ becomes available, a suitable recipient is first sought within the same region. If a suitable match is not made within the region, the computer looks at waiting lists in other regions.[19]

In 2009, the issue of priority for transplants arose when Steve Jobs, the chief executive of Apple, unexpectedly received a liver transplant some time after he had been diagnosed with pancreatic cancer, possibly because the cancer had spread to his liver. Questions were raised about whether he had jumped to the head of the waiting list because of his wealth and celebrity, as had apparently happened when Mickey Mantle had a liver transplant in 1995 after only 1 day on the list. In a *New York Times* article, transplant specialists were quoted as saying that, although jumping ahead of others would not have been allowed for Mr. Jobs, there were ways of working the system that he could have used. Because waiting times vary at different transplant centers around the country, he could have registered at more than one center and, having access to a jet, could have arrived at a center promptly when an organ became available.[20] The allocation process is a life-or-death matter because each year almost 7000 patients die while waiting for an organ.[21]

The acrimony over rationing of organs, which is unavoidable because of obvious shortages, demonstrates how difficult it is politically to make rational decisions in the allocation of medical care. Elsewhere in this text, the argument is made that rationing currently exists throughout the medical system and should be addressed openly, although very few politicians or medical professionals are willing to face this fact.

Conclusion

While public health's focus on prevention of disease aims to minimize the need for medical care, access to medical care is an important part of the assurance function of public health. Medicine has always resisted attempts to include it as part of the public health system, with considerable success. Most Americans have private health insurance provided through their employers. However, public health concerns have overcome the opposition of the medical profession on some issues.

The urgent need to control the spread of communicable diseases has led to significant government involvement at the local level in providing medical care. Governments also coordinate, and often provide, emergency services to ensure prompt response when lives are at stake. Public health clinics that provide care for the poor have been grudgingly accepted by organized medicine, but there is no general right to medical care for Americans, as there is in most other industrialized countries.

There have been repeated attempts throughout the 20th century to enact a universal health insurance system in the United States. All were defeated. However, in the 1960s, Congress created the Medicare program, which guarantees medical care for the elderly, and the Medicaid program, which provides health care for the poor. In the 1990s, a joint federal–state program called Children's Health Insurance Program (CHIP) was created to provide medical care for poor children. Now, President Obama has succeeded in persuading Congress to pass a law intended to ensure that all Americans will be covered by insurance.

Public health has a role in monitoring and ensuring the quality of medical care through licensing of physicians, nurses, and other health professionals. Healthcare institutions such as hospitals and nursing homes also must be licensed by states. By requiring institutions to be accredited in order to receive Medicare and Medicaid payment for services, the government can help to ensure that the services provided meet a standard of quality. Government involvement in medical issues also occurs in connection with ethical and legal debates about life and death—issues that impact both medicine and public health. Such questions are especially painful when they concern removal of life support from permanently unconscious patients or nontreatment of severely handicapped newborns, situations that involve the provision of costly and probably futile care, usually at the public's expense.

Public participation in medical decisions is also necessary when scarce resources other than money are distributed. When hemodialysis for kidney failure was developed, there was a shortage of dialysis machines, and committees were formed to decide which patients could have the life-saving treatments. This was such a difficult political issue that Congress decided on the expensive solution of funding treatment for all Americans with kidney failure. Currently, patients with failing livers are in similar life-and-death situations, with liver transplants being their only hope of survival. However, there is a shortage of livers available for transplant, and there is always controversy over how these organs should be distributed.

References

1. P. Starr, *The Social Transformation of American Medicine* (New York: Basic Books, 1982).
2. M. Peisert, *The Hospital's Role in Emergency Medical Services Systems* (Chicago: American Hospital Publishing, 1984).
3. D. U. Himmelstein et al., "Lack of Health Coverage Among U.S. Veterans from 1987 to 2004," *American Journal of Public Health* 97 (2007): 2199–2203.
4. L. I. Palmer, *Law, Medicine, and Social Justice* (Louisville, KY: Westminster/John Knox Press, 1989).
5. National Association of Community Health Centers, "About Our Health Centers." http://www.nachc.com/health-center-challenges.cfm, accessed November 30, 1012.
6. Centers for Medicare and Medicaid Services, "Overview: The Children's Health Insurance Program (CHIP)." http://www.cms.hhs.gov/LowCostHealthInsFamChild/, accessed September 11, 2012.
7. E. Eckholm, "Last Year's Poverty Rate Was Highest in 12 Years," *The New York Times*, September 10, 2009.
8. D. D. Kirkpatrick, "A.M.A. Endorses a Health Care Overhaul," *The New York Times*, September 9, 2009.
9. K. Schneider, "Dr. Jack Kevorkian Dies at 83; A Doctor Who Helped End Lives," *The New York Times,* June 3, 2011.

10. W. Yardley, "First Death for Washington Assisted-Suicide Law," *The New York Times*, May 22, 2009.

11. G. E. Pence, *Classic Cases in Medical Ethics: Accounts of the Cases That Have Shaped Medical Ethics*, 5th ed. (Boston: McGraw-Hill, 2008).

12. G. J. Annas, "Nancy Cruzan and the Right to Die," *New England Journal of Medicine* 323 (1990): 670–672.

13. L. O. Gostin, "Ethics, the Constitution, and the Dying Process: The Case of Theresa Marie Schiavo," *Journal of the American Medical Association* 293 (2005): 2402–2407.

14. M. Angell, "The Case of Helga Wanglie: A New Kind of 'Right to Die' Case," *New England Journal of Medicine* 225 (1991): 511–512.

15. S. H. Miles, "Sounding Board: Informed Demand for 'Non-Beneficial' Medical Treatment," *New England Journal of Medicine* 225 (1991): 512–515.

16. L. M. Kopelman, "Are the 21-Year-Old Baby Doe Rules Misunderstood or Mistaken?" *Pediatrics* 115 (2005): 797–802.

17. Institute of Medicine, *Preterm Birth: Causes, Consequences and Prevention* (Washington, DC: The National Academies Press, 2007).

18. R. D. Lamm, "Ethics of Excess," *Hastings Center Report* 24 (1994): 14.

19. UNOS: United Network of Organ Sharing, 2012. http://www.unos.org/, accessed August 8, 2012.

20. D. Grady and B. Meir, "A Transplant That Is Raising Many Questions," *The New York Times*, June 22, 2009.

21. New York Organ Donation Network, "All About Donation: Organ Donation Statistics." http://www.donatelifeny.org/about-donation/data/, accessed August 8, 2012.

Why the U.S. Medical System Needs Reform

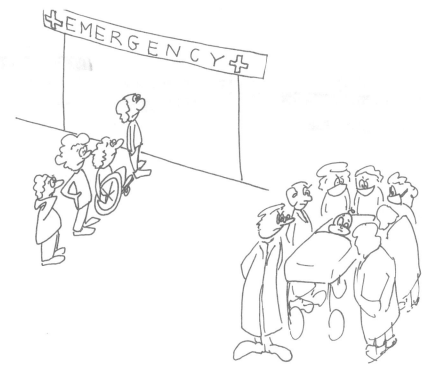

Inequalities in Access

It was obvious almost as soon as Medicare and Medicaid were enacted that the U.S. healthcare system still had problems. Medical costs in the United States, which had been rising more rapidly than general inflation, rose even more rapidly, putting a strain on all forms of health insurance. Access to medical care was difficult for many Americans because they lacked insurance. And despite the high costs, there were indications that the quality of medical care might not be as high as Americans liked to believe. A variety of attempts have been made to reform the system, aimed at controlling costs and improving access, none with significant success. The most recent attempt, described later in this chapter, is President Obama's 2010 Affordable Care Act, which is intended to take full effect in 2014.

Figure 27-1 shows the growth in medical care expenditures in the United States since 1960. In that year, approximately $27 billion was spent on medical care. In 1970, the figure had grown to $74 billion. By 2009, national health expenditures had reached $2.6 trillion dollars per year, although it remained the same in 2010 because of the recession.[1] The rate of increase averaged about 2.5 percent above the overall growth rate of the economy.[2] Because of their faster growth rate, medical costs have constituted a larger and larger percentage of the nation's gross domestic product (GDP). In 1960, medical expenditures were about 5 percent of the GDP; in 2010, they were 17.9 percent.[1]

Although expenditures on health have risen all over the world, the United States spends far more on medical care per person than any other country in the world. In 2009, an average of $7990 was spent on health costs for each American, more than twice the average of a group of 32 industrialized countries that are members of the Organization for Economic Cooperation and Development (OECD) (see Figure 27-2).[2] Spending as a percentage of GDP is also higher in the United States, amounting to 17.7 percent in 2009; the Netherlands followed at 11.9 percent; and the average for the 32 OECD countries was 9.5.

There is no evidence that Americans are healthier as a result of the greater expenditures. As measured by the common indicators of health status used for international comparisons, the United States does poorly. Of 30 OECD countries compared in 2008, the United States

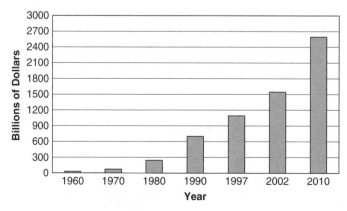

FIGURE 27-1   U.S. Health Care Expenditures Between 1960 and 2010. *Source:* Data from *Health Affairs* 13 (5) (1994): 14–31; 28 (1) (2009): 246–261; and 31 (2012): 208–219.

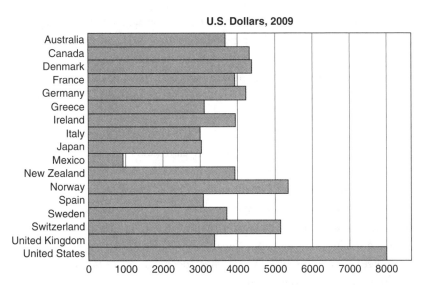

FIGURE 27-2   Per Capita Health Spending in Selected OECD Countries. *Source:* Data from *Health Affairs* 26 (5) (2007): 1481–1489.

ranked 27th in infant mortality; its life expectancy at birth was 24th for males and 25th for females. Our life expectancy at age 65, ranked 18th for males and 24th for females.[3]

Problems with Access

Despite the large expenditures, many Americans have difficulty getting access to medical care when they need it. About 49.8 million people, or 16.3 percent of the population, lacked health insurance for the entire year in 2010.[4] Many more may be uninsured for part of the year. The numbers have been increasing and were predicted to continue to rise unless the government reformed the system. It is hoped that the new Affordable Care Act will make a big difference in reducing the number of people who lack health insurance. Most of the uninsured are poor but not poor enough to qualify for Medicaid. The percentage of children who are uninsured has declined to less than 10 percent because of the Children's Health Insurance Program passed in the 1990s. But young adults are the group most likely to be uninsured: 27.2 percent of those ages 19 to 24 and 28.4 percent of those ages 25 to 34. Members of racial and ethnic minority groups are more likely to be uninsured than white Americans: about 20.8 percent of African Americans and almost 30.7 percent of Hispanics were uninsured in 2010, compared with 11.7 percent of whites.[4] Many of the uninsured are patients with chronic diseases who are closed out of the market because of policies that deny coverage for preexisting conditions or that charge exorbitant premiums for people whose health is poor.

The problem of access to medical care is closely related to the problem of its cost. As monthly premiums have risen in proportion to wages, it has become increasingly expensive for employers, especially small businesses, to provide health insurance for employees and their families. Employers have cut back on their coverage, shifting more of the costs to the employees by requiring them to pay a larger share of the premiums, higher deductibles, and higher copayments. Some low-wage workers may choose to remain uninsured because their share of the premiums is too high; yet these workers earn too much to qualify for Medicaid in most states. Nearly 83 percent of the uninsured live in families headed by workers. Uninsured workers are mostly employed in blue-collar jobs or service-sector jobs or work part-time.[5]

No other industrialized country has such large numbers of uninsured citizens as the United States. The western European countries, Japan, and Canada have national health plans that virtually guarantee coverage to all citizens. They spend less per capita and devote a smaller percentage of their economies to medical costs.

Lack of insurance clearly leads to poorer outcomes when people are sick. People who are uninsured tend to postpone seeking medical care when they need it, and they may be denied care. If they are sufficiently sick, they may go to an emergency room, which is required by law to treat them, and the cost of their care may be borne by shifting it to other payers, increasing the charges for insured patients. This is not, however, the most effective form of medical care. The uninsured are more likely to be hospitalized for preventable illnesses than insured patients, and they are less likely to survive a serious illness.[6] A study published in 2009 found that people without health insurance had a 40 percent higher risk of death than those with private insurance, leading to 45,000 deaths each year.[7]

Although Medicare has ensured that most of the elderly have access to medical care when they need it, escalating costs have had an impact here, too. Each year the program pays out more than it collects in premiums, and Congress has repeatedly tried to make adjustments to save the system from bankruptcy. In 2011, 15 percent of the federal budget went to Medicare, and spending is growing at an unsustainable rate.[8] Attempts to cut costs are politically delicate because the elderly are fiercely protective of their entitlements. Because of the overall growth of medical expenses generally, together with requirements for beneficiaries to pay deductibles and copayments, the elderly now pay on average 15 percent of their income out-of-pocket for medical care. Most have some form of supplemental insurance plan.[9]

Medicaid has never worked as well as it was expected to. Although federal law requires coverage for all children under 6 and pregnant women whose family income is below 133 percent of the federal poverty level, eligibility for the children's parents is set by the states and varies considerably. In some states, the fixed fees that the program pays to providers are so low that doctors are unwilling to participate in the program, making it difficult for families that have coverage to find someone to treat them other than poor-quality "Medicaid mills." Even so, the growing costs of Medicaid are placing a strain on many state budgets, using funds that might otherwise be used for education or other services. Although the majority of Medicaid beneficiaries are children, their parents, and pregnant women, most of the spending goes to long-term care for the elderly and disabled.

Overall, although the American medical system is the most expensive in the world, it is highly inefficient. The United States spends a higher proportion of its resources on health care than other countries; at the same time a significant proportion of the population is denied services, a situation almost unheard of in other countries. Moreover, the health status of the American population is poor in international comparisons—evidence that all the spending on medical care cannot compensate for failures in the public health system.

Why Do Costs Keep Rising?

A number of factors are responsible for the high and rising cost of medical care in the United States, some of them common to all industrialized countries, some unique to the American system. The aging of the population, for example, is a problem common to most countries. Because older people generally have a greater need for medical care, aging populations are driving up medical expenditures everywhere. In fact, several other countries have older populations than the United States.

Another factor that increases costs everywhere is the continual development of new medical technology and high-tech procedures. New instruments such as computed tomography (CT) scanners and magnetic resonance imaging (MRI) devices and new procedures such as arthroscopic and laparoscopic surgery and cardiac catheterization are expensive. They can be very effective in diagnosing and treating illness, so they are used widely—perhaps too widely. However, these technologies are available in all advanced countries, and it is not clear that they are more widely used in the United States.[10]

When inflationary factors that are unique to the American system are considered, administrative costs are one of the favorite targets of blame. According to one recent estimate, 31 percent of the American medical budget is spent on administration. Twenty-seven percent of medical workers in the United States spend most of their time on paperwork, up from 18 percent in 1968.[11] Because many different insurers pay for medical care, each with its own forms and documentation requirements, the process of billing and paying for care in the United States is much more time consuming and expensive than in countries where the government pays for everything. Moreover, some insurance companies, in trying to control costs, institute additional administrative procedures, for example requiring doctors to justify the need for certain treatments. This has the paradoxical effect of increasing paperwork and the percentage of effort and expense that goes to administration. As one eminent health economist lamented: "I look at the U.S. healthcare system and see an administrative monstrosity, a truly bizarre mélange of thousands of payers with payment systems that differ for no socially beneficial reason."[12]

Another peculiarly American characteristic that adds to medical costs is our tendency to sue for malpractice when something goes wrong. Doctors complain about the exorbitant price of malpractice insurance, and occasional news stories tell of a multimillion-dollar jury award to an unfortunate patient who was harmed by some medical procedure. Although these costs do not in themselves have a significant overall impact, the fear of malpractice suits may affect a physician's decisions. Doctors may practice "defensive medicine," ordering more diagnostic tests and medical procedures than necessary, to document in court that they did "everything possible" for the patient.

In fact, studies have shown that the whole system of malpractice compensation is inefficient and unjust. Most patients who are harmed by poor medical treatment are not compensated, and many patients who have suffered a bad outcome sue and win, even when the medical provider was not negligent.[13] However, because the United States does not have a national health plan, winning a malpractice suit may be the only way an injured patient will be able to pay for treatment of his injury.

One analysis of why medical spending in this country is higher than in other OECD countries found that the United States has higher rates of chronic diseases associated with obesity, including diabetes and heart disease. Almost two-thirds of Americans are overweight or obese, far outnumbering the prevalence in other countries, where, on average, 47 percent of the population has a BMI greater than 25.[10]

Among the most significant factors driving up medical costs are financial incentives for medical providers. In the "fee-for-service" system of payment, doctors and hospitals are motivated to provide more services in order to increase their income. Moreover, the performance of surgical procedures and the use of high-tech diagnostic equipment are more profitable than the more time-consuming practices of talking, listening, observing, and touching. Along with the growth of new medical technologies has come the growth of specialization among physicians. Fewer than 50 percent of doctors in the United States work in primary care, which includes family practice, general internal medicine, pediatrics, and obstetrics/gynecology. The majority of American physicians practice the more lucrative technological specialties such as radiology, anesthesiology, ophthalmology, cardiology, gastroenterology, and urology. Because of the relatively low pay for primary care providers, many patients looking for an internist or pediatrician may not be able to find one.[14] There is concern that the new healthcare law will exacerbate the problem.

Conspiring with providers in forcing up costs are the expectations of the medical care "consumer"—the patient. Patients with traditional insurance do not have to consider the costs of their care in making decisions on how they should be treated, because the bills will be paid by their insurance company. Thus they demand "the best" in technology, treatment by specialists, and prompt service. Economists point out that the medical marketplace is different from classical markets, which are sensitive to the price of goods and services. In the medical marketplace, the seller (the doctor) rather than the buyer (the patient) determines what the buyer needs. Sellers also set the price, and because the bill is paid by a third party (the insurance company), there is no incentive for the buyer to select less expensive options.

Approaches to Controlling Medical Costs

Of the total amount spent on medical care in the United States, 46.2 percent is paid by federal, state, and local governments. About 35 percent is paid by private health insurance sponsored by employers.[1] Thus, both governments and employers have reason to try to control costs, and they have tried a variety of approaches to achieve that goal. The first cost control effort by the federal government was the imposition of price controls by President Nixon from 1971 to 1974. Although the policy moderated cost increases temporarily, providers adapted to the lower fees paid for each service by increasing the quantity of services. Total spending continued to rise.

Another regulatory approach to cost control focused on limiting spending on new facilities and technology. This is a major strategy used by other OECD countries to control their costs. In the 1970s, the federal and some state governments tried to constrain the supply of hospital beds and high-tech equipment by establishing regional planning agencies that would assess the need for capital expenditures and issue certificates-of-need for new investments. Without limits on budgets, however, there were few incentives for state or local governments to control these expenditures. Considerable political pressure also served to force approval of new projects. In the 1980s, certificate-of-need programs were gradually abandoned as ineffective.

In the 1980s, the Medicare program tried a different approach to cost control. Because the greatest expenditures were payments to hospitals, the program devised a payment system designed to provide incentives for hospitals to limit the length of hospital stays. Medicare paid a flat fee for each hospital stay, an amount based on the illness category of the patient, or diagnosis related group (DRG), and the average cost of treating similar patients throughout the country. If a hospital could cure the patient in a shorter time than average, it could keep the extra cash. If a longer stay was necessary, the hospital had to swallow the additional cost. Hospitals, in response, began charging private insurance companies more to make up for their losses from the government; so several states adopted DRG-type rate-setting systems for all payers, forcing hospitals to accept the same rates for everyone. One result of policies limiting payments to hospitals was to move more treatment out of the hospital. Hospital stays are on average much shorter now than they were 2 decades ago, and outpatient surgery and diagnostic testing have become the rule. The DRG system was effective in reducing expenditures for hospital care, but overall costs continued to rise because there was no DRG system for outpatient care.

Managed Care and Beyond

Employer-based private insurance plans have tried a number of approaches to limiting costs by bargaining with providers—doctors and hospitals—for discounts on services. The result is a variety of plans that fall under the category of managed care. For example, in preferred provider organizations (PPOs), patients are required to seek care from participating providers who have agreed to provide services at lower rates. In some of these plans, patients are not allowed to see a specialist without a referral from a primary care physician, a strategy for limiting access to expensive high-tech care as well as for ensuring coordination of the care received by the patient from various providers. A variation on the PPO arrangement allows patients to go to nonparticipating providers but requires them to pay a higher percentage of those costs out of their own pockets.

The most stringent form of managed care is the health maintenance organization (HMO), so called because—in theory at least—the organization has a financial incentive to maintain the health of its members. An HMO acts as both insurer and provider. In return for a fixed monthly or annual payment, the HMO agrees to provide all the medical care the individual needs. Conventional HMOs hire a staff of physicians, nurses, and other healthcare workers who earn a salary and thus have no incentive to provide expensive treatments when not necessary. Moreover, HMOs have incentives to provide preventive care and health promotion programs, adopting some of the goals and objectives of public health.

Managed care flourished in the 1990s. With the continued rise of medical costs and the failure to enact President Clinton's plan for healthcare reform, employers moved to restrict the choices of their employees to plans that incorporated cost control measures. In 1995, almost three-quarters of workers covered by employer-sponsored insurance were in managed care plans.[15] States began to move Medicaid recipients into managed care plans in the hope of providing them with a higher quality of care and more continuity of care, as well as controlling Medicaid costs. The Medicare program also tried to encourage more of the elderly to enroll in managed care plans. The result was a dramatic slowing of medical inflation in the 1990s.[1] However, the slowdown did not last.

With the success of managed care came some major criticism and what was called "the HMO backlash."[16] Patients understood that the financial incentives encouraged denial of treatment, and they were outraged, even when some of the treatments denied were of unproven efficacy. Some for-profit HMOs had especially objectionable practices of giving bonuses to physicians who were most successful in denying care. Patients also objected to limits on their choice of doctors to consult. News stories told of HMO "gag rules" that forbade physicians from recommending treatments for which the HMO would not approve payment. Many state legislatures passed laws prohibiting gag rules. Similarly, states passed laws regarding "drive-through deliveries" and "drive-through mastectomies" in response to managed care plans that limited hospital stays for women giving birth or having cancer surgery. In 1996 alone, 56 laws were passed in 35 states aimed at regulating or weakening HMOs.[16] The result of such laws, together with some important decisions in federal courts that favored consumers' right to sue HMOs for denial of care, meant that managed care organizations lost much of their ability to manage medical care in a cost-conscious way.[17]

Despite the complaints about managed care, including well-publicized instances of patients' being denied expensive procedures that might have saved their lives, there is no evidence that patients are harmed by the cost-control measures overall. In many ways, managed care has an advantage over fee-for-service in providing high-quality care. The emphasis on prevention and health education may indeed help to keep members healthy. Coordination of care and use of interdisciplinary teams for disease management can help to prevent patients with chronic diseases from developing severe and costly complications. The use of primary care physicians as gatekeepers for controlling patient access to specialists may help to prevent unnecessary procedures that could put patients at risk. Managed care organizations, because of centralized recordkeeping, have the ability to monitor patients' health and to evaluate the quality of care they receive.

The result of the weakening of cost control methods used by managed care organizations was that medical spending began to grow again in the late 1990s and early 2000s, although at a slower rate. Plans became less restrictive, and PPOs became more popular because they allow more choices. Health insurance became less affordable. More of the costs are shifted to the patients. The problems of the uninsured have grown worse. When fee-for-service was the norm, hospitals could charge higher rates to insured patients to cover the costs of treating the uninsured, as they are often required to do by law. Now, however, managed care organizations, even the weaker ones, negotiate reduced payments for treatment of their members, and hospitals are less able to cost-shift, causing financial pain for the hospitals. While some states provide special payments to hospitals to cover bad debt and charity care, antitax sentiment discourages such public funding for the poor. Private hospitals select the most profitable patients, and stories of patient "dumping" have become common. Public hospitals in inner cities bear the brunt of caring for the sickest uninsured patients, and many must cut back on services or threaten to close because of lack of funding.[18]

An approach to controlling medical costs, called consumer-directed health plans, is popular among political conservatives and was encouraged during the Bush administration. The intent of these plans is to make consumers more cost-conscious when they seek medical care by providing them with information on cost and quality and requiring them to share more of the cost. The plans tend to have high deductibles, so that insurance payments do not kick in until after individuals themselves have paid for a significant amount of services, and they tend to be combined with health savings accounts, in which individuals set aside funds tax-free to be used in paying for medical expenses. A number of drawbacks have been noted with these plans, including that they are most likely to be used as a tax haven for healthy and wealthy individuals. Another difficulty is that they motivate people to avoid, skip, or delay health care because of costs, sometimes leading to more serious disease and increased risk of needing hospitalization.[19]

The Patient Protection and Affordable Care Act

In 2010, President Obama persuaded Congress to pass a healthcare reform law, aimed at addressing many of the problems with the American medical care system. One of the key components of the new law is the individual mandate, a requirement that all Americans have health insurance or pay a fine. People who already have coverage may not see any change. Many employees of large businesses already receive insurance through their employers. The new law does not require employers to provide insurance, but any business with 50 or more workers that does not provide coverage will be required to pay an assessment of $2000 per employee. Small businesses will receive tax credits to provide insurance to their workers.[20]

The individual mandate requires states to set up affordable insurance exchanges, whereby individuals can shop for a plan that meets their needs. Many states have already begun to establish an exchange. The law included a requirement to expand Medicaid, which had different eligibility rules in different states, to cover low-income adults. Some states with Republican governors have refused to follow the requirements of the law; in those states, the federal government is charged with setting up the exchanges.

Some other provisions of the law have proved popular, including an expansion of coverage for young adults on their parents' plan up to age 26. Medicare will provide older adults with preventive benefits including a yearly wellness visit and a range of no-cost screenings for cancer, diabetes, and other chronic diseases. Among the preventive services required by the law is contraception, a provision that has proven controversial. Seniors will benefit from savings in the Medicare prescription drug plan, which will gradually close the "donut hole" so that it disappears in 2010. A number of insurance company abuses, such as cancellation of policies of patients when their medical costs rise, are outlawed by the new law.[20] The law establishes a Center for Medicare and Medicaid Innovation that will begin testing new ways of delivering care aimed at improving quality of care and reducing the rate of growth in costs for Medicare, Medicaid, and the Children's Health Insurance Program. Many of the law's provisions have already implemented; many others will take effect in 2014.

The law was challenged in court by 26 states, with the individual mandate the most contested issue. The Supreme Court largely upheld the law in 2012. Chief Justice Roberts, generally a conservative, was the decisive vote in favor, ruling that the fine for not having insurance amounted to a tax, which the government has the power to impose. The decision restricted the expansion of Medicaid, allowing some states to not expand eligibility. The ultimate fate of the law depended on the outcome of the 2012 presidential election: Mitt Romney, the Republican candidate, vowed to repeal the law.[21] The reelection of President Obama ensures that the reform of the medical care system will go forward.

Rationing

In the late 1980s, the state of Oregon tried an experiment. Realizing that its Medicaid budget was not large enough to provide comprehensive coverage for all of its poor citizens, the state legislature undertook a plan to spread its resources over a larger number of people by limiting the services for which it would pay. Its first move was highly controversial. It decided not to pay for organ transplants, with the justification that the funds required for 34 transplants could provide for prenatal care and delivery for 1500 pregnant women.[22] When a young boy with acute leukemia was denied a bone-marrow transplant and died as a result, there was a national uproar.

The legislature, led by John Kitzhaber, a physician who was then president of the state senate and later became governor, decided to develop a more acceptable policy for broadening Medicaid eligibility. The new approach focused on life-saving treatments for serious conditions and tried to eliminate less effective therapies for less serious conditions. The state decided to develop a prioritized list of health services and draw a line below which treatments would not be covered. The goal was to cover all citizens whose incomes were below the poverty level, and to use managed care plans to provide medical care.

A commission was formed to develop the list by consulting as much as possible with the citizens of the state. Public hearings and town meetings were held to determine the relative value placed on various medical services by the public. The commission established 17 categories of health problems according to 13 criteria, including life expectancy, quality of life, the cost-effectiveness of a treatment, and the probable number of people who would benefit. The highest priority was placed on acute problems that could be fatal and for which treatment would provide full recovery. Surgery for appendicitis is an example of a high-priority procedure. Other highly ranked services included maternity care and preventive care for children. At the bottom of the list were treatments known to be ineffective, or those that did not improve quality of life or extend life, including some treatments for cancer and AIDS.[23]

The Oregon plan provoked opposition on legal, social, and ethical grounds. In 1991, the Department of Health and Human Services denied permission for Oregon to implement the plan on the basis that it violated the Americans with Disabilities Act, because the list under-valued the quality of life of people with disabilities. After some revisions, the plan was finally approved by the Clinton administration in 1993. More than 100,000 Oregonians were added to the Medicaid program as a result.[23]

Many critics have pointed out that the policy would be more equitable and that the decisions would be much less difficult if everyone—not just the poor—were included in the rationing proposal. The medical system as a whole is rich enough to provide necessary care for every-one; the need to ration care for the poor is a consequence of failures of the system to provide adequate and affordable care for everyone. Health policy experts have praised the Oregon plan's focus on medical necessity so that all appropriate care and no inappropriate care is covered. It called attention to the need for more research on outcomes of various treatments to permit better informed decisions on medical necessity. Some of these lessons may be useful in imple-menting President Obama's new healthcare law.

However, the Oregon Plan, while still officially in effect, is now struggling badly. In part, its difficulties stemmed from an attempt in 2002 to expand it further to include additional uninsured residents, which happened at a time when the state was undergoing an economic downturn. Oregonians, like other Americans, resisted increasing taxes to finance the program. In part, the program faltered because Governor Kitzhaber was term limited, and his successor was not such an enthusiastic defender of the plan. Also, in Oregon, as in the rest of the country, medical care costs began growing faster than the general economy, making the provision of health care for all economically and politically more and more difficult.[24]

The Oregon experiment makes many people uncomfortable. People do not like to confront the idea that rationing medical care might be necessary or desirable. In fact, however, rationing medical care has been going on all along: care has been rationed on the basis of ability to pay, but the rationing has not been explicitly admitted. When a story hits the news about an unin-sured child denied treatment for leukemia, for example, the public and politicians purport to be shocked that such a thing could happen in our society. Yet it is politically impossible to raise taxes so that such children could be provided with medical insurance or that public hospitals could afford to provide effective care.

Our society has never been willing to discuss tradeoffs between costs and quality of medical care.[25] Because third parties—usually the government or insurance companies—pay for care, people have come to believe that cost should not be considered when decisions are made about medical treatments. When asked about a particular patient or situation, people will say that no effort should be spared in trying to achieve the best possible outcome. It is an easy thing to say when they are not paying the bills. At the same time, people naturally seek out insurance plans with the lowest premiums. It is a catch-22 situation: society demands that the healthcare system maximize quality while minimizing costs, but it has placed a taboo on the consideration of cost.[25]

Rationing is a dirty word when it applies to medical care. But rationing is inevitable. In economics, "rationing is simply the process of allocating goods in the face of scarcity."[26] Since most people are unwilling to pay an unlimited amount of money to receive a small benefit, decisions are continually being made on allocation of medical services. What is needed is an open discussion on how those decisions should be made. Should kidney dialysis be denied to the elderly or to people with diabetes so advanced that they have lost their vision? Should we tolerate long waiting lists for hip replacements? Should the rich receive care and the poor be denied it? Should we allow for-profit healthcare systems that make large profits for their stockholders while refusing to care for patients with expensive chronic diseases?[27] These are difficult questions for medicine and for public health, but we need to openly discuss them and decide on a societal basis.

Conclusion

The U.S. medical care system is the most expensive in the world. At the same time, it has many faults, including lack of access for the uninsured, about 16 percent of the American population. Medical care costs have risen continuously, and the rising costs contribute to the inability of many to afford health insurance.

There are a number of reasons for the high and rising costs. An aging population needs more medical care; expensive new medical technologies are regularly developed and widely used; administrative costs are high in the United States; malpractice suits lead to defensive medicine; insured patients are shielded from consideration of costs; and financial incentives often favor overtreatment.

A number of attempts to impose cost-containment measures on medical care have been relatively unsuccessful in controlling costs. Managed care slowed the growth in healthcare costs in the 1990s and has consequently become the dominant form of employer-sponsored health insurance. Managed care organizations negotiate reduced payments to healthcare providers and employ various strategies to limit patients' access to treatments considered nonessential or too expensive for the expected benefit. Despite its successes, managed care has been unpopular with the public, and it has not improved access for the uninsured. Because of its unpopularity, managed care has suffered legislative and legal setbacks that have weakened its ability to control costs. Medical care expenditures have resumed their escalation, and it is not clear how the nation can pay for medical care in the future.

Many health policy makers believe that some form of rationing will ultimately be necessary to ensure access to high-quality medical care for the whole population. They point out that care is already rationed by cost. In Oregon, the Medicaid program, using an explicit method of ranking various treatments and cutting off access to lower priority procedures, significantly expanded the number of people covered by the plan; but the plan has faltered due to rising costs and state economic setbacks. Discussion of rationing is largely taboo in the current political climate, but if the problems of the system continue to grow, Americans may be forced to consider cost and fairness when making decisions about medical care.

President Obama set a priority on reforming the American healthcare system, and in 2010 he succeeded in persuading Congress to pass a plan that would provide health insurance to more of the population and, it is hoped, help to control costs. The law was challenged by a number of states, but it substantially was upheld by the Supreme Court. Some aspects of the law have already been implemented; many others will take effect in 2014.

References

1. A. B. Martin et al., "Growth in U.S. Health Spending Remained Slow in 2010: Health Share of Gross Domestic Product Was Unchanged from 2009," *Health Affairs* 31 (2012): 208–219.
2. Organization for Economic Cooperation and Development, "OECD iLibrary: Health: Key Tables from OECD." http://www.oecd-ilibrary.org, accessed August 12, 2012.
3. National Center for Health Statistics, *Health, United States, 2011,* Tables 20 and 21. http://www.cdc.gov/nchs/data/hus/hus11.pdf, accessed August 12, 2012.
4. C. DeNavas-Walt, B. D. Proctor, and J. C. Smith, U.S. Census Bureau, Current Population Reports, "Income, Poverty, and Health Insurance Coverage in the United States: 2010." http://www.census.gov/prod/2011pubs/p60-239.pdf, accessed August 9, 2012.
5. Employment Benefit Research Institute, "2009 Policy Resources: Facts on Benefit Issues." http://www.ebri.org/campaign, accessed August 12, 2012.
6. U.S. Institute of Medicine, *America's Uninsured Crisis: Consequences for Health and Health Care* (Washington, DC: National Academies Press, 2009).
7. A. P. Wilper et al., "Health Insurance and Mortality in U.S. Adults," *American Journal of Public Health* 99 (2009): 2289–2295.
8. Kaiser Family Foundation, "Medicare at a Glance." http://www.kff.org/medicare/upload/1066_14.pdf, accessed August 12, 2012.
9. Kaiser Family Foundation, "Medicaid Matters: Understanding Medicaid's Role in Our Health Care System." http://www.kff.org/medicaid/upload/8165.pdf, accessed August 12, 2012.
10. G. F. Anderson, B. K. Frogner, and U. E. Reinhardt, "Health Spending in OECD Countries: An Update," *Health Affairs* 26 (2007): 1481–1489.
11. S. Woolhandler, M. H. A. Campbell, and D. U. Himmelstein, "Costs of Health Care Administration in the United States and Canada," *New England Journal of Medicine* 349 (2003): 768–775.
12. H. J. Aaron, "Costs of Health Care Administration in the United States and Canada— Questionable Answers to a Questionable Question," *New England Journal of Medicine* 349 (2003): 801–803.

13. T. A. Brennan, C. M. Sox, and H. R. Burstin, "Relation Between Negligent Adverse Events and the Outcomes of Medical-Malpractice Litigation," *New England Journal of Medicine* 335 (1996): 1963–1967.

14. L. G. Sandy et al., "The Political Economy of U.S. Primary Care," *Health Affairs* 28 (2009): 1136–1144.

15. G. A. Jensen, M. A. Morrissey, S. Gaffney, and D. K. Liston, "The New Dominance of Managed Care: Insurance Trends in the 1990s," *Health Affairs* (January/February 1997): 125–136.

16. T. Bodenheimer, "The HMO Backlash—Righteous or Reactionary?" *New England Journal of Medicine* 335 (1996): 1601–1604.

17. M. G. Bloche and K. M. Studdert, "A Quiet Revolution: Law as an Agent of Health System Change," *Health Affairs* (March/April 2004): 29–42.

18. Kaiser Family Foundation, "Stresses to the Safety Net: The Public Hospital Perspective." http://www.kff.org/medicaid/upload/Stresses-to-the-Safety-Net.pdf, accessed August 12, 2012.

19. A. Dixon, J. Greene, and J. Hibbard, "Do Consumer-Directed Health Plans Drive Change in Enrollees' Health Care Behavior?" *Health Affairs* 27 (2008): 1120–1131.

20. "The Patient Protection and Affordable Care Act." http://www.healthcare.gov, accessed October 15, 2012.

21. "Health Care and the Supreme Court (Affordable Care Act)," October 2, 2012, *New York Times*. http://topics.nytimes.com/top/reference/timestopics/organizations/s/supreme_court/affordable_care_act/index.html, accessed October 15, 2012.

22. R. M. Kaplan, *The Hippocratic Predicament: Affordability, Access, and Accountability in American Medicine* (San Diego, CA: Academic Press, 1993).

23. T. Bodenheimer, "The Oregon Health Plan—Lessons for the Nation," *New England Journal of Medicine* 337 (1997): 651–655.

24. J. Oberlander, "Health Reform Interrupted: The Unraveling of the Oregon Health Plan," *Health Affairs* 26 (2007): w96–w105.

25. D. M. Eddy, "Balancing Cost and Quality in Fee-For-Service Versus Managed Care," *Health Affairs* 16 (1997): 162–173.

26. D. A. Asch and P. A. Ubel, "Rationing by Any Other Name," *New England Journal of Medicine* 336 (1997): 1668–1671.

27. J. P. Kassirer, "Our Endangered Integrity—It Can Only Get Worse," *New England Journal of Medicine* 336 (1997): 1666–1667.

Health Services Research: Finding What Works

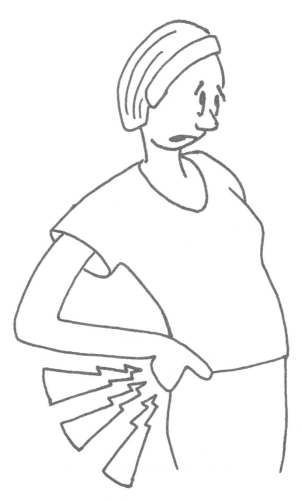

Will Back Surgery Help?

In the late 1960s and early 1970s, the medical establishment was shaken by a number of reports that documented wide variations in the way physicians treated their patients for common health problems. One study found that in Morrisville, Vermont, nearly 70 percent of the children had their tonsils removed by the time they were 15 years old, whereas in nearby Middlebury, only 8 percent of children underwent the operation. Another study in Iowa reported that more than 60 percent of the male population of one community had their prostate glands removed by age 85, whereas the rate was only 15 percent in another area. And the rates at which women underwent hysterectomy varied from 20 percent in one part of Maine to 70 percent in a city less than 20 miles away.[1]

The reasons for these differences were unclear. The populations of the comparison communities were not substantially different from one another. There was no reason to believe that the residents of one community were sicker than those of another or that their insurance coverage was more comprehensive. It seemed obvious that these procedures were being overused in some geographical areas or underused in others. However, the studies could not determine which was true or decide what the appropriate use rates should be.

This method of examining medical practice, known as small-area analysis, has been applied over the past several decades to a broad range of medical practices and procedures. Repeatedly, wide variations have been found, with no apparent reason for the differences in practice. In 1996, Dr. John Wennberg, a professor at Dartmouth Medical School and a pioneer in the field, who had conducted the studies in Vermont, Maine, and Iowa, published the *Dartmouth Atlas of Health Care*, an analysis of 1993 Medicare data.[2] (Since the Medicare program maintains files on everything it pays for, including services to virtually all Americans 65 and older, it provides valuable data for this kind of research.) All over the country, variations occur in treatments for prostate cancer, breast cancer, heart disease, and many other common conditions. Rates of surgery for low back pain were seven times higher in Provo, Utah, than in Kingsport, Tennessee. Breast-sparing surgery for women with breast cancer ranged from just over 1 percent in Rapid City, South Dakota, to 49 percent in Elyria, Ohio.

Small-area analysis called attention to the lack of scientific evidence on which doctors and patients base decisions about how various medical conditions should be treated. The surprising results of the early studies were part of a new field of research—health services research. This research attempts to understand the reasons for the observed variations in medical practice and to determine, from observations of the everyday practice of medicine, what treatments lead to the most desirable outcomes. Health services research studies the effectiveness, efficiency, and equity of the healthcare system. It is a way of trying to assess the quality of medical care. This research also may lead to insights on how to control costs and improve access.

Reasons for Practice Variations

A number of explanations have been suggested for variations in medical practice, most of which can be tested, and most of which can be shown to play a role in the observed differences. It is clear that the variability in the use of different treatments reflects the degree of uncertainty facing physicians regarding their relative efficacy. Variations in practice are far greater for some medical conditions than for others. For example, most physicians agree that surgery is the appropriate treatment for appendicitis and broken hips. Correspondingly, the geographic variability in the treatment of those conditions is much smaller than the variability in rates for tonsillitis and disorders of the uterus, on which there is much less evidence about when surgery is needed.

In many cases, doctors are unaware that their way of treating a condition is unusual, and they will change their patterns of practice when presented with evidence that they are deviating from the norm. In the early 1970s, Wennberg confronted the physicians of Morrisville, Vermont, with data showing that they were doing tonsillectomies far more frequently than other doctors in the state. The Morrisville physicians reconsidered the indications for the procedure, instituted a policy of obtaining second opinions before deciding on surgery, and ended by reducing the tonsillectomy rate to less than 10 percent of what it had been.[1]

It is easy to suspect that inappropriate use of invasive procedures is responsible for the observed variations in the frequency with which they are done. While this suspicion is supported by the Vermont experience in reducing tonsillectomy rates, other studies have found that inappropriate use explains only a small part of the wide variability observed for many procedures.

In one small-area study of three procedures commonly done on Medicare patients, panels of expert physicians examined the files of a random sample of patients who had undergone each procedure. The experts compared the indications for the procedure in a high-use area with those in a low-use area. They were asked to determine, for each patient, whether the decision to do the procedure was appropriate, equivocal, or inappropriate. Coronary angiography—used to identify blockages in the blood vessels of the heart—was performed more than twice as frequently in the high-use area as in the low-use area. Yet even in the high-use area the experts considered it inappropriate in only one-sixth of the cases. Carotid endarterectomy (CEA), which had an almost four-fold variation in frequency, was the procedure most often judged inappropriate. A risky procedure intended to remove blockages in the arteries that carry blood to the brain, CEA was deemed inappropriate in about one-third of the cases done in the high-use area. However, the procedure was considered by the experts to be inappropriate almost as frequently in the low-use area.[3]

This evidence suggests that, for many medical conditions, more than one response may be appropriate. When faced with a patient suffering from a specific illness, one physician may prefer conservative treatment using drugs and "watchful waiting," while another physician may believe that immediate surgery is indicated. These opinions tend to be shared by the physicians within a community. Wennberg has called these differences the "practice style" factor. For most of the conditions in question, there was not enough scientific evidence to determine which treatment yields a better outcome for the patient. In many cases, the choice of treatment involves weighing benefits against risks, a trade-off that different patients might evaluate differently if they are given the opportunity to choose.

The high variability and frequent inappropriate use of CEA, together with the high risks from the procedure, inspired several large randomized controlled trials, involving over 10,000 patients, to clarify the indications for and efficacy of CEA. The trials demonstrated that, among carefully selected patients and surgeons, the procedure reduced the risk of stroke and death compared with medical therapy alone. In a later analysis to determine whether the evidence provided by the trials changed medical practice, researchers in New York State conducted a cohort study of all Medicare patients who had had a CEA over an 18-month period in 1998 and 1999. The results were a great improvement over the earlier study: overall 87.1 percent of the procedures had been done for appropriate reasons; 4.3 percent had been done for uncertain reasons; and 8.6 percent had been done for inappropriate reasons.[4]

As for coronary angiography, another procedure studied earlier, no such randomized trials have been done to determine appropriateness. It is still a high-variability procedure: a recent study comparing rates in different states found a 53 percent higher rate in Florida than in Colorado. The rate depended in part on the density of specialists in the area.[5]

The Field of Dreams Effect

One factor that has consistently been shown to influence practice styles is the availability of services in a community, as shown in the rates of coronary angiography discussed above. The presence of a greater number of surgeons is accompanied by the performance of a larger number of surgeries; higher numbers of hospital beds lead to higher rates of hospitalization. This effect was dramatically illustrated in Maine during the early 1980s, when two neurosurgeons moved to a community and devoted themselves to performing laminectomies—disc surgery for low back pain. The number of laminectomies for the whole state nearly doubled as a result of the work of these two surgeons, although only 20 percent of the population of Maine lived in that community and the adjacent referral area.[6] This high rate of surgery, like the tonsillectomies in Vermont, came down after the surgeons were confronted with data on practice patterns in other communities.

Research has consistently demonstrated an influence of supply on usage when hospital beds are concerned. A study done in the 1980s comparing Boston, Massachusetts, with New Haven, Connecticut, found that Boston had 4.5 hospital beds per thousand people, whereas New Haven had only 2.9 beds per thousand. Approximately the same percentage of beds was filled in the two cities, meaning that the population of Boston was hospitalized at a higher rate than that of New Haven. When Wennberg and his colleagues interviewed physicians in the two cities, they found that New Haven doctors were not purposely trying to ration care and that neither group of doctors was aware that they hospitalized patients more or less frequently than average.[6] Mortality rates and other measures of quality of care were almost the same in the two cities. In the 1990s, when managed care came to both cities, hospitalization rates fell, but by about the same percentages, so that Boston doctors still hospitalized their patients much more frequently than New Haven doctors.[7]

The Dartmouth researchers' analysis of Medicare data found that the number of hospital beds in a community significantly influences the kind of care received by dying elderly people.[8] Medicare patients in New York City, Newark, New Jersey, and Memphis, Tennessee, are much more likely to spend their final days in a hospital, often in an intensive-care unit, than elderly patients in Portland, Oregon, or Salt Lake City, Utah, who are more likely to die at home. Based on 1994 and 1995 data, the rates at which Medicare patients die in the hospital correlate closely with the number of hospital beds per thousand residents in their community. Researchers call this correlation the "Field of Dreams Effect," after the line in the 1989 movie about a baseball field: "If you build it, they will come."

While there is little evidence to show that patients are helped or harmed by the more intensive care they receive in Boston, Miami, and other high-use areas of the country, the differences in use have a major impact on medical care costs. For example, the average hospital bill for each Medicare enrollee's final 6 months of life was $16,571 in the New York City borough of Manhattan, as opposed to an average of only $6793 in Portland, Oregon.[8] In the Boston–New Haven comparative study, Boston's per capita hospital expenditures were about double those of New Haven.[9] Wennberg calculated that overall hospital expenditures for the 685,000 residents of Boston were $300 million higher in 1982 than they would have been if the usage rates of New Haven applied.

Wennberg does not specifically argue that conflict of interest or pecuniary motives enter into decisions that determine use rates of medical services. However, many studies suggest that financial considerations may enter into some physicians' medical decision making. For example, there is evidence that when physicians stand to profit from the performance of diagnostic tests, they are much more likely to order such tests. Until the practice was outlawed by Congress, physicians who owned an interest in clinical laboratories were more likely to refer patients for laboratory tests than similar physicians who referred patients to labs in which they had no financial interest.[10] Similarly, physicians who own diagnostic imaging equipment are more likely to use it than comparable physicians who must refer patients elsewhere for such examinations.[11] A recent surge in complex spinal-fusion operations has been linked to the high rates Medicare will pay to surgeons and hospitals, although there is no evidence that the procedure is more effective at curing back pain than laminectomies or even less invasive approaches.[12]

Outcomes Research

As we have seen, variations in medical care are greatest for medical conditions for which the least is known about the effectiveness and appropriateness of various diagnostic and treatment approaches. The solution to the uncertainties raised by small-area analysis, therefore, is to study outcomes of these various diagnostic and treatment approaches in order to determine what works. Many policymakers believe that such research will allow the development of guidelines for medical practice, leading not only to more effective medical care but also to cost savings through the elimination of unnecessary care.

Outcomes research is the epidemiologic study of medical care. Whereas epidemiology usually examines the disease-causing effects of exposure to agents such as viruses and toxic chemicals, medical care epidemiology examines the health effects of exposure to medical interventions. Controlled clinical trials are one form of medical care epidemiology, but there are practical, financial, and ethical barriers that prevent conducting controlled trials aimed at answering many important questions about medical care. Outcomes research collects and analyzes data generated by the everyday practice of medicine in order to reach conclusions on benefits and risks of various interventions for various types of patients.

One of the early questions John Wennberg's group looked into was prostatectomy, the surgical removal of men's prostate glands. It was a high-variation procedure; in some parts of Maine, 60 percent of the men had their prostates removed by age 80; in other parts, less than 20 percent had.[13] The procedure is used as a treatment for cancer of the prostate and for benign prostatic hyperplasia (BPH), a common condition in older men that causes difficulties with urination. Other treatments are available for both conditions, including watchful waiting, since many cases of prostate cancer never progress to become life threatening. For BPH, proponents of the surgical procedure argued that it could reduce symptoms and improve the quality of men's lives. Skeptics point out that surgery often has unwelcome side effects.

Wennberg and his colleagues conducted a major analysis of Medicare records to determine outcomes of surgery for BPH. They found that published reports significantly overstated the benefits of prostatectomy and understated the complications. Although only about 1 percent of men died in the hospital, 2 to 5 percent of the patients died in the weeks following the surgery. Moreover, within 4 years of the surgery, almost half of the patients had required further treatment for urinary tract problems. After 8 years, about 1 in 5 had needed a second prostatectomy.[6] Having the surgery did not increase life expectancy, and the effect on quality of life was mixed: it improved urinary tract symptoms, but it had a negative impact on sexual function.[13]

The results of these studies indicate a need for better informing patients about their choices and about the probable outcomes of each choice.[14] Feelings about symptoms, willingness to accept risks of the surgery, and personal assessment of the possible outcomes vary substantially among individuals. Outcomes research should enable these patients to make informed decisions based on their own values. As Wennberg has pointed out, "current rates of use of invasive high-technology medicine could well be higher than patients want.... Given an option, patients will on average select less invasive strategies than physicians."[7(p.1203)] Effective drug therapies have been developed for BPH, and the number of surgeries performed for this condition declined in the 1990s, perhaps due in part to evidence contributed by outcomes research.[15]

The number of prostatectomies for cancer has increased, however, due in part to the develop ment of a new screening method that became widely used in the 1990s. The test measures prostate-specific antigen (PSA) in the blood, levels of which have been correlated with the presence of cancer. However, low-grade prostate cancer is very common in older men, and many cases never progress to cause a problem. The follow-up testing and treatment of men whose PSA levels are elevated is invasive and may have undesirable side effects. The problem with the use of PSA screening is that there is no evidence that it reduces mortality from prostate cancer.

In a study conducted by the Dartmouth researchers, Medicare data were used to compare two cohorts of men who lived in areas with different practice patterns for screening and treatment. In the Seattle–Puget Sound area, men were tested at a rate 5.39 times the rate in Connecticut. The researchers found that more than twice as many men in the Seattle area, compared with Connecticut men, were subjected to biopsies of the prostate to confirm the presence of cancer. The Seattle area men were over five times more likely to have a prostatectomy than the Connecticut men. However, after 11 years of follow-up, there was no significant difference in the mortality rates from prostate cancer between the two groups of men.[16] This finding was confirmed in 2009 with the publication of results from two clinical trials that followed a total of 259,000 men in the United States and Europe for 7 to 10 years. In both trials, men were randomly assigned to groups with and without PSA screening, and there was little difference in mortality between the two groups.[17] In 2011, the U.S. Preventive Services Task Force, an independent panel of experts appointed and funded by the Agency for Healthcare Research and Quality (see discussion later in this chapter), reviewed the findings from these trials as well as other studies and recommended against routine PSA screening. The panel concluded that PSA screening resulted in small or no reduction in mortality from the disease and is associated with unnecessary harms.[18] The problem with finding prostate cancers through screening is that there is no good way to determine which ones are likely to progress rapidly and cause harm and which are indolent and can be left alone.

Inspired in part by Wennberg's work, Congress in 1989 established the federal Agency for Health Care Policy and Research (AHCPR), hoping that studies such as those on BPH would encourage a reduction in high-technology medicine and save money on medical costs, especially for Medicare and Medicaid. The agency was mandated to examine the reasons for the wide variations in healthcare practices around the country, develop guidelines for treatment, and find effective ways to disseminate its research findings and guidelines.[19] However, the agency—and Congress—discovered to their surprise that the research results were not always welcome.

One of the health conditions that the AHCPR tackled early was low back pain. It is a widespread problem, ranking second only to the common cold as a reason that people go to the doctor. Treatment of low back problems cost over $20 billion a year in the United States. Surgery for low back pain is a high-variability procedure, ranging from a low in the Northeast to a rate in the Northwest that is more than three times higher. The guidelines developed by AHCPR's panel of experts and released in December 1994 recommended treating most acute, painful low back problems with nonprescription painkillers and mild exercise, followed in about 2 weeks by conditioning exercises. Surgery benefits only about 1 in 200 people with acute low back problems, according to the chairman of the panel, a professor of orthopedic surgery at the University of Washington School of Medicine.[20]

Back surgeons responded with rage and political action. With the Republican Congress intent on budget cutting in 1995, legislators were sympathetic to claims by the back surgeons' lobbying group that AHCPR was a waste of money, that the government should not be telling doctors how to practice medicine, and that the agency should be eliminated.[21] Defenders of the AHCPR pointed out that the guidelines could save billions of dollars and accused back surgeons of merely trying to protect their incomes. When the federal budget was finally approved that year, AHCPR had survived, although its budget was cut substantially. Its leaders decided that developing clinical guidelines was too dangerous politically, but the agency continued collecting evidence that allowed other organizations to do so, and it maintains a national clearinghouse of evidence-based clinical guidelines developed by other organizations. A new emphasis on quality of care and patient safety was implemented, and the agency's name was changed to the Agency for Healthcare Research and Quality (AHRQ). Four years after its "near-death experience," AHRQ had regained all the funding it lost, and by 2002 the budget had grown to more than double its pre-1995 level.[22] Wennberg has argued for an expanded role for AHRQ, noting that outcomes research has the potential to restrain wasteful spending and could help to control costs.[13]

In fact, the federal government is increasingly interested in supporting comparative effectiveness research to evaluate, for example, the efficacy of competing drugs, or to compare the effectiveness of different treatment options. In 2009, it announced plans to provide $1.1 billion to the AHRQ, the National Institutes of Health, and the Department of Health and Human Services to conduct the research, and it also provided funds to the Institute of Medicine to recommend priorities for spending the money.[23] The new Patient Protection and Affordable Care Act, passed in 2010, includes the establishment of a Patient Centered Outcomes Research Institute aimed at helping patients to make better-informed healthcare decisions.[24] It is not clear how this agency will differ from AHRQ.

As for treatment of low back pain, surgery rates in the Medicare population increased by 220 percent between 1988 and 2001, and the rates vary dramatically across geographic areas.[25] To determine what an appropriate rate might be, a prospective study was conducted in Maine, where surgery rates were four times higher in some areas than in others. The researchers followed all patients who had surgery to see whether their symptoms improved after the operation. They found that the best outcomes occurred in the areas where the rates were lowest; and the worst outcomes occurred in the areas with the highest rates. The evidence suggested that surgeons in the low-use area used more stringent criteria for recommending surgery. In these areas, patients with more severe disease were more likely to benefit, and those with less severe disease avoided the risks of surgery, which are significant. The authors concluded: "Outcomes research has the potential to provide information that will enable each patient to better understand the outcomes, risks and benefits of an operation and other treatment."[26(p.761)]

Quality

The AHCPR drama came at a time when there had been a series of highly publicized medical errors. A 39-year-old health reporter for *The Boston Globe* died after receiving an overdose of a chemotherapy drug while being treated for breast cancer at one of the most prestigious hospitals in the country. A 51-year-old diabetic man had the wrong leg amputated in a Florida hospital. And an 8-year-old boy in another Florida hospital died due to a drug mix-up during "minor" surgery.

A number of studies were published in the 1990s documenting that preventable medical errors occurred in 1.5 to 2 percent of hospitalizations, and that many of these errors caused the patient's death. The Institute of Medicine was asked to investigate the issue and recommend a strategy that would lead to improvements in quality of care. The study led to the publication in 1999 of a report, *To Err Is Human: Building a Safer Health System.*[27] The report estimated that 44,000 to 98,000 deaths per year in the United States were caused by medical errors, more than motor vehicle accidents, breast cancer, or AIDS, placing medical errors among the top 10 causes of death.

Before the Institute of Medicine report was published, medical errors were blamed on failures by individual doctors and nurses; practitioners who made mistakes were sued for malpractice, and some had even been prosecuted as criminals. The report shifted the blame to the medical care system—or nonsystem, according to some critics—characterizing it as decentralized and fragmented, rife with confusion, miscommunication, and lack of incentives for improvements in safety. The Institute of Medicine committee compared the medical care industry unfavorably with other high-risk industries that had been much more successful at improving safety and preventing injury, especially the commercial airline industry. The report made a number of recommendations, beginning with the creation of a Center for Patient Safety within the AHRQ, which would set national goals, track progress, develop a research agenda, evaluate methods for identifying and preventing errors, and disseminate information. Another recommendation was that, as in the airline industry, accidents and near-misses should be reported so that errors could be investigated, leading to an understanding of the underlying factors that contribute to them. A mandatory, nonpunitive system should be developed that encourages providers to learn from their mistakes.[28]

Recognizing that many adverse events involve medication errors, the report recommended that the Food and Drug Administration (FDA) should require that drug naming, packaging, and labeling be designed to minimize confusion. Because of doctors' notoriously poor handwriting, procedures should be developed to ensure accurate communication of prescriptions and other orders.

In 2009, Consumers Union (CU), the nonprofit agency that publishes *Consumer Reports*, published an evaluation of progress in implementing the Institute of Medicine report's recommendations 10 years later.[29] The report gave the country a failing grade in implementing procedures they believe necessary to create a healthcare system free of preventable medical harm. In particular, CU reported that few hospitals had adopted measures to prevent medication errors and that the FDA rarely intervened. Computerized prescribing and dispensing systems have not been widely adopted, despite evidence that they make patients safer. There is no national system of reporting medical errors and, where there is reporting, it is generally confidential, meaning that patients do not have access to information on how to compare the performance of doctors and hospitals, and there is little pressure for them to improve. Another Institute of Medicine recommendation was to raise standards for competency of doctors, nurses, and other healthcare professionals by requiring them to periodically pass examinations demonstrating skills, knowledge, and use of best-practice care in order to maintain their certification. Most specialty boards now have this requirement but, according to the CU report, there is no mechanism in place to ensure the competency of the 15 percent of physicians not certified by one of these boards, as well as those "grandfathered" prior to the adoption of the standards.[28]

The CU report, as an example of medication errors, described the widely publicized incident in which the twin babies of actor Dennis Quaid and his wife were given 1000 times the prescribed dose of the blood thinner heparin because the different doses were packaged in similar vials with similar blue labels. The twins survived, but even though a similar mix-up had caused the deaths of three infants the previous year in an Indianapolis hospital, the packaging had not been changed.

An example of a system that works, described in the CU report, was instituted in 2004 in 103 Michigan intensive care units to prevent catheter-associated bloodstream infections. It consisted of a short checklist of best practices related to catheter use; nurses were empowered to ensure that doctors were following these practices. Researchers tracked catheter-associated infections and found that the incidence dropped to less than 20 percent of what it had been before the procedures were implemented. The Centers for Disease Control and Prevention has estimated that hospital-acquired infections kill 99,000 people each year.

The CU report argues that among the most important of the Institute of Medicine recommendations is "increased accountability through mandatory, validated and public reporting of preventable medical harm, including healthcare-acquired infections." According to the report, "It is a fundamental principle of quality control that if a process cannot be measured, it cannot be improved."[28(p.6)]

Medical Care Report Cards

The rise of managed care contributed to an increasing interest in the measurement of the quality and efficiency, or cost-effectiveness, of medical care. Managed care's focus on cutting costs, however, conflicted with the common assumption that, when it comes to medical care, more is better—an assumption that is challenged by outcomes research that suggests that sometimes less may be better as well as less expensive.[29] However, many people are suspicious that managed care companies, which have a financial incentive to do less for their patients, may have an inherent conflict of interest. The suspicion is especially strong in the case of for-profit managed care plans, which have an obligation to maximize profits for their investors, perhaps at the expense of the patients.

In the medical care marketplace, where economic factors are becoming increasingly significant, outcomes research has an important role to play in evaluating the quality and efficiency of different medical plans. In theory, when given enough information, customers—both the employers who choose which plans to offer and the employees who must choose among the plans that are offered—can make informed decisions, weighing quality and cost.[30] Moreover, patients are increasingly becoming more active participants in their own care. In part because of growing distrust of the medical system, patients want information on risks and benefits of available treatments and, if possible, on the competence of their physicians and other medical providers. Outcomes research provides some of this information.

Although managed care is often regarded with skepticism, it is more easily evaluated than the traditional fee-for-service form of medical practice. The organization of services that allows care to be "managed" also makes it possible for those services to be assessed in a formal way, something that is not realistic when each medical provider acts independently. Through an accreditation process conducted by the nonprofit National Committee for Quality Assurance (NCQA), it is possible to rate managed care plans on their performance with respect to a number of standards. Information on the accreditation status of a plan can influence a business's decision about whether to offer the plan to its employees, and the information can be used by employees to choose among plans offered. In its 2011 State of Health Care Quality report, 1042 health plans covering more than 118 million Americans provided data to NCQA on 48 different measures of healthcare quality. NCQA reported that most of the health plans had improved on most of the measures. There was significant geographical variation in how well the plans had measured up, with several states in the Northeast and Midwest doing well, while some South Central states did worse than average. Although in the past, health maintenance organizations (HMOs) did better than preferred provider organizations (PPOs), the performance of PPOs is catching up with that of HMOs.[31] Consumers can access "report cards" of plans on the NCQA website and compare their performances.

Many of the most easily measured standards used by NCQA focus on preventive care: for example, whether children receive a full set of immunizations and whether women get mammograms and Pap tests. Other standards evaluate how a plan manages care for patients with common diseases. The findings of outcomes research can be used, for example, to measure performance of an HMO in treating elderly heart attack victims. Research supported by AHCPR found that patients 65 years of age and older were 43 percent less likely to die after a heart attack if they were treated with beta blockers than if they did not receive these drugs.[32] Using that information, NCQA established, as one of its standards for evaluating a plan, the use of beta blockers for treatment of heart attacks. Since the agency began reporting on this measure, the percentage of heart attack patients who received the drugs went from 60 percent to well over 90 percent.[33]

Outcomes research can also be used in some circumstances to evaluate the performance of individual medical providers. The findings offer a basis not only for patients to choose where to go for treatment, but also for providers to compare their performance with that of their peers. Since 1989, New York State has measured the outcomes of coronary artery bypass surgery for treatment of blocked arteries in the heart, monitoring each of the 31 hospitals where the operations are performed. Mortality rates in 1989, adjusted for patients' risk factors such as age, diabetes, and hypertension, ranged between 0.88 percent and 10.02 percent.[34] Data have also been collected on outcomes achieved by individual surgeons.

One of the study's findings was that hospitals that perform large volumes of coronary surgery have better outcomes than those that perform few of the operations, a result that has also been found true of other types of surgery. The New York study also found that surgeons who perform more than 150 bypass operations per year have only half the patient mortality rate of surgeons who perform fewer than 50. The publicity that followed release of the 1989 data on individual hospitals led to a dramatic decline (41 percent) statewide in mortality rates associated with the surgery over the next 3 years.[35] Data collection and analysis continues, and mortality rates have continued to fall. By 1992, New York had the lowest risk-adjusted mortality rates of any state in the nation, and New York's rates continued to be lower than other states', at least through 1999. Thus, the information provided by outcomes research led to improved quality of surgical care statewide. An analysis of how the improvements were accomplished show that hospitals identified as performing poorly reacted strongly, for example, by restricting the surgical privileges of some low-volume surgeons whose patients were more likely to die from the operation.[36] Several other states including Pennsylvania, California, Massachusetts, and New Jersey now maintain similar datasets for coronary surgery in their hospitals.[37]

Despite the successes, health services research has a long way to go before it can be widely used to help people make decisions about health care based on quality. Most of the indicators of managed care quality measured by accrediting agencies focus on preventive care for the healthy. Although this approach is important from a public health perspective, what matters most to patients is the quality of care they receive when they are ill.[27] Detailed analyses of providers' performance are available for only a limited number of procedures in New York and the few other states that carry out such ambitious programs. The New York State Health Department publishes annual reports on its cardiac surgery data (available at http://www.health.state.ny.us/statistics/diseases/cardiovascular); until recently it appeared that neither managed care companies nor patients used the information to choose hospitals and surgeons.[36] However, it has become clear that the data is being used: Managed care organizations are more likely to contract with surgeons who have lower risk-adjusted mortality rates, and surgeons who are rated poorly are more likely to discontinue performing the procedures.[37]

Inequities in Medical Care

Health services research has shed light on an unpleasant reality that pervades the American medical care system. Not only is care rationed by ability to pay, but there are racial inequities in how care is delivered even when individuals are able to pay for it. As documented in a 2002 Institute of Medicine report, *Unequal Treatment: What Healthcare Providers Need to Know about Racial and Ethnic Disparities in Healthcare*,[38] African Americans and Hispanics are less likely than whites to receive the most effective treatments for heart disease, human immunodeficiency virus (HIV) infection, asthma, breast cancer, and many other conditions, even when their income and insurance status are equal to whites.

Regarding heart disease, for example, the work of the New York State researchers described above has also found racial differences in access to coronary artery bypass surgery. It seems that physicians are less likely to recommend surgery to patients from ethnic minority groups than to comparable white patients. Studying files of patients who had undergone diagnostic testing in eight New York hospitals, and using guidelines developed by the RAND Corporation for "appropriateness" and "necessity" of the operation, the researchers selected 1261 patients who would benefit from a coronary artery bypass. Returning to the files 3 months later, the researchers found that African-American and Hispanic patients were significantly less likely to have had the surgery than comparable white patients. It was not that the blacks and Hispanics had decided against the surgery; for the overwhelming majority, their physicians had not recommended it.[39]

Childhood asthma is a chronic disease that can usually be kept under control by providing patients and their families with prescriptions for inhaled medications and education on how to use them. A study that examined records of young children hospitalized for asthma found that racial minorities were less likely than whites to have taken the most effective medications before they were hospitalized and were less likely to be given prescriptions for such medications when they were discharged. Thus, African-American and Hispanic patients received poorer quality care than whites, an observation that was especially disturbing because the prevalence of asthma in minority children is higher than in whites—25 percent higher.[40]

According to the American Cancer Society, African Americans have the highest death rate and the shortest survival of any racial and ethnic group in the United States for most cancers. Although the overall racial disparity in cancer death rates is decreasing, the death rate for all cancers combined is 32 percent higher in black men and 16 percent higher in black women than in white men and women, respectively.[41] Blacks are less likely to survive 5 years after diagnosis, most likely due to a later stage at diagnosis, when the disease has spread. Blacks are also less likely to receive timely and high-quality treatment.

Blacks and Hispanics who are infected with HIV are less likely to receive antiretroviral therapy than nonminorities with HIV. Even after adjusting for insurance status, CD4 cell count, and other factors, minorities were 24 percent less likely than whites to receive protease inhibitors or other advanced drugs.[38]

These studies provide evidence that inequities in medical care extend significantly beyond disparities in health insurance status and the corresponding financial barriers to care common in members of minority groups. The Institute of Medicine report concluded that "although myriad sources contribute to these disparities, some evidence suggests that bias, prejudice, and stereotyping on the part of healthcare providers may contribute to differences in care."[38] However, more recent analyses indicate that the situation is more complex. Health services research by the Dartmouth group, discussed above, has found evidence that some of the differences are due more to geographic variations than racial disparities within the same area. Some of the disparities in treatment may be due to blacks living disproportionately in regions with low rates for all patients. Others may be due to higher-than-average surgery rates among whites rather than lower-than-average rates among blacks.[42]

Other analysts remind us that the causes of disparities in health are not limited to disparities in health care. For example, there is a threefold difference in diabetes mortality rates between college graduates and those with only a high school education. No diabetes drug makes such a difference. It is clear that diabetes would be less of a problem in the United States if our society promoted education reform as avidly as it emphasizes healthcare reform.[43]

The Relative Importance of Medical Care for Public Health

Health services research, in addition to studying medical care epidemiology, has tried to answer questions about the proper place for medical care in the public health system. To what extent does medical care contribute to improving the health of the population as a whole? Some skeptics have argued that medicine's effectiveness is limited and that its impact on health is marginal at best. Much of the improvement in life expectancy over the past century resulted more from public health measures and improvements in the population's economic status than from improvements in medical interventions.

In focusing on the population perspective, analysts weigh the contribution of medical care with other factors that contribute to people's health (see Figure 28-1). There is little agreement on the relative importance of the various factors, which include genetics, lifestyle, and the environment, in addition to medical care. However, any consideration of these factors calls attention

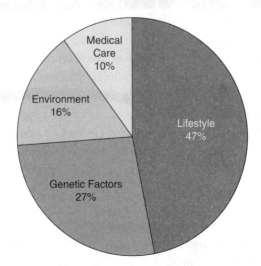

FIGURE 28-1   Contribution of Medical Care to Health. *Source:* Data from P. R. Lee, & C. L. Estes, eds. *The Nation's Health.* (Sudbury, MA: Jones & Bartlett Learning, 2001), p. 50.

to the fact that, in the United States, resources devoted to medical care are far out of proportion to its contribution to health. In fact, the enormous American investment in medical care uses up resources that would otherwise be available to address other factors that affect health, such as education, housing, and the environment. In that sense, it may be that the greater the expansion of the medical care system, the more negative the impact on the population's health.[44]

Evidence from small-area comparisons in the United States, as well as comparative studies of industrialized nations, has clearly indicated that health is not correlated with resources devoted to medical care. This was true, for example, in Wennberg's comparison of healthcare costs and the population's health status in Boston and New Haven. Similarly, international studies of mortality rates in developed nations have found no consistent relationship with levels of medical care resources.[45] The United States has higher rates of chronic disease prevalence and mortality than other OECD countries, despite its high spending on medical care. The fact that more medical care does not lead to better health is supported by a 2003 study by Wennberg's group that looked at patients with heart attacks, hip fractures, or colorectal cancer who lived in geographical areas with high Medicare spending compared with similar patients in areas with lower spending. The researchers found that patients in the high-spending areas had more physicians' visits, more tests and procedures, and spent more time in the hospital than those in the low-spending areas, but the outcomes were not better and, in fact, included a small increase in the risk of death. Apparently, the higher-intensity practice patterns caused harm to patients.[46]

The United States does not get its money's worth for the resources allocated to medical care. Health services research that focuses on the efficiency of the healthcare system can offer evidence on how the nation could keep costs under control while achieving better health. A number of studies have investigated the effects of different methods of paying for care on the use of care and on health outcomes. One influential study was the RAND Health Insurance Experiment.[47] This study compared use of services, expenditures, and health outcomes among several groups of consumers who were assigned randomly to receive free care or to pay copayments of varying amounts. The evidence showed, not surprisingly, that higher copayments discouraged patients from seeking care. The more consumers had to pay, the less medical care they consumed, and the free-care group used services costing 50 percent more than those who had to pay the most. For most of the participants, the extra services were not found to have any impact on their health status. Thus, many healthcare services provided to Americans with generous insurance policies may be wasted in that they do not contribute to better health.

However, for those who were poor and chronically ill, free care did provide significant benefits in health status. These are the people most likely to lack access to medical care because of financial barriers. They are the ones who may need care the most, but may be least likely to get it. This is the tragedy of the American health system, which, despite the highest rate of healthcare spending in the world—much of it probably unnecessary—leaves 16 percent of the population uninsured.

Now that the president and Congress have succeeded in making significant reforms in the American medical care system, there is a great deal to be learned from health services research. The research thus far has demonstrated that a significant proportion of the resources spent on medical care in the United States does not contribute to better health in the population. If the reformed system can be made much more efficient and equitable than it is today, then the health of the American population can be significantly improved.

Conclusion

One hope for reducing costs of medical care and improving its quality is health services research, which studies the effectiveness, efficiency, and equity of the healthcare system. Small-area analysis, a form of health services research, has found that physicians in different geographical areas vary widely in how they treat common health problems. This observation suggests that for some conditions, decisions on treatment are somewhat arbitrary, and that different treatments may be equally valid—or invalid. Large variations are most likely when there is no clear evidence on which treatments are most effective.

The observed differences may be due in part to the varying availability of services in a community. Larger amounts of surgery are done in communities with higher numbers of surgeons. More people are hospitalized in communities with higher per capita numbers of hospital beds. Other variations seem to be merely variations in practice style, which tends to be shared by all physicians in a community. Comparisons of high-usage areas with low-usage areas have not found significant differences in health status, indicating that the variations are not caused by greater severity of illness in some areas, and there is no evidence that high usage helps or harms people's health. However, medical costs are proportionately high in the high-usage areas, suggesting that adopting the practices of low-usage areas could save substantial sums.

Outcomes research, the epidemiologic study of the everyday practice of medicine, holds hope for reaching conclusions on the benefits and risks of various treatments for high-variation conditions. For example, prostatectomy for benign prostatic disease is a common surgery performed on older men. However, it is not always effective in relieving symptoms, and it can have undesirable complications such as impotence and incontinence. Results of outcomes research have made it clear that people should be informed of the risks of surgery and the possible outcomes before they make choices about their treatment. Surgery for BPH is now used less often than in the past. PSA screening for prostate cancer is also of questionable value since it leads to many biopsies and prostatectomies but does not appear to lower mortality rates.

The federal agency formerly called AHCPR got into political trouble in the 1990s when it published evidence recommending less use of back surgery for low back pain. Now known as AHRQ, the agency has regained its funding and more, and healthcare reformers are hoping that its comparative effectiveness research will help save money for the American healthcare system.

Outcomes research can be used to evaluate the quality of managed care plans, assessing whether plans provide services that have been demonstrated to be effective. The research can also be used to compare the performance of hospitals and surgeons. New York State has done this research, an exercise that has resulted in improved quality of coronary surgery in that state.

Health services research has documented extensive evidence that the delivery of medical care is inequitable and that ethnic and racial minorities receive poorer quality care than do white Americans. This is true even after differences in health insurance status have been taken into consideration.

Although health services research has been proven capable of improving the quality of medical care, it also shows that medical care is a less important influence on people's health than some other factors, including education, housing, and the environment. In fact, health services research suggests that if the United States spent less on medical care, and instead invested the savings in these other services, the population's health might be improved.

References

1. J. E. Wennberg, "Dealing with Medical Practice Variations: A Proposal for Action," *Health Affairs* 3 (1984): 6–32.
2. J. E. Wennberg and M. M. Cooper, eds. *Dartmouth Atlas of Health Care 1996* (Chicago, IL: American Hospital Publishing, 1996).
3. M. R. Chassin et al., "Does Inappropriate Use Explain Geographic Variations in the Use of Health Care Services? A Study of Three Procedures," *Journal of the American Medical Association* 258 (1987): 2533–2537.
4. E. A. Halm et al., "Has Evidence Changed Practice? Appropriateness of Carotid Endarterectomy After the Clinical Trials," *Neurology* 68 (2007): 187–194.
5. E. L. Hannan, C. Wu, and M. R. Chassin, "Differences in Per Capita Rates of Revascularization and in Choice of Revascularization Procedure for Eleven States," *BMS Health Services Research* 6 (2008): 35.
6. J. E. Wennberg, "Small Area Analysis and the Medical Care Outcome Problem," in L. Sechrest, E. Perrin, and J. Bunker, *Conference Proceedings: Research Methodology: Strengthening Causal Interpretations of Nonexperimental Data, AHCPR.* (May 1990): 177–201.
7. G. Kolata, "In the U.S., All Medicine Is Local," *The New York Times*, February 4, 1996.
8. J. E. Wennberg and M. M. Cooper, eds. *Dartmouth Atlas of Health Care 1998* (Chicago, IL: American Hospital Publishing, 1998).
9. J. E. Wennberg, "Outcomes Research, Cost Containment, and the Fear of Health Care Rationing," *New England Journal of Medicine* 323 (1990): 1202–1204.
10. M. Waldholtz and W. Bogdanich, "Warm Bodies: Doctor-Owned Labs Earn Lavish Profits in a Captive Market," *Wall Street Journal*, March 1, 1989.
11. B. J. Hillman et al., "Frequency and Costs of Diagnostic Imaging in Office Practice—A Comparison of Self-Referring and Radiologist-Referring Physicians," *New England Journal of Medicine* 323 (1990): 1604–1608.

12. R. Abelson and M. Petersen, "An Operation to Ease Back Pain Bolsters the Bottom Line, Too," *The New York Times*, December 31, 2003.

13. F. Mullan, "Wrestling with Variation: An Interview with Jack Wennberg," *Health Affairs Web Exclusive* (2004): VAR-71-80.

14. F. J. Fowler et al., "Symptom Status and Quality of Life Following Prostatectomy," *Journal of the American Medical Association* 259 (1988): 3018–3022.

15. J. H. Wasson et al., "Transurethral Resection of the Prostate among Medicare Beneficiaries: 1984–1997. For the Patient Outcomes Research Team for Prostatic Diseases," *Journal of Urology* 164 (2000): 1212–1215.

16. G. Lu-Yao et al., "Natural Experiment Examining Impact of Aggressive Screening and Treatment on Prostate Cancer Mortality in Two Fixed Cohorts from Seattle Area and Connecticut," *British Medical Journal* 325 (2002): 740–746.

17. M. J. Barry, "Screening for Prostate Cancer—The Controversy That Refuses to Die," *New England Journal of Medicine* 360 (2009): 1351–1354.

18. R. Chou et al, "Screening for Prostate Cancer: A Review of the Evidence for the U.S. Preventive Services Task Force," *Annals of Internal Medicine* 155 (2011): 762–771.

19. J. Kosterlitz, "Cookbook Medicine," *National Journal* (March 9, 1991): 574–577.

20. Agency for Health Care Policy and Research, "AHCPR Releases Low Back Pain Guideline" *Research Activities* (January 1995): 15–16.

21. N. A. Lewis, "Agency Facing Revolt After Report: Enraged Back Surgeons Recruiting Republicans for a Battle," *The New York Times*, September 14, 1995.

22. B. H. Gray, M. K. Gusmano, and S. R. Collins, "AHCPR and the Changing Politics of Health Services Research," *Health Affairs* (June 25, 2003), Web exclusive.

23. M. Mitka, "Studies Comparing Treatments Ramp Up," *Journal of the American Medical Association* 301 (2009): 1975.

24. Kaiser Family Foundation, "Health Reform Source." http://healthreform.kff.org/en/the-basics.aspx, accessed August 15, 2012.

25. R. A. Deyo et al., "Overtreating Chronic Back Pain: Time to Back Off?" *Journal of the American Board of Family Medicine* 22 (2009): 62–68.

26. R. B. Keller et al., "Relationship Between Rates and Outcomes of Operative Treatment for Lumbar Disc Herniation and Spinal Stenosis," *Journal of Bone and Joint Surgery* 81-A (1999): 752–762.

27. Institute of Medicine, *To Err Is Human: Building a Safer Health System* (Washington, DC: National Academy Press, 1999).

28. Consumers Union, *To Err Is Human—To Delay Is Deadly*. http://www.safepatientproject.org/pdf/safepatientproject.org-to_delay_is_deadly-2009_05.pdf, accessed August 15, 2012.

29. C. R. Gaus and L. Simpson, "Reinventing Health Services Research," *Inquiry* 32 (1995): 130–133.

30. M. Angell and J. P. Kassirer, "Quality and the Medical Marketplace—Following Elephants," *New England Journal of Medicine* 335 (1996): 883–885.

31. National Committee for Quality Assurance, "2011 State of Health Care Quality Report." http://www.ncqa.org/tabid/836/Default.aspx, accessed August 15, 2012.

32. S. B. Soumerai et al., "Adverse Outcomes of Underuse of Beta-Blockers in Elderly Survivors of Acute Myocardial Infarction," *Journal of the American Medical Association* 277 (1997): 115–121.

33. National Committee for Quality Assurance, "The Basics: Performance Measurements." http://www.ncqa.org/tabid/441/Default.aspx, accessed September 27, 2012.

34. E. L. Hannan et al., "Improving the Outcomes of Coronary Bypass Surgery in New York State," *Journal of the American Medical Association* 271 (1994): 761–766.

35. E. L. Hannan et al., "Decline in Coronary Artery Bypass Graft Surgery Mortality in New York State: The Role of Surgeon Volume," *Journal of the American Medical Association* 273 (1995): 209–213.

36. M. R. Chassin, "Achieving and Sustaining Improved Quality: Lessons from New York State and Cardiac Surgery," *Health Affairs* (July/August 2002): 40–51.

37. E. L. Hannan et al., "The New York State Cardiac Registries: History, Contributions, Limitations, and Lessons for Future Efforts to Assess and Publicly Report Healthcare Outcomes," *Journal of the American College of Cardiology* 59 (2012): 2309–2316.

38. Institute of Medicine, *Unequal Treatment: What Healthcare Providers Need to Know About Racial and Ethnic Disparities in Healthcare* (Washington, DC: National Academy Press, 2002).

39. E. L. Hannan et al., "Access to Coronary Artery Bypass Surgery by Race/Ethnicity and Gender Among Patients Who Are Appropriate for Surgery," *Medical Care* 37 (1999): 68–77.

40. J. A. Finkelstein et al., "Quality of Care for Preschool Children with Asthma: The Role of Social Factors and Practice Setting," *Pediatrics* 95 (1995): 389–394.

41. American Cancer Society, "Cancer Facts and Figures for African Americans 2011–2012." http://www.cancer.org/acs/groups/content/@epidemiologysurveillance/documents/document/acspc-027765.pdf, accessed August 18, 2012.

42. K. Baicker et al., "Who You Are and Where You Live: How Race and Geography Affect the Treatment of Medicare Beneficiaries," *Health Affairs* (October 7, 2004): Web exclusive.

43. S. H. Woolf, "Social Policy as Health Policy," *Journal of the American Medical Association* 301 (2009): 1166–1169.

44. R. G. Evans and G. L. Stoddart, "Producing Health, Consuming Health Care," *Social Science and Medicine* 31 (1990): 1347–1363.

45. G. F. Anderson, B. K. Frogner, and U. E. Reinhardt, "Health Spending in OECD Countries in 2004: An Update," *Health Affairs* 26 (2007): 1481–1489.

46. E. S. Fisher et al., "The Implications of Regional Variations in Medicare Spending. Part 2: Health Outcomes and Satisfaction with Care," *Annals of Internal Medicine* 138 (2003): 288–298.

47. L. A. Aday, *Evaluating the Medical Care System: Effectiveness, Efficiency, and Equity* (Ann Arbor, MI: Health Administration Press, 1993).

Public Health and the Aging Population

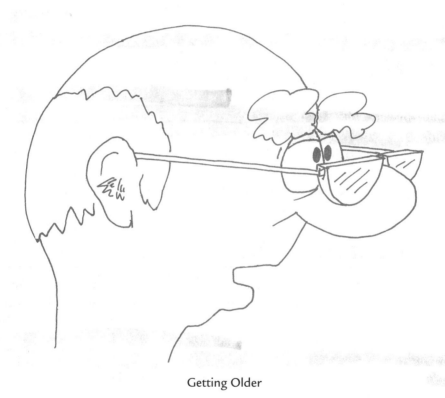

Getting Older

The U.S. population is getting older. The "baby-boom" generation, the oldest of whom have passed 65, is already beginning to retire. The prospect is causing great alarm among health planners because of the increasing pressure it will place on medical costs. Medicare spending has grown dramatically since the program began, both because of growing medical care costs and because of the aging population. Politicians know that they must do something to remedy the situation, but there is no agreement on how or on what should be done. Present trends are unsustainable: if growth in Medicare and Social Security continued at the present rate, together they would consume the entire federal budget by 2070.[1]

Older people tend to be in poorer health than younger ones. They tend to have more chronic illness, and they are more likely to suffer limitations on their ability to participate fully in the activities of their community. These truths have two unhappy consequences: the quality of life of the elderly is, on average, poorer than that for younger people, and their medical costs are higher. Both issues are of great concern for public health.

Quality of life in later years depends significantly on lifestyle in youth and middle age. Therefore, to the extent that public health succeeds in promoting healthy behavior throughout life, there is a payoff in improved health and quality of life for older people. Public health must also address the inevitability that there will be limits to society's willingness to pay the medical costs of the aged. Although the Medicare program was created in the hope of enabling all older people to receive adequate care, financial barriers are increasing and, like the system as a whole, medical care for the elderly is being rationed. The challenge for public health is twofold: first, to improve the health of older people by prevention of disease and disability; and second, to confront the issue of how costs can be controlled in an equitable and humane way. Although these public health goals for older people are no different from those for other age groups, there is special urgency in the case of the elderly because society has made a unique commitment to this group through the Social Security and Medicare programs, a commitment that is now under stress.

The Aging of the Population—Trends

The population is getting older by a number of measures. The median age of the American population—the age at which half the population is younger and half older—increased from 22.9 in 1900 to 37.2 in 2010 and is predicted to reach 39.0 by 2030.[2,3] In 2010, 13 percent of the population was 65 and over. As the baby-boom cohort grows rapidly, the number of people over 65 will double in size, reaching 72 million, or 20 percent of the population by 2030. The increased number of older people was accompanied by an increase in life expectancy at birth, from 47.3 in 1900–1902 to 78.5 in 2009. Centenarians have increased from 37,000 in 1990 to more than 53,000 in 2010.[3]

As people are living longer, most people aged 65 —the traditional retirement age—are still relatively vigorous. To reflect this reality, the elderly are categorized into three component groups, which have quite different characteristics and needs: the "young old," ages 65 to 74; the "aged," who are 75 to 84; and the "oldest old," those 85 and older. In 2010, there were 5.5 million oldest-old people in the United States, and this is the fastest growing age group in the population other than the baby boomers.[3] The Census Bureau predicts that there will be about 9.6 million people age 85 and older by the year 2030.[2] Obviously these projections have important implications for the Social Security and Medicare systems, because the numbers of working-age people—who will be expected to pay to support the elderly—are growing at much slower rates.

Figure 29-1 shows the age distribution of the population in 2000 and 2010. The baby-boom generation—those born between 1946 and 1964—is making its way through the age groups like the proverbial pig through a python and accounts for an explosive increase in the numbers of elderly that began in 2011. Predictions of future population size depend both on the birth rate—which is currently fairly stable—and immigration rates, which are somewhat unpredictable and depend on federal policies.

Females increasingly outnumber males in older age groups. Among the oldest old, there are more than twice as many women as men. This is a consequence of the fact that women have a longer life expectancy than men, although the difference is decreasing. After the age of 75, most women are widowed and live alone, while most men are married and live with their wives. Racial and ethnic diversity among the elderly is expected to increase: non-Hispanic whites constituted 80 percent of the older population in 2010, but that proportion is projected to shrink to 58 percent in 2050. The proportion of Hispanics will grow to 20 percent; blacks will be 12 percent; and Asians will be 8.5 percent. As in younger age groups, older whites are in better health than older people of racial and ethnic minorities. Life expectancy at age 65 is 1.6 years longer for whites than for blacks. However, racial differences in health grow smaller in the oldest populations, and African Americans who survive to join the oldest-old category have a slightly longer life expectancy than whites of the same age.[4]

Social Security and Medicare have helped most of the older population to stay out of poverty. The percentage of people 65 and older living in poverty declined from 15 percent in 1974 to about 9 percent in 2010. Elderly women (11 percent) were more likely to be poor than elderly men (7 percent). Poverty rates were higher for older blacks (18 percent) and Hispanics (18 percent) than for whites (7 percent).[4] The percentage of the general population that have a high school diploma increased from 24 percent in 1965 to 80 percent in 2010; college graduates increased from 5 percent to 22 percent. This increased level of education is generally expected to be correlated with greater health.

Health Status of the Older Population

The greatest public health concern for Americans over 65 is long-term chronic illness, disability, and dependency. The majority of the older population, especially those in the younger groups, are in good health. In national surveys of noninstitutionalized persons, about 82 percent of the young old who are white consider their health to be good to excellent, as do about 76 percent of those 75

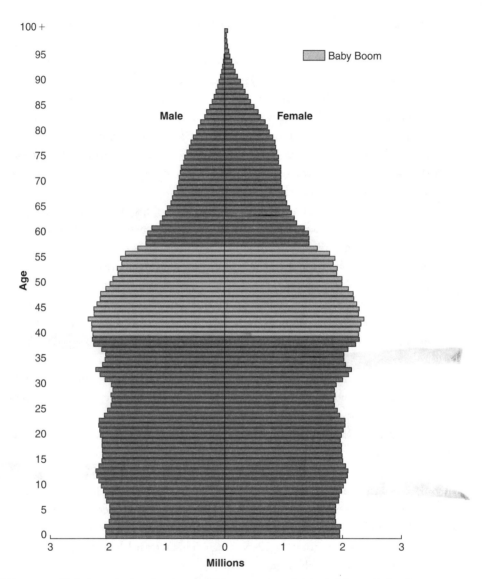

FIGURE 29-1   U.S. Population by Age and Sex, 2000 and 2010. Note: Baby-Boom population bulge at ages 46–64 in 2010. *Source:* Reproduced from U.S. Census Bureau, "2010 Census Briefs: Age and Sex Composition: 2010," Figure 2, May 2011. www .census.gov/prod/cen2010/briefs/c2010br-03.pdf, accessed October 10, 2012.

to 84 and 69 percent of those 85 and over. Blacks and Hispanics report poorer health than whites. With more advanced age, many older people have chronic conditions that cause them to require assistance with the activities of daily living. Overall, less than 1 percent of people 65 to 75 live in nursing homes, but that proportion increases to about 12 percent of the oldest old.[4]

The causes of death of older people are pretty much the same as the causes of death in the overall population, with cardiovascular disease and cancer leading the list (Figure 29-2). Motor vehicle crashes and suicide are also significant causes of death, among older men far more than older women. Men are likely to die at a younger age, whereas older women are more likely to suffer from chronic, disabling diseases. Heart disease, cancer, and stroke, in addition to killing people, can contribute to chronic health problems and dependency. Many of the elderly, especially women, suffer from arthritis, diabetes, osteoporosis, and Alzheimer's disease, conditions that limit their independence and may force them into nursing homes.

A still unanswered question with very important implications for public health is whether longer life expectancy means more healthy years for most people or, alternatively, if it leads to longer periods of chronic illness and disability. The financial solvency of the Medicare system will be highly dependent on the answer. Experts on aging agree that the trend of the 20th century has been a "compression of mortality," shown in Figure 29-3, meaning that deaths are increasingly concentrated in a relatively short age range at about the biological limit of life span. What is less certain is whether the compression of mortality will be accompanied by a compression of morbidity—the rates of chronic disease and

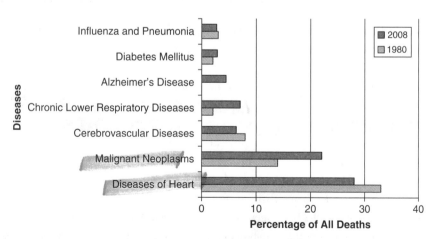

FIGURE 29-2 Leading Causes of Death, Individuals 65 Years and Older.
Source: Data from National Center for Health Statistics, *Health, United States*, 2011. Table 27.

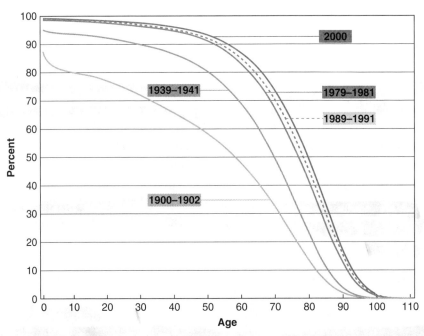

Note: The reference population for these data is the resident population. Data for 1900–1902 and 1939–1941 also include deaths of nonresidents of the United States.

FIGURE 29-3   Compression of Mortality. *Source:* Reproduced from U.S. Census Bureau, "65+ in the United States, 2005," Figure 3-1. www.census.gov/prod/2006pubs/p23-209.pdf, accessed October 10, 2012.

disability. Ideally most people would prefer to live a long, healthy life and then suddenly drop dead, like the "wonderful one-hoss shay," a scenario that would also save massive amounts of Medicare money.

Evidence is beginning to emerge that a compression of morbidity is indeed taking place.[5] An ongoing national survey of Medicare recipients indicates that disability rates among those over 65 declined steadily, from 26.5 percent in 1982 to 19.0 percent in 2004.[6] Other national surveys have had similar findings. Surveys by the Centers for Disease Control and Prevention (CDC) have shown that the percentage of older people living in nursing homes has declined significantly since 1977.[7] The Framingham Heart Study, which tracked the health of a cohort of original participants and their offspring, found that the younger generation had less disability than their parents at the same ages.[8] On the other hand, the prevalence of many diseases has increased in the older population. For example, cardiovascular disease has become more prevalent as deaths from cardiovascular disease have declined. Having a disease appears to be less disabling than in the past.[9]

General Approaches to Maximizing Health in Old Age

There is still a great deal to learn about how public health can continue to achieve a compression of morbidity, improving quality of life for those who benefit from the compression of mortality that has already occurred. Although a variety of factors might influence the risk of disability in old age, health-related behavior is one important variable that would be expected to make a difference. A study that tracked 1741 older alumni of the University of Pennsylvania found that, indeed, a healthy lifestyle reduced not only their risk of dying but also their disability in later years. The study subjects, who had attended the University in 1939 and 1940, were surveyed on their smoking habits, body-mass index (BMI), and exercise patterns and, beginning in 1986, chronic conditions, use of medical services, and extent of disability. The alumni were classified into three risk groups, the highest risk belonging to obese, inactive smokers. Those in the highest risk group had twice the cumulative disability of those with low risks, and the onset of disability was postponed by almost 8 years in the low-risk group.[5,10]

This evidence indicates that, as in younger age groups, the behaviors that most significantly affect health in older people are smoking, obesity, and physical inactivity.[5] However, the recently observed compression of morbidity cannot entirely be explained by improvements in these factors. The reduced prevalence of smoking over the past several decades is no doubt responsible in part for the fact that the elderly are healthier than they used to be. But the increased prevalence of overweight, obesity, and physical inactivity would be expected to have the opposite effect, leading to increased disability in older people.

Smoking is always a major risk factor for cardiovascular disease and cancer, still the leading causes of death in those over 65. Chronic obstructive pulmonary disease is caused almost entirely by smoking. Osteoporosis and disorders of the mouth are also made worse by smoking. It is significant that prevalence of smoking drops off with increasing age, in part because many older people have succeeded in quitting and in part because many smokers die before they reach old age. In 2010, only 9.7 percent of American men aged 65 and over smoked. The rate among older women was 9.3 percent.[4]

Nutrition and physical activity are the other most important determinants of health in old age. Diet and exercise affect the risk of cardiovascular disease and cancer. Overweight and obesity, the result of overnutrition and lack of exercise, increase the risk not only of the leading killers, but also of diabetes and arthritis of the weight-bearing joints. Interestingly, the percentage of the population that is overweight and obese decreases after age 75, as seen in Figure 29-4. The reason for this is not known, but one theory is that, like cigarette smokers, obese people die at an earlier age. This may explain in part the apparent paradox between the obesity epidemic and the trend toward better health in the older population. Because obese people are more likely

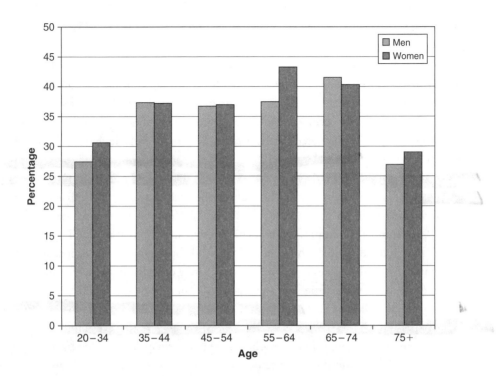

FIGURE 29-4   Percentage of Population Obese by Age and Sex, 2007–2010.
Source: Data from National Center for Health Statistics, *Health, United States*, 2011.
Table 74.

to report poor health than people of normal weight, it is likely that the compression of morbidity seen in recent years will be reversed unless the obesity epidemic can be halted.[11] However, some studies suggest that the health effects of obesity in older people may be less harmful.[6]

Obesity is not the only outcome of poor diet and lack of exercise. Elderly individuals need physical activity to maintain muscle strength, balance, and cardiovascular fitness, which protect them against osteoporosis and falls. The special nutritional needs of the elderly are not well understood, but adequate calcium and vitamin D are clearly important for the strength of bones and teeth. There is little evidence about the special effects of other nutrients in protecting against the diseases of the elderly, and the best advice is, as for younger people, to eat a varied diet low in fat and rich in fruits and vegetables.

Through the 1990s, more and more evidence appeared suggesting that hormone replacement therapy (HRT) might have broad health advantages for older women in addition to its well-known efficacy in fending off the symptoms of menopause. A number of epidemiologic studies, including the cohort of 60,000 women in the Nurses' Health Study, showed that estrogen therapy was associated with lower rates of heart disease and osteoporosis and perhaps Alzheimer's as well. On the other hand, the hormone increases the risk of breast and uterine cancer. In a 1997 publication, the investigators concluded that HRT reduced women's overall risk of dying as long as they took the hormones.[12] The hopes for estrogen's anti-aging effects were crushed, however, with the publication of the clinical trial conducted as part of the Women's Health Initiative. The trial found that although HRT helped to prevent osteoporosis and the symptoms of menopause, it actually increased the risk of heart disease, strokes, and even Alzheimer's disease. It seems that the apparent benefits of estrogen were caused by the confounding factor that women who chose HRT were healthier and more likely to have a healthy lifestyle than those who chose not to use the hormone.[13]

Other aspects of medical care have probably contributed to reductions in disability among the elderly. For example, secondary prevention such as the use of drugs to treat diabetes, high blood pressure, and high cholesterol have undoubtedly reduced morbidity and mortality in many older people. The number of total knee replacements for arthritis and cataract surgeries has doubled over the past 2 decades, greatly reducing disabilities and improving quality of life. Still, there are concerns about shortages of healthcare workers, especially those with education and training in caring for older adults.[14] According to a 2008 report of the Institute of Medicine, older adults, 12 percent of the population, account for approximately 26 percent of all physician office visits, 35 percent of hospital stays, 34 percent of prescriptions, and 38 percent of emergency medical service responses. The Institute of Medicine predicts that the current workforce is not large enough to meet the needs of the growing number of elderly.

Preventing Disease and Disability in Old Age

Much of the disease and disability common in later life is linked to unhealthy behavior in earlier years. However, there are preventive measures that the elderly and their caregivers can take to improve their quality of life and prospects for independence even after health has begun to fail. Some of these measures are well known and easily available, such as vaccination against pneumonia and influenza. Some are beneficial and appropriate for people of any age, such as smoking cessation and blood pressure control. Others are not widely recognized or well understood. Research is needed on how to prevent many of the debilitating conditions and how to minimize their impact on quality of life for the elderly. In a 1990 report, the Institute of Medicine identified a number of the most common problems of the elderly and made recommendations for combating them.[15] These problems commonly and uniquely afflict the elderly and have a severe impact on their quality of life but are not among the leading causes of death. Despite the passage of more than 20 years since the Institute of Medicine report, these difficulties are still causing trouble for older people.

Medications

Although chronic conditions that afflict many of the elderly can be helped by prescription drugs, some of these treatments have unwanted side effects that may seriously impair health and quality of life. Little is known about how the body's ability to metabolize drugs changes with age. Kidney and liver function are often impaired in older people, leading to increased sensitivity to drugs. In older bodies, a higher percentage of body weight is fat, which metabolizes drugs less actively, causing an increased risk of overdoses. Moreover, older people often take a number of medications for various chronic conditions. This could lead to unexpected interactions between drugs, including over-the-counter drugs, because patients tend not to inform their doctors about these medications.

Reducing the risks from adverse drug reactions requires education and vigilance by everyone involved. Elderly patients' needs for medications should be reassessed regularly. In some cases, the potential benefit provided by a drug—for example, improved heart function—may not be worth the damage it could cause to other aging organs, for example, the brain. According to the Institute of Medicine, there is an urgent need for more research on risk versus benefit of various types of drugs in the elderly. There is also a need for better coordination and monitoring of medical care, a need that might be better filled by managed care than by fee-for-service care, which currently dominates in serving the Medicare population.

Osteoporosis

Bone loss is common with age, especially in women. This loss leads to osteoporosis—"porous bones," which tend to break easily. Bone loss among women is greatest in the years following menopause. Smoking and alcohol consumption increase the risk of osteoporosis; obesity reduces the risk (one of the few health benefits of being overweight). White women have the greatest risk for the condition; black men have the lowest, and Asians have intermediate risk. A number of medications commonly used by older people cause bone loss. Some diseases also cause bone loss. The degree of osteoporosis depends on bone density earlier in life, which is determined by a number of factors including genetics, diet, and physical activity. Thus, drinking milk and exercising during youth can protect women against osteoporosis in old age. Unfortunately, girls tend to not take the threat seriously when these habits could do them the most good. Surveys have found that the average amount of calcium women obtain in their diet is significantly below the recommended amount.[16]

Osteoporosis itself has no symptoms, and most older people are unaware that they have the problem until they suffer a broken bone. Hip fractures are the most serious consequence of osteoporosis; there is a significant risk that a hip fracture might lead to substantial disability and death. Of those aged 65 or older who suffer a hip fracture, about 20 percent die within a year.[16] About 20 percent of the survivors end up in nursing homes because they are unable to walk or care for themselves. Wrist fractures are also a frequent result of osteoporosis, but there is little data on their frequency. Fractures of the vertebrae, even more common, might go unrecognized but often lead to progressive loss of height and the curvature of the upper spine called "dowager's hump." Some osteoporotic fractures are untreatable and cause chronic, debilitating pain. A Surgeon General's report on bone health, published in 2004, estimated that about 1.5 million people per year suffer a bone fracture related to osteoporosis, and the cost of caring for these patients is up to $18 billion per year.[16]

Considerable research has been done on how to prevent osteoporosis. The Framingham Study, among others, found that taking estrogen after menopause can protect women from bone loss and reduce the risk of hip fracture.[17] However, HRT is no longer recommended for older women. The Surgeon General's report makes a number of recommendations for preventing osteoporosis. These include getting adequate amounts of calcium (1000 milligrams [mg] per day for adults under 50 years and 1200 mg for those over 50) and vitamin D (200 mg per day for everyone up to 50 years, 400 mg for those 51 to 70, and 600 mg for those over 70). Good sources of calcium are milk, leafy green vegetables, soybeans, yogurt, and cheese. Vitamin D is produced in the skin by exposure to the sun and is found in fortified milk and other foods. Other recommendations include being physically active at least 30 minutes per day for adults and 60 minutes per day for children, including weight-bearing activities, which have been shown to increase bone strength.[16]

Bone scan tests can screen for risk of osteoporosis, and the Surgeon General's report recommends that the test be used to screen all women over 65 and younger men and women who have risk factors, including previous fractures. When the test shows bone thinning, drugs are available that help to prevent further loss of bone mass. The drugs have been found to reduce the fracture rate by about 50 percent.

Falls

Most osteoporotic fractures occur when elderly people fall. Thus, in addition to osteoporosis prevention, public health efforts focus on preventing falls. More than one-third of people 65 and older fall each year; many of them fall repeatedly. About 1 fall in 10 results in a serious injury, such as a fracture or head injury. Many older people have a high risk of falls because of medical conditions that affect their mobility, such as arthritis, stroke, and Parkinson's disease. Other risk factors include vision impairment, muscular weakness, problems with balance, and the side effects of medications. The use of four or more prescription drugs is considered a risk factor for falls. Psychoactive drugs such as antidepressants, tranquilizers, and sleeping pills are especially dangerous.[17]

The CDC recommends five measures older people can take to prevent falls. They should exercise regularly. Muscle strengthening exercises can significantly increase their mobility, strength, and balance. People should have their medications reviewed, as discussed above, to reduce drug interactions and side effects. They should have yearly eye exams. They should improve the lighting in their homes, and they should reduce fall hazards in the home. The environment can be fall-proofed by such means as covering floors with tacked-down carpets, keeping walkways clear of obstacles, equipping bathrooms with grab bars around toilets and tubs, keeping stairways well lit, and using night lights.[18]

Clinical trials have shown that vitamin D supplements can reduce the risk of falls independently of their value in osteoporosis prevention. The vitamin appears to directly improve muscle strength.[19]

Impairment of Vision and Hearing

Loss of vision and hearing are among the most prevalent conditions among elderly Americans. Either condition may be disabling, limiting the individual's ability to interact with the environment and communicate with others. Loss of vision increases the risk of falls and other injuries. It may restrict the individual's ability to drive, a significant handicap in many parts of the country. Impairment of either vision or hearing is likely to lead to social isolation, a risk factor for poor health at any age and an even greater risk factor in the elderly. Sensory loss also is associated with depression and cognitive impairment in the elderly.

The leading causes of visual impairment among the elderly are cataracts, glaucoma, macular degeneration, and diabetic retinopathy. Cataracts—clouding of the lens—are the most prevalent cause of eye disease; by age 80, more than half of Americans either have a cataract or have had cataract surgery. Exposure to sunlight contributes to the lens damage, so wearing sunglasses and hats with brims can help protect the eyes. Smoking increases the risk of cataracts, as does diabetes. Most cataracts can be effectively corrected by surgery in which the clouded lens is removed and replaced with a synthetic lens.[20]

Glaucoma is a gradual increase in pressure within the eye that causes damage to the optic nerve. It is not known why this occurs or how it can be prevented. It is a common cause of blindness, especially in African Americans and Hispanics. People with a family history of the disease have an increased risk. Secondary prevention is the best approach to controlling glaucoma: regular eye checkups can catch the increase in pressure before it causes harm, and the pressure can be reduced with medication in the form of eye drops.[20]

Macular degeneration involves the breakdown of the light-sensing cells in the macula, the central part of the retina. The risk of macular degeneration increases with age. People with a family history have a greater risk. Whites are at greater risk than blacks, and women have a higher risk than men. Smoking may increase the risk. The cause of macular degeneration is not well understood, and there is no known way to prevent the disease. Progression of some forms of the disease can be slowed by drugs that are injected into the eye. Researchers are studying whether certain vitamins and minerals might help to slow the progress of the disease.[20]

There is some evidence that high levels of vitamin D in the blood may protect against macular degeneration.[21]

Diabetic retinopathy is a common complication of diabetes that poses a major risk to vision. The condition occurs when high blood sugar damages the tiny blood vessels in the retina. Strict blood sugar control helps to reduce the extent of this damage, and the condition can be treated with laser surgery.[20]

The most common form of hearing loss among the elderly is characterized by reduced sensitivity to higher frequency tones and, therefore, difficulty in comprehending speech. This pattern is similar to that associated with exposure to excessive noise. In fact, populations living in relatively noise-free environments are less likely to suffer age-related hearing loss. The proportion of Americans affected by hearing impairment ranges from about 30 to 35 percent of individuals 65 to 74 to half of those 85 and older, and that proportion is expected to increase with the aging of generations that thrive on rock concerts and iPods. Many products can help people to hear better, including hearing aids, telephone amplifying devices, and assistive listening devices in public places such as movie theaters, churches and synagogues, and auditoriums.[22]

One barrier that limits the access of many older individuals to services and devices that correct the effects of sensory loss, such as glasses and hearing aids, is that Medicare does not cover them.[15]

Oral Health

As people age, they suffer increasingly from diseases and impairments of the mouth, including tooth loss, dental caries, periodontal disease, salivary dysfunction, cancer and precancerous conditions, and chronic pain. Such problems can have a severe impact on quality of life. They may impair the individual's ability to chew, taste, and swallow, thereby posing a threat to physical health and nutrition far beyond the anatomical parts that are primarily affected. Like sensory impairments, disorders of the mouth may diminish social functioning by affecting speech, facial esthetics, and self-esteem. Oral health in old age, like overall health, depends on healthy behaviors throughout life, but older people can improve their health status by instituting healthier habits at any time. They can quit smoking, use better oral hygiene self-care practices, and use professional dental services. Unfortunately, many of the elderly do not have access to dental services for financial reasons, and Medicare does not cover them.[15]

Alzheimer's and Other Dementias

Alzheimer's disease is one of the most dreaded afflictions of old age. It robs the individual of memory and individuality, and eventually reduces him or her to the helplessness of an infant. Caring for someone with Alzheimer's imposes a crushing emotional, physical, and financial burden on a family. Dementia among the elderly is a major public health problem, currently affecting an estimated 5.4 million people in the United States at a cost of more than $200 billion per year; much of this cost is for long-term care in nursing homes.[23]

Alzheimer's is the most common cause of dementia in the elderly, although there is no definitive diagnostic test for the disease, which can be identified for certain only on autopsy. The risk of dementia increases with age, becoming especially high in the oldest age group. The Alzheimer's Association estimates that 2.9 percent of white Americans aged 65 to 74 have the disease. From age 75 to 84, prevalence is 10.9 percent, and among those 85 and older, it is 20.2 percent. African Americans are twice as likely to develop Alzheimer's than whites and the prevalence among Hispanics is 1.5 that of whites. With the rapid increase in the oldest-old population, it is estimated that by the middle of the 21st century, between 11 and 16 million Americans could be suffering from Alzheimer's disease unless a way can be found to prevent or effectively treat the disease.[23]

While a few types of dementia are treatable, there is no cure for Alzheimer's. Until recently, virtually nothing was known about its cause or how the disease could be prevented. However, the magnitude of the problem has stimulated a great deal of research. Biomedical scientists have learned much about the changes in the brain that are typical of Alzheimer's disease. These changes include characteristic tangles of fibers within brain cells and deposits of the protein beta-amyloid, called plaques, in extracellular spaces. These changes lead to the loss of connections between nerve cells, which eventually die, and the brain atrophies. Several genes have been identified that influence the risk that an individual will develop Alzheimer's disease. Much of what is known about the disease has come from studies of a rare early-onset form of the disease, which is largely determined by genetics.[24] In some families, this form is inherited as an autosomal dominant mutated gene, causing symptoms to appear between ages 30 and 60. An animal model of Alzheimer's has been developed by genetically engineering a mouse with a mutant human gene so that it produces amyloid plaques and develops memory loss as it ages. These animals can be used to study methods of preventing plaque formation.[24]

Risk for the more common late-onset form of Alzheimer's is also affected by genes, a few of which have been identified. However, nongenetic factors play a significant role in the development of the late-onset form. This offers hope that it will be possible to prevent, or at least postpone, the onset of the disease. Some experts predict that merely delaying the onset of Alzheimer's by an average of 5 years could reduce the number of cases by half, because many potential victims are nearing the end of their lives for other reasons. Factors that have been found to increase the risk of Alzheimer's include risk factors for cardiovascular disease. This suggests that preventive measures against heart disease, such as weight control, physical activity, avoidance of smoking, treatment of high blood pressure and cholesterol, and aspirin, might help against dementia as well.[24] Diabetes increases the risk of Alzheimer's as it does cardiovascular disease.

A number of studies have followed cohorts of people to try to determine what factors might influence their risk of developing Alzheimer's. Several of these studies have found that formal education seems to protect the brain, providing people with "cognitive reserve." According to this theory, when aging begins to cause pathology in the brain, people with a larger reserve would be better able to function normally. This theory is supported by evidence from the Swedish Twin Registry of 109 pairs of identical twins in which one twin had been diagnosed with dementia and the other had not. The twin with the dementia had significantly less education than the healthy one.[25]

However, a different theory comes from the Nun Study of 678 Sisters of Notre Dame, who had similar lifestyles and medical care throughout their lives. The nuns, all born before 1917, had been required to write an autobiographical essay when they entered the convent. It turned out that the nuns who had demonstrated the lowest linguistic skills in their essays, written in their early 20s, were most likely to develop Alzheimer's as they aged. This evidence suggests that the sisters with higher linguistic ability were more resistant to developing brain pathology in the first place.[25]

Other studies have suggested that all forms of mental activity—reading, puzzles, cards, board games, crafts, playing a musical instrument—are protective. On the other hand, watching television is correlated with an increased risk. It is not clear, however, whether less participation in intellectually demanding activities is merely an early symptom rather than a cause of the disease.

Physical exercise has been found in a number of studies to protect against Alzheimer's. The Nurses' Health Study, for example, found that women who got the most exercise showed less cognitive decline over the years than less active women. This is consistent with evidence, discussed above, that the brain is protected by the same factors that protect the heart. Participating in social activities also appears to help protect people's brains.[25]

A number of medical approaches are being tested to treat or prevent Alzheimer's disease. Vaccines against beta-amyloid have been tested in humans with mixed results. Drugs that act on the neurotransmitters—chemicals that carry signals between nerve cells—have been shown to delay progression of some symptoms, and these drugs have been approved by the Food and Drug Administration.[24] There was great hope that HRT would protect against Alzheimer's, as discussed earlier in this chapter, but the Women's Health Initiative found evidence to the contrary.

There is some evidence that taking nonsteroidal anti-inflammatory drugs (NSAIDs) could reduce the risk or Alzheimer's disease. Arthritis patients who take regular doses of these drugs—such as aspirin, ibuprofen, naproxen—to control their pain have been observed to have an unusually low risk of dementia.[26] Inflammation is found in the brains of Alzheimer's patients, further supporting the approach of treating them with NSAIDs. However, in December 2004, the National Institutes of Health halted a major clinical trial testing whether Celebrex—one of a new type of NSAIDs called COX-2 inhibitors—could prevent Alzheimer's. When Vioxx, another COX-2 inhibitor, was pulled from the market for increasing the risk of heart disease, questions were raised about other drugs of the same type. A number of studies testing this group of NSAIDs for cancer prevention were also halted as a result of the new data on risk to the heart. COX-2 inhibitors had been thought safer than the older NSAIDs because they were less likely to cause bleeding in the digestive tract. Now, there is uncertainty about the safety even of some of the older NSAIDs.[27] Since the older people who have the greatest risk for Alzheimer's are also likely to have a greater risk for heart disease, the wisdom of treating them long-term with anti-inflammatory drugs now seems questionable.

Medical Costs of the Elderly

Medicare, the federal program that pays medical bills for elderly Americans, is already feeling the strain of the aging population. The number of people enrolled for Medicare coverage has more than doubled since 1966, from 19 million then to 50 million in 2012, and the numbers will continue to swell much more rapidly as the baby boomers retire.[28] The number of workers whose earnings contribute to the system is growing at a much slower pace. The same problem applies to Social Security, the retirement system for the elderly. In 2010, there were 2.9 workers supporting every retiree; by the year 2029, only 2.1 workers will be expected to support each retiree.[29] The government projects that, at the current rate, the system went into the red in 2010, but the Social Security trust fund will keep the program solvent until 2036.[29] Medicare's problems are worse than Social Security's, however, because its costs are less predictable. Not only is the number of people enrolled growing, but the cost per enrollee is also rising, even faster than healthcare cost inflation overall. The average annual expenditure for each Medicare enrollee rose from about $1200 in 1980 to $9,083 in 2007.[30] If present trends continue, Medicare spending is projected to nearly double from $477 billion in 2009 to $903 billion in 2020.[31]

Despite the large expenditures that threaten Medicare's solvency, the program pays only about half of the healthcare costs of its enrollees.[30] About 1 in 5 beneficiaries purchase "Medigap" insurance policies that help pay for expenses not covered by Medicare. Employer-sponsored retiree health plans provide supplemental coverage for about a third of beneficiaries. Medicaid, with funding provided jointly by federal and state governments, acts as a Medigap policy for the poor elderly. The Medicaid program, which was intended to serve the poor, and poor children in particular, has increasingly been called on to pay for services for the elderly that Medicare does not provide, especially nursing home care and home health care. Because of the high costs, most nursing home patients rapidly deplete their savings and become poor enough to qualify for Medicaid, which does cover such care. Almost half of all nursing home costs are paid by Medicaid, which like Medicare, has seen its budget mushroom, from $25.8

billion in 1980 to $401.4 billion in 2010.[28] While the elderly constitute only 10 percent of the persons enrolled in Medicaid, they consume 25 percent of the Medicaid budget.[32] This aspect of the crisis in healthcare costs for the elderly has received less attention than the problems of Medicare.

Past efforts to rein in the growth of government expenditures for the elderly's medical bills have meant that these patients bear a higher percentage of the costs through higher premiums and copayments. Half of all Medicare beneficiaries have annual incomes less than $22,000.[31] Beneficiaries pay an average of 15 percent of their household income on medical expenses, and 1 in 4 spends 30 percent or more.[30,31] This trend threatens the Medicare population with rationing by ability to pay, a matter of great concern to them.

Another approach to controlling growth of costs has been to reduce reimbursement to medical providers, a strategy that, it is feared, could induce some providers to refuse treatment to Medicare patients. In 1997, Congress tried to control Medicare costs by providing incentives for the elderly to enroll in managed care plans, an approach that had been successful in younger groups. However, over the next few years, there were many problems with the plans, in part because of Congress's efforts to control costs. The plans raised premiums and reduced benefits; providers withdrew from the plans; and a large number of plans withdrew from the Medicare program. The 2003 legislation that established prescription drug benefits also contained provisions meant to encourage the use of private managed care plans, now called "Medicare Advantage" plans. Some of these plans offer supplemental benefits, such as vision or hearing or prescription drugs. In 2011, 25 percent of Medicare beneficiaries were in Medicare Advantage plans. These plans have been criticized because they cost the government more money than regular fee-for-service Medicare.[33,34] One provision of the Affordable Care Act is that government payments to Medicare Advantage plans will be reduced.

The Medicare prescription drug plan, or Medicare Part D, which became effective in 2006, was inspired by news stories of old folks having to choose between drugs and food. The plan has indeed helped many old people to pay for their medicines, but it has many drawbacks and sources of confusion. In contrast to traditional Medicare, Part D is optional and is offered exclusively through private plans. These vary widely, offering different choices of drugs, with widely varying premiums, a situation that can be very confusing to the elderly. Most bizarre, the benefit structure features the so-called "donut hole," which was instituted to prevent the new benefit from costing more than Congress wanted to spend. Each year, beneficiaries must pay for the first $295 of their drug costs; then the plan covers 75 percent of their costs up to $2700 in total expenses. At that point individuals must pay 100 percent of their prescription costs until their total expenditures have reached $3454, at which catastrophic coverage kicks in. When the coverage gap has been reached, the elderly are back in the situation they were in before Part D took effect, and many find it hard to afford the cost of their medicines. By

2009, nearly 60 percent of Medicare beneficiaries were enrolled in Part D; another 30 percent had prescription coverage through employers' retiree health plans or other sources such as the Veterans Administration.[35] The program adds to the growth in Medicare costs, amounting to 12 percent of Medicare spending in 2011.[30]

On the Medicaid side, costs for the program have increased faster than those of Medicare, putting immense strain on state budgets. About 34 percent of Medicaid spending is for long-term care, not only for the elderly, but also for the disabled.[32] Many states set low reimbursement rates for long-term care providers in order to save money. Some states try to control costs through regulations limiting the number of available nursing home beds. In response, nursing homes tend to preferentially admit patients who can pay their own bills, usually at higher rates than allowed by Medicaid. Consequently, there is a large and growing unmet need among the less affluent elderly for nursing home care.

Unless the baby-boom generation turns out to be significantly healthier and more independent than the aged and oldest old of today, their need for nursing homes and other forms of long-term care is likely to reach critical proportions. In the past, and even today, most elderly Americans who need help with the activities of daily living have been cared for by their families, with primary responsibility borne by a daughter or daughter-in-law. A number of trends make these arrangements less feasible in the future. Baby boomers have fewer children to share the burden of caring for them in old age than did previous generations. The increased divorce rate has led to more complicated family arrangements, which may make it more difficult for the younger generation to take their parents into their homes. A more mobile society means that many children live far away from their parents. Moreover, most women work outside the home. Thus, just as the government is reducing social services for the elderly, old people may be less able to depend on their families for the help they need.

Proposals for Rationing

As it has become obvious that the growth in healthcare costs for the elderly has become unsustainable, various proposals have been made for controlling the costs through a systematic process that would be fair and equitable, such as rationing. Richard Lamm, a former governor of Colorado, was one of the first to draw attention to the idea by suggesting in 1984 that older persons have a duty to die and get out of the way.[36] His concern was that, as the elderly consume increasing amounts of medical care, society is cutting back on care for children and working people, jeopardizing their future and the productivity of society as a whole. Moreover, as medical costs—largely for the elderly—consume an increasing proportion of the national budget, the government is making cutbacks in other social programs, such as education or food programs targeted for the young, which are important for the future health and prosperity of the country.

Most of the proposals for rationing involve denying expensive life-prolonging technology to people over a set age, which seems unfair because it appears to punish people who have taken care of their health, or denying it to people who are not expected to achieve a substantial improvement in quality of life from the treatment, an approach that has many defenders. In some cases, expensive treatments are denied to people who are seen as causing their own medical problems through unhealthy behavior; for example, liver transplants are often denied to alcoholics who cannot or will not stop drinking, justified because the new scarce organ is likely to be similarly destroyed.

Considering how the nation should care for its increasing numbers of elderly citizens requires examination of our ethics and values as a society. The questions raised are difficult to answer and most people would prefer not to think about them. However, refusal to take responsibility for solving the problems that will inevitably face us will lead to desperation among the elderly and those who must care for them, especially people who do not have the resources to pay for needed care.

The current interest in assisted suicide is one consequence of ill and elderly patients' fear that they will not receive humane care as they lose control and independence. Euthanasia is only a step further, and its widespread use would certainly cut the costs of caring for the dying, an incentive feared by its opponents. Desperate families might increasingly resort to "granny dumping"—abandoning in a public place an unidentified elderly person, most often someone with Alzheimer's disease—when they feel they can no longer cope with caring for a difficult dependent.

Although Governor Lamm's statement outraged some, evidence says his suggestion makes sense. He explained his reasoning by saying that he was referring to the terminally ill, that they should not attempt to prolong their lives by artificial means, generating high medical costs and often adding to their suffering. John Wennberg and the Dartmouth research group have found that geographical variations in end-of-life care demonstrate that a significant amount of the spending is wasted. The work also shows that more aggressive care is not necessarily better quality care.

The Dartmouth group compared the care of patients dying of chronic diseases, such as cancer and heart failure, in different geographical areas. The studies confirmed that there are wide variations in Medicare spending, determined largely by the aggressiveness of care. Patients in high-spending areas spent more time in the hospital, more time in intensive care, and had more visits to physician specialists. These patients do not have better survival. In fact, there is evidence that the higher-intensity pattern of care may have worse outcomes.[37] Examples of expensive care that could be considered futile are kidney dialysis for frail nursing home residents with end-stage renal disease, which offers little benefit for most of them, and burdensome interventions in Alzheimer's patients' last 3 months of life, when hospice or "comfort" care would have been more appropriate.[38,39] As Dr. Wennberg is quoted as saying, "Some chronically ill and dying Americans are receiving too much care—more than they and their families actually want or benefit from."[40] The Dartmouth researchers note that Medicare costs could be greatly reduced, and end-of-life care might be more humane, if all parts of the country used the same patterns of care as the low-cost areas.

Applying lessons from the study of regional variations is not what is usually considered rationing. It is merely common sense. It requires patients and their families to consider what they want at the end of their lives and discuss it with their families and doctors. The issue is still highly controversial, however. During the 2009 debate over healthcare reform, a proposal calling for Medicare reimbursement for doctors who counseled patients about end-of-life care provoked accusations that President Obama was advocating "death panels."

Perhaps the greatest hope for reducing costs in an aging population is the possibility of improved health for the elderly, the compression of morbidity that most people would wish for as they look forward to longer lives. This is a realistic hope in that the baby-boom generation is relatively well educated as compared to preceding generations, and more education correlates with better health in the elderly as in other age groups. A consortium of opinion leaders has proposed that this goal could be more readily achieved through a conscious policy of integrating public health and medical services with the aim of reducing the need and demand for medical care.[41] The advocates include James F. Fries, author of the University of Pennsylvania alumni study described earlier in this chapter, who has long argued that compression of morbidity is already occurring, and former Surgeon General C. Everett Koop. Fries and Koop propose that the goal of an integrated healthcare system should be to postpone the onset of chronic infirmity—which accounts for the bulk of illness in the population—by reducing risk factors such as smoking, dietary fat intake, lack of exercise, and failure to wear seat belts, measures that would reduce the need for medical care. In addition, they suggest that demand for medical care could be reduced by educating individuals to assume more responsibility for their own health, including self-management of chronic disease. The Fries–Koop consortium's proposal is in effect an integration of the missions of public health and medicine, a "doubly positive policy goal," they write; "it promises better health for the individual and lowering of the medical costs that now consume a dangerously high share of our nation's productivity."[41(p.82)]

Conclusion

The American population is aging. Because older people tend to use medical services more than younger people, there are fears that the reliance of an increasing percentage of the population on Medicare to pay for their medical costs will overwhelm the system.

Factors that increase the risk of chronic disability in the elderly—and thus drive up medical costs—are similar to those that cause premature mortality in younger people. These include smoking, poor diet, physical inactivity, and unsafe driving practices. Public health aims to prevent the major killers, such as cardiovascular disease, cancer, diabetes, and injuries, but it also has a role in secondary and tertiary prevention of a number of problems common in elderly patients that can adversely affect their independence and quality of life. These include overmedication, osteoporosis, falls, impairment of vision and hearing, impairments of the mouth, and Alzheimer's and other dementias.

A key question in planning for the future is whether the compression of mortality—the increasing probability that people will survive until the biological limit of life span—will be accompanied by a compression of morbidity, permitting people to remain healthy until shortly before they die. As medical costs of the elderly have grown, and as the baby-boom generation has begun to retire, it has become clear that current trends would cause the system to be overwhelmed. Various proposals for rationing medical care have been put forward. Evidence on geographical variations on end-of-life care intensity and cost suggests that care could be delivered much more efficiently without sacrificing quality. The best hope for avoiding the need for rationing, and at the same time for improving quality of life for the elderly, would be to devise a way of integrating public health measures with the medical system to prevent chronic disease in the elderly, thereby reducing the need and demand for medical care.

References

1. M. W. Serafini, "The Real Medicare Crisis Ahead," *National Journal* (June 5, 2004).
2. U.S. Bureau of the Census, "2010 Census Briefs: Age and Sex Composition." http://www.census.gov/prod/cen2010/briefs/c2010br-03.pdf, accessed August 18, 2012.
3. National Center for Health Statistics, "*Health, United States, 2011*," May 2012. http://www.cdc.gov/nchs/data/hus/hus11.pdf, accessed August 19, 2012.
4. Federal Interagency Forum on Aging-Related Statistics, "Older Americans: 2012: Key Indicators of Well-Being." http://www.agingstats.gov/agingstatsdotnet/Main_Site/, accessed August 19, 2012.
5. J. F. Fries, "Measuring and Monitoring Success in Compressing Morbidity," *Annals of Internal Medicine* 139 (2003): 456–459.
6. K. G. Manton, "Recent Declines in Chronic Disability in the Elderly U.S. Population: Risk Factors and Future Dynamics," *Annual Review of Public Health* 29 (2008): 91–113.
7. U.S. Centers for Disease Control and Prevention, "Nursing Home Residents, U.S., 1977–2004. http://205.207.175.93/HDI/TableViewer/tableView.aspx?Reportid=175, accessed August 19, 2012.
8. S. H. Allaire et al., "Evidence for Decline in Disability and Improved Health Among Persons Aged 55 to 70 Years: The Framingham Heart Study," *American Journal of Public Health* 89 (1997): 1678–1683.
9. E. M. Crimmins, "Trends in the Health of the Elderly," *Annual Review of Public Health* 25 (2004): 79–98.

10. A. J. Vita, R. B. Terry, H. B. Hubert, and J. F. Fries, "Aging, Health Risks, and Cumulative Disability," *New England Journal of Medicine* 338 (1998): 1035–1066.

11. R. Sturm, J. S. Ringel, and T. Andreyeva, "Increasing Obesity Rates and Disability Trends," *Health Affairs* 23 (March/April 2004): 199–205.

12. F. Grodstein et al., "Postmenopausal Hormone Therapy and Mortality," *New England Journal of Medicine* 336 (1997): 1769–1775.

13. National Institutes of Health, "Menopausal Hormone Therapy Information." http://www.nih.gov/PHTindex.htm, accessed October 9, 2012.

14. U.S. Institute of Medicine, *Retooling for an Aging America: Building the Health Care Workforce* (Washington, DC: National Academies Press, 2008).

15. U.S. Institute of Medicine, *The Second 50 Years: Promoting Health and Preventing Disability* (Washington, DC: National Academy Press, 1990).

16. U.S. Department of Health and Human Services, *Bone Health and Osteoporosis: A Report of the Surgeon General* (Washington, DC: Government Printing Office, 2004).

17. M. E. Tinetti, "Preventing Falls in Elderly Persons," *New England Journal of Medicine* 348 (2003): 42–49.

18. Centers for Disease Control and Prevention, "Falls Among Older Adults: An Overview." http://www.cdc.gov/HomeandRecreationalSafety/Falls/adultfalls.html, accessed October 9, 2012.

19. H. A. Bischoff-Ferrari et al., "Effect of Vitamin D on Falls: A Meta-Analysis," *Journal of the American Medical Association* 291 (2004): 1999–2006.

20. National Eye Institute, "Eye Health Information." http://www.nei.nih.gov/health/, accessed September 29, 2012.

21. N. Parekh et al., "Association Between Vitamin D and Age-Related Macular Degeneration in the Third National Health and Nutrition Examination Survey, 1988 Through 1994," *Archives of Ophthalmology* 125 (2007): 661–669.

22. National Institute on Deafness and Other Communication Disorders, "Hearing, Ear Infections and Deafness." http://www.nidcd.nih.gov/health/hearing/, accessed September 29, 2012.

23. Alzheimer's Association, "2012 Alzheimer's Disease Facts and Figures," *Alzheimer's and Dementia: The Journal of the Alzheimer's Association* 8 (2012): 131–168.

24. National Institute on Aging, "Alzheimer's Disease: Unraveling the Mystery." http://www.nia.nih.gov/sites/default/files/alzheimers_disease_unraveling_the_mystery.pdf, accessed August 27, 2012.

25. J. Marx, "Preventing Alzheimer's: A Lifelong Commitment?" *Science* 309 (2005): 864–866.

26. L. Helmuth, "Protecting the Brain While Killing Pain?" *Science* 297 (2002): 1262–1263.

27. J. Couzin, "FDA Panel Urges Caution on Many Anti-Inflammatory Drugs," *Science* 307 (2005): 1183–1184.

28. U.S. Department of Health and Human Services, "CMS Fast Facts." http://www.cms.gov/fastfacts, accessed August 20, 2012.

29. Social Security Administration, "Fast Facts & Figures About Social Security, 2011." http://www.ssa.gov/policy/docs/chartbooks/fast_facts/2011/fast_fact.11.pdf, accessed August 20, 2012.

30. Kaiser Family Foundation, Fact Sheet: "Medicare at a Glance." http://www.kff.org/medicare/upload/1066-14.pdf, accessed August 20, 2012.

31. Kaiser Family Foundation, Fact Sheet: "Medicare Spending and Financing." http://www.kff.org/medicare/upload/7305-06.pdf, accessed August 20, 2012.

32. Kaiser Family Foundation, "Medicaid: A Primer," June 2010. http://www.kff.org/medicaid/upload/7334-04.pdf, accessed August 26, 2012

33. B. Biles, G. Dallek, and L. H. Nicholas, "Medicare Advantage: Déjà vu All Over Again?" *Health Affairs*, Web exclusive. http://content.healthaffairsorg/egi/reprint/hlthaff.w4.586v1.

34. Kaiser Family Foundation, Fact Sheet: "Medicare Advantage." http://www.kff.org/medicare/upload/2052-12.pdf, accessed September 29, 2012.

35. P. Neuman and J. Cubanski, "Medicare Part D Update—Lessons Learned and Unfinished Business," *New England Journal of Medicine* 361 (2009): 406–414.

36. Associated Press, "Gov. Lamm Asserts Elderly, If Very Ill, Have 'Duty to Die,'" *The New York Times*, March 29, 1994.

37. D. C. Goodman et al., "Trends and Variations in End-of-Life Care for Medicare Beneficiaries with Severe Chronic Illness." http://www.dartmouthatlas.org/downloads/reports/EOL_Trend_Report_0411.pdf, accessed August 26, 2012.

38. R. M. Arnold and M. L. Zeidel, "Dialysis in Frail Elders—A Role for Palliative Care," *New England Journal of Medicine* 361 (2009): 1597–1598.

39. G. A. Sachs, "Dying from Dementia," *New England Journal of Medicine* 361 (2009): 1595–1596.

40. R. Pear, "Researchers Find Huge Variations in End-of-Life Treatment," *The New York Times*, April 7, 2008.

41. J. F. Fries et al., "Beyond Health Promotion: Reducing Need and Demand for Medical Care," *Health Affairs* (March/April 1998): 70–84.

The Future of Public Health

Emergency Preparedness, Post-9/11

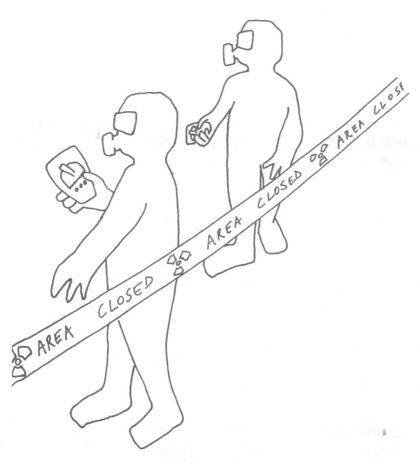

Emergency Response

The events of September 2001 confronted the United States with a new awareness of vulnerability. The attacks on the World Trade Center and the Pentagon made clear that the nation was threatened by enemies who wished to terrorize it using nonconventional weapons and that military and intelligence agencies were unprepared to defend against them. The anthrax-containing letters sent through the mail, while causing only minimal loss of life, exposed a threat from another nonconventional weapon, suggesting the equally terrifying possibility of epidemics for which health agencies were unprepared. The successes and, mostly, the failures of the nation's response to these events forced national soul-searching and mobilization of resources to ensure that the United States would not again be caught unprepared. However, the nation again proved to be unprepared in August 2005, when New Orleans and the surrounding areas were hit with a natural disaster in the form of Hurricane Katrina. Despite extensive planning for emergencies by federal, state, and local governments, especially after 9/11, it became apparent during and after the hurricane that important segments of the New Orleans population had not been considered in the plans, with tragic consequences.

The plane crashes and the intentional spread of pathogenic bacteria required law-enforcement responses aimed at identifying responsibility, punishing the perpetrators, and preventing further harmful actions. These events also prompted public health responses to deal with the consequences of the incidents and to prevent further injury and illness. In responding to natural disasters, such as hurricanes, public health has always had an important role. However, important lessons have been learned from the failures of Katrina, and it is hoped that further planning will better prepare the nation to deal with future emergencies of all kinds.

Types of Disasters and Public Health Responses

Disasters cause death, injury, disease, and property damage on a scale beyond the routine emergencies to which the health system is accustomed. However, many natural disasters are predictable—for example, hurricanes, blizzards, and forest fires—and vulnerable areas generally have plans to deal with them—although the adequacy of these plans may not be obvious until they are put to the test. These plans usually include prior evacuation of the population in affected areas to minimize negative health effects and loss of life. Other natural disasters may be unpredictable, like earthquakes, but even these unpredictable disasters tend to occur in specific geographic areas—California, for example—and therefore allow communities to be prepared through strict building codes, requirements that appliances be secured, easy turn-off of gas and electricity, and so on.

Manmade or technological disasters are generally unpredictable, although the potential can sometimes be identified and the possibility minimized through government regulation and community planning. Typical technological disasters include industrial explosions, hazardous material releases, building or bridge collapses, and transportation crashes that may also cause a chemical or radioactive release. The presence of an industrial facility or a nuclear power plant should prompt a community to conduct emergency planning appropriate to the facility and the possible exposures. Detailed planning is more complicated for plane crashes and crashes of trains or trucks carrying hazardous materials, which may occur at unforeseen sites. Most terrorist events fall into the category of technological disasters. An act of bioterrorism could cause a disaster, but it would be expected to mimic a natural disease outbreak and demand the same public health response that a natural epidemic would require.

Most disasters, natural or manmade, cause immediate injury to many residents of the affected area. Sometimes specially trained and equipped rescue personnel are needed to locate and extricate people buried in the rubble of collapsed buildings or to move people out of harm's way in fires or floods. Police and firefighters are often on the front line in combating a disaster. The injured require emergency medical care and transportation to hospitals. If hazardous materials are involved, measures must be taken to protect the rescuers and medical personnel. The situation can get even more complex when volunteers join the rescue efforts. In some cases, family members might be wandering around anxiously searching for loved ones. These individuals may also need protection from hazards in the affected environment. When there are many deaths, procedures must be established to identify victims and to communicate with their families. In situations such as this, there is a critical need for coordination of activities.

Disasters create conditions that cause health risks for the survivors. These tend to be amplifications of the general environmental hazards that public health deals with routinely: contamination of air, water, and food; exposure to toxic chemicals or radioactivity; and injury hazards such as fallen power lines and unstable buildings. The survivors need food and potable water; some people with chronic diseases may urgently need medications such as insulin or cardiac drugs. People may be left homeless by the disaster, or they may be displaced and need temporary shelter.

What is the role of public health in all these activities? One of its most important functions is planning in advance of the emergency, working with other agencies to ensure coordination of all the activities of the responders. Local public health authorities should be knowledgeable about the community and its resources because they have the responsibility to protect the health of the survivors. One of the outcomes of the 9/11 attacks was the recognition of weaknesses in coordination and communication of the emergency responders. This led to a concerted effort, organized by the federal government, to ensure that all communities have disaster response plans in place so that any future attack may be met by an effective response. This planning process is intended to have the added benefit of preparing the nation to deal with other natural or manmade disasters. In fact, many private and public organizations actively promote the need for "all-hazard planning." Unfortunately, the response by all levels of government to Hurricane Katrina demonstrated the weaknesses in the previous planning.

New York's Response to the World Trade Center Attacks

When two jet planes hit the World Trade Center towers at 8:46 and 9:02 A.M., New York City police, firefighters, and emergency medical workers rushed to the site. The firefighters and police launched rescue and evacuation efforts, and emergency medical workers set up temporary medical posts to treat injured survivors. The city's Office of Emergency Management (OEM) began directing activities from its headquarters nearby at 7 World Trade Center. Ambulances came from all over the city, and hospitals in all five boroughs prepared to receive large numbers of casualties.

Between 13,000 and 15,000 people were successfully evacuated from the towers before the south tower collapsed at 9:59 A.M. and the north tower at 10:28 A.M.[1] Tragically, 2801 people died, including 149 passengers on the planes.[2] The fact that so many people survived the disaster showed that, in many ways, the emergency response efforts were successful. Subsequent to the 1993 bombing at the World Trade Center, improvements in fire safety measures had been established, including better lighting in the stairways and evacuation drills. However, many things went wrong on September 11. The building housing OEM headquarters was severely damaged by the collapse of the north tower soon after the attack and had to be evacuated, significantly undermining OEM's ability to coordinate the rescue efforts. Moreover, OEM's communication depended on an antenna located on the roof of the north tower.[3] The Police Department and the Fire Department each had its own radio communications system, but they used different frequencies and could not communicate with each other. Poor communication led to confusion for some evacuees when some stairways were blocked, and they were not informed of alternative routes down. Doors to the roof were locked, trapping people who worked above the impact sites and tried to escape by climbing upward. Tragically, the Fire Department radios worked only sporadically in the high-rise buildings, so, despite attempts to warn them, at least 121 of the 343 firefighters who died were in the north tower when it collapsed. They had not realized that the south tower had fallen.[4]

After the buildings collapsed, the air was filled with dust, soot, and smoke, posing a threat to the thousands of rescue workers, cleanup workers, and later, residents and people who worked in downtown Manhattan, who were allowed to return to their homes and offices. An estimated 5000 tons of asbestos had been released into the air due to the destruction of the buildings.[5] Lead, other metals, dioxin, and PCBs were also detected in the soot, as fires continued to burn for months after the disaster. Although workers at the site should have been wearing respirators to protect their lungs, few of them did in the early days, and many of them developed the notorious "World Trade Center cough." It was not clear which agencies were responsible for determining when the area was safe. A priority at the highest levels of government was to get the downtown area back in business, especially Wall Street, which was reopened only 6 days after the collapse. Politicians rushed to reassure New Yorkers that the environment was safe, but there was no scientific basis for these reassurances, and their statements were received with appropriate skepticism.[6] The Environmental Protection Agency was accused of covering up the risk.

The Departments of Health of New York City and New York State had the responsibility to carry out routine public health functions, under not-so-routine conditions, during the period after the disaster. They issued death certificates and burial permits. They monitored food and drinking water served to emergency workers to ensure that it was safe. They cleaned up food in abandoned restaurants at the site to prevent outbreaks of rodents. Because there was concern that the attack might have included biological agents, the Centers for Disease Control and Prevention (CDC) sent officers to monitor hospital emergency rooms for patients with unusual symptoms. Later ongoing surveillance activities included sampling of dust and debris near the site to assess risk and monitoring of symptoms of cleanup workers and area residents. In addition to respiratory symptoms, insomnia, headaches, and dizziness, millions of survivors and workers suffered from psychological distress suggestive of post-traumatic stress disorder. Mental health agencies arranged for counseling. Victim location services were established for families with missing relatives, and shelters for displaced residents were set up. At least 19 city, state, and federal government agencies, as well as several academic, medical, and other organizations, were involved in the public health and medical response to the disaster.[2]

Response to Hurricane Katrina

Hurricane Katrina was not a surprise. Hurricanes regularly make landfall along the Gulf Coast, frequently threatening Louisiana. Parts of New Orleans were flooded by Betsy in 1965, and the city was threatened by Camille in 1969, Andrew in 1992, and Ivan in 2004.[7] Some 80 percent of New Orleans is below sea level and the city is essentially surrounded by water, bordered by the Mississippi River on the south and Lake Ponchartrain on the north, which is connected with the Gulf of Mexico on the East.[8] The city is kept dry by levees, built by the Army Corps of Engineers, that have long been known to be inadequate to withstand a major storm; funds for planned upgrades have been repeatedly cut from the federal budget.

Tropical Storm Katrina was identified and named on Wednesday, August 24, 2005, while it was in the vicinity of the Bahamas. On Thursday, August 25, the storm was upgraded to a category one hurricane as it passed through Florida into the Gulf. The Federal Emergency Management Agency National Coordination Center was activated. On Friday, the National Hurricane Center forecasted that the hurricane would strike east of New Orleans, and Louisiana Governor Kathleen Blanco declared a state of emergency. On Saturday, Katrina was upgraded to category three and several parishes and coastal areas were ordered to evacuate. Contraflow traffic was instituted on all highways in southeastern Louisiana, allowing outgoing travel only. Governor Blanco called into duty 4000 National Guard troops. Early Sunday morning, Katrina was upgraded to a category four storm; a few hours later it was upgraded to category five, with winds of 160 miles per hour. At 10:00 A.M., the governor and New Orleans Mayor Ray Nagin ordered mandatory evacuation.[7,9]

On Sunday morning, the Superdome opened as a shelter of last resort. Cars were leaving Greater New Orleans at the rate of 18,000 per hour, and the highways were clogged. By the end of the day, an estimated 80 percent of the city's population of 458,000 had left, but over 100,000 people did not have a car and were unable or unwilling to evacuate. About 10,000 people were in the Superdome, and an unknown number were waiting in houses and other buildings in the region. Rain began to fall in the city around 9:00 P.M.

By early Monday morning, New Orleans was being pounded by wind and rain; power and telephone service had failed, and some of the levees had been breached. Generators provided dim light to the Superdome, but no air conditioning, and the air was stifling and stinking. Two holes opened up in the roof of the Superdome, which was a cesspool of human waste and garbage, lacking food, water, and medicines. In various parts of the city the water was 4 to 15 feet deep. People were trapped in attics and clinging to rooftops. The Coast Guard and the Louisiana Department of Wildlife and Fisheries began going around in boats, rescuing people and taking them to the Convention Center, which did not have food, water, or other provisions for sheltering people. As the day progressed, the hurricane began to move away from the city.[7,9]

As of Tuesday morning, there were 20,000 people in the Convention Center. Patients and staff members were stranded in New Orleans hospitals, all but one of which were without power, and conditions were deteriorating. There were dead bodies in the street, floating in polluted water, people drowned in their beds because they were old or disabled and could not get up and go to higher ground; others drowned in their attics because there was nowhere higher to go. In one nursing home that did not evacuate, 35 elderly or handicapped people died in the flood; 5 more died within a week, probably from the stress of the ordeal. Although some hospitals evacuated before the storm and others were on high enough ground to escape flooding, three of the poorest hospitals suffered through the storm in primitive conditions, in stifling heat, without electricity to run ventilators or other medical equipment; some ran out of food and medicines.[7,9]

As of Wednesday morning, 26,000 people were in the Superdome. Secretary of Health and Human Services Michael Leavitt declared that a public health emergency existed in the states affected by Katrina. At 2:00 P.M., buses began evacuating seriously ill and disabled people from the Superdome. On Thursday through Sunday, patients and medical personnel were evacuated from hospitals by helicopter or boat to a makeshift field hospital at the airport. Many patients did not survive that long.[7,9]

An accurate death toll from Katrina will probably never be known. According to a report by the National Hurricane Center, it was more than 1800.[10] Most of them were poor and African American. In fact, 68 percent of the pre-Katrina population of New Orleans were African American; 23 percent were below the poverty level; and 21 percent lacked a vehicle, all factors that contributed to the high death toll.[11] The majority of the fatalities were people who did not or could not evacuate ahead of the storm. This raises the question, why did so many people apparently ignore orders to evacuate?

Later surveys of survivors from New Orleans who were evacuated after the storm to shelters elsewhere found several common themes in people's decisions. One study analyzed the findings according to the Health Belief Model (HBM).[12] On the first factor in the HBM, the extent to which people felt susceptible to the threat, many long-time residents felt they could survive because they had survived many previous hurricanes without serious problems. Another source of optimism was religious faith; many people believed God would take care of them. The second factor in the HBM, the perceived severity of the threat, many interviewees reported that they were confused about the messages from the governor and the mayor. The early evacuation orders were not mandatory, and residents interpreted this to mean the threat was not severe. By the time the officials made the order mandatory, they said, it was too late to leave. The third factor in the HBM, the barriers to action, poor African Americans perceived many barriers, financial, logistical, and community. Orders to evacuate were not clear on how or where to go. Even families that had a car may have lacked money for gas or worried about paying for necessities while traveling, or their family might have been too large to fit comfortably in the car. Family members who were old or had health problems made it difficult for the whole family to evacuate. Some people were reluctant to leave their homes without their pets, making it difficult even to go to a shelter. Some people were afraid they would lose their jobs if they left the city. Others felt they needed to stay behind to protect their property from looters.[12,13,14]

Many of those who stayed in New Orleans during the storm felt they were victims of racism. The feeling was reinforced by incidents in which residents of black neighborhoods were prevented by police from entering richer, white neighborhoods when they tried to get to safer ground. A rumor was going around that levees in poorer areas had been purposely dynamited to protect whiter, richer areas of the city.[9] One later survey found that 68 percent of survivors thought that government would have responded more quickly if more New Orleans residents had been wealthy and white.[13]

The scale of the disaster was well beyond the coping ability of a single city or even a single state. Not only was 80 percent of New Orleans flooded, but widespread destruction occurred throughout southern Louisiana, Mississippi, Alabama, and Florida. Katrina turned out to be the deadliest hurricane since 1928 and the costliest natural disaster on record in the United States.[15] Then, 26 days later, Hurricane Rita made landfall near the Texas–Louisiana border, interfering with hurricane-response activities in New Orleans and forcing evacuation of coastal regions of Louisiana and Texas, including some areas where New Orleans evacuees had taken shelter.

In New Orleans there was a desperate need for help from outside the city, a need that should have been filled by the Federal Emergency Management Agency (FEMA) and the National Guard. Help from these fronts was tragically inadequate, for a number of reasons. Governor Blanco called up the Louisiana National Guard on Friday before the storm struck, but the ranks were depleted because 35 to 40 percent of them had been called to active duty in Iraq and Afghanistan along with much of their equipment. The troops patrolled the streets of the city, provided security at the Superdome and the Convention Center, and delivered what food and water were available. Eventually, National Guard troops from other states were sent to New Orleans to help with evacuation and cleanup.[7,9]

FEMA was a weaker agency than it had been during the Clinton administration, when it was a cabinet-level agency with a professional disaster-relief professional as a director. Under President Bush, FEMA had been incorporated into the Department of Homeland Security, where the focus was on terrorism; its budget had been repeatedly cut, and it had lost many of its experienced staff.[9,16] Moreover, its director, Michael Brown, was a political crony of Bush, clearly incompetent for the job. Despite the notoriously untrue Bush remark on his visit to New Orleans Friday, September 2—"Brownie, you're doing a heck of a job"—Brown was severely criticized in the press, by Congress, and within the administration, and he resigned in mid-September.[9]

President Bush himself was mostly absent from the early days of the crisis. He had been on an extended vacation at his ranch in Crawford, Texas throughout August, and he had not seemed to pay much attention to the hurricane as it developed. On Tuesday, August 30, he delivered a speech on Iraq in San Diego, making only brief, reassuring comments on Katrina. He returned to Washington on Wednesday, declaring that he was cutting his vacation 2 days short. Vice President Cheney was on vacation in Wyoming.[9]

Hurricanes Katrina and Rita left many public health problems in New Orleans and the surrounding area, some of which are still unaddressed. Because most of the city's population, estimated at 485,000 in 2000, was evacuated either before or after the hurricanes, it stood at fewer than several thousand by the end of the first week in September, 2005. A study found that, as of December, approximately 91,000 people had returned to their homes, and it was estimated that that number would rise to about 198,000.[17] The population has continued to grow, and the 2010 Census found the population to be 343,829 with somewhat smaller proportions of whites and African Americans, more Hispanics and Asians, and fewer children than before the storm.[18] New Orleans evacuees were still living in communities throughout the country.

Many homes were destroyed by the floods and many damaged houses remain, especially in the poorer areas of the city that were badly inundated. Housing problems account for some health problems among hurricane survivors. FEMA had supplied trailers for people whose homes had been destroyed, and it later became apparent that the air in these trailers was contaminated with unhealthy levels of formaldehyde. Mold, common in many homes that had been under water during the floods, caused respiratory problems in people with allergies. Wells had been contaminated. Mosquito-borne diseases were a threat, as well as home invasions by rodents and snakes. An estimated 50 percent of survivors are expected to suffer from persistent psychological trauma and post-traumatic stress disorder.[19] The full extent of the health consequences of the disaster may never be known.

Principles of Emergency Planning and Preparedness

The evident weaknesses in the response to the 9/11 attacks called attention to the need for advance planning for possible future disasters. After 9/11, the federal government funded planning efforts throughout the nation, but obviously the results were not adequate to be ready for Hurricane Katrina. Two essential ingredients of an emergency plan missing in both New York and New Orleans were coordination and communication. The lack of these functions in New York resulted in part from the fact that the emergency management headquarters and communication antenna were disabled in the event. In New Orleans also, communication was disabled by the loss of electricity and telephones throughout the region. This situation highlights the importance of emergency system redundancy. A backup plan for managing the crisis in the absence of these resources should have been in place in both places. Redundancy in the communication system would have ensured, for example, that critical information about evacuation routes could have been shared with everyone in the World Trade Center towers. In New Orleans, an unambiguous message to evacuate did not come until too close to the time the hurricane struck for it to be acted on by the most vulnerable of the population. The situations were aggravated in New York by a history of competition between police and fire departments and the OEM and in New Orleans by the lack of a competent federal official with whom the governor and mayor could coordinate.

Because any disaster will require a coordinated response from a number of different agencies, the basic principle used in the immediate response to an emergency is the Incident Command System (ICS).[20] This approach puts a single person, who has responsibility for managing and coordinating the response, in charge at the scene. Disaster response is generally managed by authorities from local government agencies, because the response must be immediate and local authorities are closest to the scene and know the territory. The lead agency is often the fire department or the police department. The state and federal government provide technical assistance and backup resources.

Agencies involved in the ICS might include an emergency operations center, the fire department, the police department, the emergency medical system, the public health agency, the American Red Cross, the electric company and gas company, and, sometimes, the highway department or, as in the case of the World Trade Center, the Port Authority and the manager of the buildings. Most of these agencies would know their responsibilities in an emergency and would have practiced them as part of their planning and preparedness process. Different agencies might have different communications networks, but it is critically important that all communication be integrated. The public health agency, in coordination with emergency medical services and hospitals, is responsible for directing patients to the appropriate level of care and for dispatching ambulances according to the availability of appropriate resources such as operating rooms and intensive care units. On September 11, one nearby hospital was swamped with "walking wounded" and critical patients, while a trauma center only 3 miles away sat idle.[3] In New Orleans, hospitals and nursing homes lacked plans for evacuating their patients, and governments were not prepared to assist. FEMA has now developed a system called the National Incident Management System, which standardizes the organizational structures, processes, and procedures that communities should employ in planning for an emergency. It also provides guidelines and protocols for integration of all levels of government and the voluntary and private sectors in coping with a disaster.[21]

In a guide to public health management of disasters published by the American Public Health Association, the author lists 12 tasks or problems likely to occur in most disasters.[20] All of these tasks depend on effective interorganizational coordination and should be sorted out and practiced ahead of time.

- Sharing information: Two-way radios are often the most reliable way to communicate, but it is important to choose a common frequency.
- Resource management: personnel should identify themselves at a check-in area and should be given an assignment and a radio; arrival of equipment and supplies should be logged in and they should be distributed where they are most needed.
- Warnings should be issued and evacuations ordered by the appropriate agencies. The warnings should be delivered, usually by the mass media, in a manner that will prompt appropriate action by the population.
- Warnings must be unambiguous and consistent and must include specific information about who is at risk and what actions should be taken.
- Search and rescue operations should be coordinated so that casualties are entered into the emergency medical services system and the healthcare system.
- The mass media should be used to warn the public about health risks after the disaster as an effective public health measure.

- Triage, a method for sorting survivors by severity of their injury and need for treatment, should be established at the scene by trained medical personnel.
- Casualty distribution: Protocols should be established to ensure that patients are distributed among available hospitals or other facilities.
- Tracking of patients and other survivors is difficult but, to the extent it is possible, should be done in order to avert later difficulties.
- Establishing methods to care for patients with all levels of need should be part of the advance planning. Many survivors seek care for minor injuries or may need prescription medications for chronic medical conditions. Backup arrangements should be made for care of patients when hospitals and other healthcare centers are damaged, including backup supplies of power and water and plans to evacuate to alternative sites.
- Management of volunteers and donations should be planned for; resources should be collected, organized, and distributed at a site outside the disaster area to not disrupt ongoing emergency operations.
- Expect the unexpected. Be ready to respond to unanticipated problems.

The plan should be practiced at least once, and preferably once per year. The exercises can be desktop simulations, field exercises, or drills. The time for partners to meet each other is before, not after, the disaster strikes.

After September 11, the federal government has provided substantial resources to states and major metropolitan areas for public health preparedness, including preparedness for natural disasters, bioterrorism, and chemical and radiological disasters. Since 2002, the CDC has invested more than $9 billion in state, local, tribal, and territorial public health departments to upgrade their ability to respond to a range of pubic heath threats.[22] The money is used for planning, training, improving communication and coordination, strengthening hospitals and laboratories, and improving epidemiology and disease surveillance in state and local areas. A Strategic National Stockpile includes medical supplies, antibiotics, vaccines, and antidotes for chemical agents. In the event of an emergency, federal personnel can deliver these supplies to the people who need them anywhere in the United States within 12 hours.

An evaluation of the progress made by 12 metropolitan areas between September 11, 2001, and May 2003 found that emergency preparedness had improved, but gaps still remained. The researchers highlighted three communities of different sizes that they found to be especially strong in their level of preparedness: Syracuse, New York, Indianapolis, Indiana, and Orange County, California.[23] The success of these three communities is credited in part to previous experience with public health threats. Syracuse, for example, has a nuclear power plant nearby, which had stimulated the population's concern about a nuclear accident or a terrorist attack. Indianapolis has done extensive planning over the years for the annual Indianapolis 500 auto races and other large sporting events. Orange County has experience in disaster planning because of the ongoing threat of earthquakes and fires; a nuclear power plant is also located nearby. Other factors that contribute to readiness, the researchers concluded, are strong leadership, successful collaboration, and adequate funding.[23]

Congressional hearings on the response to Hurricane Katrina, however, noted in early 2006 that whatever improvements had been made to our capacity to respond to natural or manmade disaster, 4.5 years after 9/11, U.S. disaster preparedness remained dangerously inadequate. A report by a bipartisan committee of the House of Representatives identified failures at all levels of government. "All the little pigs built houses of straw," the report wrote. "Katrina was a national failure, an abdication of the most solemn obligation to provide for the common welfare."[24] Whether the nation would be better prepared today will not be known until the next emergency.

Bioterrorism Preparedness

The anthrax letters attack of fall 2001 constituted a terrorist attack just as surely as the hijacking and plane crashes, and similarly spread terror in the American population, although it caused few deaths. The anthrax letters were recognized to be a terrorist attack in part because of the heightened alertness created by the events of 9/11, and in part because anthrax is such a rare pathogen in humans. Anthrax had been identified as a possible agent of biowarfare in the planning that the federal government had been carrying out during the late 1990s. If a less conspicuous pathogen had been used, the attack might not have been recognized as quickly. For example, the 1984 *Salmonella* outbreak in Oregon was not recognized as a deliberate attack until much later, when the cult members quarreled publicly about the attack, and a criminal investigation was launched.[25]

Bioterrorism requires a very different kind of preparedness strategy than the response needed for dramatic disasters such as a hurricane or the attack on and collapse of the World Trade Center towers. The greatest challenge in bioterrorism preparedness might be the ability to recognize that an attack is underway. Accordingly, the CDC coordinated extensive efforts throughout the nation to improve the public health infrastructure, understanding that the response to a biological attack must be the same as that for a natural disease outbreak. As Dr. Julie Gerberding, then director of the CDC said, "We are building . . . capacity [to handle biological terrorism] on the foundation of public health, but we are also using the new investments in [combating] terrorism to strengthen the public health foundation" because "these two programs are inextricably linked."[26]

The CDC has listed pathogens most likely to be used in a terrorist attack. Category A agents, shown in Table 30-1, include smallpox, anthrax, Ebola, and other hemorrhagic fever viruses. These agents can be easily disseminated or transmitted person-to-person and cause high mortality, with potential for major public health impact. Recommendations for preparing for biological attacks are shown in Table 30-2.

Table 30-1   Category A Bioterrorism Agents and Diseases

Category A

The U.S. public health system and primary healthcare providers must be prepared to address varied biological agents, including pathogens that are rarely seen in the United States. High-priority agents include organisms that pose a risk to national security for the following reasons:

· They can be easily disseminated or transmitted person-to-person.

· They cause high mortality, with potential for major public health impact.

· They might cause public panic and social disruption.

· They require special action for public health preparedness.

Category A Agents/Diseases

· Anthrax (*Bacillus anthracis*)

· Botulism (*Clostridium botulinum toxin*)

· Plague (*Yersinia pestis*)

· Smallpox (*Variola major*)

· Tularaemia (*Francisella tularensis*)

· Viral hemorrhagic fevers (filoviruses [e.g., Ebola, Marburg] and arenaviruses [e.g., Lassa, Junin])

Source: Reproduced from U.S. Centers for Disease Control and Prevention, "Emergency Preparedness and Response." emergency.cdc.gov/agent/agentlist-category.asp, accessed October 10, 2012.

Table 30-2   Steps in Preparing for Biological Attacks

· Enhance epidemiologic capacity to detect and respond to biological attacks.

· Supply diagnostic reagents to state and local public health agencies.

· Establish communication programs to ensure delivery of accurate information.

· Enhance bioterrorism-related education and training for healthcare professionals.

· Prepare educational materials that will inform and reassure the public during and after a biological attack.

· Stockpile appropriate vaccines and drugs.

· Establish molecular surveillance for microbial strains, including unusual or drug-resistant strains.

· Support the development of diagnostic tests.

· Encourage research on antiviral drugs and vaccines.

Source: Reproduced from U.S. Centers for Disease Control and Prevention, *Morbidity and Mortality Weekly Report* 49 (2000): RR-4:5.

The public health capacities that are being strengthened to improve recognition of a disease outbreak include (1) educating physicians and other medical workers to recognize unusual diseases, (2) monitoring emergency rooms for certain patterns of symptoms, (3) opening new laboratories with the capability of identifying unusual viruses and bacteria, and (4) improving communication between public health agencies at the local, state, and federal level and the professionals and facilities most likely to first encounter affected patients. Surveillance activities include emergency room visits, calls to 911 and poison control centers, and pharmacy records to detect increased use of antibiotics and/or over-the-counter drugs. (One early indication of the 1993 cryptosporidiosis outbreak in Milwaukee was that pharmacies were selling out of medications for diarrhea.) Similar measures are important for recognizing chemical attacks as well, and the CDC coordinates an integrated network of state, local, federal, military, and international public health laboratories that can respond to both bioterrorism and chemical terrorism.[27] The Department of Agriculture is similarly conducting surveillance for animal diseases and other agricultural threats. Animal health is an important component of homeland security, both because of the need to protect the food supply and because many animal diseases are also a threat to humans. Seventy-five percent of emerging infections that have recently been identified in humans originate in animals—for example, bird flu, SARS, hantavirus, mad cow disease, and *E. coli* O157:H7.[28] Computer networks serve to alert public health officials about significant or unusual findings from surveillance data. In addition to public health efforts to improve the ability to recognize a bioterrorist attack and identify the agent, the CDC has taken steps to improve response to the event, including the Strategic National Stockpile, as previously described.

The spread of West Nile encephalitis across the country provided an opportunity and a challenge for the public health and medical care systems to develop and practice response to a new infectious disease. When West Nile virus first appeared in 1999 in New York City, bioterrorism was considered as one possible explanation for its origin. That hypothesis was soon discarded, but the disease has been closely monitored as it spreads to areas where it is unfamiliar. The mechanisms used to deal with the spread of West Nile virus are the same as those that would be used in a bioterrorist event.

The prospect of bioterrorism has raised other issues that affect the nation's ability to respond effectively. Among the most important of these is that public health officials need to have the legal power to take action to protect the public and contain an outbreak of an infectious disease. For example, the officials have to be able to isolate and quarantine people. Public health activities are, for the most part, controlled by state law, and the public health laws in many states predate modern scientific understanding of disease. The laws may be outdated, inadequate, and inconsistent. For example, some states have laws that prevented sharing of surveillance information with other states; private property laws might prevent destruction of contaminated property or the imposed distribution of drugs and medical supplies to where they are needed; privacy laws might interfere with public health agencies' ability to obtain information from hospitals or pharmacies; quarantine laws might be challenged by affected individuals and thus prevent prompt action.[29]

After the anthrax attacks of 2001, the CDC requested a group of legal and public health scholars to develop a Model State Emergency Health Powers Act that state legislatures could follow to update their laws. The suggested provisions include measures to encourage planning for emergencies; surveillance; managing property to ensure availability of vaccines, pharmaceuticals, and hospitals; powers to compel vaccination, testing, treatment, isolation, and quarantine when necessary; and provision of information to the public. These measures would be activated when a public health emergency is declared and would include legal safeguards to protect personal rights while promoting the common good.[29] The model act was released in December 2001, and most states have passed at least some of the measures. The CDC has a public health law program that seeks to improve the understanding and use of law as a public health tool, to develop CDC's capacity to apply law to achieve public health goals, and to develop the legal preparedness of the public health system to address public health priorities.[30]

Another issue that has been raised but not so readily addressed is the problem of the 50 million Americans who lack health insurance. If the first individuals to be exposed to an infectious agent are uninsured, they may choose not to seek medical care or may delay visiting an emergency room, thus spreading the pathogen and delaying the recognition that an outbreak is under way. "Their lack of insurance is a known risk to their own health, but it must now also be recognized as a risk to the nation's health," noted two public health experts.[31] The problem is compounded by the federal law, passed in 1996, that prohibits federally funded medical clinics from treating illegal immigrants. Unless it is made clear to the whole population that everyone with symptoms of a contagious illness should seek treatment and that they will not suffer legal or financial consequences from presenting themselves for a medical evaluation, the United States will be vulnerable to bioterrorism in a way different from any other developed country. The Affordable Care Act will help to address this problem by reducing the number of uninsured Americans, but the problem of treating illegal immigrants remains because they are not covered by the Act.

While the CDC is taking a major role in planning for bioterrorism, the Department of Homeland Security has been developing technological methods of detecting biological and chemical attacks, in the hope of recognizing an attack faster, even before people begin developing symptoms, and of identifying the biological or chemical agent. Monitoring devices with sensors that detect bacteria, viruses, and toxins were used at the Salt Lake City Olympics in 2002, and these devices have been installed in more than 30 major American cities. The devices suck air through filters, which are periodically changed, and the filter paper taken to a laboratory for testing. It is not clear how effective these detectors would be in an attack, and many scientists are skeptical about the value of the monitoring systems. The Department of Homeland Security is supporting research to develop more sophisticated systems for environmental monitoring.[32]

Smallpox is the most dreaded of the possible bioterrorism agents, and after the initial shock of the anthrax events in 2001, a great deal of government planning efforts were devoted to the possibility of a bioterrorist attack using smallpox. There were concerns that, although smallpox was officially eradicated in the 1970s, rogue nations might have obtained stocks of the virus from the former Soviet Union. A smallpox attack would be devastating. The disease is highly contagious, and there is no effective treatment. About 30 percent of those infected die. Virtually everyone in the world is susceptible to some extent, because immunizations have not been given in 35 years. A tabletop exercise, assuming that anonymous terrorists covertly sprayed smallpox virus in three shopping malls, had predicted 3 million hypothetical cases of the disease, of whom 1 million died.[33] Lessons learned from the exercise, which was conducted in June 2001 by policy scholars and former senior government officials, included that such an attack could cause breakdowns in essential institutions, disruption of democratic processes, civil disorder, loss of confidence in government, and reduced U.S. strategic flexibility. One of the participants testified to Congress that the exercise taught us that public health is a major national security issue.[34]

During the prelude to the war in Iraq, which was believed to have biological weapons, the Bush administration sponsored development of large quantities of vaccine. Members of the military were required to be vaccinated before the invasion. The administration planned to vaccinate public health and medical workers also, to be ready for a biological attack, but very few civilians agreed to be vaccinated. After Iraq was found not to have weapons of mass destruction after all, the concern about smallpox died down.

Pandemic Flu

Since the emergence of the avian flu in Asia in the 1990s, there has been concern about the possibility of its turning into a pandemic. The virus had had a frighteningly high mortality rate among people who had been infected. Thus far, it has not had the capability to be transmitted easily from one human to another. The prospect of a mutated avian flu virus easily spread within the population has prompted governments to make plans for how to respond if this should occur. Measures that would be needed include rapid development and manufacture of a vaccine targeted to the specific pandemic strain, surveillance of the virus's spread, and stockpiling of antiviral drugs and antibiotics to combat the secondary bacterial infections that killed many of the victims of the 1918 flu. In part due to bioterrorism planning, the CDC has intensified its surveillance activities, and the Strategic National Stockpile would be as useful in a flu pandemic as it would in the event of a bioterrorism attack. Producing vaccines is still a very slow process. The technology involves growing viruses in eggs, which requires huge numbers of eggs. Most seasonal flu vaccines require 1 egg for every 3 or 4 doses. Research on developing methods to produce vaccines using cells grown in culture is under way, but has not yet led to any approved vaccines. Current methods require about 6 months to produce an adequate supply.[35,36]

Other concerns in planning for a severe pandemic include hospital capacity and the need for mechanical respirators. Symptoms of the 1918 flu were similar to those of the SARS epidemic, which required intensive care for those affected. It is assumed that more lives of flu patients could be saved by modern medical treatments than was possible in 1918. However, because flu spreads much more readily than SARS, the medical system would be quickly overwhelmed by a flu epidemic of the severity that occurred in 1918. Planning for pandemic flu has included discussions of how to allocate scarce medical resources when not everyone can be helped.

Unexpectedly, the pandemic that appeared in 2009—the first flu pandemic since the Hong Kong flu of 1968—was not the avian flu but a swine flu, H1N1 instead of H5N1, that turned out to be much less severe than avian flu. The United States was relatively prepared to put its plans into effect. The H1N1 pandemic emerged in the spring, at the end of the normal influenza season, and a public health emergency was declared. The virus was quickly isolated and provided to manufacturers, who were encouraged to begin producing vaccines. Immunizations began in October, but production of the vaccine was slower than expected. The regular seasonal flu vaccine was expected not to provide protection against H1N1 flu; so both immunizations were necessary for complete protection. Because of vaccine shortages, however, public health officials advised limiting the H1N1 vaccine to those at highest risk:

- Pregnant women, because they are at highest risk of complications and because immunizing them potentially protects their infants who cannot be vaccinated.
- Household contacts and caregivers of infants under 6 months old.
- Healthcare workers and emergency services personnel, because they could be a source of infection for vulnerable patients, and because increased absenteeism in this population would weaken the healthcare system.
- Anyone 6 months to 24 years of age, because they are often in close contact in daycare and school.
- Anyone older than 24 who has underlying health problems that might make them susceptible to influenza-related complications.

As of mid-October 2009, H1N1 was the predominant strain of flu throughout the United States, and it was widespread all over the country. People age 65 and older seem to be less susceptible to the H1N1 strain, probably because it is similar to strains they have been exposed to earlier in their lives. The H1N1 strain was incorporated into the 2010–2011 seasonal flu vaccine, further reducing the threat of swine flu as a deadly epidemic, at least in the United States.[37,38]

Conclusion

Public health has an important role in preparing for and responding to all kinds of emergencies and disasters, natural and manmade. The immediate response to a disaster must include emergency medical care for the injured and evacuation of survivors. In cases where the disaster can be predicted, such as a hurricane, the safest response is to evacuate people in advance. Later there is the need to ensure that air, water, and food are not contaminated and that injury hazards such as fallen power lines and unstable buildings are eliminated. Generally the disaster response is carried out by a number of agencies, and coordination among them is very important. After 9/11, the federal government provided funding for all communities to develop disaster plans, in which all the relevant agencies should participate.

The response in New York to the World Trade Center attacks demonstrated a number of weaknesses, offering lessons that should be incorporated in planning for any future emergencies. The most serious problem was poor communication among response agencies. The city's emergency management center was damaged by the attack, as well as the antenna it used for communication, and the fire department and police department could not communicate with each other. Although more than 13,000 people escaped from the towers, some of the 2801 deaths could have been prevented by better communication and coordination. The air in lower Manhattan was contaminated for months after the attacks, and many of the cleanup workers at the site did not use respiratory protection devices. Critics complained that government agencies were more intent on reassuring the population than on telling them the truth about health risks.

The response to Hurricane Katrina was inadequate at all levels of government. The New Orleans mayor and the Louisiana governor hesitated before ordering a mandatory evacuation, and they did not provide information or the means for the most vulnerable of the population to evacuate. The federal government agency that should have been providing assistance and resources, FEMA, had been weakened by its incorporation into the new Department of Homeland Security; its budget had been severely cut; and its director had no knowledge or experience of emergency planning or response.

There are well-established principles for management of disasters that should be understood by all medical and safety responders. All agencies involved should participate in planning; all responders should be familiar with the plans; and the response should be practiced at least once a year. Since 9/11, the federal government has invested more than $3.7 billion in strengthening the public health infrastructure. The preparations were intended to improve the nation's ability to respond not only to disasters, but also to naturally occurring disease outbreaks and other public health emergencies. However, Katrina demonstrated that more planning is needed.

Preparedness for bioterrorism requires that the public health system carry out its normal surveillance functions. A biological attack might be recognized only after patients start showing up in hospitals and doctors' offices; even their symptoms may not be unusual—most of the pathogens that might be used as bioweapons first cause flu-like symptoms. The CDC has provided funding for states and major cities to develop surveillance of hospital emergency rooms, 911 calls, calls to poison control centers, and pharmacies. The CDC has also opened new laboratories capable of testing for biological and chemical agents, and it maintains a Strategic National Stockpile of medical and emergency supplies. The Department of Agriculture conducts surveillance for animal diseases. While much of the concern about bioterrorism has subsided since the war in Iraq proved that Saddam Hussein did not have weapons of mass destruction, some of this planning and surveillance have proved useful in dealing with the flu pandemic of 2009.

Pandemic flu has caused concern since the late 1990s, when a lethal strain of avian flu appeared in Asia. Although avian flu is not easily transmitted person-to-person, public health authorities fear that it could mutate and turn into a deadly pandemic. However, the first pandemic since 1968, which struck in 2009, turned out to be a milder swine flu strain, H1N1. Thanks in part to preparation for bioterrorism, the United States has seemed to cope successfully with the new pandemic.

References

1. U.S. Centers for Disease Control and Prevention, "Preliminary Results from the World Trade Center Evacuation Study—New York City, 2003," *Morbidity and Mortality Weekly Report* 53 (2004): 815–817.
2. S. Klitzman and F. Freudenberg, "Implications of the World Trade Center Attack for the Public Health and Health Care Infrastructures," *American Journal of Public Health* 93 (2003): 400–406.
3. R. Simon and S. Teperman, "World Trade Center Attack: Lessons for Disaster Management," *Critical Care* 5 (2001): 317–319.
4. J. Dwyer, K. Flynn, and F. Fessenden, "9/11 Exposed Deadly Flaws in Rescue Plan," *The New York Times*, July 7, 2002.
5. J. Shufro, "Perspective on the Tragedy at the World Trade Center," *American Journal of Medicine* 42 (2002): 557–559.
6. G. D. Thurston and L. C. Chen, "Risk Communication in the Aftermath of the World Trade Center Disaster," *American Journal of Industrial Medicine* 42 (2002): 543–544.
7. D. Brinkley, *The Great Deluge: Hurricane Katrina, New Orleans, and the Mississippi Gulf Coast* (New York: William Morrow, 2006).
8. J. Travis, "Scientists' Fears Come True as Hurricane Floods New Orleans," *Science* 309 (2005): 1545–1548.
9. M. E. Dyson, *Come Hell or High Water: Hurricane Katrina and the Color of Disaster* (New York: Basic Books, 2006).
10. R. D. Knabb, J. R. Rhome, and D. P. Brown, "Tropical Cyclone Report: Hurricane Katrina." http://www.nhc.noaa.gov/pdf/TCR-AL122005_Katrina.pdf, accessed August 29, 2012.

11. Kaiser Family Foundation, "Key Facts—States Most Affected by Hurricane Katrina." http://www.kff.org/uninsured/upload/7395-02.pdf, accessed September 29, 2012.

12. K. Elder et al., "African Americans' Decisions Not to Evacuate New Orleans Before Hurricane Katrina: A Qualitative Study," *American Journal of Public Health* 97 (2007): S124–S129.

13. M. Brodie et al., "Experiences of Hurricane Katrina Evacuees in Houston Shelters: Implications for Future Planning," *American Journal of Public Health* 96 (2006): 1402–1408.

14. D. P. Eisenman et al., "Disaster Planning and Risk Communication with Vulnerable Communities: Lessons from Hurricane Katrina," *American Journal of Public Health* 97 (2007): S109–S115.

15. Centers for Disease Control and Prevention, "Public Health Response to Hurricanes Katrina and Rita—United States, 2005," *Morbidity and Mortality Weekly Report* 55 (2006): 229–231.

16. D. Rosner and G. Markowitz, *Are We Ready? Public Health Since 9/11* (Berkeley: University of California Press, 2006).

17. K. F. McCarthy et al., "Repopulation of New Orleans after Hurricane Katrina," 2006. http://www.rand.org/pubs/technical_reports/TR369, accessed August 28, 2012.

18. Greater New Orleans Community Data Center, "What Census 2010 Reveals About Population and Housing in New Orleans and the Metro Area," March 17, 2011. https://gnocdc.s3.amazonaws.com/reports/GNOCDC_Census2010PopulationAndHousing.pdf, accessed August 28, 2012.

19. M. A. Mills, D. Edmondson, and C. L. Park, "Trauma and Stress Response Among Hurricane Katrina Evacuees," *American Journal of Public Health* 97 (2007): S116–S123.

20. L. Y. Landesman, *Public Health Management of Disaster: The Practice Guide*, 2nd ed. (Washington, DC: American Public Health Association, 2005).

21. Federal Emergency Management Agency, "National Incident Management System (NIMS)." http://www.fema.gov/national-incident-management-system, accessed August 28, 2012.

22. U.S. Centers for Disease Control and Prevention, Office of Public Health Preparedness and Response, "Funding and Guidance for State and Local Health Departments." http://www.cdc.gov/phpr/coopagreement.htm, accessed August 28, 2012.

23. M. McHugh, A. B. Staiti, and L. E. Felland, "How Prepared Are Americans for Public Health Emergencies? Twelve Communities Weigh In," *Health Affairs* (May/June 2004): 201–209.

24. S. S. Hsu, "Katrina Report Spreads Blame," *The Washington* Post, February 12, 2006.

25. T. J. Torok et al., "A Large Community Outbreak of Salmonellosis Caused by Intentional Contamination of Restaurant Salad Bars," *Journal of the American Medical Association* 278 (1997): 389–395.

26. L. K. Altman, "Disease Control Center Bolsters Terror Response," *The New York Times*, August 28, 2002.

27. Centers for Disease Control and Prevention, "Laboratory Response Network: Partners in Preparedness." http://emergency.cdc.gov/lrn, accessed August 28, 2012.

28. N. Marano and M. Pappiaoanou, "Historical, New, and Reemerging Links Between Human and Animal Health," *Emerging Infectious Diseases* 10 (2004): 2065–2066.

29. L. O. Gostin et al., "Model State Emergency Health Powers Act: Planning for and Response to Bioterrorism and Naturally Occurring Infectious Diseases," *Journal of the American Medical Association* 288 (2002): 622–628.

30. Centers for Disease Control and Prevention, "Public Health Law Program." http://www.cdc.gov/phlp/about.html, accessed August 28, 2012.

31. M. K. Wynis and L. Gostin, "Bioterrorist Threat and Access to Health Care," *Science* 296 (2002): 1613.

32. D. A. Shea and S. A. Lister, "The Biowatch Program: Detection of Bioterrorism," Congressional Research Service Report No. RL 32152. http://www.fas.org/sgp/crs/terror/RL32152.htm#_1_3, accessed August 29, 2012.

33. T. O'Toole, M. Mair, and T. V. Inglesby, "Shining Light on 'Dark Winter,'" *Clinical Infectious Diseases* 34 (2002): 972–983.

34. "Avoiding a Dark Winter," *The Economist*, October 25, 2001. http://www.economist.com/node/835123, accessed August 29, 2012.

35. M. T. Osterholm, "Preparing for the Next Pandemic," *New England Journal of Medicine* 358 (2005): 1839–1842.

36. A. Pollack and D. G. McNeil, Jr., "Road to Flu Vaccine Shortfall, Paved with Undue Optimism," *The New York Times*, October 26, 2009.

37. U.S. Centers for Disease Control and Prevention, "2009 H1N1 Flu." http://www.cdc.gov/h1n1flu/, accessed August 29, 2012.

38. U.S. Centers for Disease Control and Prevention, "Key Facts About Seasonal Flu Vaccine." http://www.cdc.gov/flu/protect/keyfacts.htm, August 29, 2012.

Public Health in the Twenty-First Century: Achievements and Challenges

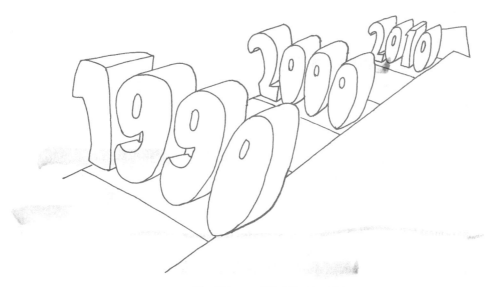

The Future of Public Health

The United States in the 20th century saw great progress in public health. As a field of practice, public health has advanced in knowledge and methodology. Biomedical scientists have identified many of the organisms that cause infectious diseases and have developed methods to control them. Epidemiologists have recognized risk factors that lead to many chronic diseases, information that can be used to reduce people's risk of illness. Efforts to clean up the environment have resulted in air and water that are much safer than they were a half-century ago. Intensive health education efforts have even persuaded Americans to improve some health-related behaviors, leading to reductions in tobacco use and drunk driving. The ability to assess the state of the public's health and to evaluate the impact of medical and public health interventions has also advanced dramatically because of vast stores of health-related data and computer software capable of analyzing them. These achievements have greatly improved the health of Americans. The average lifespan has increased by 30 years since 1900 (when it was 47), and 25 of those years are attributed to improvements in public health.[1]

In 1999, the Centers for Disease Control and Prevention (CDC) published a "top ten" list of great public health achievements of the 20th century.[1] These accomplishments were chosen for the positive impact they have had and will continue to have in reducing deaths, illnesses, and disabilities in the United States. Following is the CDC's list (not in order of importance).

- Routine use of vaccination has resulted in a dramatic reduction in infectious diseases, including the eradication of smallpox; the elimination of polio in the Americas; and control of measles, rubella, tetanus, diphtheria, and a number of other infectious diseases in the United States and other parts of the world.
- Improvements in motor vehicle safety have contributed to large reductions in motor vehicle-related deaths. This has been achieved through engineering efforts to make vehicles and highways safer and through success in persuading people to adopt healthier behaviors, such as using seat belts, child safety seats, and motorcycle helmets, and to not drink and drive.
- Safer workplaces have resulted in a dramatic reduction in fatal occupational injuries—down 90 percent since 1933—and illness. This achievement results from improvements in safety in mines and in the manufacturing, construction, and transportation industries.
- Control of infectious diseases has been achieved by (in addition to vaccination) improved sanitation, cleaner water, safer food, the discovery of antibiotic drugs, and methods of epidemiologic surveillance and follow-up.
- A decline in deaths from heart disease and stroke has resulted from the identification of risk factors and people's significant success in changing their behavior to reduce cholesterol levels and to stop smoking. Secondary prevention methods, such as early detection and treatment of high blood pressure, also contribute to the lower number of deaths.
- Safer and healthier foods have almost eliminated major nutritional deficiency diseases such as rickets, goiter, and pellagra in the United States. Microbial contamination of food has been reduced, and nutritional supplementation and labeling have made possible a healthier diet.
- Healthier mothers and babies are the result of better hygiene and nutrition; availability of antibiotics; greater access to health care, including prenatal care; and technologic advances in medicine. Since 1900, there has been a 90 percent reduction in the infant mortality rate and a 99 percent reduction in the maternal mortality rate.

- Access to family planning and contraceptive services has contributed to healthier mothers and babies through smaller family size and longer intervals between the birth of children; increased opportunities for preconception counseling and screening; and improved control of sexually transmitted diseases.
- Fluoridation of drinking water has reduced tooth decay in children by 40 percent to 70 percent, and tooth loss in adults has been reduced by 40 percent to 50 percent.
- Recognition of tobacco use as a health hazard and subsequent public health antismoking campaigns have helped to prevent people from beginning to smoke, have promoted quitting, and have reduced exposure to environmental (second-hand) tobacco smoke. The resulting decrease in the prevalence of smoking among adults has prevented millions of smoking-related deaths.

Challenges for the Twenty-First Century

In the early 21st century, public health faces many challenges, both old and new. There are renewed threats from infectious diseases, such as AIDS, antibiotic resistance, and foodborne pathogens. The global economy has increased Americans' vulnerability to many of the health threats faced by residents of less developed nations, brought about by international travel and by imported agricultural products. Paradoxically, past successes have led to new threats, such as climate change caused by overpopulation and economic development, and rising costs of medical care for the aging population. The challenge of understanding and altering human behavior—the factor that now contributes most substantially to premature mortality—remains to be confronted by the public health practitioners of the 21st century. The decline in cigarette smoking has slowed; rates of alcohol and illicit drug use among adolescents are largely unchanged over the past decade; physical inactivity and unhealthy diets contribute to the increasing prevalence of obesity among Americans; and injury is still a major cause of death.[2]

Ironically, the successes of public health in the 20th century led to cutbacks in resources and support for preventive activities. During the second half of the century, the medical approach—curing health problems rather than preventing them—gained acceptance. Public health's many achievements, including those described above, were taken for granted while rapidly increasing resources were devoted to medical care. This problem was recognized in the Institute of Medicine's (IOM's) 1988 report, *The Future of Public Health*.[3] This report prompted public health agencies, policy makers, and academic institutions to initiate a national discussion on the role of public health and the steps necessary to strengthen its capacity to fulfill its role. Attempts were made to coordinate public health efforts at various levels of government, to develop public–private partnerships in communities, and to undertake strategic planning aimed at achieving defined goals and objectives. The IOM undertook a new analysis in 2003 to follow up on the 1988 report and made recommendations for enhancing understanding of public health and developing a framework for assuring the public's health in the new century.[4]

The events of fall 2001, particularly the bioterrorist attacks using anthrax, brought new attention to the American public health system and revealed the weaknesses in the public health infrastructure—workforce, information systems, laboratories, and other organizational capacity—which was suffering from neglect. It became clear to policy makers and the public that the public health system is the front line of defense in protecting the population from bioterrorism and other threats. Concerns about preparedness led to a flow of federal funds into public health agencies and activities. These funds have helped state and local agencies to begin strengthening their capacity to respond to public health challenges; however, public health officials are concerned whether the efforts can be sustained. Budget deficits at the federal and state levels threaten to derail the upgrades just when their importance is being recognized. The IOM's report, *The Future of the Public's Health in the 21st Century*, was published in 2003 and includes lessons learned from the 2001 attacks.[4]

The 2003 report stated that, "the public health system that was in disarray in 1988 remains in disarray today."[4(p.100)] It noted that the United States was not meeting its potential in the area of population health, in part because of the nation's emphasis on (1) medical care rather than preventive services and (2) biomedical research rather than prevention research. It also noted the serious and persistent disparities in health status among various population groups, according to race and ethnicity, gender, and socioeconomic status. The report recommended that the public health workforce needs better education and training, that changes are needed in public health laws to bring them up-to-date and to ensure better coordination among states and territories, and that advances in information technology should be used more effectively to provide adequate surveillance and communication. Although the resources to rectify some of the deficiencies have been provided in the wake of 9/11, the IOM report stressed the need for these efforts to be sustained for the long term.

In 2009, the IOM again considered the state of public health in the United States and produced a report called, *For the Public's Health: Investing in a Healthier Future*, concluding that the health system's failure to develop and deliver effective prevention strategies continues to take a toll on the economy and society. Public health departments should be the backbone of the health system, the report said, but they need adequate funding to do so. The report recommended that all public health agencies develop a minimum package of public health services that all health departments should deliver, and that Congress should authorize a dedicated, stable, and long-term financing structure to generate the revenue required to deliver this minimum package of services. As a source of this revenue, the report suggested a tax on all healthcare transactions.[5]

Strategic Planning for Public Health

With so many different agencies at so many different political and organizational levels involved in implementing public health's mission, it became apparent some time ago that there was a need for planning and coordination. Beginning in 1979, the Public Health Service adopted "management by objectives," a process that was becoming increasingly widespread in the private sector. This technique requires that managers jointly define a set of measurable goals, use these goals as a guide to their actions, and regularly measure progress toward achieving them. The management-by-objectives approach is especially useful in decentralized organizations, where many different actors must coordinate their efforts, and thus is well suited to the needs of the public health system.[6]

To develop goals for the year 1990, the Public Health Service enlisted a broad range of participants from both within and outside of government to specify a set of health status objectives. The national goals, published as *Healthy People: The Surgeon General's Report on Health Promotion and Disease Prevention*,[7] set targets for reducing mortality rates in different age groups, with specific objectives designed to meet each target. For example, to achieve the goal of a 25 percent death rate reduction for ages 25 through 64, progress had to be made in reducing the prevalence of cigarette smoking, high blood cholesterol, and high blood pressure among adults. Any state, community, or research group that applied for federal funds for a public health program had to justify its request by showing how its project would contribute to achieving one or more of the *Healthy People* goals. When the results of the first planning cycle were tallied in 1990, the numerical mortality goals were met for three of the four age groups: infants, children, and adults aged 25 through 64. Only targets for adolescents and young adults were not met, because of continued high rates of fatal motor vehicle injuries, homicides, and suicides.[6]

The Healthy People planning process encourages states and local communities to use the national objectives as a basis for developing objectives of their own. One problem that became obvious during the first decade of the program was a lack of data systems that could track progress, especially at the local level.

In 1987, the Public Health Service began the process of setting objectives for the following decade. *Healthy People 2000*, a 692-page book sets three overall goals, with over 300 measurable objectives divided into 22 priority areas.[8] As in the previous *Healthy People* publication, these objectives set targets for individual behavioral change, environmental and regulatory protections, and access to preventive health services. *Healthy People 2000* also addressed the problem of inadequate data, which had hindered evaluation of progress toward the 1990 objectives. Implementing, tracking, and reporting on the goals and objectives involved many agencies of the federal government, as well as hundreds of state agencies, national organizations, academic institutions, and business groups. Most states developed their own year 2000 objectives. The individual states' objectives either paralleled or modified the national objectives to suit the states' own needs and priorities.

In 2001, a final review was published that evaluated the nation's progress in meeting the *Healthy People* objectives.[9] Progress was achieved on over 60 percent of the objectives. Targets were met in reducing deaths from coronary heart disease and cancer, reducing AIDS incidence, and reducing homicide, suicide, and firearm-related deaths. Tobacco-related mortality targets were met. Goals for infant mortality and the number of children with elevated blood lead levels were nearly met. There was progress toward reducing health disparities. However, for 15 percent of the *Healthy People 2000* objectives, the nation moved away from the report's targets. Notably, these included the prevalence of overweight and obesity, especially among adolescents, an ominous sign for the future health of Americans.

Healthy People 2010, launched in January 2000, set public health goals and objectives even higher.[2] *Healthy People 2010* has two overall goals:

1. Increase quality and years of healthy life, and
2. Eliminate health disparities.

These are similar to the goals of *Healthy People 2000*, except that the first goal places a new focus on quality of life, and the second goal no longer sets different targets for racial and ethnic minorities, aiming to ensure that all groups in the United States will be equally healthy.

Healthy People 2010 is organized into 28 focus areas, many of which are the same as the priority areas in Healthy People 2000. In addition, a set of 10 leading health indicators, shown in **Box 31-1**, were chosen as areas of special focus. These indicators were based on their ability to motivate action, the availability of data to measure their progress, and their relevance as broad public health issues.

A final review of Healthy People 2010 was published in 2011, assessing progress in achieving the objectives in each of the 28 focus areas, as well as a summary of progress for the leading health indicators and the two goals. Also, for each objective, the review summarizes disparities by race and ethnicity, sex, education level, income, geographic location, and disability status whenever data is available.[10]

For eight of the focus areas, more than 75 percent of the objectives moved toward, met, or exceeded their 2010 targets. These areas included health communication, heart disease and stroke, immunization and infectious diseases, occupational safety and health, and tobacco use. For five of the focus areas, more than 30 percent of the objectives could not be assessed because of lack of data. Two focus areas—arthritis, osteoporosis, and chronic back conditions, and nutrition and overweight—moved toward or achieved less than 25 percent of their targets.

Box 31-1   Healthy People 2020 Framework

The Mission, Vision, Goals, and Topic Areas of *Healthy People 2020*

The vision, mission, and overarching goals provide structure and guidance for achieving the *Healthy People 2020* objectives. While general in nature, they offer specific, important areas of emphasis where action must be taken if the United States is to achieve better health by the year 2020. Developed under the leadership of the Federal Interagency Workgroup (FIW), the *Healthy People 2020* framework is the product of an exhaustive collaborative process among the U.S. Department of Health and Human Services (HHS) and other federal agencies, public stakeholders, and the advisory committee.

Vision—A society in which all people live long, healthy lives.
Mission—*Healthy People 2020* strives to:

- Identify nationwide health improvement priorities;
- Increase public awareness and understanding of the determinates of health, disease, and disability and the opportunities for progress;
- Provide measurable objectives and goals that are applicable at the national, state, and local levels;
- Engage multiple sectors to take actions to strengthen policies and improve practices that are driven by the best available evidence and knowledge; and
- Identify critical research, evaluation, and data collection needs.

Overarching Goals

- Attain high-quality, longer lives free of preventable disease, disability, injury, and premature death.
- Achieve health equity, eliminate disparities, and improve the health of all groups.
- Create social and physical environments that promote good health for all.
- Promote quality of life, healthy development, and healthy behaviors across all life stages.

Topic Areas

The Topic Areas of Healthy People 2020 identify and group objectives of related content, highlighting specific issues and populations. Each Topic Area is assigned to one or more lead agencies within the federal government that is responsible for developing, tracking, monitoring, and periodically reporting on objectives.

1. Access to Health Services
2. Adolescent Health
3. Arthritis, Osteoporosis, and Chronic Back Conditions
4. Blood Disorders and Blood Safety
5. Cancer
6. Chronic Kidney Disease
7. Dementias, Including Alzheimer's Disease
8. Diabetes
9. Disability and Health
10. Early and Middle Childhood
11. Educational and Community-Based Programs
12. Environmental Health
13. Family Planning
14. Food Safety
15. Genomics
16. Global Health
17. Healthcare-Associated Infections
18. Health Communication and Health Information Technology
19. Health-Related Quality of Life and Well-Being
20. Hearing and Other Sensory or Communication Disorders
21. Heart Disease and Stroke
22. HIV
23. Immunization and Infectious Diseases
24. Injury and Violence Prevention
25. Lesbian, Gay, Bisexual, and Transgender Health
26. Maternal, Infant, and Child Health
27. Medical Product Safety
28. Mental Health and Mental Disorders
29. Nutrition and Weight Status
30. Occupational Safety and Health
31. Older Adults
32. Oral Health

33. Physical Activity

34. Preparedness

35. Public Health Infrastructure

36. Respiratory Diseases

37. Sexually Transmitted Diseases

38. Sleep Health

39. Social Determinants of Health

40. Substance Abuse

41. Tobacco Use

42. Vision

Source: Reproduced from *Healthy People 2020*. healthypeople.gov/2020/
TopicsObjectives2020/pdfs/HP2020_brochure_with_LHI_508.pdf, page 5 and 6,
November 2010, accessed October 10, 2012.

In assessing the first goal of Healthy People 2010—quality and years of healthy life—years of life continue to improve, especially in the older population, but measures of quality yielded mixed results. There were slight improvements in "years in good or better health" and "expected years free of activity limitations." However, "expected years free of selected chronic conditions" declined. The second goal, eliminating health disparities, did not show evidence of systematic improvement. Status on the objectives was improving for most populations, but the differences among the groups were generally not declining.[10]

As 2010 approached, the public health community mobilized to launch the process for *Healthy People 2020*. An organizing framework, including vision, mission, and goals was released in 2009, with public comment invited. There were four overarching goals:

- Attain high-quality, longer lives free of preventable disease, disability, injury, and premature death.
- Achieve health equity, eliminate disparities, and improve the health of all groups.
- Create social and physical environments that promote good health for all.
- Promote quality of life, health development, and health behaviors across all life stages.

Final 2020 goals and objectives were released in December 2010.[11] Healthy People 2020 included 42 topic areas, including 13 that were not part of Healthy People 2010 (see Box 31-1). Inspired by the IOM reports and the success of the Public Health Service's planning initiative, and recognizing that most public health activities take place at a local level, a group of public health associations began working on ways to help local public health agencies apply the management-by-objective approach. The participating organizations—the CDC, the Public Health Foundation, the American Public Health Association, the Association of State and Territorial Health Officials, the National Association of Local Boards of Health—developed guidelines for local public health agencies to conduct their own strategic planning process, involving all sectors of the community in both planning and implementation.[12] With funding from the Robert Wood Johnson Foundation, the participating organizations developed a program called "Turning Point: Collaborating for a New Century in Public Health."[13] Turning Point created partnerships with 21 state and local public health and community-based organizations to serve as models for a more effective and responsive public health system. Although the project has now closed, it created materials and resources that can be used by communities and public health organizations to achieve public health goals. One of the outcomes has been the Turning Point Leadership Development National Excellence Collaborative, which developed a curriculum that is used by public health leadership institutes throughout the United States to train public health leaders to create learning organizations that work in collaborative environments.[14]

Dashed Hopes for the Integration of Public Health and Medical Practice

Because of the high and continuously rising cost of medical care, managed care became more prevalent in the 1990s. Managed care moves the incentives of medicine closer to the mission of public health—keeping people healthy. While traditional fee-for-service medicine focuses on people who seek care, offering financial rewards to doctors for providing services to patients, managed care organizations (MCOs) are responsible for all their members, yielding financial rewards when the need for expensive medical services is averted. This shift in medicine's perspective has a number of implications for public health.

The incentives for MCOs to keep their patients healthy encourage medical plans to use public health strategies to prevent disease and to promote healthy behaviors among members. The financial incentives also make medicine economically dependent on public health's effectiveness in preventing unnecessary disease in the community. Public health failures can be expensive. The 1993 cryptosporidiosis outbreak in Milwaukee, for example, caused $15.5 million in medical costs.[15] Thus, the changes in how medical care is financed and delivered encourage the medical sector to support adequate funding for the public health sector.

With managed care, medicine is driven by the same kind of measurable goals and objectives that public health has been developing. MCOs are required to collect data on the effectiveness of their services and the health status of their members. They are evaluated on their success in achieving the same kinds of goals and objectives detailed in the Healthy People process. These common goals provide medicine and public health with strong incentives to work together.

Unfortunately from the standpoint of public health, managed care has lost its popularity since the late 1990s. There was a backlash against many of its cost-control measures, and the benefits that come from incentives to keep MCO members healthy were not obvious to the public. State Medicaid programs continue to rely heavily on managed care, however.

For the majority of Americans, whose health insurance is provided by their employers or through Medicare, the future is uncertain. The cost of medical care is again rising rapidly, and the trend is economically unsustainable. Employers are shifting the costs to their employees, who are paying an increasing share through higher premiums and copayments. The number of Americans who lack health insurance continues to rise. As the 2003 IOM report comments, "the loss of trust in the idea of managed care is also the loss of a great opportunity to improve quality and restrain costs."[4(p.241)]

President Obama's reform of the healthcare system, the Affordable Care Act, with the goals of increasing access to health insurance and controlling costs, includes a number of prevention and wellness measures. Insurers will be required to cover preventive benefits such as screening and counseling for obesity, tobacco use, sexually transmitted diseases, cancer, high cholesterol, and HIV, as well as recommended immunizations. Medicare is required to provide many of these preventive services at no cost to the beneficiaries. Preventive services for women including well-woman visits and contraception are required free of charge; the latter is particularly controversial with Republicans. Preventive services for children include recommended immunizations, lead screening for those at risk, and regular monitoring of development throughout childhood.[16]

Information Technology

Advances in information technology offer extraordinary opportunities for collaboration between public health and medical care. For example, epidemiologic surveillance using the Internet would allow a system linking state and local health departments, public health laboratories, hospitals, and doctors' offices to collect data in real time and rapidly analyze it to detect unusual disease patterns. Such a system could simultaneously disseminate the information among all participants. However, at this time, there is no single system. Instead, there are multiple systems that do not necessarily communicate with each other.

One important system is the CDC's Public Health Information Network (PHIN), a national initiative to increase the capacity of public health agencies to electronically exchange data and information across organizations and jurisdictions. The PHIN promotes the use of standards and defines functional and technical requirements for management and public health information exchange. Using such information exchange systems, the CDC facilitates a number of programs, including, for example, biosurveillance, outbreak management, and national notifiable disease surveillance.[17] The biosurveillance program, called BioSense, integrates data from the Department of Veterans Affairs and the Department of Defense, as well as over 100 hospitals across the country, to enhance national situational awareness by real-time disease detection and monitoring.[18] The Outbreak Management System assists public health workers in the management of outbreaks by enabling the integration of data on demographics, case investigations, laboratory results, exposures and relationships between persons, and other factors relevant to an outbreak. The National Notifiable Diseases Surveillance Program is a state-based system that facilitates exchange of data between public health, laboratories, and clinical providers about conditions designated as nationally notifiable.[17]

Another program linked with PHIN is the National Environmental Public Health Tracking Network (EPHT), in which the CDC funds health departments in 23 states and one city to build local tracking networks. Other partners include the Environmental Protection Agency, the American Public Health Association, and the National Aeronautics and Space Administration. The EPHT Network was established in 2002 to improve environmental public health surveillance by tracking and reporting environmental hazards and the health problems that may be related to them. It allows scientists, health professionals, and members of the public to see where these hazards and health problems are occurring and how they are changing over time. The network is currently focusing on data regarding noninfectious diseases or other conditions: poisoning by carbon monoxide or lead, asthma, cancers, and heart attacks; the concentrations of certain chemicals inside people's bodies, for example, lead levels in the blood of children; and hazardous contaminants and pollutants that may be found in air and water.[18]

As the 2003 IOM report noted, the anthrax attacks of fall 2001 demonstrated the weaknesses of public health communication and information systems being used at the time. Only half of the nation's state, local, and territorial health departments had Internet capability. Another 20 percent of these health agencies lacked e-mail.[4] Federal funding for bioterrorism preparedness has helped to bring many of the local health departments up to modern standards of information technology, and by 2006 93 percent had continuous, high-speed Internet access.[19]

In addition to being used in epidemiologic surveillance, information technology is already transforming the assessment and evaluation activities that are so important to the practice of public health and that promise also to improve outcomes in the practice of medicine. States and some counties maintain electronic databases on vital statistics, notifiable diseases, chronic diseases, hospital discharges, and immunizations; many of these are tied into the PHIN. Billing records on patients covered by the Medicare program have proven useful in assessing outcomes of medical care.

Information networks are also being developed by MCOs and other nongovernmental providers of health services. Giant healthcare companies have streamlined procedures for storing and exchanging data on medical tests, procedures, costs, and outcomes. However, as noted by Paul Starr, historian of the relationship between medicine and public health, "National policy has yet to resolve two of the most fundamental questions about computerized health information: how to keep private what ought to be private, and how to make public what ought to be public."[20(p.103)]

President Obama's reform of the healthcare system, includes incentives for physicians, hospitals, and other medical providers to use health information technology to improve the efficiency and quality of medical care for all American citizens. A uniform system of electronic medical records for all patients would help to overcome the fragmentation of medical care, which, for example, leads to duplication of services when doctors do not have information about procedures and testing a patient has received during previous visits to other doctors. A uniform system of billing could also reduce some of the administrative costs that contribute to the high medical expenditures in the United States.

An investment of $19.5 billion for health information technology was passed by Congress in early 2009, and President Obama appointed a national coordinator to lead the implementation of a nationwide interoperable, privacy-protected health information technology infrastructure. The Department of Health and Human Services has developed software that is available to hospitals, physicians' offices, pharmacies, labs, insurance companies, and other components of the healthcare system, to enable them to connect to each other and to share data. The Department also published guidelines on securing health information by making it unreadable by unauthorized individuals.[21,22,23]

A federal law passed by Congress in 1996, which became effective in 2003, was designed to protect the privacy of medical records. The Health Insurance Portability and Accountability Act (HIPAA) forbids "wrongful disclosure of individually identifiable health information." While this provision helps to eliminate some abuses, it has raised concerns that the privacy measures obstruct the use of medical data for many useful purposes. For example, researchers have complained that they cannot conduct outcomes studies, such as comparisons of different treatments for cancer.[24] The privacy rules also have discouraged the creation of public databases that consumers could use to make optimal decisions concerning their health and health care.[20]

The rise of the Internet presents major new opportunities and challenges for individuals who wish to understand and make choices concerning their personal health. People have access to vast quantities of health information—and misinformation—on the Internet. Many state and federal public health agencies provide the latest and most accurate information about health issues on their Web pages. Many nongovernmental sites also offer good advice and information, which can raise people's awareness of health risks, provide them with motivation and skills to reduce these risks, offer a helpful sense of connection to others who are in similar situations, and furnish information about difficult choices. However, caution is necessary in using the information presented on Web sites that lack authoritative sponsors. This information may be biased because of the Web site creators' commercial interests, distrust of science, or ignorance.

The Internet poses challenges to government agencies charged with regulating medical care because of the lack of accountability on the part of those who create Web sites. For example, doctors set up Web sites to diagnose and prescribe for patients' ills without examining the patients. Prescription drugs are sometimes sold over the Internet to people without valid prescriptions. Drugs that are not approved in the United States can be ordered from foreign markets. Even prescription drugs that are available in the United States may cost more here than in other countries, including Canada, and many people choose to buy them over the Internet in order to save money. The traditional role of the Food and Drug Administration (FDA) and other governmental agencies—to protect consumers from fraudulent and irresponsible medical practice—is made much more difficult by the free-wheeling culture of Internet commerce. At the same time, the FDA's opposition to importing cheaper drugs from Canada has begun to seem like a ploy to protect the American drug industry's profits, generating skepticism about the integrity of the agency's mission.

The widespread use of smart phones provides opportunities for people to receive health information and monitor their behaviors. For example, a program called "Sweet Talk," was successful in supporting young people with type 1 diabetes. Participants were sent text messages tailored to their self-management goals and could use the system to submit data and ask questions.[25] A study of young smokers who wanted to quit found that, after 6 weeks, participants who received regular, personalized text messages providing smoking cessation advice, support, and distraction were twice as likely to not be smoking than members of a control group.[26]

The CDC has a text-messaging program that allows people to sign up to get emergency alerts, new research and reports, and health tips. People with diabetes, for example, can receive tips and reminders on how to manage their diet and exercise. In the event of an emergency, people in the affected zip codes can be alerted and instructed on how to respond.[27]

The FDA in 2011 issued a declaration that it intends to apply its regulatory authority to the oversight of mobile medical apps that may or may not yet be in use. These include apps that allow a doctor or nurse, for example, to view medical images such as electrocardiograms on a mobile platform, or to monitor vital signs measurements of patients at home.[28]

The Challenge of Biotechnology

Biotechnology promises to solve many medical problems with new drugs and procedures that will contribute to the spiraling costs of medical care. Information from the Human Genome Project, for example, allows the detection of individual differences in people's response to various drugs, with the promise that doctors can choose among medications to prescribe for a patient based on genetic tests. Discoveries in cancer genomics offer to provide information on individual tumors that will allow treatments specifically targeted toward a single patient. These promises of "personalized medicine" come with a caveat, however: At a time when medical costs are spiraling out of control, and when a significant proportion of the American population does not have access to even the most basic health care, who will have access to these expensive treatments? Public health should have a voice in deciding how many of these "miracles" our society can afford, and how priorities should be set when resources are limited.

Biotechnology offers even more unprecedented possibilities, such as that of choosing the characteristics of future children through genetic engineering and cloning or of slowing the aging process. These developments will raise many legal and ethical issues, which will have to be faced through public debate and difficult policy choices.

The Ultimate Challenge to Public Health in the Twenty-First Century

"If public health's mission is to fulfill society's interest in assuring conditions in which people can be healthy (The *Future of Public Health* definition), public health has yet to succeed in fostering a national debate on the relative return on investment to improve population health."[29(p.xxiii)] As Jonathan E. Fielding noted, in a review of public health in the 20th century, the enormous expansion of the medical care system—a system that is largely inaccessible to much of the population that needs it most—occurred without consideration of whether this investment could have yielded more benefits to health if invested elsewhere. Public health agencies are chronically starved for funding to carry out essential public health services that are clearly cost-effective in raising the health status of communities.[29]

Health is determined by the social, physical, and economic environments; health behaviors; and genetics. Health is affected only marginally by medical interventions. The challenge for public health continues to be educating the public and policymakers about the role of these nonmedical factors in determining people's health and convincing people of the importance of the core public health functions in protecting and promoting the health of the entire population. As it becomes increasingly apparent that advances in high-technology medical care have become economically unsustainable, the nation must focus on assuring conditions in which people can be healthy—the mission of public health —in the 21th century.

Conclusion

The United States has made great progress in public health during the 20th century. The threat of infectious diseases has been greatly reduced, risk factors for some chronic diseases are well understood, the environment has been substantially cleaned up, and a great deal has been learned about how health is affected by behavior. The ability to assess the state of the public's health and to evaluate the impact of medical and public health interventions has advanced dramatically because of the existence of vast stores of health-related data and computer software capable of analyzing it.

During the 20th century, the life expectancy of Americans has been extended by 30 years. Much of this improvement came from 10 great public health achievements identified by the CDC: vaccination, motor vehicle safety, safer workplaces, control of infectious diseases, decline in deaths from coronary heart disease and stroke, safer and healthier foods, healthier mothers and babies, family planning, fluoridation of drinking water, and recognition of tobacco use as a health hazard.

Still, public health faces many challenges in the 21st century. Some of these challenges come from new forms of familiar public health problems such as infectious diseases and environmental pollution. Others are posed by efforts to change people's unhealthy behavior, the factor that now contributes the most to premature mortality.

A trend toward decentralizing governmental responsibilities and authority has prompted public health to adopt a planning process called "management by objectives." This process involves setting measurable goals and objectives and periodically assessing progress. The federal government has led this planning process over the past 3 decades, and involvement has expanded to include state, county, and local communities. The result has been substantial progress toward achieving public health goals, but the goals must be constantly reset.

The trend toward managed care as a strategy for controlling medical care costs moved the incentives of medical practice closer to the mission of public health. However, the unpopularity of managed care and the failure to communicate the health benefits it offers led to a backlash. Consequently medical costs have resumed their upward spiral, raising concerns that medical care will become even less affordable in the 21st century, and the number of uninsured will continue to rise.

Advances in information technology have led to great improvements in public health surveillance capabilities. The bioterrorism attacks of fall 2001 stimulated a flow of federal funds to state and county health departments for preparedness, allowing improvements in information systems at all levels of government. Information technology also makes possible much of the assessment and evaluation activity that is becoming important to the practice of public health and medicine. President Obama has identified integrated health information systems as a priority in his efforts to reform the healthcare system. The rise of the Internet as a source of information and commerce also poses challenges to individual consumers on how to evaluate the information and to government regulators on how to protect consumers from fraudulent and irresponsible medical practice.

Perhaps the most important challenge faced by public health in the 21st century will be to encourage a society-wide debate on how public resources should be allocated to most effectively improve the health of the population as a whole.

References

1. U.S. Centers for Disease Control and Prevention, "Ten Great Public Health Achievements—United States, 1900–1999," *Morbidity and Mortality Weekly Report* 48 (1999): 241–243.

2. U.S. Department of Health and Human Services, *Healthy People 2010: Understanding and Improving Health*, 2nd ed. (Washington, DC: U.S. Government Printing Office, November 2000).

3. U.S. Institute of Medicine, *The Future of Public Health* (Washington, DC: National Academy Press, 1988).

4. U.S. Institute of Medicine, *The Future of the Public's Health in the 21st Century* (Washington, DC: National Academy Press, 2003).

5. U.S. Institute of Medicine, *For the Public's Health: Investing in a Healthier Future*, April 10, 2012. http://www.iom.edu/Reports/2012/For-the-Publics-Health-Investing-in-a-Healthier-Future.aspx, accessed August 29, 2012.

6. J. M. McGinnis and D. R. Maiese, "Defining Missions, Goals, and Objectives," in F. D. Scutchfield and C. W. Keck, eds., *Principles of Public Health Practice* (Albany, NY: Delmar, 1997), pp. 131–146.

7. U.S. Department of Health, Education, and Welfare, *Healthy People: Surgeon General's Report on Health Promotion and Disease Prevention* (Washington, DC: PHS publication 79–55071, 1979).

8. U.S. Department of Health and Human Services, *Healthy People 2000: National Health Promotion and Disease Prevention Objectives* (Washington, DC: PHS publication 91–50212, 1990).

9. National Center for Health Statistics, *Healthy People 2000 Final Review* (Hyattsville, MD: Public Health Service, 2001).

10. U.S. Centers for Disease Control and Prevention, *Healthy People 2010 Final Review*. http://www.cdc.gov/nchs/healthy_people/hp2010/hp2010_final_review.htm, accessed August 30, 2012.

11. U.S. Department of Health and Human Services, "HHS Announces the Nation's New Health Promotion and Disease Prevention Agenda." http://healthypeople.gov/2020/about/DefaultPressRelease.pdf, accessed September 29, 2012.

12. M. F. Katz and M. W. Kreuter, "Community Assessment and Empowerment," in F. D. Scutchfield and C. W. Keck, eds., *Principles of Public Health Practice* (Albany, NY: Delmar, 1997), pp. 147–157.

13. Robert Wood Johnson Foundation, "*About Turning Point.*" http://www.turningpointprogram .org/Pages/about.html, accessed August 31, 2012.

14. C. D. Lamberth and L. Rowitz, "Leadership in Public Health Practice," in F. D. Scutchfield and C. W. Keck, eds., *Principles of Public Health Practice*, 3rd ed. (Clifton Park, NY: Delmar, 2009), pp. 418–444.

15. R. Lasker, *Medicine and Public Health: The Power of Collaboration* (New York: New York Academy of Medicine, 1997), p. 37.

16. "Prevention and Wellness." http://www.healthcare.gov/prevention/index.html, accessed August 31, 2012.

17. U.S. Centers for Disease Control and Prevention, "Public Health Information Network." http://www.cdc.gov/phin/, October 6, 2009, accessed October 30, 2009.

18. U.S. Centers for Disease Control and Prevention, "The National Environmental Public Health Tracking Network." http://ephtracking.cdc.gov/showHome.action, accessed August 31, 2012.

19. C. J. Leep, G. Gorenflo, and P. M. Libbey, "The Local Health Department," in F. D. Scutchfield and C. W. Keck, eds., *Principles of Public Health Practice* (Clifton Park, NY: Delmar, 2009), pp. 207–231.

20. P. Starr, "Smart Technology, Stunted Policy: Developing Health Information Networks," *Health Affairs* 16 (3) (1997): 103.

21. U.S. Department of Health and Human Services, Press Release: "HHS Names David Blumenthal as National Coordinator for Health Information Technology." http://www.hhs .gov/news/press/2009pres/03/20090320b.html, accessed August 31, 2012.

22. U.S. Department of Health and Human Services, Press Release: "Federal Health Architecture Delivers Free, Scalable Solution Helping Organizations Tie Health IT Systems into the NHIN," April 6, 2009. http://www.hhs.gov/news/press/2009pres/04/20090406a.html, accessed August 31, 2012.

23. U.S. Department of Health and Human Services, Press Release, "HHS Releases Guidance for Securing Health Information and Preventing Harm from Breaches." http://www.hhs .gov/news/press/2009pres/04/20090417a.html, accessed August 31, 2012.

24. J. Kaiser, "Privacy Rule Creates Bottleneck for U.S. Biomedical Researchers," *Science* 305 (2004): 168–169.

25. V. L. Franklin et al., "Patients' Engagement with 'Sweet Talk'—a Text Messaging Support System for Young People with Diabetes," *Journal of Medical Internet Research* 10 (2008): e20.

26. A. Rodgers et al., "u smoke after txt? Results of a Randomised Trial of Smoking Cessation Using Mobile Phone Text Messaging," *Tobacco Control* 14 (2005): 255–261.

27. U.S. Centers for Disease Control and Prevention, "Text Messages & Health Tips," July 17, 2012. http://www.cdc.gov/mobile/textmessaging/, accessed September 20, 2012.

28. U.S. Food and Drug Administration, "Medical Devices: Draft Guidance for Industry and Food and Drug Administration Staff–Mobile Medical Applications." http://www.fda.gov/ MedicalDevices/DeviceRegulationandGuidance/GuidanceDocuments/ucm263280.htm#a, accessed September 20, 2012.

29. J. E. Fielding, "Public Health in the Twentieth Century: Advances and Challenges," *Annual Review of Public Health* 20 (1999): xiii–xxx.

Glossary

Access to health care: The potential for timely use of medical services to achieve the best possible health outcomes.

Acquired immune deficiency syndrome (AIDS): The most severe phase of infection with the human immunodeficiency virus (HIV). People infected with HIV are said to have AIDS when they get certain opportunistic infections or when their CD4+ cell count drops below 200.

Adjusted rate: A way of comparing two groups that differ in some important variable (e.g., age) by mathematically eliminating the effect of that variable.

Aerosol: A suspension of liquid particles in the air; many infectious diseases of the respiratory system are transmitted by pathogen-containing aerosols released when an infected person coughs or sneezes.

Age-adjusted rate: A rate calculated to reflect a standard age distribution.

Alzheimer's disease: A degenerative disease of the brain characterized by mental deterioration. It is the most common cause of dementia in the elderly, and its prevalence increases with age.

Antibody: A protein produced by cells of the immune system that reacts specifically with invading antigens.

Antigens: Proteins on the surface of a pathogen that stimulate the development of antibodies to destroy the pathogen.

Anxiety disorder: A mental illness characterized by intense fear or dread lacking an unambiguous cause or a specific threat.

Arthritis: Inflammation of the joints that often causes limitations of activity due to pain and stiffness. Its prevalence increases with age.

Assessment: One of the three core functions of public health as specified by *The Future of Public Health*. The process by which a public health agency regularly and systematically collects, assembles, analyzes, and makes available information on the health of a community, including statistics on health status, community health needs, and epidemiologic and other studies of health problems.

Association: The relationship between two or more events or variables. Events are said to be associated when they occur more frequently together than one would expect by chance. Association does not necessarily imply a causal relationship.

Assurance: One of the three core functions of public health as specified by *The Future of Public Health*. The process by which a public health agency ensures its constituents that services necessary to achieve agreed-upon goals are provided, either by encouraging actions by other entities (private or public sectors), by requiring such action through regulation, or by providing services directly.

Asthma: A lung disease with recurrent exacerbation of airway constriction, mucous secretion, and chronic inflammation of the airways, resulting in reduced airflow that causes symptoms of wheezing, cough, chest tightness, and difficulty breathing.

Attention deficit hyperactivity disorder (ADHD): A common childhood disorder with symptoms including difficulty staying focused and paying attention, difficulty controlling behavior, and over-activity.

Autism: A group of developmental brain disorders, characterized by a wide range of symptoms, skills, and levels of impairment, generally including social impairment, communication difficulties, and repetitive and stereotyped behaviors.

Bacteria: One-celled microorganisms of the plant kingdom. Only a few cause disease.

Benign: Not cancerous; does not invade nearby tissue or spread to other parts of the body.

Bias: The influence of irrelevant or even spurious factors or associations—commonly called confounding variables—on a result or conclusion.

Biomedical science: The study of the biological basis of human health and disease, including genetics, immunology, infectious diseases, chronic diseases, and molecular approaches to treatment.

Biopsy: The removal of a sample of tissue that is then examined under a microscope to check for cancer cells.

Biostatistics: Statistics applied to the analysis of biological and medical data.

Bipolar disorder (manic-depressive illness): A brain disorder that causes unusual shifts in mood, energy, activity levels, and the ability to carry out day-to-day tasks.

Birth defect: An abnormality in structure, function, or body metabolism that is present at birth, such as cleft lip or palate, phenylketonuria, or sickle cell disease.

Blinding: A method of keeping subjects and, if possible, researchers unaware of which subjects are in an experimental group (those getting a new drug, for example) and which are in a control group (those getting an older drug or a placebo).

Cancer: Diseases in which abnormal cells divide without control. Cancer cells can invade nearby tissue and can spread through the bloodstream and lymphatic system to other parts of the body.

Carcinogen: A substance or agent that is known to cause cancer.

Cardiovascular disease: Disease of the heart and blood vessels, most commonly caused by atherosclerosis, deposits of fatty substances in the inner layer of the arteries. Coronary heart disease affects the arteries of the heart and may lead to a heart attack. Cerebrovascular disease affects the arteries of the brain and may lead to a stroke.

Carrying capacity: The limit of population size that the environment can support without being degraded.

Case control study: An epidemiologic study that compares individuals affected by a disease with a comparable group of persons who do not have the disease to seek possible causes or associations.

Centers for Disease Control and Prevention (CDC): The main assessment and epidemiologic agency for the nation, directly serving the population as well as providing technical assistance to states and localities.

Chronic disease: A disease that is marked by long duration or frequent recurrence, usually incurable but not immediately fatal. Common diseases that are considered chronic include cardiovascular disease, cancer, diabetes, Alzheimer's disease, and, recently, acquired immune deficiency syndrome (AIDS).

Chronic obstructive pulmonary disease (COPD): A disease characterized by the presence of airflow obstruction due to chronic bronchitis and emphysema, two diseases that often coexist.

Clinical trial: At its best, a study of the effect of some treatment on two (or more) comparable, randomly selected groups (e.g., an experimental group that is treated and an untreated or otherwise treated control group).

Cohort study: A study of a group of people, or cohort, followed over time to see how some disease or diseases develop.

Communicable disease: Infectious disease that spreads directly from one person to another.

Community: A specific group of people, often living in a defined geographical area, who share a common culture, values, and norms and are arranged in a social structure according to relationships the community has developed over a period of time.

Confounding variable: Another factor or explanation that may affect a result or conclusion.

Congenital: Present at birth.

Contraception (birth control): The means of pregnancy prevention. Methods include permanent methods (i.e., male and female sterilization) and temporary methods (i.e., barrier, hormonal, and behavioral).

Control group (controls): A group of individuals used by an experimenter as a standard for comparison—to see the effect of changing one or more variables in an experimental group.

Copayment: A modest fixed fee for each medical visit, charged to patients who have health insurance. The remainder of the bill is paid by the health insurance company or the managed care organization.

Core functions of public health: Three basic tasks performed by public health agencies to ensure conditions in which people can be healthy. As defined by *The Future of Public Health*, these tasks are assessment, policy development, and assurance.

Correlation: The extent to which two or more variables in an association are related—for example, the extent to which one variable changes in response to change in another.

Cost benefit analysis: An economic analysis in which all costs and benefits are converted into monetary values and results are expressed as dollars of benefit per dollar expended.

Cost-effectiveness analysis: An economic analysis assessed as health outcome per cost expended.

Crude rate: The actual rate of events (births, deaths, cases of a disease or injury, etc.) in a population, without adjustment.

Developmental disabilities: A broad spectrum of impairments characterized by developmental delay and/or limitation in personal activity, such as mental retardation, cerebral palsy, epilepsy, hearing and other communication disorders, and vision impairment.

Diabetes: A chronic disease due to insulin deficiency and/or resistance to insulin action and associated with high levels of sugar in the blood. Over time, unless properly treated, organ complications related to diabetes develop, including heart, nerve, foot, eye, and kidney damage and problems with pregnancy.

Disability: Reduction of a person's capacity to function in society.

Dose-response relationship: The relationship between the dose of some agent, or the extent of some exposure, and a physiological response. A dose-response effect means that the effect increases with the dose.

Ecological model of health behavior: A way of considering individual behavior in the context of the social environment, including influences at the interpersonal, organizational, community, and public policy levels. The ecological model is useful in designing interventions to promote healthy behavior; the most effective programs intervene at several levels of influence.

Effectiveness: The improvement in health outcome that a strategy can produce in typical community-based settings. Also, the degree to which objectives are achieved.

Emerging infectious diseases: Infectious diseases whose incidence in humans has increased within the past two decades or threatens to increase in the near future. Emerging diseases may be caused by microorganisms previously unknown to be human pathogens, foodborne pathogens not expected to occur in particular foods, or pathogens that are dramatically increasing in prevalence.

Endemic level: The usual prevalence of a disease within a given geographic area.

Environmental health: Those aspects of human health, diseases, and injury that are determined or influenced by factors in the environment. This includes the study of the direct pathological effects of various chemical, physical, and biological agents as well as the effects on health of the broad physical and social environment, which includes housing, urban development, land use and transportation, industry, and agriculture.

Environmental Protection Agency (EPA): The federal agency responsible for prevention and cleanup of water pollution and air pollution, control of toxic substances, and other issues of environmental contamination.

Epidemic: The occurrence in a community or geographic area of a disease at a rate that clearly exceeds the normally expected rate.

Epidemiology: The study of populations to seek the causes of health and disease. The study of the distribution and determinants of disease frequency in human populations.

Experimental group: The treated group in a study, in contrast to an untreated or more conventionally treated control group.

False negative: A mistaken identification of persons as healthy or unaffected when, in fact, they have the disease or condition being tested for.

False positive: A mistaken identification of persons as affected by some disease or condition when, in fact, they are unaffected by the disease or condition being tested for.

Family planning: The process of establishing the preferred number and spacing of one's children, selecting the means by which this plan is best achieved, and effectively using that means.

Fee for service: In contrast with managed care, a method of paying for medical care in which each visit to a doctor or hospital and each procedure is billed and paid for separately.

Food and Drug Administration (FDA): The federal agency that ensures the safety and nutritional value of the food supply; evaluates all new drugs, food additives, and colorings; and regulates medical devices, vaccines, diagnostic tests, animal drugs, and cosmetics.

Gene: A unit of hereditary information passed from parents to offspring; the totality of genetic information, contained in DNA (except for some viruses that use RNA), determines the way the offspring develops.

Genetic disorders: The group of health conditions that result from genes passed to the embryo from the parents.

Greenhouse gas: A gas that absorbs radiation of specific wavelengths within the infrared spectrum of radiation emitted by the earth's surface and clouds. The effect is a local trapping of part of the absorbed energy and a tendency to warm the earth's surface. Water vapor, carbon dioxide, nitrous oxide, methane, and ozone are the primary greenhouse gases in the earth's atmosphere.

Gross Domestic Product (GDP): The market value of the goods and services produced by labor and property located in a country.

Health: As defined by the World Health Organization, a state of physical, mental, and social well-being and not merely the absence of disease and infirmity.

Health education: Instruction that promotes healthy behaviors by informing and educating individuals through the use of materials and structured activities.

Health maintenance organization: An organization that manages both the financing and provision of health services to enrolled members.

Health outcomes: Results of healthcare interventions.

Health promotion: Any planned combination of educational, political, regulatory, and organizational supports for actions and conditions of living conducive to the health of individuals, groups, or communities.

Health services research: The study of the effectiveness, efficiency, and equity of the health care system.

Health status indicators: Measurements of the state of health of a specified individual, group, or population. Health status may be measured by proxies such as people's subjective assessments of their health; by one or more indicators of mortality and morbidity in the population, such as longevity or maternal and infant mortality; or by the incidence or prevalence of major diseases (communicable, chronic, or nutritional).

Human immunodeficiency virus (HIV): The virus that causes acquired immune deficiency syndrome (AIDS).

Immune system: The body's natural defense system, which works to eliminate pathogens.

Immunization: Stimulating immunity to an infectious disease by exposing an individual to a weakened or inactivated pathogen or a portion of the pathogen.

Incidence: A measure of the number of new cases reported in a given amount of time, usually a year.

Incubation period: The time between infection of an individual by a pathogen and the manifestation of the disease it causes.

Infant mortality: Number of live-born infants who die before their first birthday per 1,000 live births.

Infectious disease: Disease caused by a microorganism (such as bacteria, protozoans, fungi, or viruses) that enters the body and grows and multiplies there.

Injection drug use: The use of a needle and syringe to inject illicit drugs (e.g., heroin). This practice places the user at great risk for contracting the human immunodeficiency virus (HIV).

Injury: Unintentional or intentional damage to the body resulting from acute exposure to thermal, mechanical, electrical, or chemical energy or from the absence of such essentials as heat or oxygen.

Intervention: A generic term used in public health to describe a program or policy designed to have an impact on a health problem.

Intervention study: An epidemiologic study in which the impact of some intervention on one group of subjects is compared with the effect of a placebo or conventional therapy on a control group; for example, a clinical trial.

Life expectancy: The number of additional years of life expected at a specified point in time, such as at birth or at age 45.

Low birth weight (LBW): Weight at birth of less than 2,500 grams. Very low birth weight means a weight at birth of less than 1,500 grams.

Major depressive disorder: A combination of symptoms that interfere with a person's ability to work, sleep, study, eat, and enjoy once pleasurable activities.

Mammogram: An x-ray of the breast. Mammograms screen for breast cancer.

Managed care: A system of administrative controls intended to reduce costs through managing the utilization of health services.

Maternal death: Death of a woman while pregnant or within 42 days of the end of pregnancy from any cause related to or aggravated by the pregnancy or its management, but not from accidental or incidental causes.

Medicaid: A federally aided, state-operated and -administered program that provides medical services to eligible low-income populations.

Medicare: A national health insurance program for persons over age 65 and certain younger persons who are disabled.

Minamata: Village in southern Japan made famous by the poisoning of its population in the 1950s by mercury released into the bay by a plastics factory. Most severely affected were children born with severe brain damage to mothers who had been exposed while pregnant.

Morbidity: The term often used to mean illness or disease.

Mortality rate: The incidence of deaths per unit of time, most often per year, in a population.

National Institutes of Health (NIH): The primary federal agency for biomedical research. The NIH has its own laboratories and also provides funding to biomedical scientists at universities and research centers.

Notifiable disease: A disease that the law requires to be reported to public health authorities as part of the public health surveillance system.

Occupational Safety and Health Administration (OSHA): The federal agency, part of the Department of Labor, responsible for occupational health and the prevention of occupational injury.

Opportunistic infections: Infections that take advantage of the opportunity offered when a person's immune system has been weakened by the human immunodeficiency virus (HIV). At least 25 medical conditions, including cancers and bacterial, fungal, and viral infections, are associated with HIV infection.

Osteoporosis: Reduction of bone mass and a deterioration of the microarchitecture of the bone leading to bone fragility.

Outbreak: A sudden increase in the incidence of a disease.

Pap test: Microscopic examination of cells collected from the cervix. The Pap test is used to detect changes that may be cancer and can show noncancerous conditions, such as infection or inflammation.

Parasite: An organism that lives off another organism (called a host) but does not contribute to the welfare of the host.

Parts per million (ppm): A measure of very low concentrations of pollutants in air, water, or soil (e.g., 1 ppm of an air pollutant is one particle of the pollutant for every million molecules of air). Parts per billion is similarly used for even smaller concentrations of pollutants.

Pathogen: A microorganism that causes illness.

Placebo: A supposedly ineffective pill or agent used in a control group to gauge the effect of an actual treatment in another group. Experimenters often must allow for a placebo effect, a response caused by suggestion.

Policy development: One of the three core functions of public health as specified by *The Future of Public Health*. The process by which a public health agency exercises its responsibility to serve the public interest in the development of comprehensive public health policies by promoting use of scientific knowledge in decision making about public health and by leading in developing public health policy. Agencies must take a strategic approach, developed on the basis of a positive appreciation for the democratic political process.

Polychlorinated biphenyls (PCBs): A group of chemicals that are common environmental pollutants.

Post-traumatic stress disorder (PTSD): An anxiety disorder that some people get after seeing or living through a dangerous event.

Premature birth: Birth occurring before 37 weeks of pregnancy.

Prenatal care: Pregnancy-related healthcare services provided to a woman between conception and delivery. The American College of Obstetricians and Gynecologists recommends at least 13 prenatal visits in a normal 9-month pregnancy: a visit each month for the first 28 weeks of pregnancy, a visit every 2 weeks until 36 weeks, and then weekly visits until birth.

Prevalence: Proportion of persons in a population who have a particular disease or attribute at a specified point in time or during a specified time period.

Primary care: The provision of integrated, accessible healthcare services by clinicians who are accountable for addressing a large majority of personal healthcare needs, developing a sustained partnership with patients, and practicing in the context of family and community.

Primary prevention: Activities that are intended to prevent the onset of a disease or injury.

Probability: A calculation of what may be expected, based on what has happened in the past under similar conditions.

Psychosis: Any severe mental disorder characterized by deterioration of normal intellectual and social functioning and by partial or complete withdrawal from reality.

Public health: As defined by *The Future of Public Health*, organized community efforts to ensure conditions in which people can be healthy. Activities that society undertakes to prevent, identify, and counter threats to the health of the public.

p value: The probability that an observed result or effect could have occurred by chance if there had actually been no real effect.

Quality of health care: The degree to which health services for individuals increase the likelihood of desired health outcomes and are consistent with current professional standards.

Randomization: Division of a sample into two or more comparable groups by some random method that eliminates biased selection.

Random variation: The way a coin will successively turn up heads or tails if flipped in just the same way.

Rate: The proportion of some disease or condition in a group per unit of time, with a numerator and denominator (stated or implied) indicating "so many per so many per year or other unit of time."

Relative risk: A comparison of two morbidity or mortality rates using a calculation of the ratio of one to the other.

Reportable disease: See notifiable disease.

Reservoir: A place where a pathogen lives and multiplies before invading a noninfected person. Some pathogens infect only humans; some have animal reservoirs and infect humans only occasionally. Contaminated water or food may serve as a reservoir for waterborne or foodborne diseases.

Risk assessment: A quantitative estimate of the degree of hazard to a population presented by some agent or technology or decision. A risk–benefit assessment attempts to weigh possible risks against possible benefits.

Risk factor: A characteristic that has been demonstrated statistically to increase a person's chance of developing a disease or being injured.

Schizophrenia: A chronic, severe, and disabling brain disorder with symptoms that may include hearing voices that other people do not hear and belief that other people are reading their minds, controlling their thoughts, or plotting to harm them.

Screening: Checking for a disease when there are no symptoms.

Secondary prevention: Activities intended to minimize the risk of progression of or complications from a disease or to minimize damage from an injury.

Self-efficacy: People's sense that they are in control of their lives. High self-efficacy is beneficial to health.

Sensitivity: The ability of a test to avoid false negatives; its ability to identify a disease or condition in those who have it.

Sexually transmitted diseases (STDs): Infections caused by bacteria or viruses that are primarily transmitted through sexual activity. Examples of bacterial STDs are syphilis, gonorrhea, and chlamydia. Viral STDs include the human immunodeficiency virus (HIV), genital herpes, and the human papilloma virus.

Significance: In an experiment or clinical trial, statistical significance means there is only a small statistical probability that the same result could have been found by chance and that the intervention had no real effect.

Social support: Emotional and practical help provided by family and friends; social support helps people cope with stress.

Socioeconomic status (SES): A concept that includes income, education, and occupational status; a strong determinant of health.

Specificity: The ability of a test to avoid mistaken identifications—false positives.

Statistics: As a scientific discipline or method, a way of gathering and analyzing data to extract information, seek causation, and calculate probabilities.

Stress: A psychological and emotional state of tension; "a state that occurs when persons perceive that demands exceed their ability to cope."

Stroke: A loss of blood flow to part of the brain caused by a blood vessel bursting or becoming clogged by a blood clot or some other particle.

Substance abuse: The problematic consumption or illicit use of alcoholic beverages, tobacco products, and drugs, including misuse of prescription drugs.

Sudden infant death syndrome (SIDS): Sudden, unexplained death of an infant from an unknown cause.

Surveillance: The ongoing and systematic collection, analysis, and interpretation of health data essential to the planning, implementation, and evaluation of public health practice, closely integrated with the timely dissemination of these data to those who need to know. The final link in the surveillance chain is the application of these data to prevention and control.

Teratogen: A substance or agent that causes birth defects.

Tertiary prevention: Activities intended to minimize disability caused by a disease or injury. Rehabilitation is one tertiary prevention activity.

Unintended pregnancy: A general term that includes pregnancies that a woman states were either mistimed or unwanted at the time of conception (and not at the time of birth).

Vector: An animal or insect that transmits a pathogen to a human host.

Virus: A very small pathogen that is not capable of independent metabolism and can reproduce only inside living cells.

Vital statistics: Systematically collected statistics on births, deaths, marriages, divorces, and other life events. More broadly, the statistics of life, health, disease, and death—the statistics that measure progress, or lack of it, against disease.

Years of potential life lost (YPLL): A measure of the impact of disease or injury in a population, YPLL is years of life lost before a specific age (usually age 75). This approach places additional value on deaths that occur at earlier ages.

Index

Note: Italicized page locators indicate figures; tables are noted with t.

B

G